FRÉDÉRIC DELAVIER

STRENGTH TRAINING ANATOMY

FOURTH EDITION

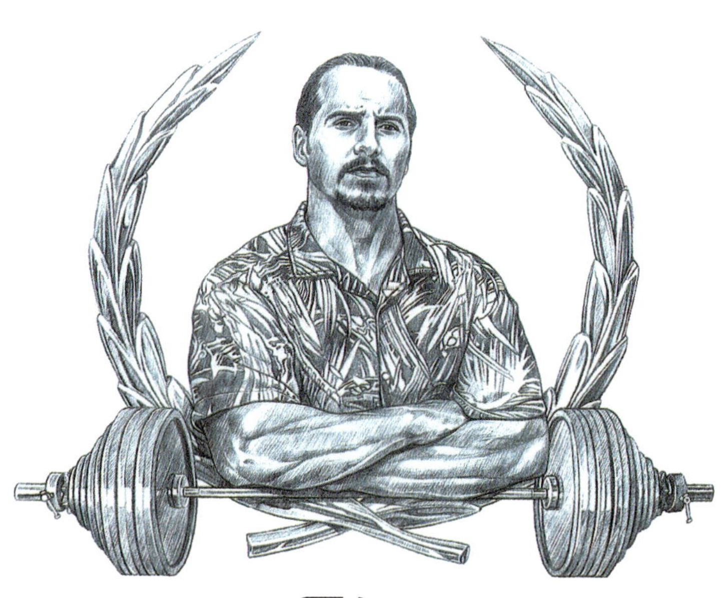

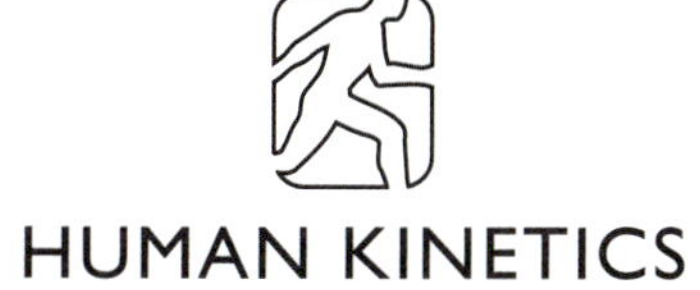

HUMAN KINETICS

FOR MY FATHER.

Library of Congress Cataloging-in-Publication Data

Names: Delavier, Frédéric, author.
Title: Strength training anatomy / Frédéric Delavier.
Other titles: Guide des mouvements de musculation. English
Description: Fourth Edition. | Champaign, IL : Human Kinetics, [2023] | 3rd
  edition: 2010.
Identifiers: LCCN 2022004789 | ISBN 9781718214866 (Print)
Subjects: LCSH: Muscles--Anatomy. | Weight training. | Muscle strength.
Classification: LCC QM151 .D454 2023 | DDC 611/.73--dc23/eng/20220207
LC record available at https://lccn.loc.gov/2022004789

ISBN: 978-1-7182-1486-6 (print)

This book is a revised edition of *Guide des Mouvements de Musculation Approche Anatomique, 6th Édition*, published in 2021 by Éditions Vigot.

Illustrator: Frédéric Delavier

Printed in France by Pollina

10   9   8   7   6   5   4   3   2

Human Kinetics
1607 N. Market Street
Champaign, IL 61820
USA

United States and International
Website: **US.HumanKinetics.com**
Email: info@hkusa.com
Phone: 1-800-747-4457

Canada
Website: **Canada.HumanKinetics.com**
Email: info@hkcanada.com

Human Kinetics' authorized representative for product safety in the EU is Mare Nostrum Group B.V., Mauritskade 21D, 1091 GC Amsterdam, The Netherlands.
Email: gpsr@mare-nostrum.co.uk

E8794

CONTENTS

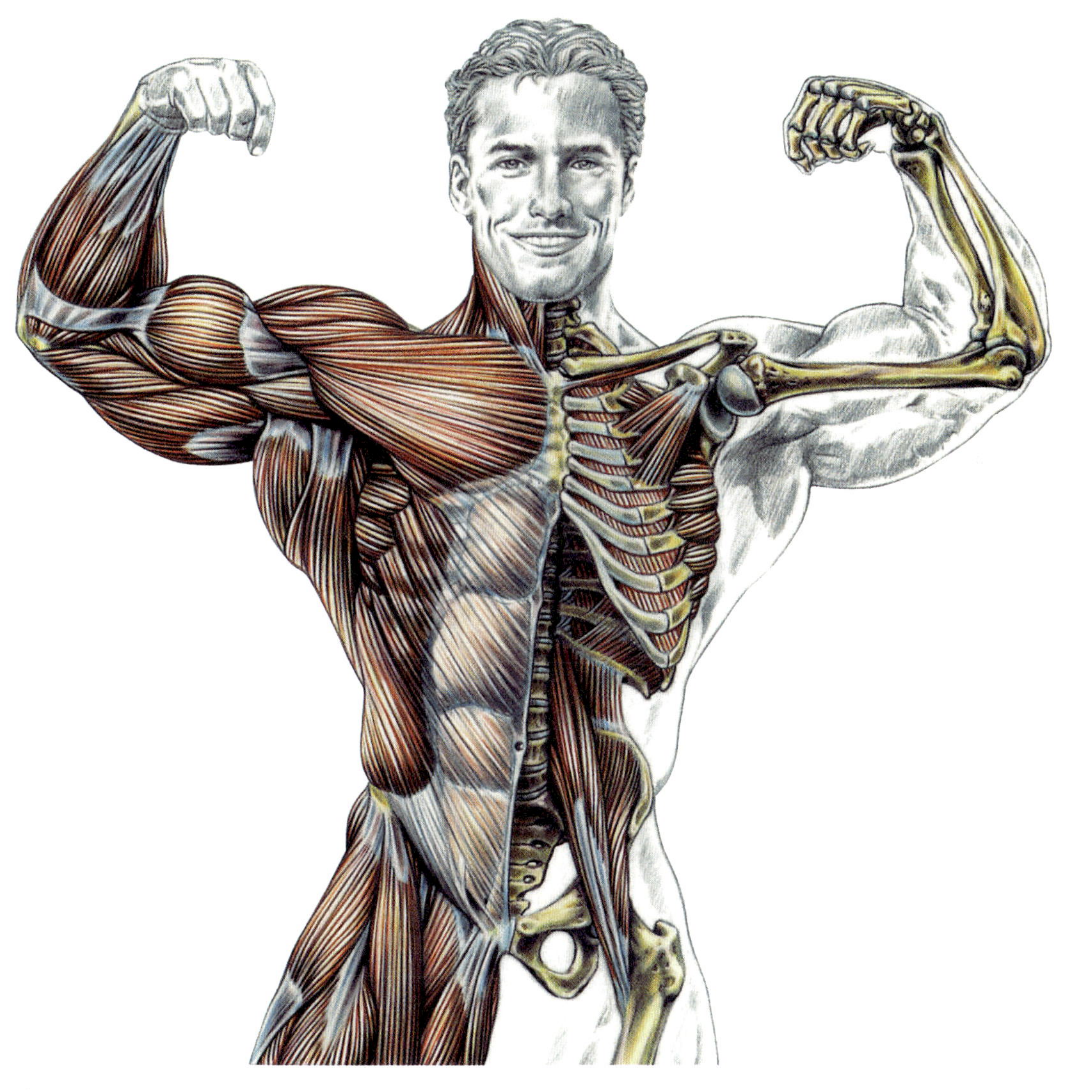

BODYBUILDER: FRONT VIEW

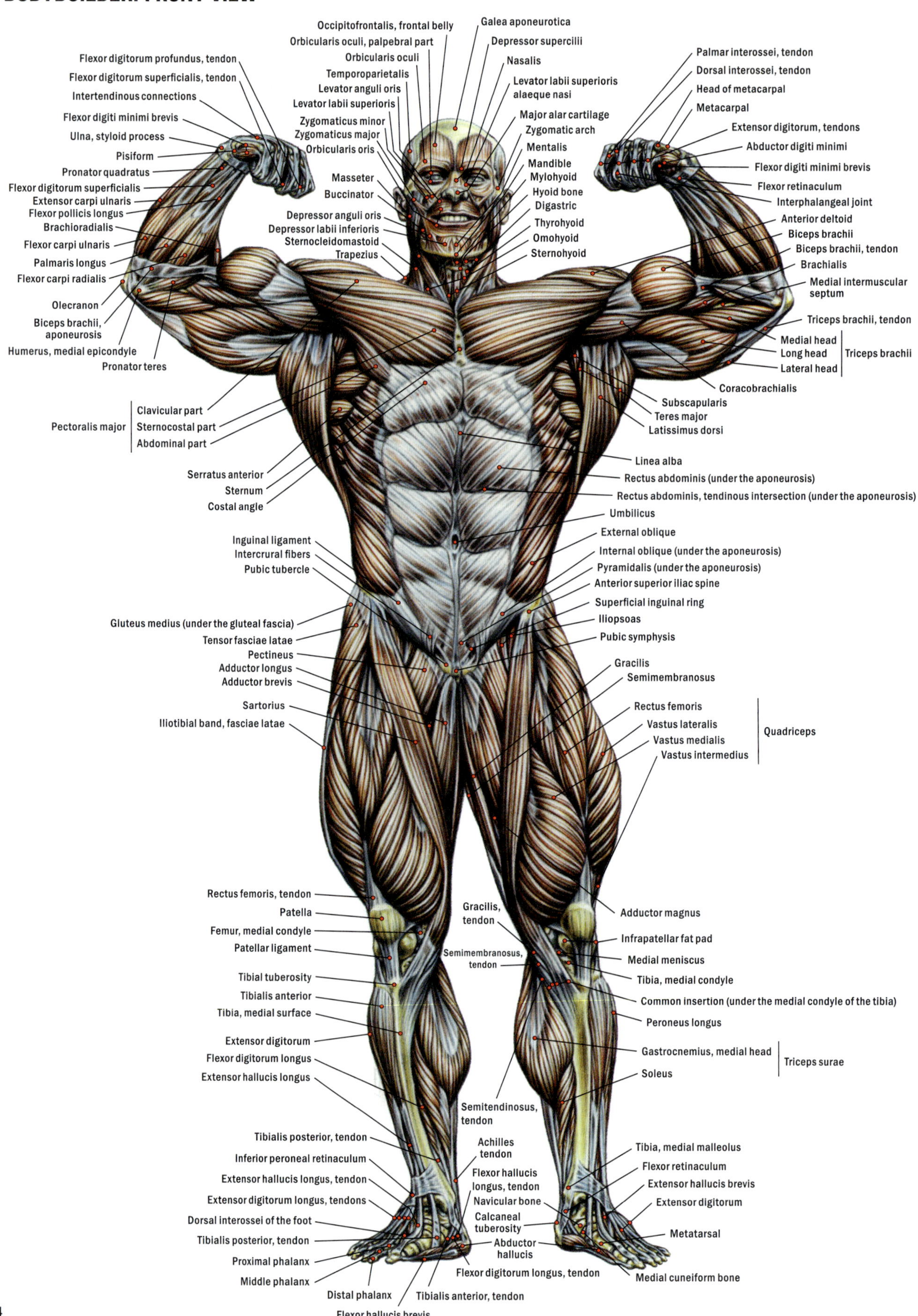

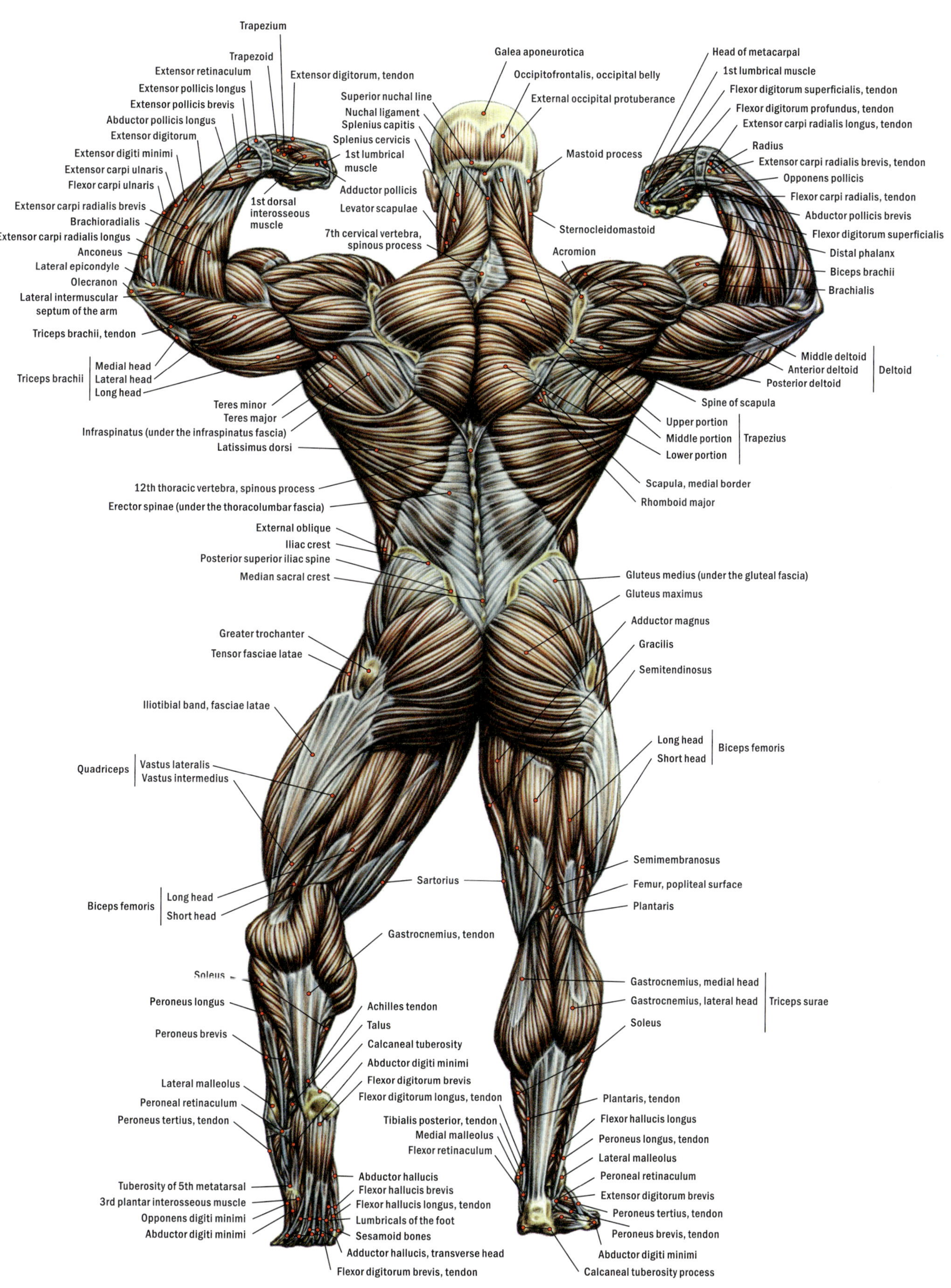

Trapezium
Trapezoid
Extensor retinaculum
Extensor pollicis longus
Extensor pollicis brevis
Abductor pollicis longus
Extensor digitorum
Extensor digiti minimi
Extensor carpi ulnaris
Flexor carpi ulnaris
Extensor carpi radialis brevis
Brachioradialis
Extensor carpi radialis longus
Anconeus
Lateral epicondyle
Olecranon
Lateral intermuscular septum of the arm
Triceps brachii, tendon
Triceps brachii
Medial head
Lateral head
Long head
Teres minor
Teres major
Infraspinatus (under the infraspinatus fascia)
Latissimus dorsi
12th thoracic vertebra, spinous process
Erector spinae (under the thoracolumbar fascia)
External oblique
Iliac crest
Posterior superior iliac spine
Median sacral crest
Greater trochanter
Tensor fasciae latae
Iliotibial band, fasciae latae
Quadriceps
Vastus lateralis
Vastus intermedius
Biceps femoris
Long head
Short head
Soleus
Peroneus longus
Peroneus brevis
Lateral malleolus
Peroneal retinaculum
Peroneus tertius, tendon
Tuberosity of 5th metatarsal
3rd plantar interosseous muscle
Opponens digiti minimi
Abductor digiti minimi
Extensor digitorum, tendon
Superior nuchal line
Nuchal ligament
Splenius capitis
Splenius cervicis
1st lumbrical muscle
Adductor pollicis
1st dorsal interosseous muscle
Levator scapulae
7th cervical vertebra, spinous process
Galea aponeurotica
Occipitofrontalis, occipital belly
External occipital protuberance
Mastoid process
Sternocleidomastoid
Acromion
Head of metacarpal
1st lumbrical muscle
Flexor digitorum superficialis, tendon
Flexor digitorum profundus, tendon
Extensor carpi radialis longus, tendon
Radius
Extensor carpi radialis brevis, tendon
Opponens pollicis
Flexor carpi radialis, tendon
Abductor pollicis brevis
Flexor digitorum superficialis
Distal phalanx
Biceps brachii
Brachialis
Middle deltoid
Anterior deltoid
Posterior deltoid
Deltoid
Spine of scapula
Upper portion
Middle portion
Lower portion
Trapezius
Scapula, medial border
Rhomboid major
Gluteus medius (under the gluteal fascia)
Gluteus maximus
Adductor magnus
Gracilis
Semitendinosus
Long head
Short head
Biceps femoris
Semimembranosus
Femur, popliteal surface
Plantaris
Sartorius
Gastrocnemius, tendon
Gastrocnemius, medial head
Gastrocnemius, lateral head
Triceps surae
Soleus
Achilles tendon
Talus
Calcaneal tuberosity
Abductor digiti minimi
Flexor digitorum brevis
Flexor digitorum longus, tendon
Tibialis posterior, tendon
Medial malleolus
Flexor retinaculum
Plantaris, tendon
Flexor hallucis longus
Peroneus longus, tendon
Lateral malleolus
Peroneal retinaculum
Extensor digitorum brevis
Peroneus tertius, tendon
Peroneus brevis, tendon
Abductor digiti minimi
Calcaneal tuberosity process
Abductor hallucis
Flexor hallucis brevis
Flexor hallucis longus, tendon
Lumbricals of the foot
Sesamoid bones
Adductor hallucis, transverse head
Flexor digitorum brevis, tendon

01 ARMS

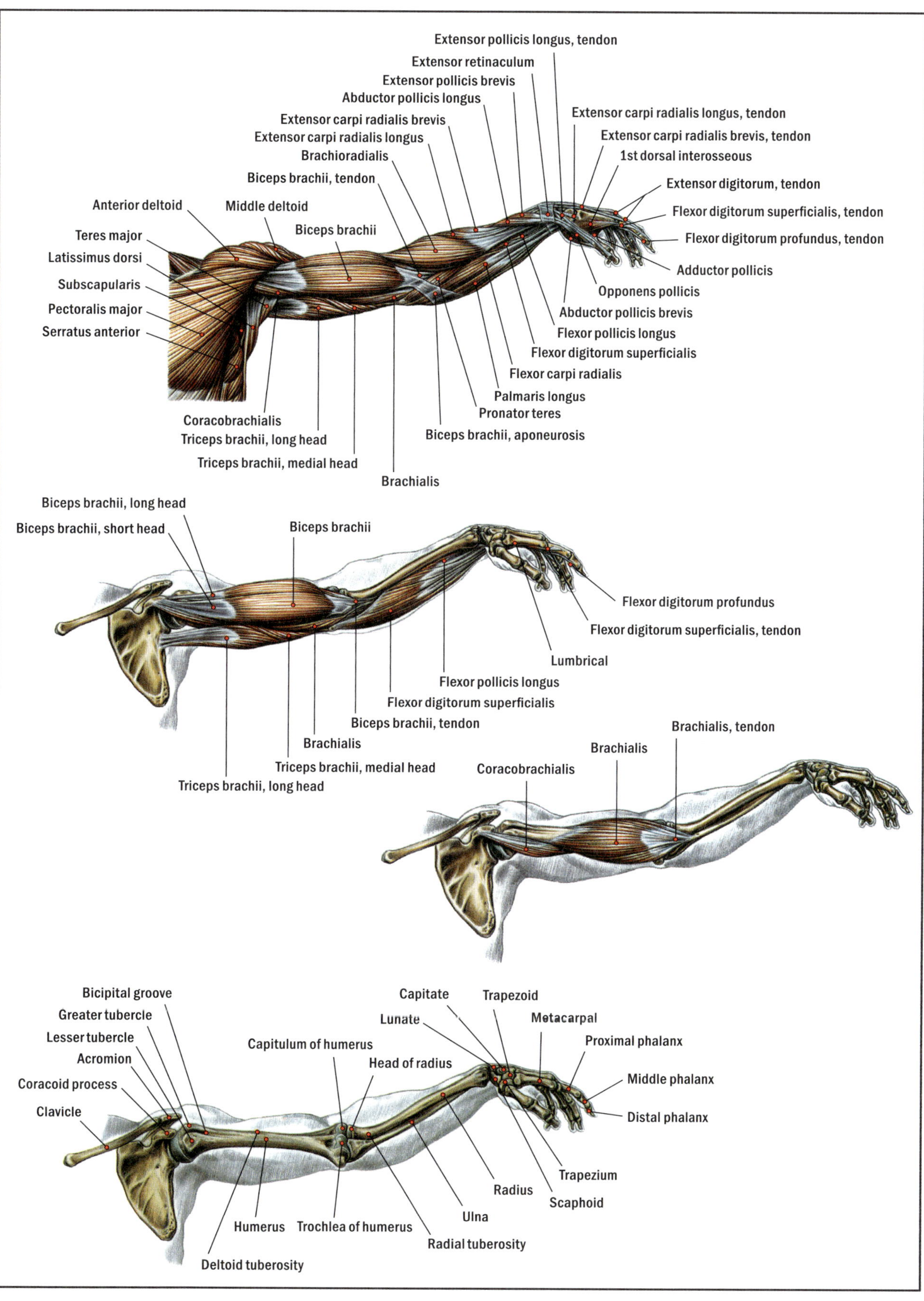

Extensor pollicis longus, tendon
Extensor retinaculum
Extensor pollicis brevis
Abductor pollicis longus
Extensor carpi radialis brevis
Extensor carpi radialis longus
Brachioradialis
Biceps brachii, tendon
Anterior deltoid
Middle deltoid
Biceps brachii
Teres major
Latissimus dorsi
Subscapularis
Pectoralis major
Serratus anterior
Extensor carpi radialis longus, tendon
Extensor carpi radialis brevis, tendon
1st dorsal interosseous
Extensor digitorum, tendon
Flexor digitorum superficialis, tendon
Flexor digitorum profundus, tendon
Adductor pollicis
Opponens pollicis
Abductor pollicis brevis
Flexor pollicis longus
Flexor digitorum superficialis
Flexor carpi radialis
Palmaris longus
Pronator teres
Biceps brachii, aponeurosis
Coracobrachialis
Triceps brachii, long head
Triceps brachii, medial head
Brachialis
Biceps brachii, long head
Biceps brachii, short head
Biceps brachii
Flexor digitorum profundus
Flexor digitorum superficialis, tendon
Lumbrical
Flexor pollicis longus
Flexor digitorum superficialis
Biceps brachii, tendon
Brachialis
Triceps brachii, medial head
Triceps brachii, long head
Brachialis, tendon
Brachialis
Coracobrachialis
Bicipital groove
Greater tubercle
Lesser tubercle
Acromion
Coracoid process
Clavicle
Capitate
Lunate
Capitulum of humerus
Head of radius
Trapezoid
Metacarpal
Proximal phalanx
Middle phalanx
Distal phalanx
Trapezium
Scaphoid
Radius
Ulna
Radial tuberosity
Humerus
Trochlea of humerus
Deltoid tuberosity

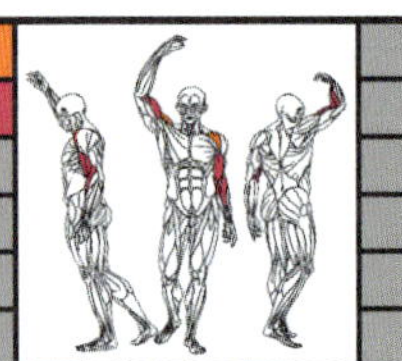

Flexor carpi ulnaris

Biceps brachii

Pectoralis major, clavicular head

Trapezius

Anterior deltoid

Middle deltoid

Posterior deltoid

Deltoid

Flexor carpi radialis

Palmaris longus

Pronator teres

Brachialis

Triceps brachii

Medial head

Long head

Biceps brachii

Triceps brachii, lateral head

Brachialis

Brachioradialis

Extensor carpi radialis longus

Anconeus

Extensor carpi radialis brevis

Extensor digitorum

Extensor carpi ulnaris

Extensor digiti minimi

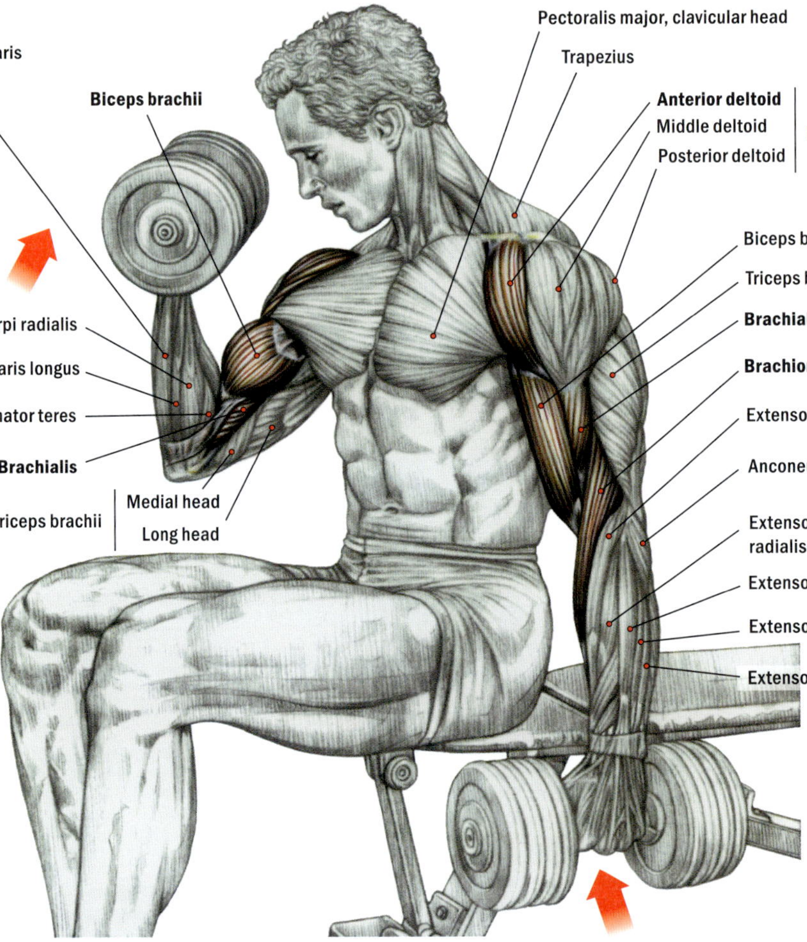

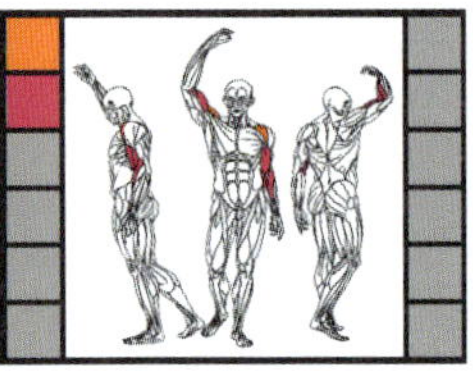

Sit holding a dumbbell in each hand with the arms hanging down and the palms of your hands facing your body:

- Inhale and bend your elbow, rotating your palm up before your forearm reaches a horizontal position.

- Continue by raising your elbow; exhale at the end of the movement.

This exercise primarily uses the brachioradialis (long supinator), brachialis, biceps brachii, anterior deltoid, and, to a lesser extent, the coracobrachialis and clavicular head of the pectoralis major.

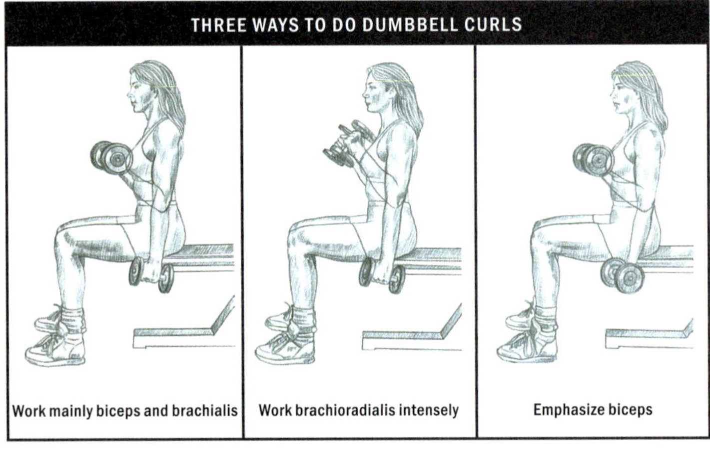

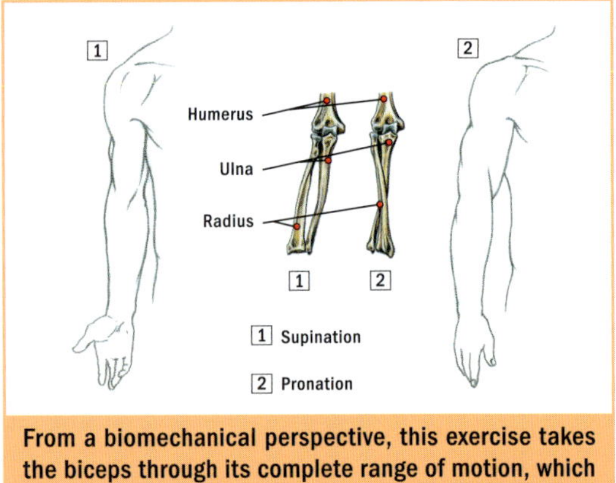

From a biomechanical perspective, this exercise takes the biceps through its complete range of motion, which includes flexion, protraction, and, above all, supination.

CONCENTRATION CURLS 02

ENDING POSITION

BRACHIALIS MUSCLE

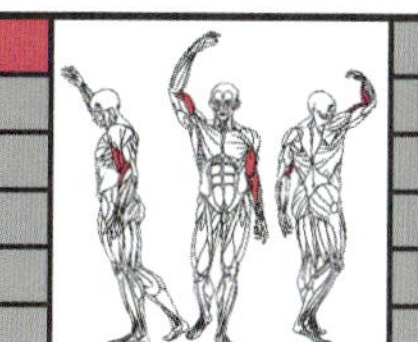

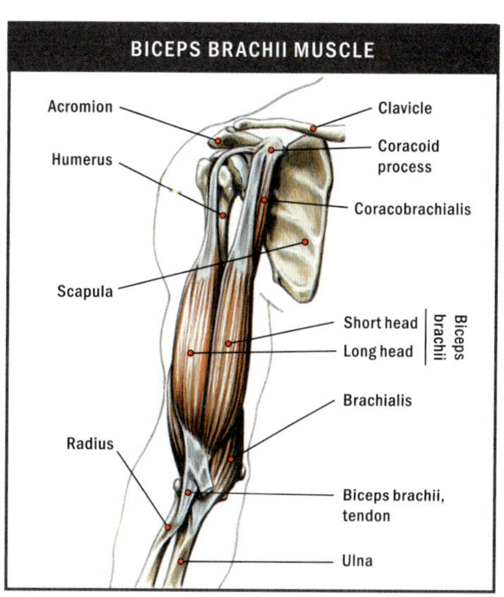

Sit holding a dumbbell with your palm facing forward and your elbow resting against your inner thigh:

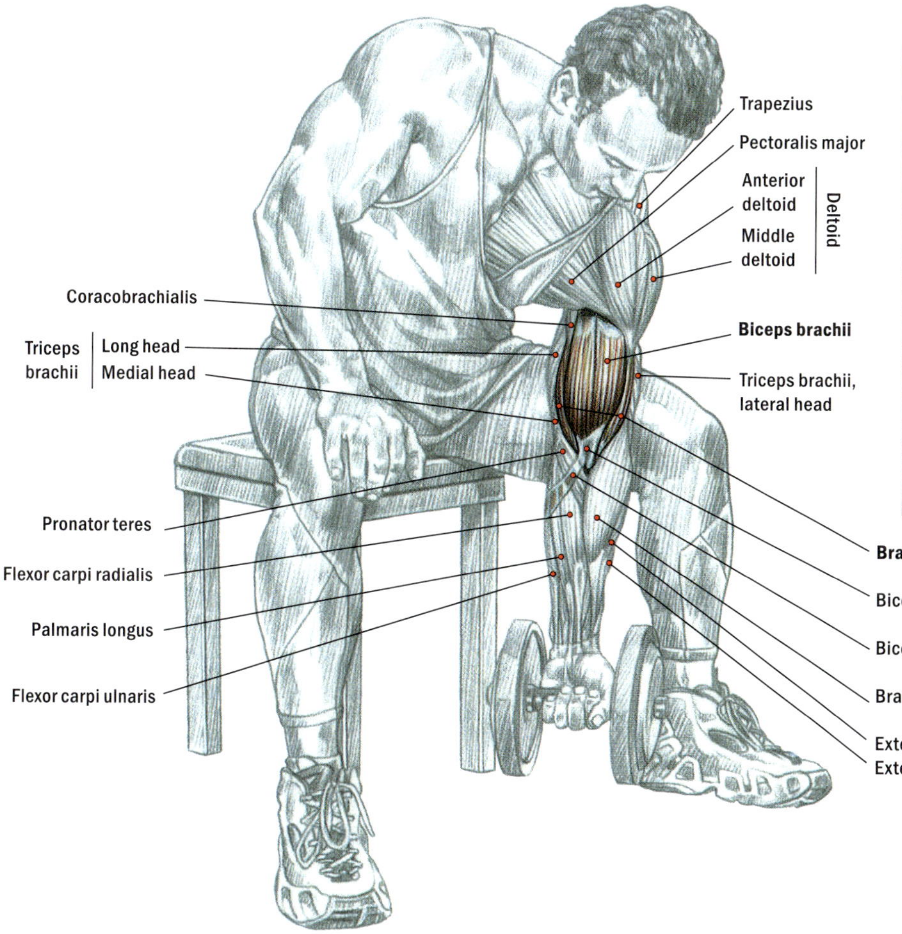

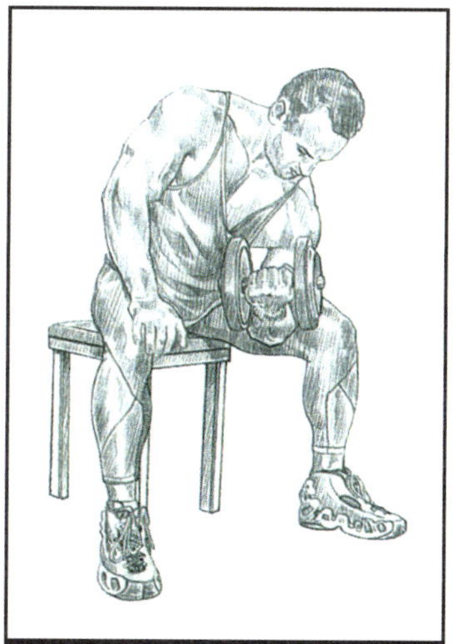

- Inhale and lift your forearm by bending the elbow.
- Exhale at the end of the effort.

This isolation exercise allows you to control the range of motion, speed, and form of the movement. It mainly works the biceps brachii and brachialis.

BICEPS BRACHII MUSCLE

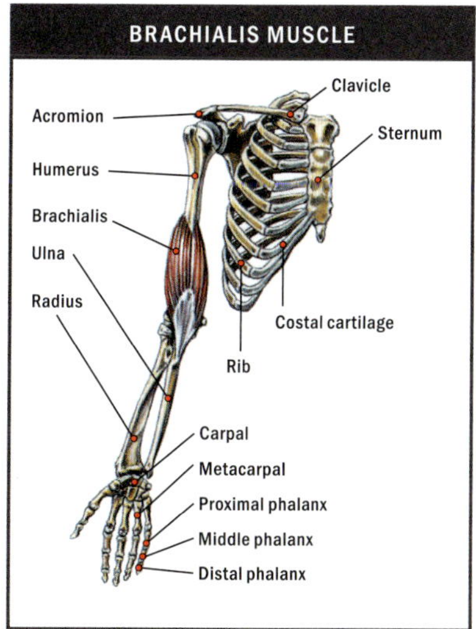

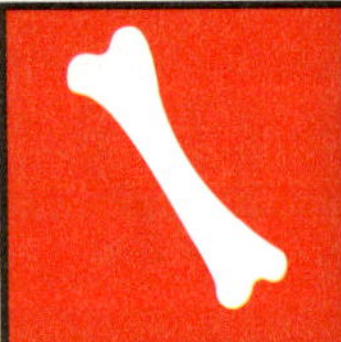

LONG MUSCLE, SHORT MUSCLE

The longer the lever arm, the thinner the biceps muscle is, and, therefore, less strength is required of the muscle producing the movement to move the same load over the same distance. But the longer the lever arm is and the longer the muscle contracts over a greater distance, the slower the movement of the load will be.

SHORT BICEPS BRACHII WITH THE DISTAL BICEPS TENDON INSERTION NEAR THE ELBOW JOINT

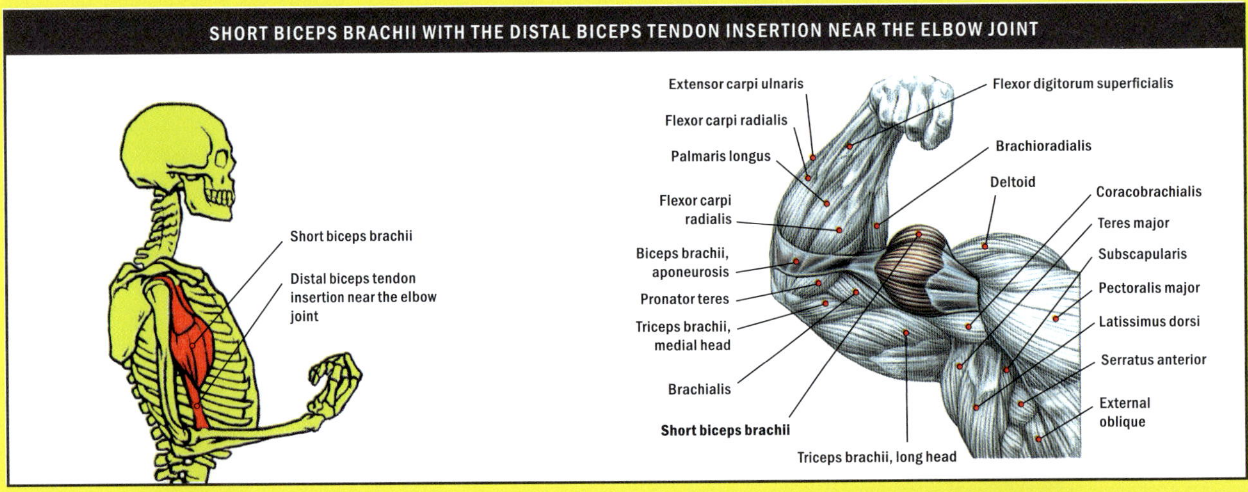

LONG BICEPS BRACHII WITH THE DISTAL BICEPS TENDON INSERTION AWAY FROM THE ELBOW JOINT

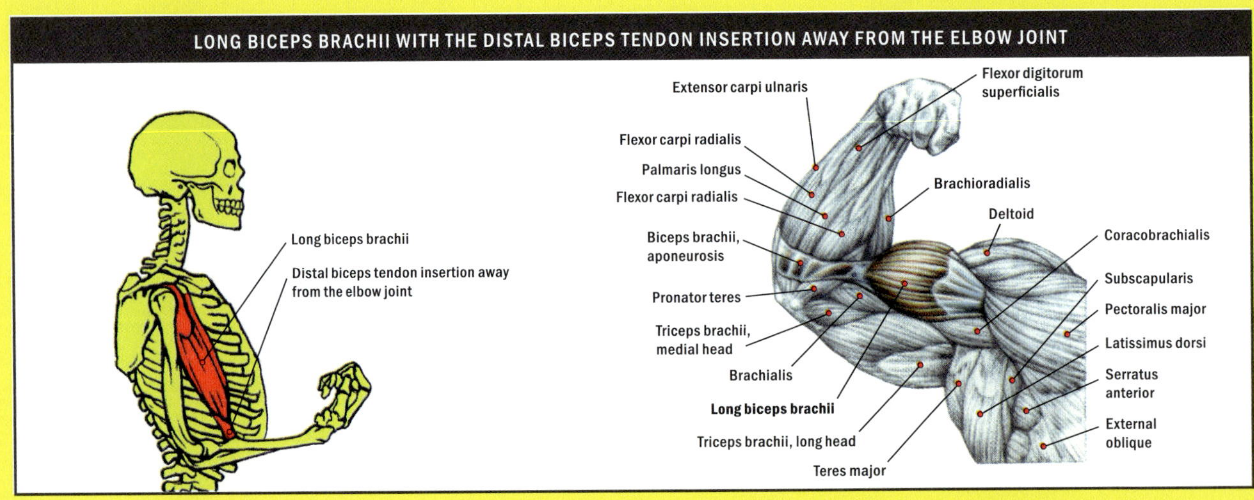

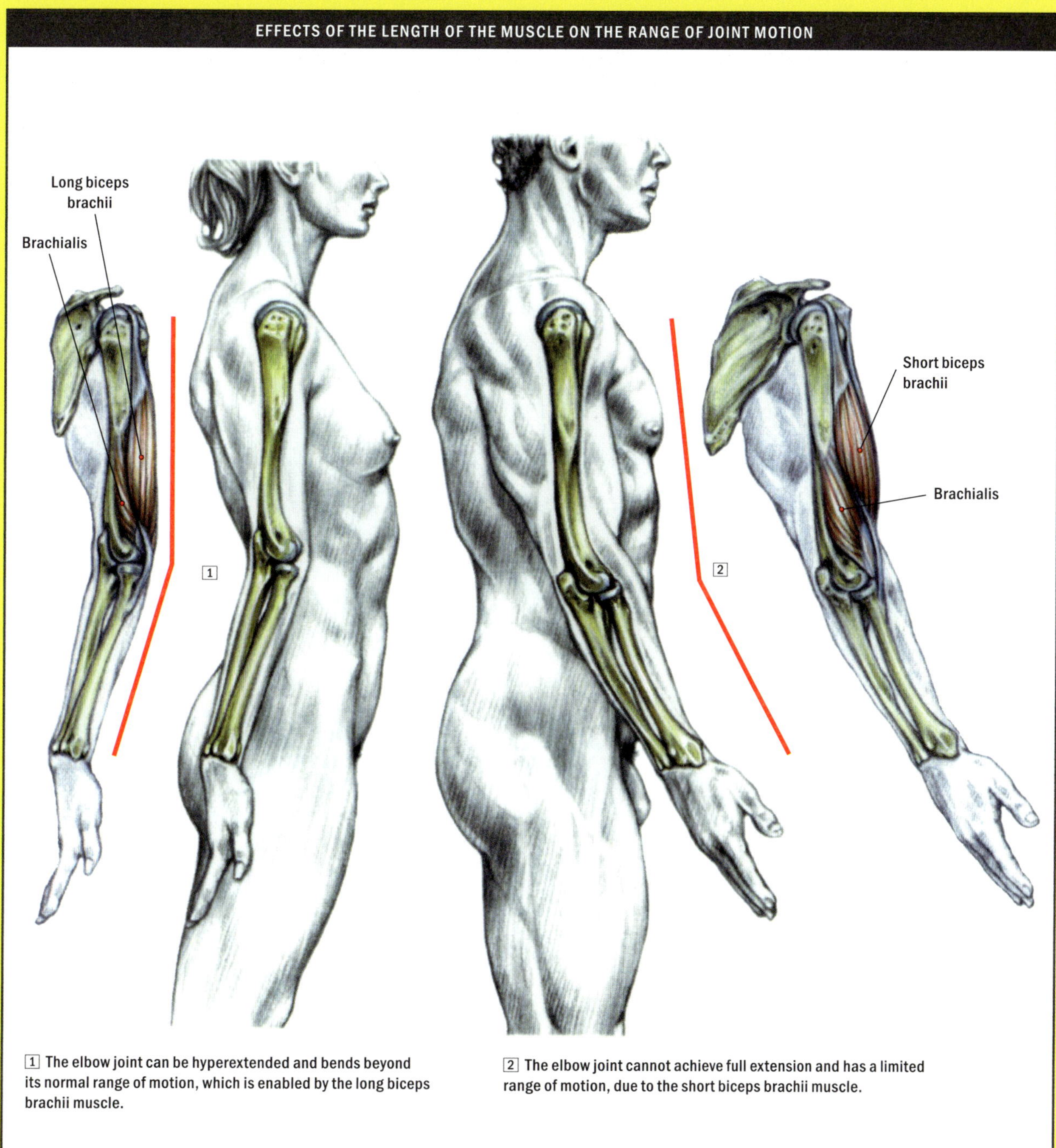

1 The elbow joint can be hyperextended and bends beyond its normal range of motion, which is enabled by the long biceps brachii muscle.

2 The elbow joint cannot achieve full extension and has a limited range of motion, due to the short biceps brachii muscle.

You don't have to train with full range of motion to increase biceps muscle size. Lifting heavy weights generally promotes muscle growth, but to avoid muscle tears and tendon ruptures, it is crucial to limit the elbow range of motion during the stretching phase when the weights get heavy. At the same time, to maintain healthy elbow joint motion, it is essential to practice movements using light weights with full range of motion at the start of the workout.

Over time, if the joint is not fully mobilized, it risks losing its mobility, which will cause the muscles, tendons, or ligaments to shorten. This is known as *contracture*, a phenomenon that gives this knotted appearance to the elderly and disabled. To train your biceps muscles, develop them, and maintain joint mobility, you need to lift light weights with full range of motion and gradually limit the range of motion as the weights get heavier.

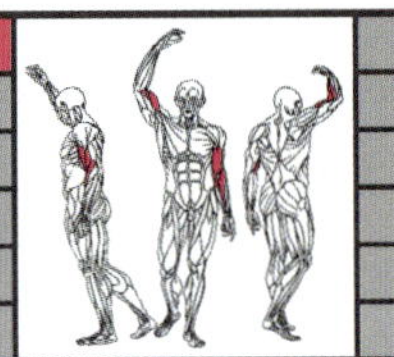

STARTING POSITION

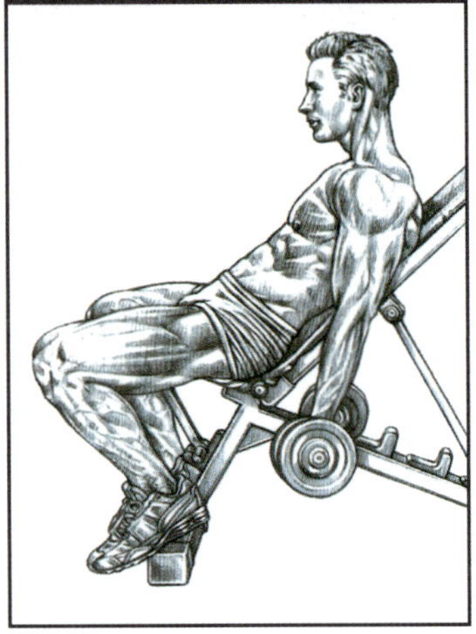

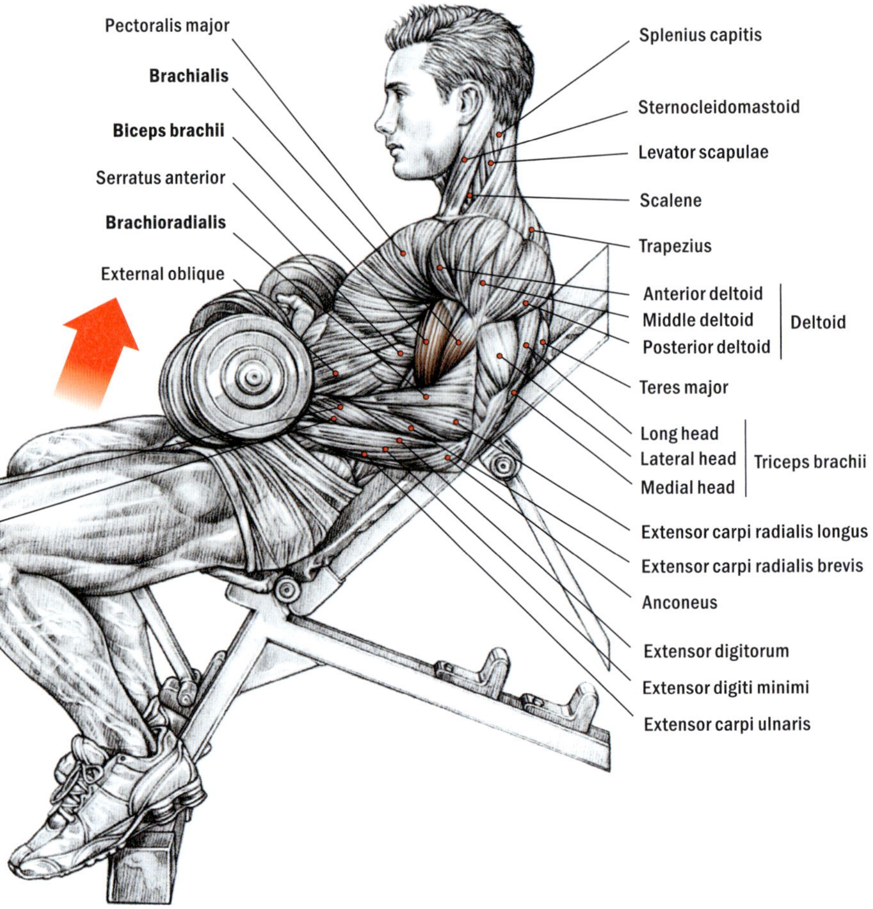

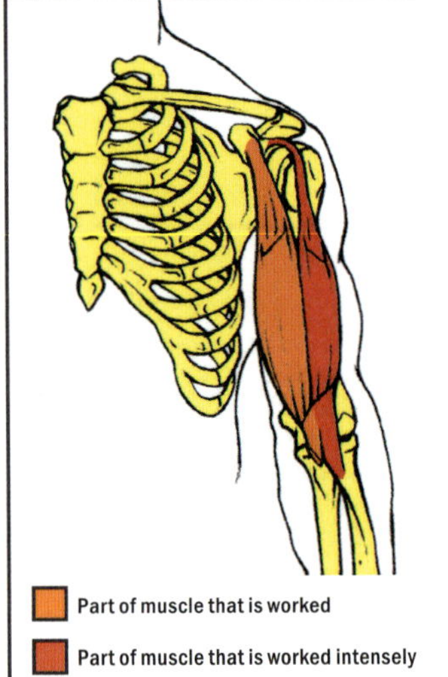

Sit on an incline bench with your back leaning against the support. In each hand, hold a dumbbell with a semipronated grip:

- Inhale and bend your arms while externally rotating your wrists, stopping before your forearms reach a horizontal position. At the end of the movement your hands are supinated (thumbs facing the outside).
- Exhale at the end of the exercise.

This exercise targets the long head of the biceps (the lateral part of the muscle), which is stretched as the forearm begins to flex due to the inclined position of the chest. This exercise also works the brachioradialis and the brachialis.

Variations
You can alternate arms when doing dumbbell curls. You can also increase the intensity of the biceps' work by starting the exercise with an underhand grip.

Part of muscle that is worked

Part of muscle that is worked intensely

Adjust the angle of the bench based on your shoulder flexibility. (This will vary among different people.) If your arm is too far back, the long head of the biceps will experience excessive friction in the bicipital groove of the humerus, and this could cause inflammation or strain the tendon.

THE FRAGILITY OF THE LONG HEAD OF THE BICEPS

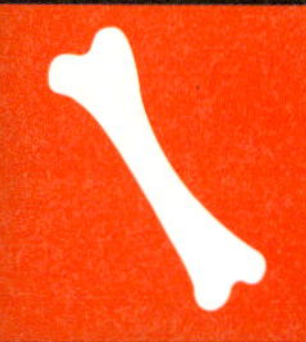

COMPARING THE UPPER BODY OF AN OCCASIONALLY BIPEDAL CHIMPANZEE TO THAT OF A TOTALLY BIPEDAL HUMAN

Whether they are moving through trees or on the ground, chimpanzees' arms rarely hang next to their bodies. This means that the long head of the biceps brachii tendon is not subject to much friction. Unlike humans, chimpanzees' tendons are rarely damaged by wear and tear.

With totally bipedal locomotion, humans' arms constantly hang at the sides of the body. The long head of the biceps brachii is, therefore, subject to intense friction against the humerus. The surface of the tendon that is in contact with the bone is covered with cartilage to limit wear and tear, but this makes the tendon even more vulnerable to space constraints.

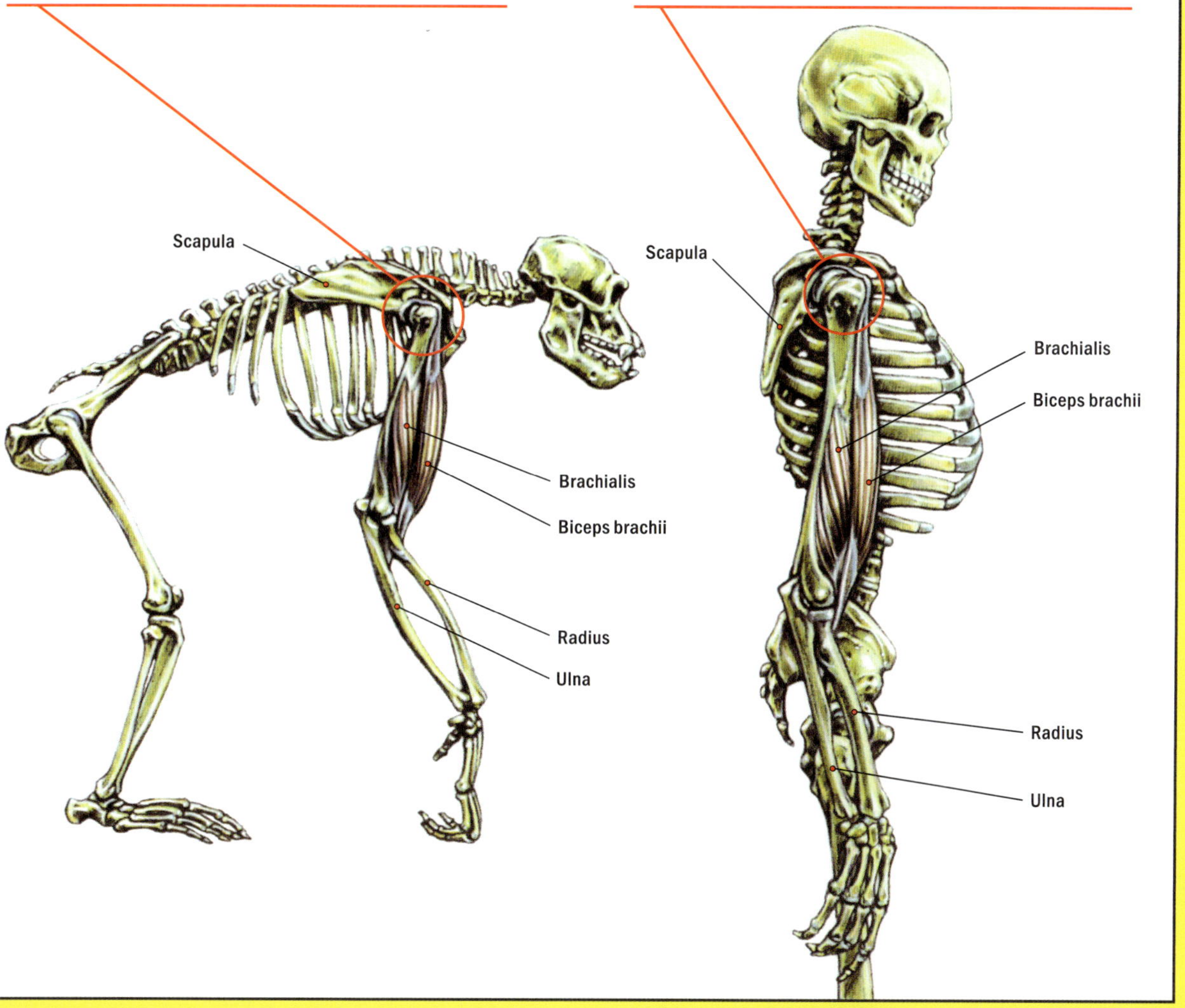

The long head of the biceps tendon is highly vulnerable and often the source of inflammatory wear and tear injuries. This is because the way our ancestors moved about completely changed during evolution. The long head of the biceps tendon was perfectly adapted when our ancestors walked with four legs. But the quick switch to bipedalism upset this mechanism, causing it to adopt a winding path that increases the friction and, over time, produces more overuse injuries, ranging from inflammation to total rupture of the tendon.

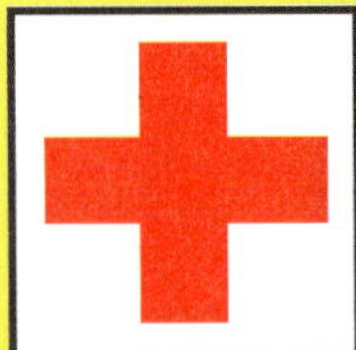

DIAGRAM SHOWING THE LONG HEAD OF THE BICEPS BRACHII, WHOSE TENDON IS A COMMON SITE OF OVERUSE INJURIES

In strength training, the upper part of the long head of the biceps brachii is a particularly vulnerable area; it is a common source of overuse injuries due to repetitive movements, ranging from inflammation to total rupture of the tendon. Injuries to the long head of the biceps brachii are often painful; they are felt during shoulder and chest workouts and during some biceps exercises such as incline dumbbell curls.

Since the long head of the biceps tendon passes under the anterior part of the deltoid muscle, injuries to the long head of the biceps are often confused with pain in the anterior deltoid. From an anatomical perspective, the long head of the biceps tendon passes through a deep bone groove called the *bicipital groove* or *intertubercular sulcus* of the humerus, covered by the synovial sheath and the subscapularis tendon. These structures keep the biceps tendon in place. At the upper end of this tunnel, the long head of the biceps tendon bends as it passes through the glenohumeral joint and attaches to the scapula and the labrum surrounding the glenoid cavity.

This bending of the long head of the biceps tendon as it passes through the shoulder joint means that as the arm moves, the tendon experiences pressure and friction on the underside, where it contacts the humerus. So, during exercises like the bench press, dips, and particularly incline dumbbell curls, the long head of the biceps tendon is strongly pressed into the bicipital groove in the bend formed by the head of the humerus, which increases the amount of friction. This can cause inflammation of the tendon, premature wear and tear, and even, over time, its rupture. However, this wear and tear is limited by the tendon's structure, which is adapted to withstand friction and compression since the part of the tendon in contact with the humerus is covered by fibrocartilage that is resistant to abrasions from friction.

But this specific resistance to friction makes the long head of the biceps tendon much less flexible than most other tendons. The process of aging makes the tendon more vulnerable during sudden tension from a movement done too quickly or from lifting a heavy weight, which is also a cause of tendon rupture. This most often affects individuals after the age of 40.

If you start to feel pain from inflammation in this tendon, it is important to avoid all movements that cause discomfort or pain to limit the risk of overuse injuries and rupture of the long head of the biceps tendon. Look for exercises with ranges of motion and working angles that do not cause any pain. You should also avoid exercises where the humerus moves backward, such as incline dumbbell curls, for a while. This is because they increase the friction of the long head of the biceps tendon in the bicipital groove, and this friction is what causes inflammation and, in the long run, a possible rupture.

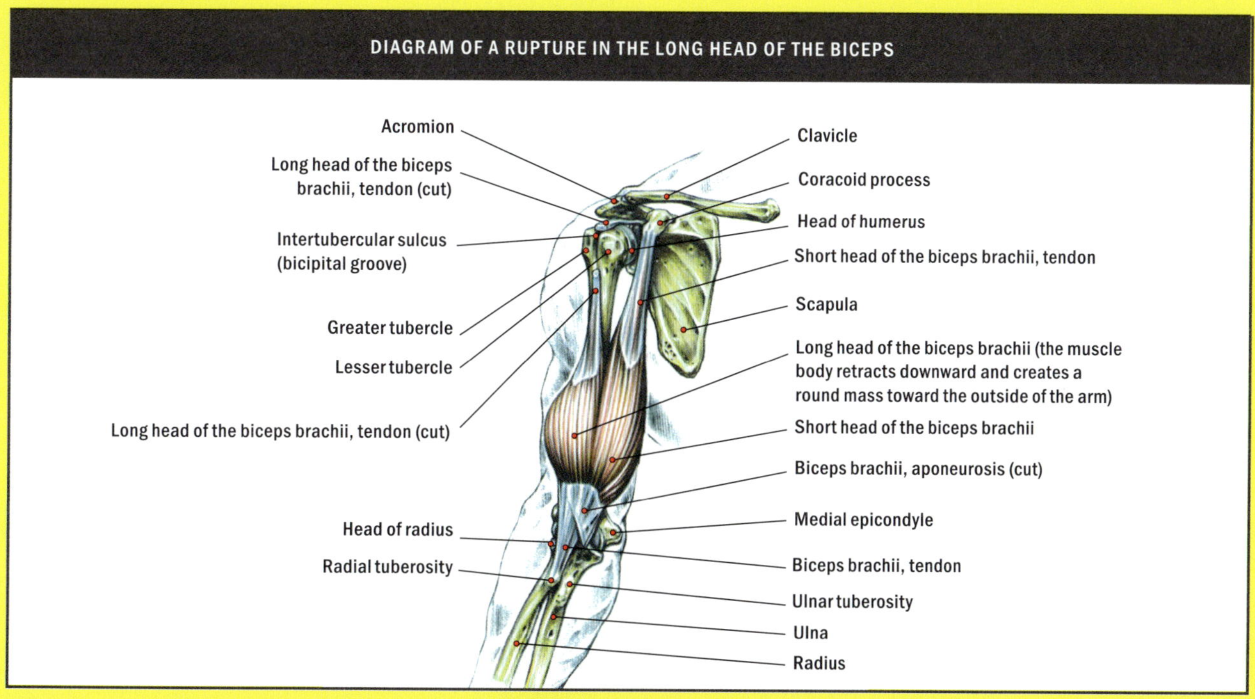

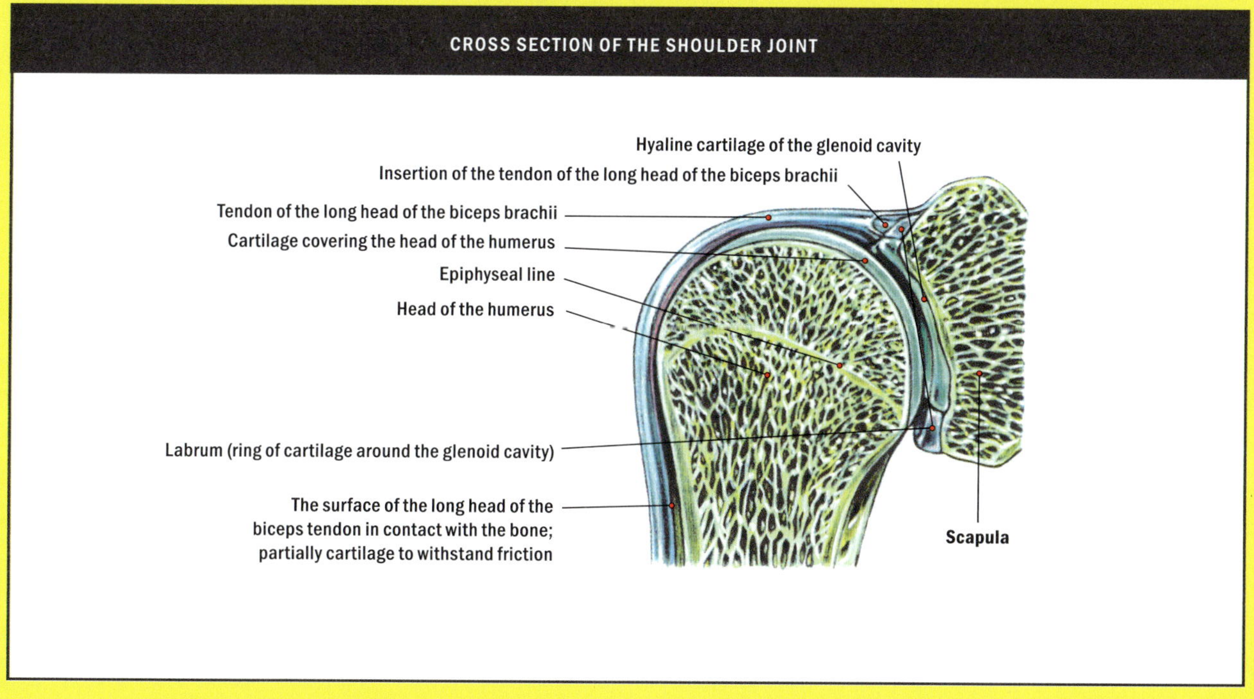

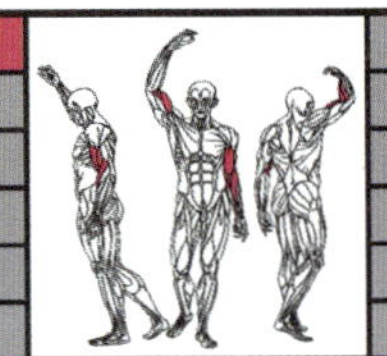

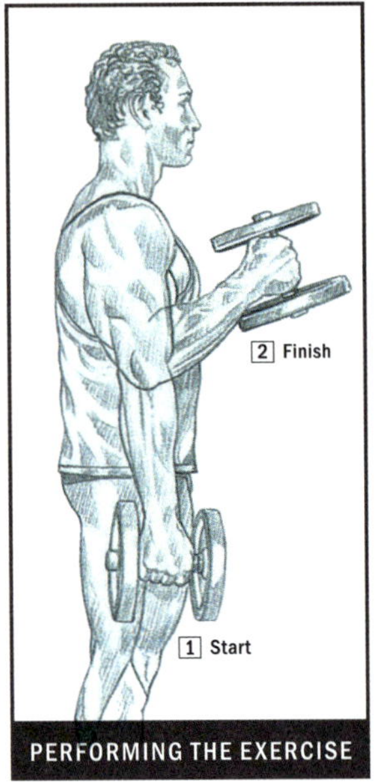

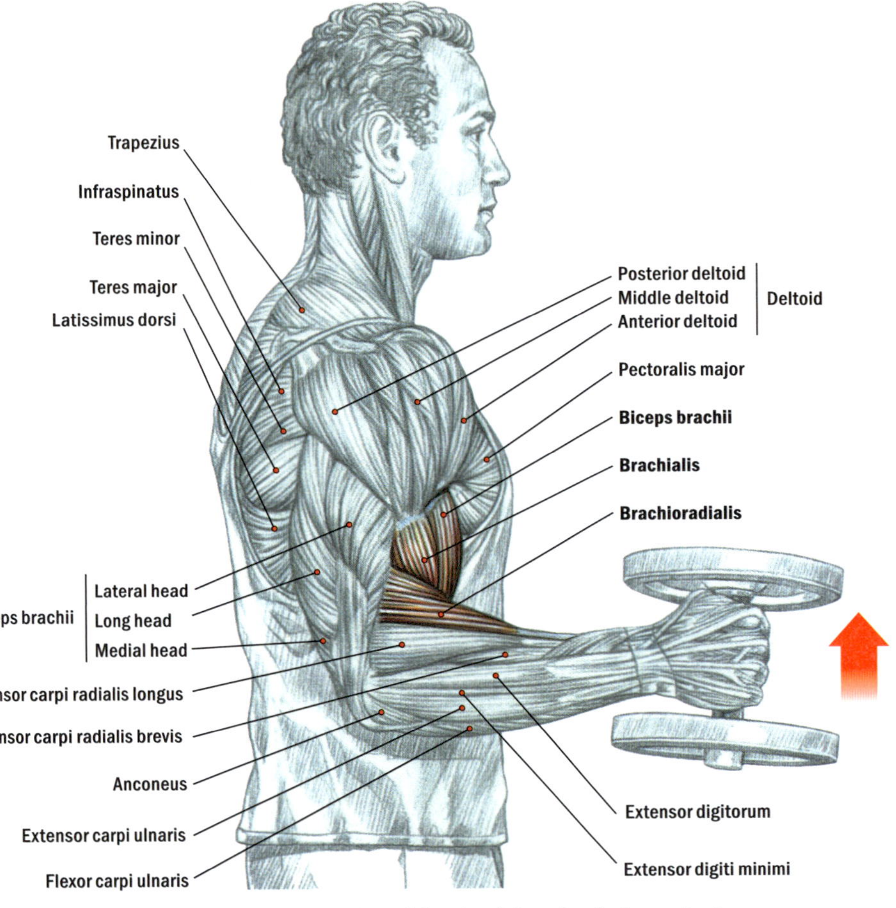

Stand or sit with a dumbbell in each hand and the palms facing each other:

- Inhale and raise your forearms at the same time; you can also alternate.
- Exhale at the end of the exercise.

This is the best exercise for developing the brachioradialis. It also develops the biceps brachii, brachialis, and, to a lesser degree, the extensor carpi radialis brevis and longus.

BRACHIORADIALIS MUSCLE

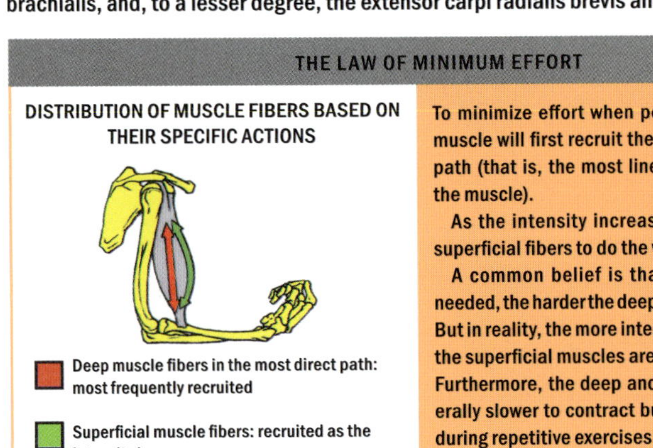

THE LAW OF MINIMUM EFFORT

DISTRIBUTION OF MUSCLE FIBERS BASED ON THEIR SPECIFIC ACTIONS

To minimize effort when performing an exercise, a muscle will first recruit the fibers in the most direct path (that is, the most linear path located deep in the muscle).

As the intensity increases, the muscle recruits superficial fibers to do the work.

A common belief is that the greater the force needed, the harder the deep part of the muscle works. But in reality, the more intense the effort is, the more the superficial muscles are recruited to do the work. Furthermore, the deep and linear muscles are generally slower to contract but have better endurance during repetitive exercises than the lateral muscles, which are more curved and longer.

DIAGRAM SHOWING THE ROTATION OF THE RADIUS AROUND THE ULNA DURING PRONATION AND SUPINATION

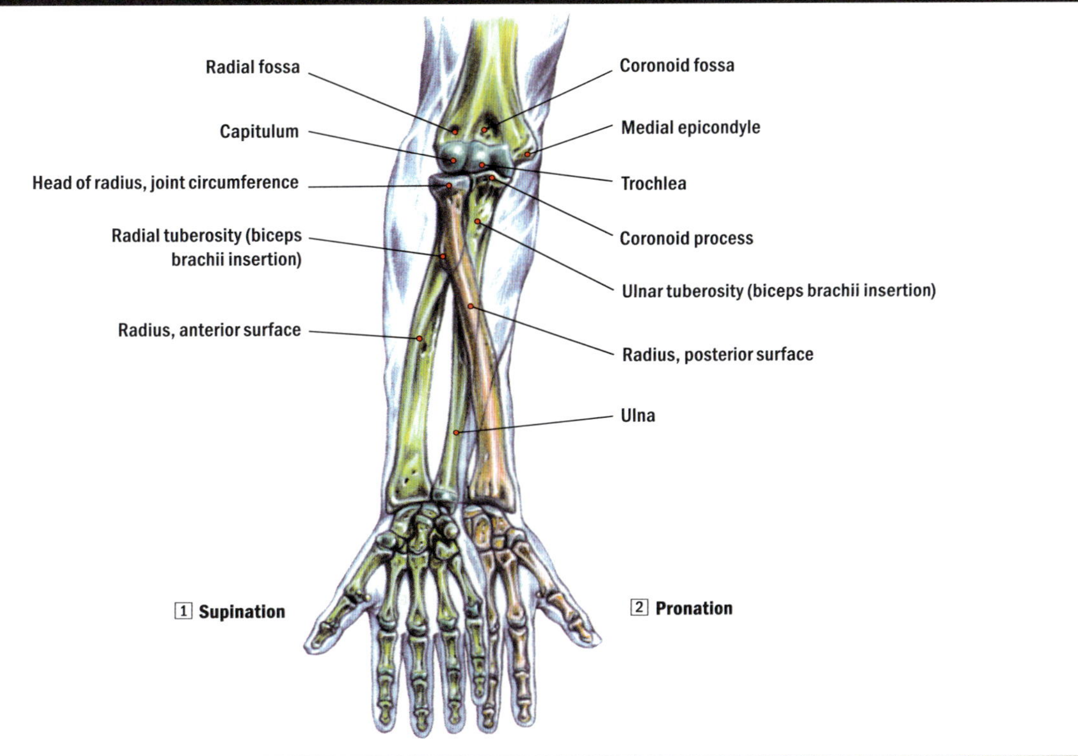

PRACTICAL APPLICATION OF PRONATION AND SUPINATION: WHY DO WE TWIST FROM LEFT TO RIGHT?

MUSCLES INVOLVED IN PRONATION AND SUPINATION

Because we are stronger when moving from a pronated to a supinated position than from a supinated to a pronated position, it is easier for a right-handed person to turn a screw clockwise. When it is time to remove the screw, it is obvious how much weaker the arm is when moving from a supinated to pronated position (counterclockwise).

This difference is mainly because the biceps brachii is the most powerful supinator and is assisted by the supinator muscle of the forearm. Pronation is mainly performed by smaller muscles (pronator teres, pronator quadratus).

DIAGRAM OF THE BRACHIORADIALIS MUSCLE SHOWING ITS SPIRAL SHAPE

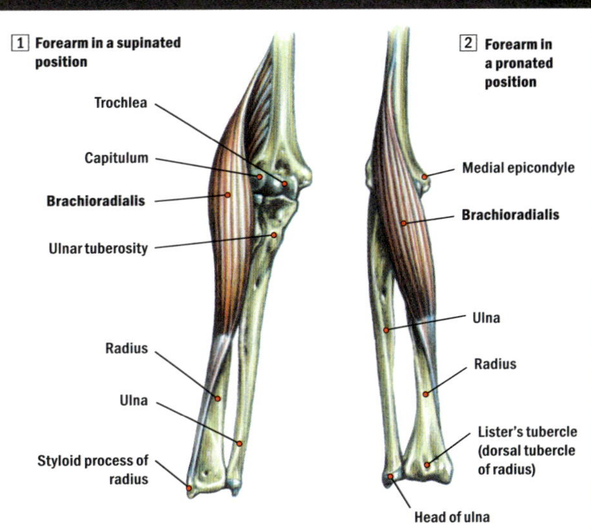

The brachioradialis brings the forearm from a supinated position to a neutral position and from a pronated position to a neutral position. It is, therefore, a pronator and a supinator.

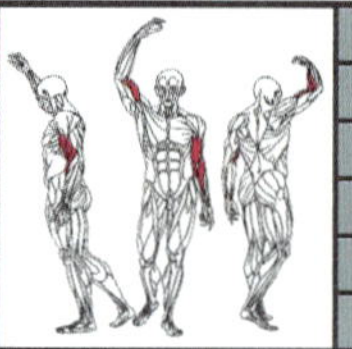

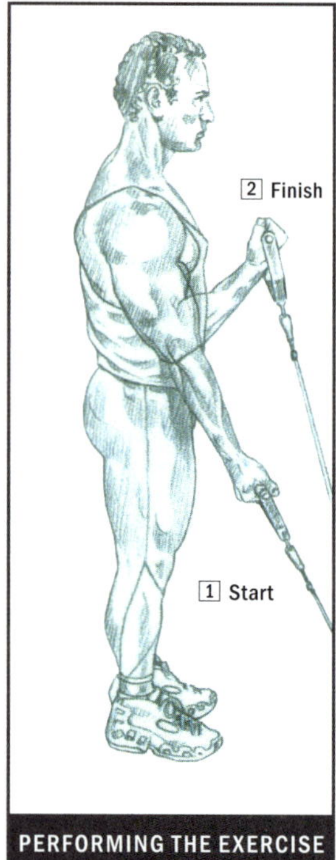

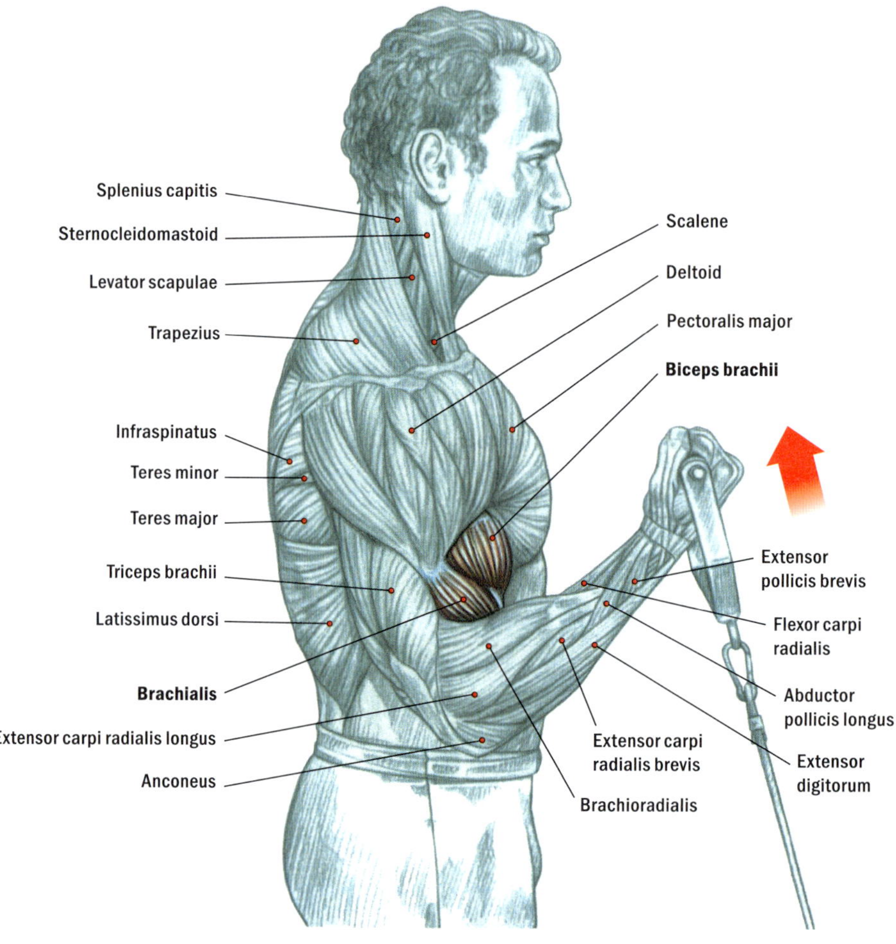

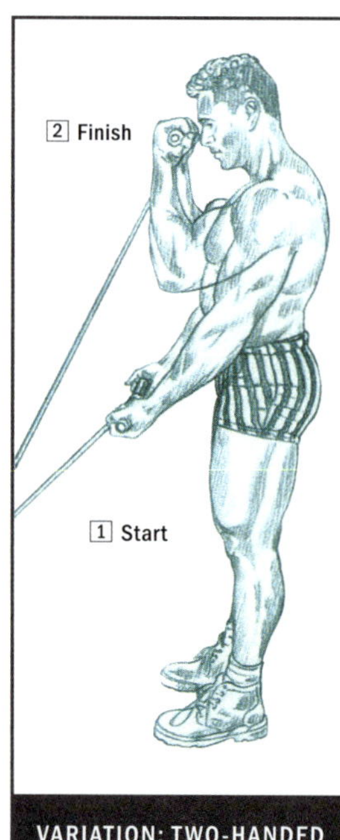

Stand facing the machine. Grasp the handle with an underhand (supinated) grip:

- Inhale and bend your elbow to raise your forearm.
- Exhale at the end of the exercise.

This exercise focuses the work on the biceps brachii and promotes intense blood flow to the muscle.

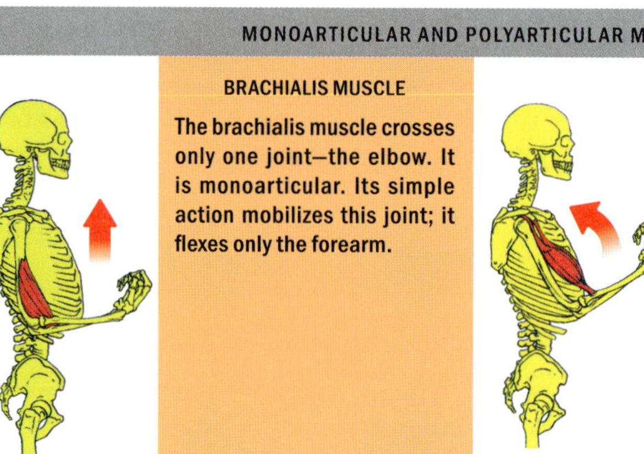

MONOARTICULAR AND POLYARTICULAR MUSCLES

BRACHIALIS MUSCLE

The brachialis muscle crosses only one joint—the elbow. It is monoarticular. Its simple action mobilizes this joint; it flexes only the forearm.

BICEPS BRACHII MUSCLE

The biceps brachii muscle crosses more than one joint: the elbow and the shoulder. It is polyarticular. This means that it mobilizes more than one joint, and its action is more complex than that of the brachialis. The biceps brachii can bend the elbow, raise the elbow, bring the arm to the thorax, and place the forearm into supination (underhand grip).

HIGH-PULLEY CURLS 06

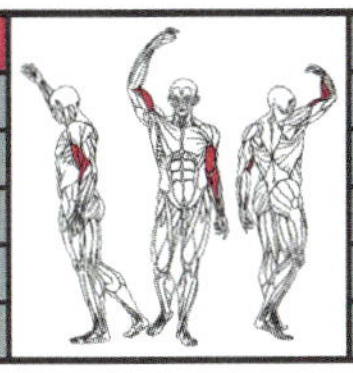

Flexor digitorum superficialis
Flexor carpi ulnaris
Palmaris longus
Flexor carpi radialis
Pronator teres
Sternocleidomastoid
Aponeurotic expansion of biceps brachii
Triceps brachii, medial head
Brachialis
Biceps brachii
Triceps brachii, long head
Coracobrachialis
Teres major
Latissimus dorsi
Serratus anterior
Ulna
Radius
Brachialis
Humerus
Long head
Short head
Biceps brachii
Clavicle
Scapula
Sternum
Rib
Pectoralis major

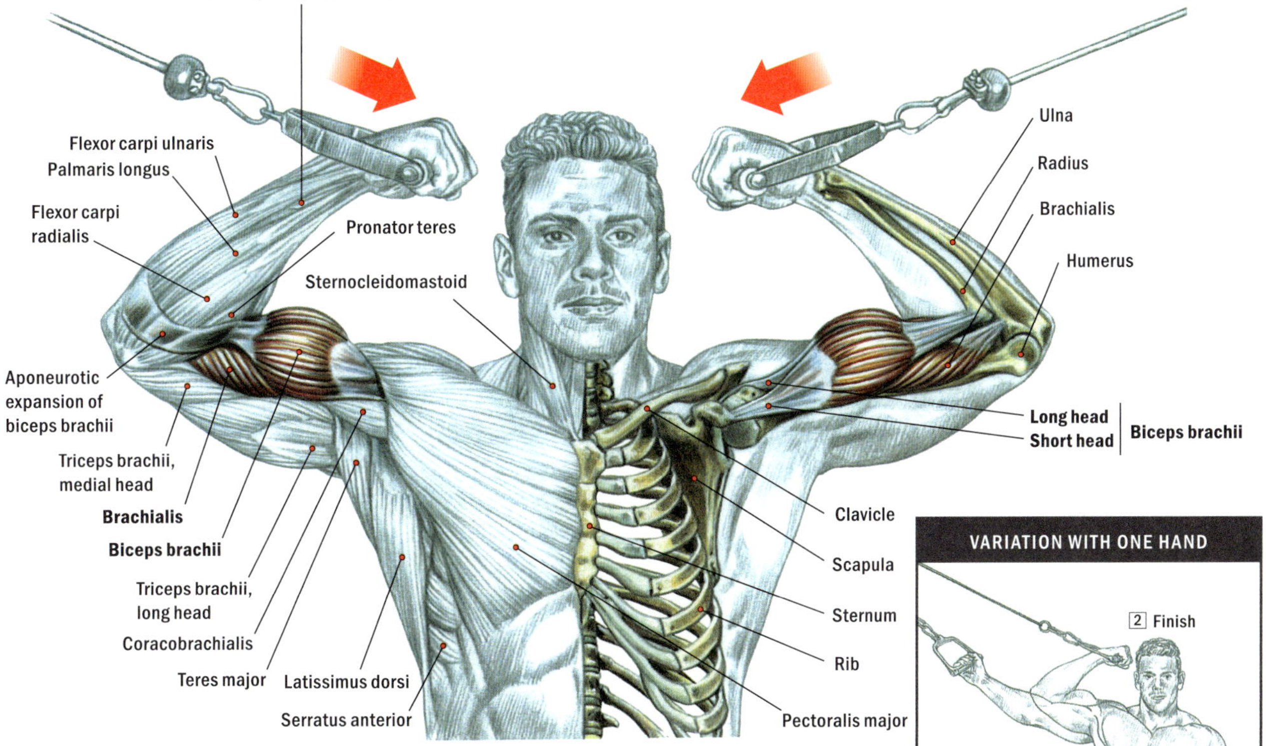

Stand between the pulleys with your arms apart and grasp the handles of the high pulleys with an underhand grip:

- Inhale and bend your arms.
- Exhale at the end of the exercise.

This exercise, which is most often performed as a cool-down at the end of an arm session, focuses the work on the short head of the biceps brachii, which has been stretched and put under tension because of the arms' extended position at the start. This exercise also works the brachialis, the monoarticular elbow flexor.

Do this exercise with light weights so that you can concentrate and feel the contraction of the internal part of the biceps brachii. Sets with a high number of reps give the best results.

VARIATION WITH ONE HAND

2 Finish
1 Start

Phalanx
Metacarpal
Carpal
Radius
Ulna
Humerus
Biceps brachii tendon, partially wrapped around the radius
Biceps brachii tendon, partially unwrapped and stretched around the radius

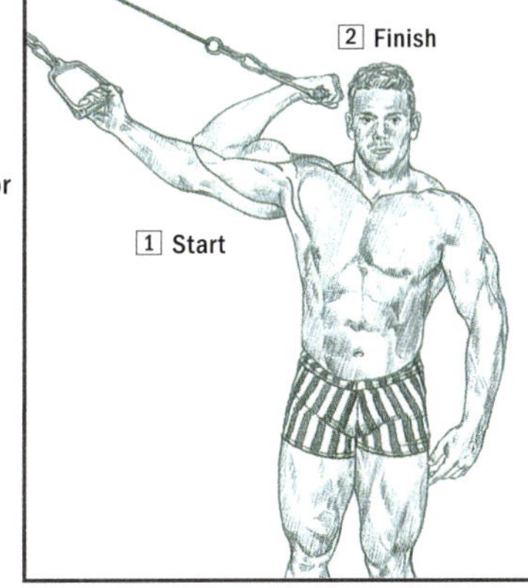

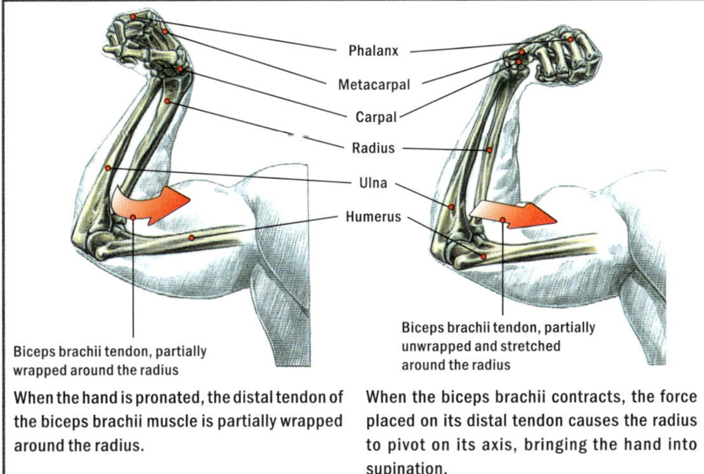

When the hand is pronated, the distal tendon of the biceps brachii muscle is partially wrapped around the radius.

When the biceps brachii contracts, the force placed on its distal tendon causes the radius to pivot on its axis, bringing the hand into supination.

Extensor carpi ulnaris
Flexor carpi ulnaris
Palmaris longus
Flexor carpi radialis
Biceps brachii, aponeurosis
Pronator teres
Triceps brachii, medial head
Brachialis
Biceps brachii
Triceps brachii, long head
Flexor digitorum superficialis
Brachioradialis
Deltoid
Coracobrachialis
Teres major
Subscapularis
Pectoralis major
Latissimus dorsi
Serratus anterior
External oblique

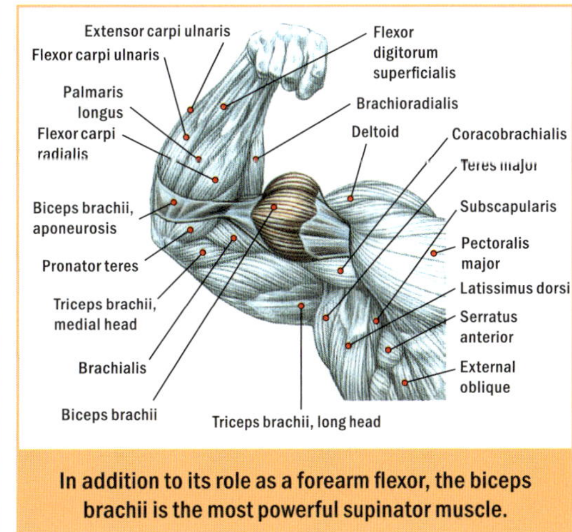

In addition to its role as a forearm flexor, the biceps brachii is the most powerful supinator muscle.

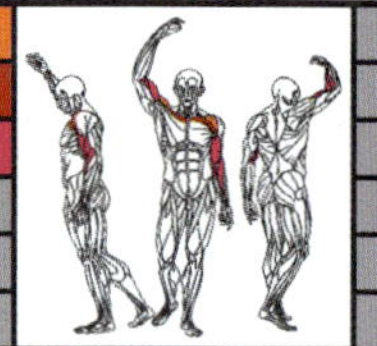

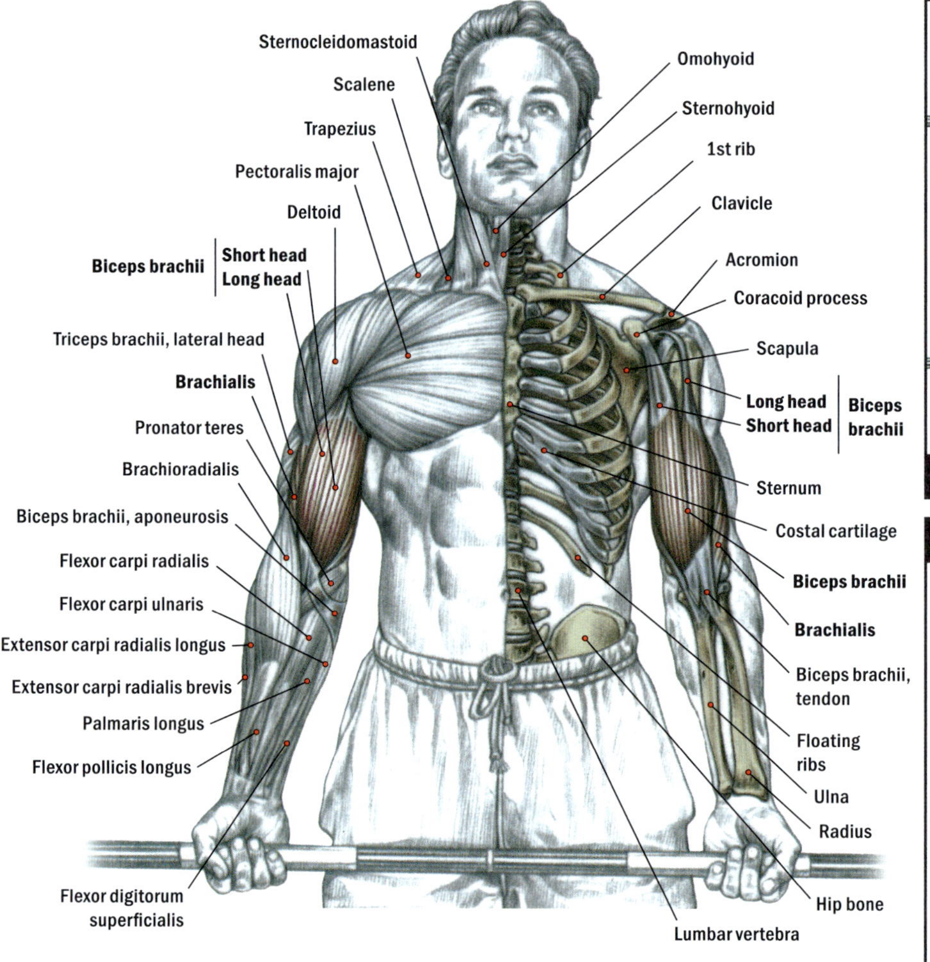

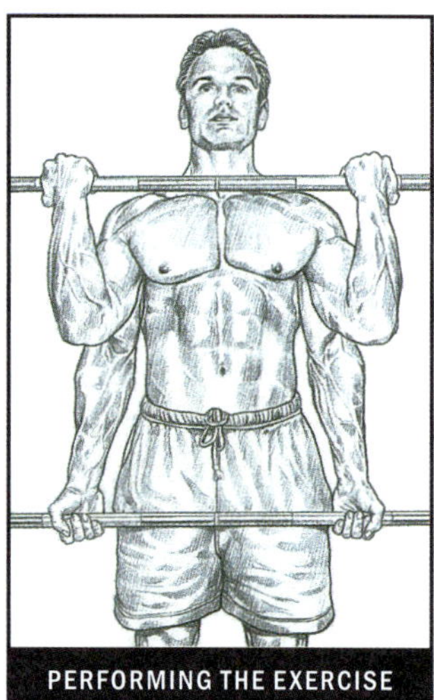
PERFORMING THE EXERCISE

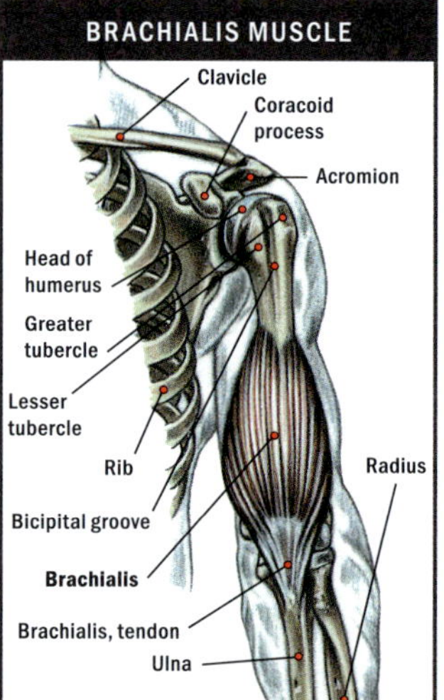
BRACHIALIS MUSCLE

Stand with your back straight. Grasp the barbell with an underhand grip and hands slightly wider than shoulder-width apart:

- Inhale and flex your forearms, taking care to stabilize your torso and spine by isometrically contracting your gluteus muscles, abdominal muscles, and spinal muscles.
- Exhale at the end of the exercise.

This exercise mainly works the biceps brachii, the brachialis, and, to a lesser degree, the brachioradialis, the pronator teres, and the wrist and finger flexor muscles.

Variations

- Vary the width of the grip to work different parts of the muscle more intensely:
  - Place your hands very far apart to isolate the short head of the biceps brachii.
  - Place your hands very close together to isolate the long head of the biceps brachii.
- Lifting both elbows after they are flexed increases the contraction of the biceps brachii and contracts the anterior deltoid.
- To make the exercise more difficult, press your back against a wall so that your shoulder blades do not come off of the wall.
- You can also lift more weight and gain strength by leaning your torso backward to help lift the bar. However, use this technique cautiously to avoid injury; among other things, it requires well-developed abdominal and lumbar muscles.

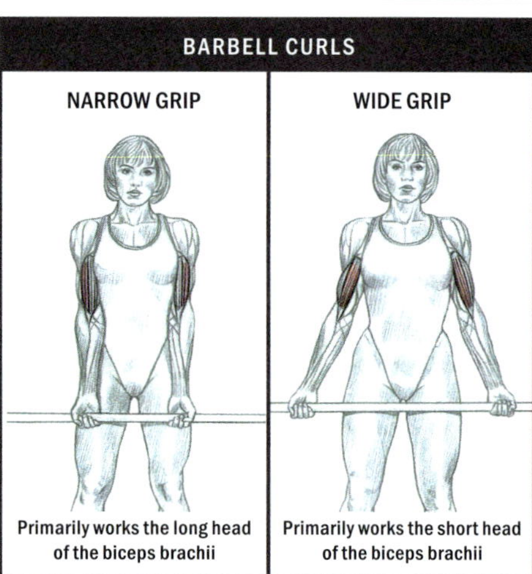
BARBELL CURLS

Primarily works the long head of the biceps brachii

Primarily works the short head of the biceps brachii

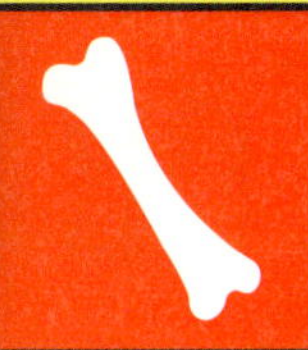

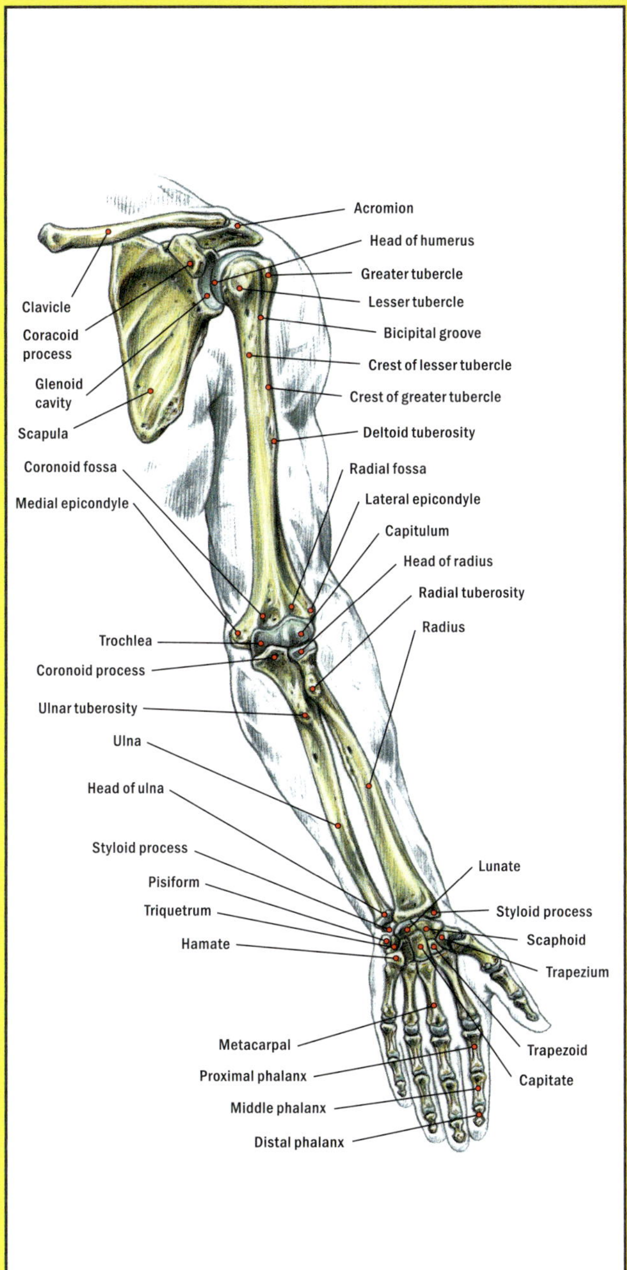

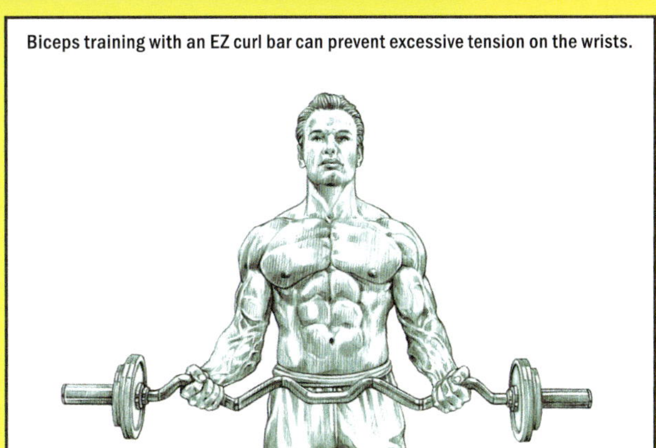

Biceps training with an EZ curl bar can prevent excessive tension on the wrists.

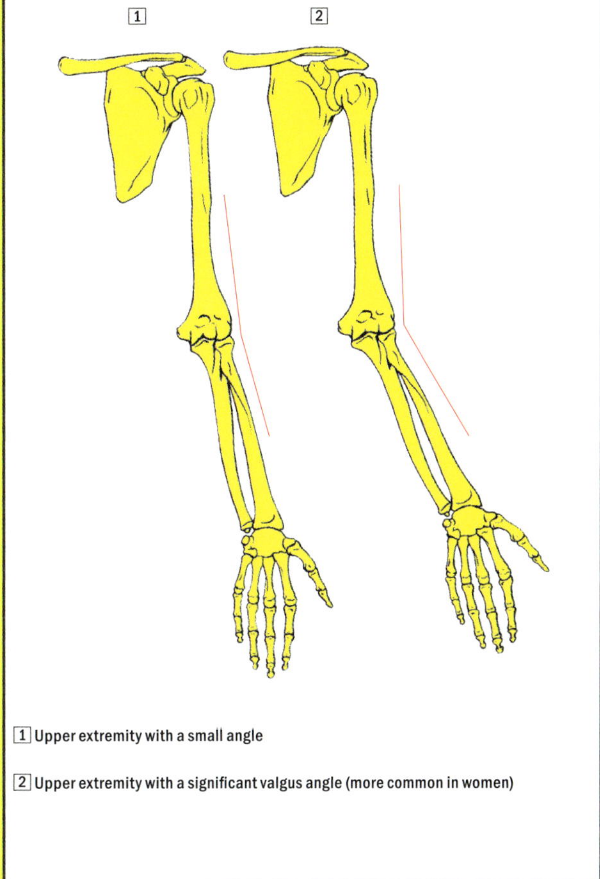

1 Upper extremity with a small angle

2 Upper extremity with a significant valgus angle (more common in women)

When working the biceps brachii using a barbell, it is important to consider individual differences in morphology. The angle at the elbow between the upper arm and the forearm varies from person to person. Some people have a large angle at the elbow when their arms are hanging at their sides with the palms facing forward and thumbs to the outside. The forearm is in a valgus position, clearly pointing outward. Because of this angle, they will have to bend their wrists inward when using a bar to do curls. This can make strength training painful. To alleviate this problem, it is best to use an EZ curl bar to spare their wrists.

Valgus of the elbow is usually more pronounced in women.

08 MACHINE CURLS

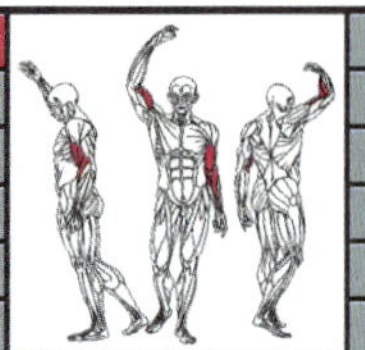

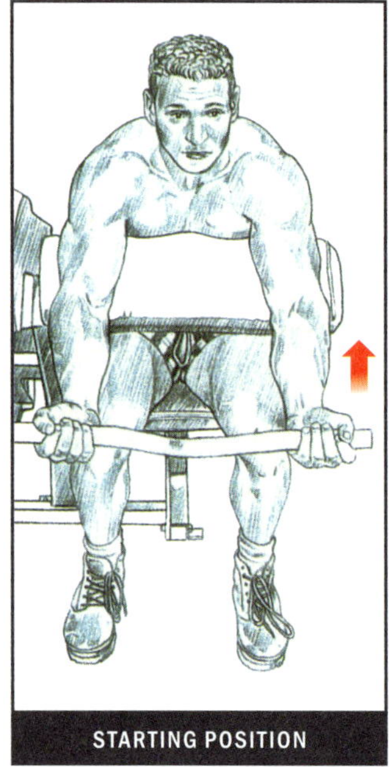

STARTING POSITION

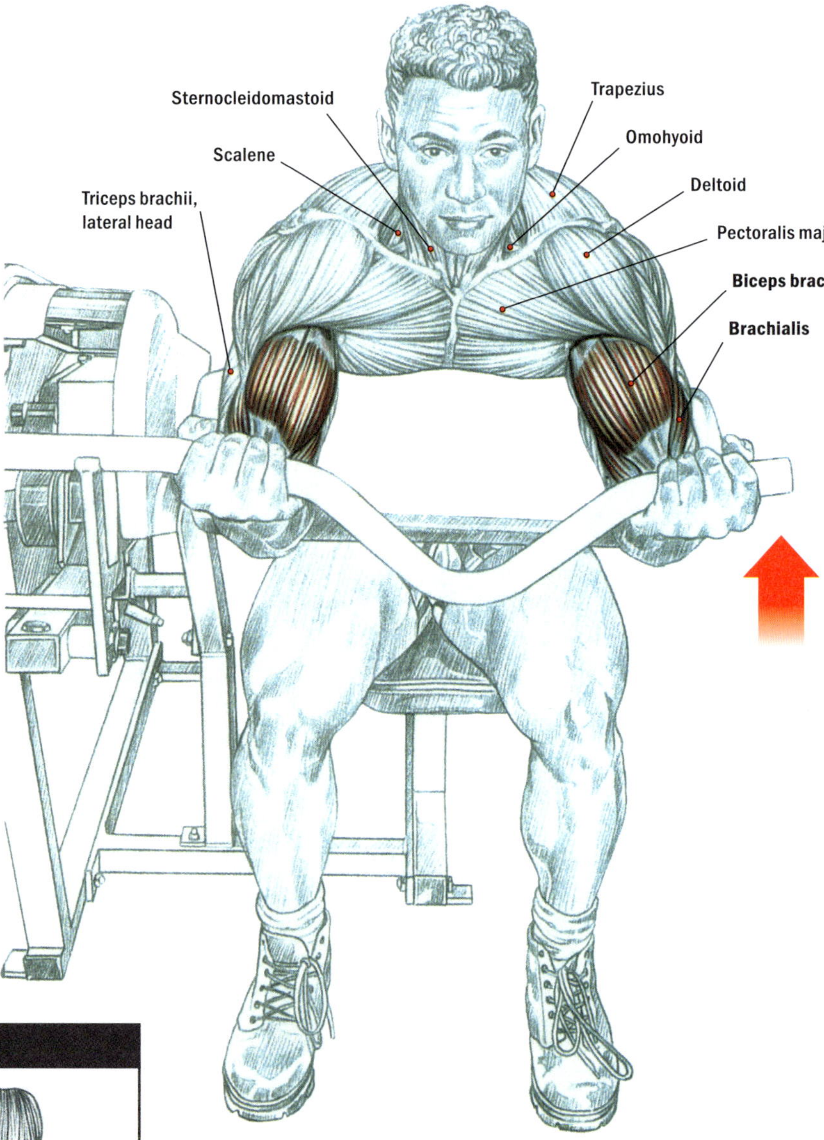

VARIATION

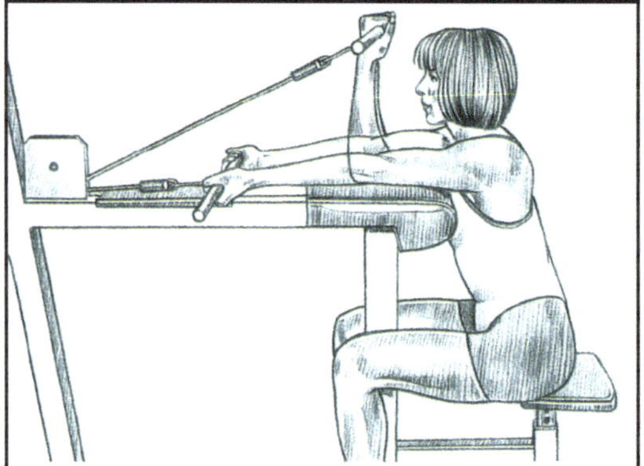

Doing Atlas curls with a pulley is a great way to pump up the muscle.

Sit at the machine and grasp the bar with an underhand grip and with your arms extended and resting on the support:

- Inhale and raise your forearms.
- Exhale at the end of the exercise.

This is one of the best exercises for working the biceps brachii. Fixing the arms against the support makes it impossible to cheat.

At the beginning, the muscle tension is intense, so be sure to warm up properly using light weights. To avoid the risk of tendinitis, do not completely straighten your arms.

This movement also works the brachialis and, to a lesser extent, the brachioradialis and pronator teres.

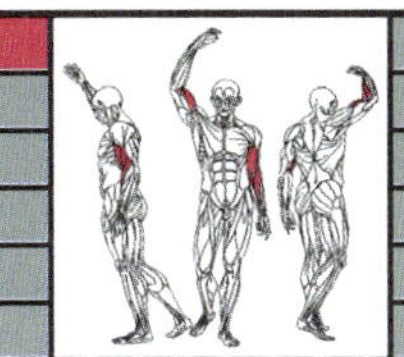

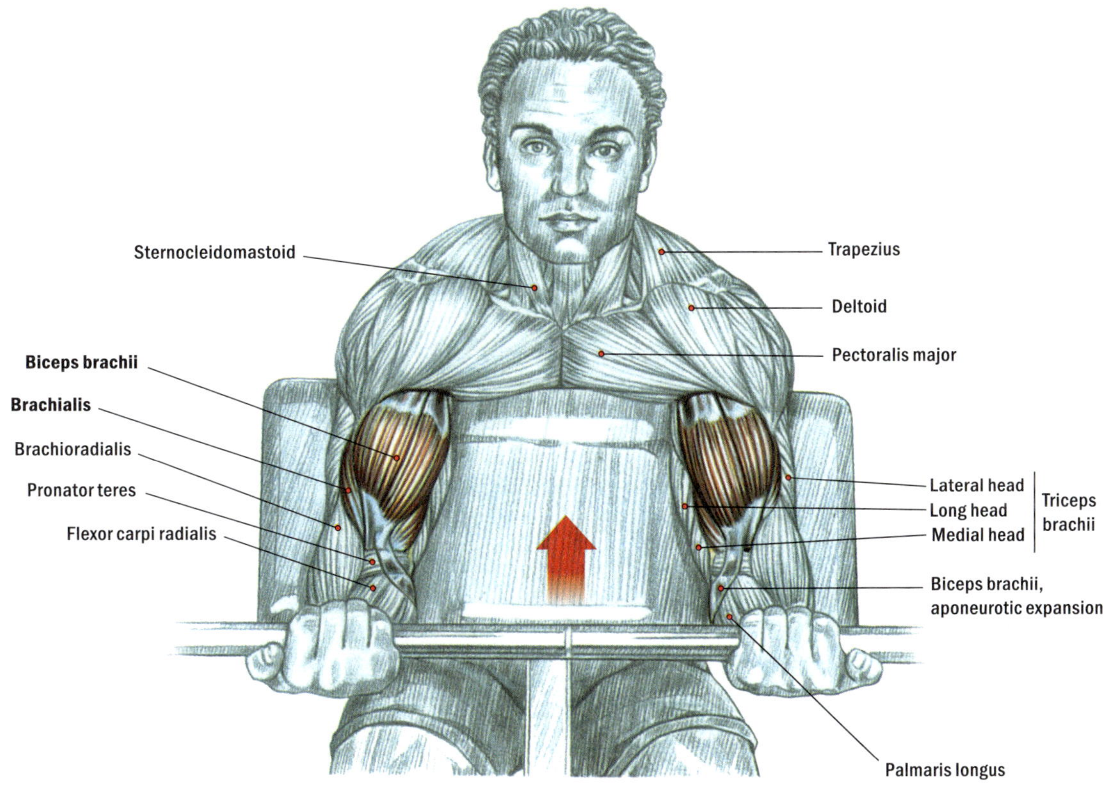

Sit with your arms resting on the support pad and grasp the bar with an underhand grip:

- Inhale and raise your forearms.
- Exhale at the end of the exercise.

This is one of the best exercises for focused work on the biceps.

⚠

The angle of the support pad places significant tension on the forearms when the arms are completely extended. Therefore, warm up the muscles properly and begin with lighter weights.

MUSCLE ANATOMY

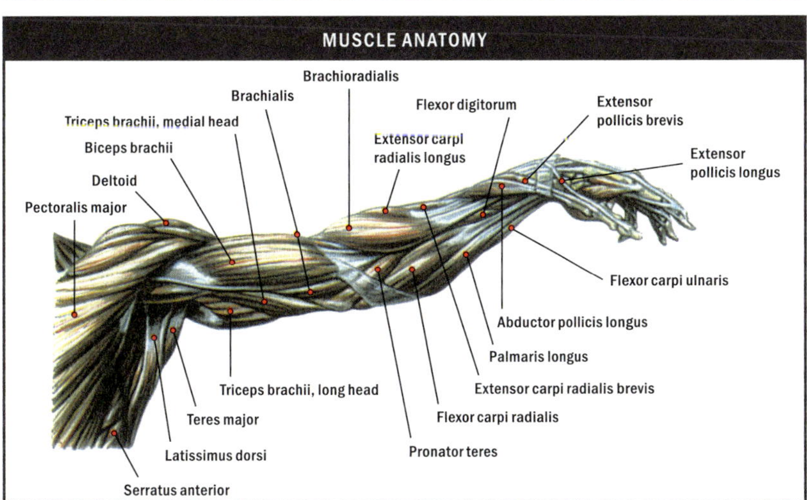

PERFORMING THE EXERCISE

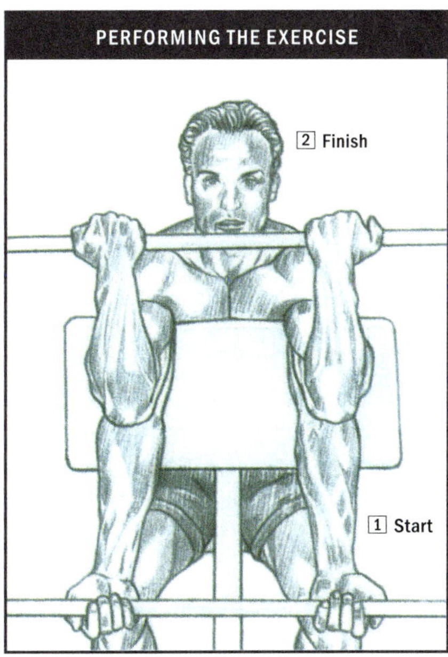

10 STANDING REVERSE WRIST CURLS

ENDING POSITION

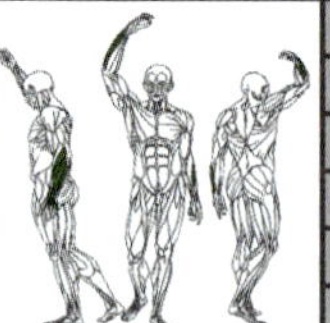

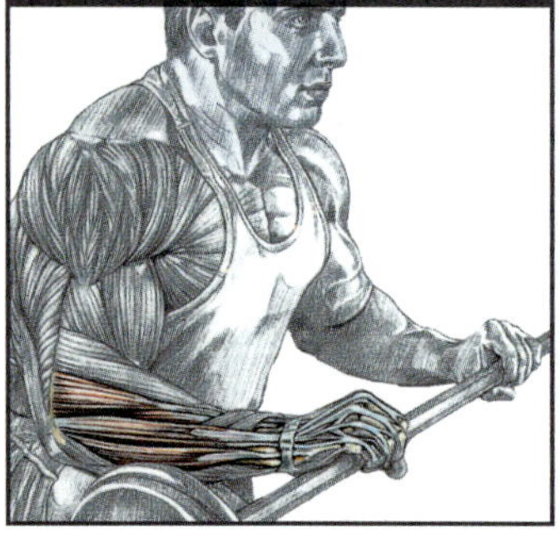

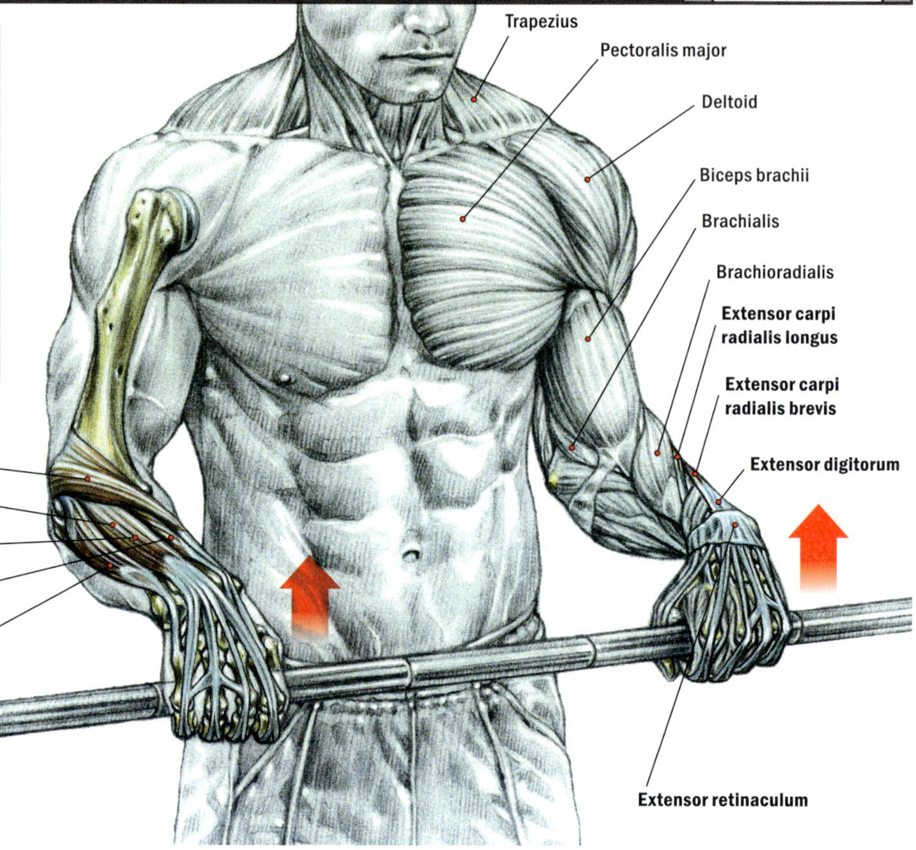

Stand with your forearms in a horizontal position and grasp the bar with an overhand grip, keeping your wrists relaxed:

- Inhale and lift your hands.

This exercise works the extensor carpi radialis longus and brevis, extensor digitorum, extensor digiti minimi, and extensor carpi ulnaris.

This exercise is excellent for strengthening the wrist extensors, which are often underdeveloped because of a focus on developing the wrist flexors. High-repetition sets of 10 to 50 reps will strengthen the wrist extensors and can reduce wrist pain, which is common in these joints.

BONE ANATOMY

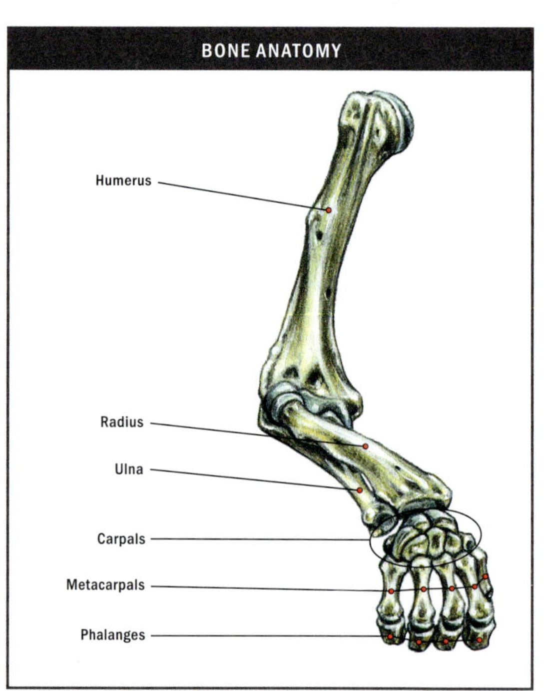

SEATED REVERSE WRIST CURLS 11

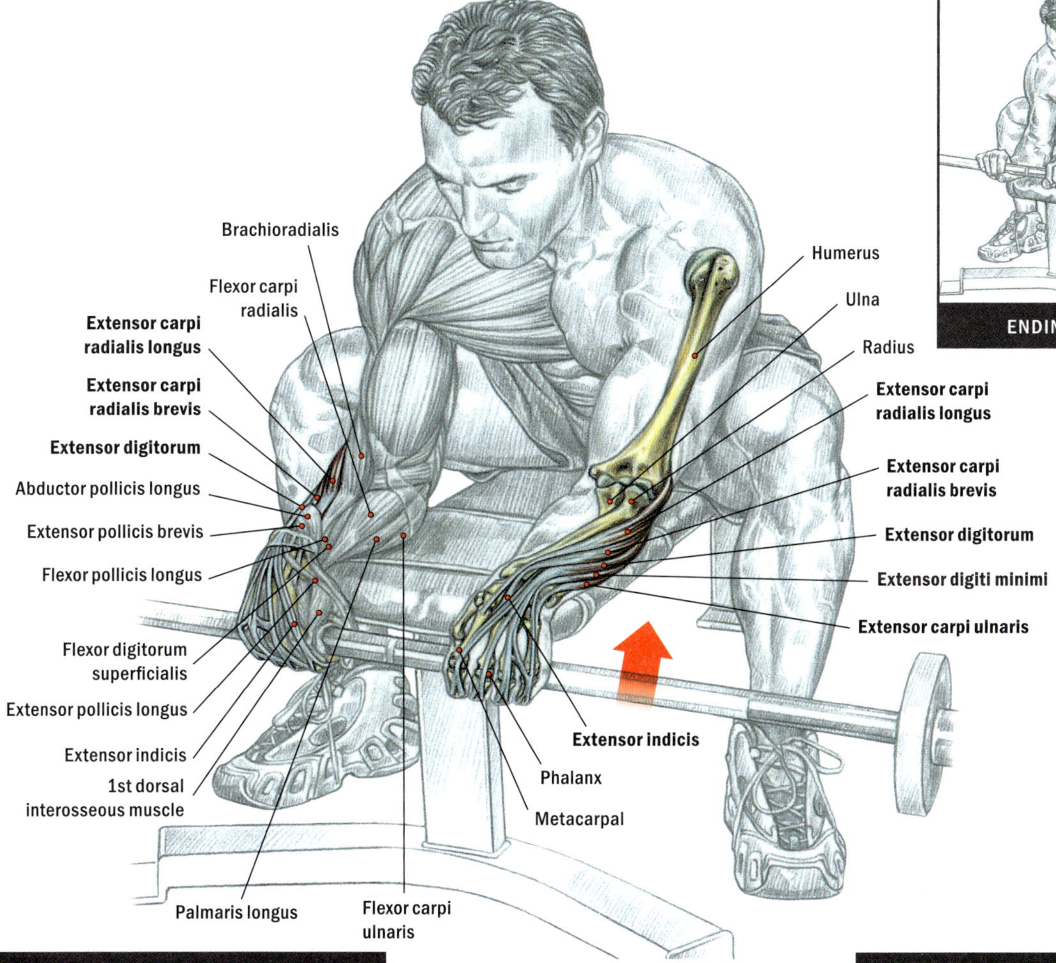

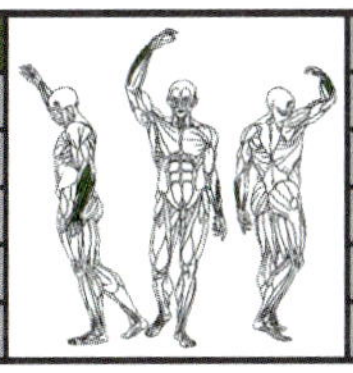

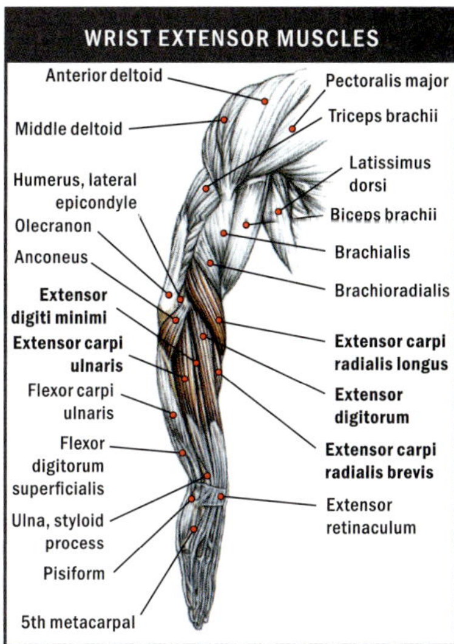

Brachioradialis
Flexor carpi radialis
Extensor carpi radialis longus
Extensor carpi radialis brevis
Extensor digitorum
Abductor pollicis longus
Extensor pollicis brevis
Flexor pollicis longus
Flexor digitorum superficialis
Extensor pollicis longus
Extensor indicis
1st dorsal interosseous muscle
Palmaris longus
Flexor carpi ulnaris
Humerus
Ulna
Radius
Extensor carpi radialis longus
Extensor carpi radialis brevis
Extensor digitorum
Extensor digiti minimi
Extensor carpi ulnaris
Extensor indicis
Phalanx
Metacarpal

ENDING POSITION

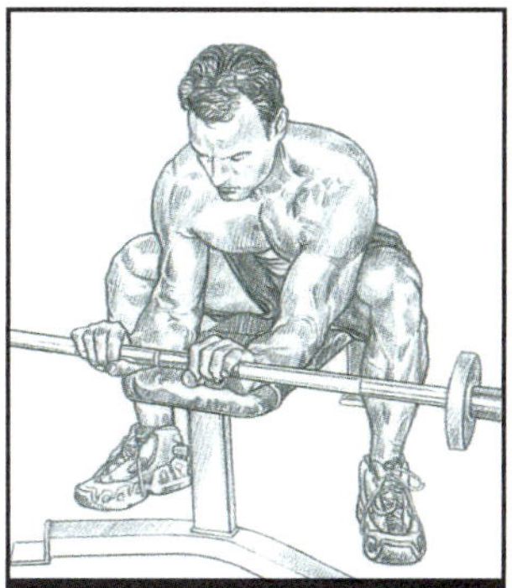

WRIST EXTENSORS

Humerus
Medial epicondyle
Olecranon
Extensor carpi radialis longus
Extensor digitorum
Extensor carpi ulnaris
Extensor carpi radialis brevis
Ulna
Head of ulna
Extensor digiti minimi
Radius
Carpal
Metacarpal
Proximal phalanx
Middle phalanx
Distal phalanx
Extensor indicis

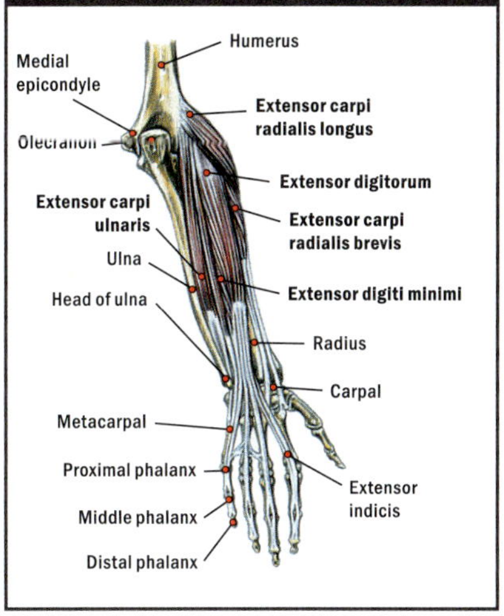

Sit with your forearms resting on your thighs or on a bench and grasp the bar with an overhand grip, keeping your wrists relaxed:

- Inhale and lift your hands.

This exercise contracts the extensor carpi radialis longus and brevis, extensor digitorum, extensor digiti minimi, and extensor carpi ulnaris.

This exercise strengthens the wrists, which are often vulnerable because of weak wrist extensor muscles.

WRIST EXTENSOR MUSCLES

Anterior deltoid
Middle deltoid
Humerus, lateral epicondyle
Olecranon
Anconeus
Extensor digiti minimi
Extensor carpi ulnaris
Flexor carpi ulnaris
Flexor digitorum superficialis
Ulna, styloid process
Pisiform
5th metacarpal
Pectoralis major
Triceps brachii
Latissimus dorsi
Biceps brachii
Brachialis
Brachioradialis
Extensor carpi radialis longus
Extensor digitorum
Extensor carpi radialis brevis
Extensor retinaculum

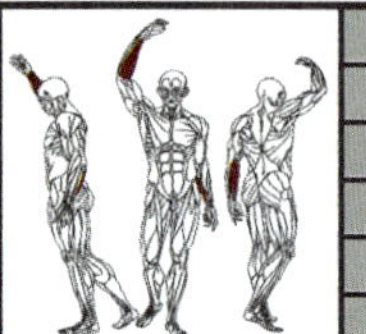

Deltoid

Biceps brachii

Triceps brachii, long head

Brachialis

Triceps brachii, medial head

Pronator teres

Brachioradialis

Flexor carpi radialis

Palmaris longus

Pisiform

Flexor digitorum superficialis and profundus

Flexor carpi ulnaris

Pectoralis major

Humerus

Ulna

Radial tuberosity

Radius

Pisiform

Trapezium

Metacarpal

Flexor digitorum superficialis, covering the flexor digitorum profundus

Flexor pollicis longus

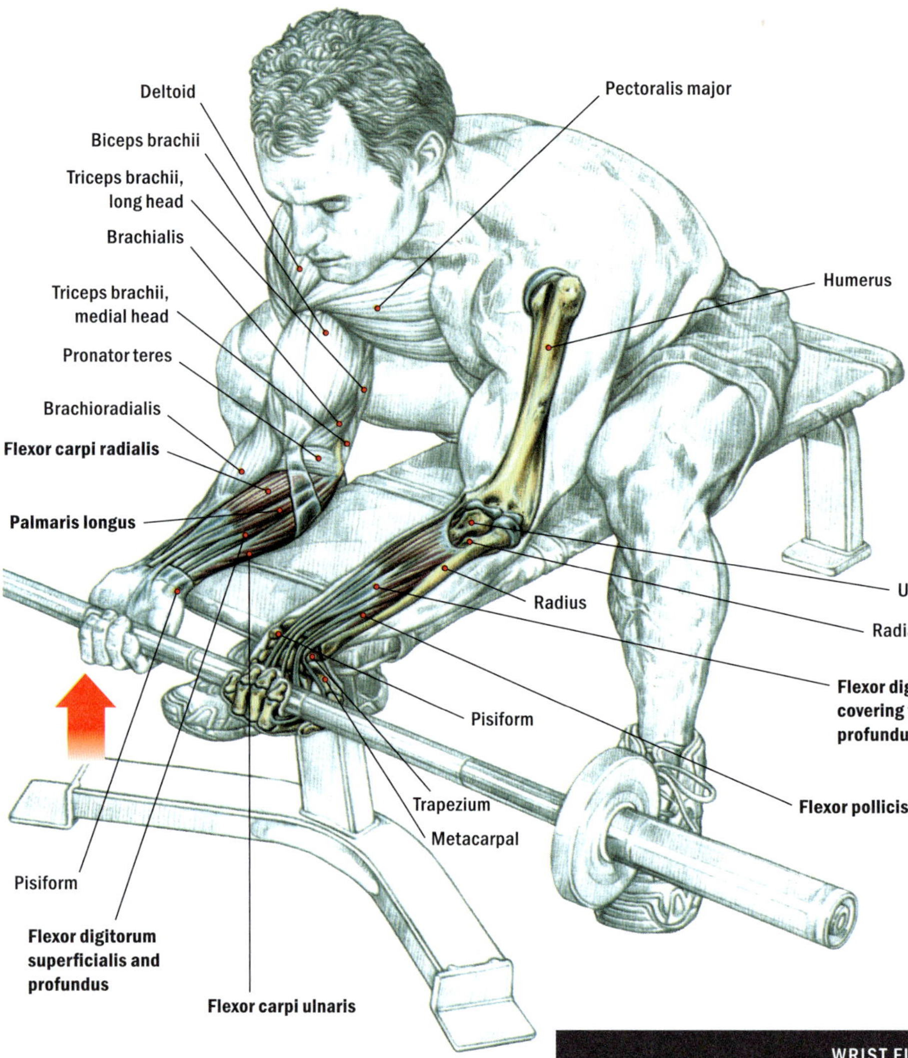

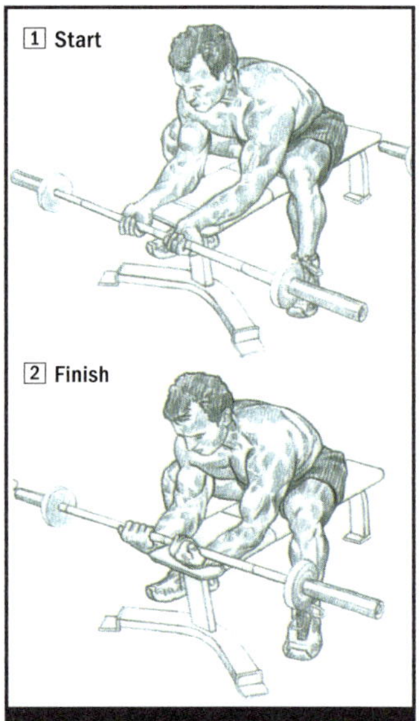

PERFORMING THE EXERCISE

1 Start

2 Finish

Sit with your forearms resting on your thighs or on a bench and grasp the bar with an underhand grip and with the wrists relaxed:

• Inhale and raise your hands.

This exercise works the flexor carpi radialis, palmaris longus, flexor carpi ulnaris, flexor digitorum superficialis, and flexor digitorum profundus. The latter two muscles, although located deep in the wrist, make up most of the mass of the wrist flexors.

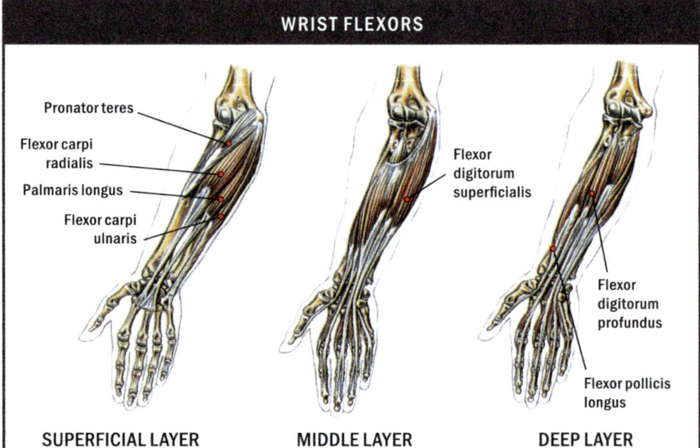

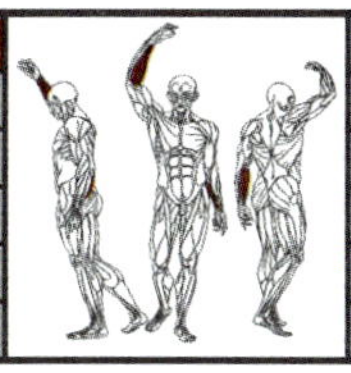

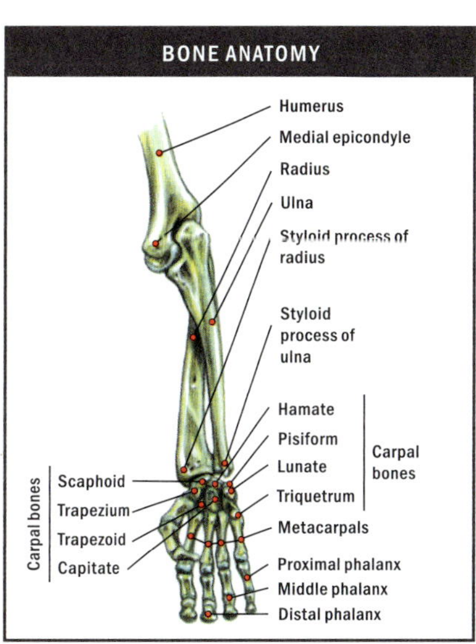

Trapezius
- Upper portion
- Middle portion
- Lower portion

Spine of scapula
Acromion
Posterior deltoid
Infraspinatus
Teres minor
Rhomboid
Teres major

Triceps brachii
- Long head
- Lateral head
- Medial head

Brachioradialis
Biceps brachii
Brachialis
Flexor carpi ulnaris
Flexor digitorum muscles
Anconeus
Antebrachial fascia

Extensor carpi ulnaris
Flexor carpi radialis
Palmaris longus
Brachioradialis, tendon

Flexor pollicis longus

Abductor digiti minimi
Opponens digiti minimi
Aponeurosis palmaris

Abductor pollicis brevis
Flexor pollicis brevis
Flexor retinaculum

Sternocleidomastoid
Splenius capitis
Levator scapulae
4th cervical vertebra
Splenius capitis
Clavicle
Acromion
Head of humerus
Scapula
Deltoid tuberosity
Humerus

Latissimus dorsi

Flexor digitorum superficialis

Flexor retinaculum covering the carpal tunnel

Flexor digitorum superficialis, tendons

Flexor digitorum profundus, tendons

Lumbricals

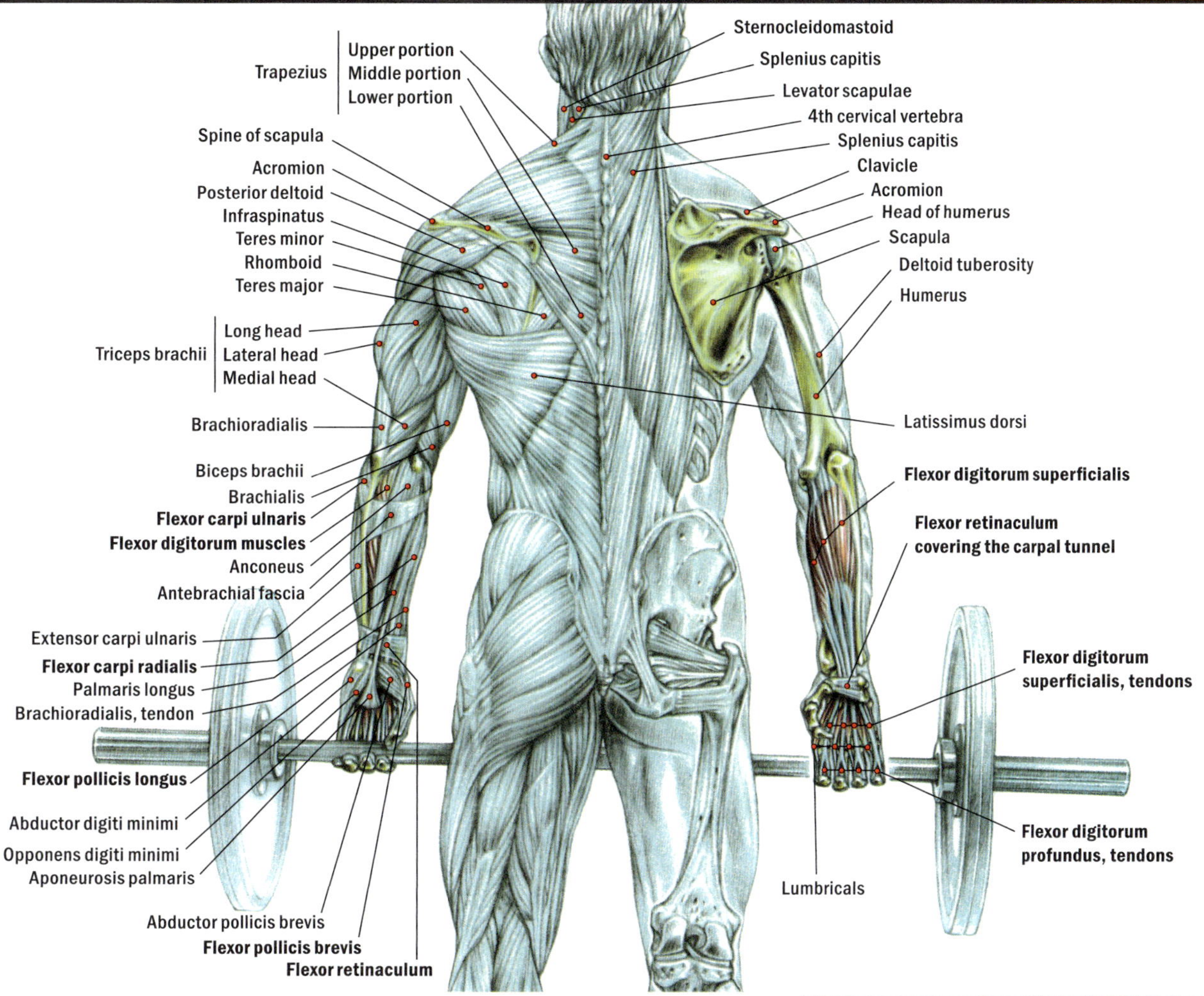

Stand and grasp the bar with an overhand grip:

- Roll the bar to the end of your fingers.
- Bend your fingers to bring the bar back into the palm of your hands.

This exercise works the deep and superficial finger flexor muscles; these muscles are used to grasp objects and to make a strong fist.

This exercise is helpful for strengthening the grip, allowing you to hold barbells and dumbbells better and, therefore, to lift heavier weights. It also helps improve your grip on the bar during pull-ups.

This is an excellent complementary exercise for combat sports such as judo and wrestling in which the power of the grip is key to grabbing and pulling an opponent. Sets of 10 to 30 reps give very good results.

BONE ANATOMY

Humerus
Medial epicondyle
Radius
Ulna
Styloid process of radius
Styloid process of ulna

Hamate
Pisiform
Lunate
Triquetrum
Metacarpals

Carpal bones

Scaphoid
Trapezium
Trapezoid
Capitate

Carpal bones

Proximal phalanx
Middle phalanx
Distal phalanx

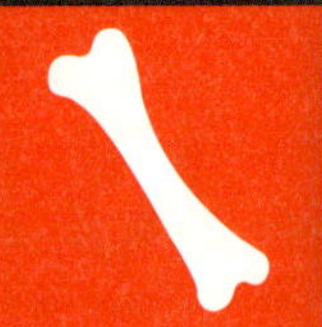

EVOLUTION OF THE HAND

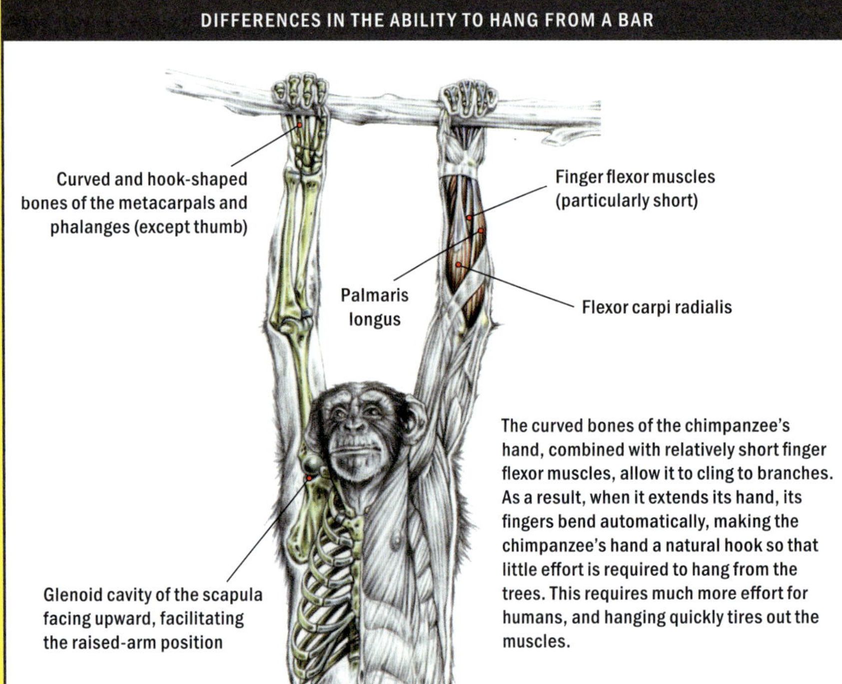

The curved bones of the chimpanzee's hand, combined with relatively short finger flexor muscles, allow it to cling to branches. As a result, when it extends its hand, its fingers bend automatically, making the chimpanzee's hand a natural hook so that little effort is required to hang from the trees. This requires much more effort for humans, and hanging quickly tires out the muscles.

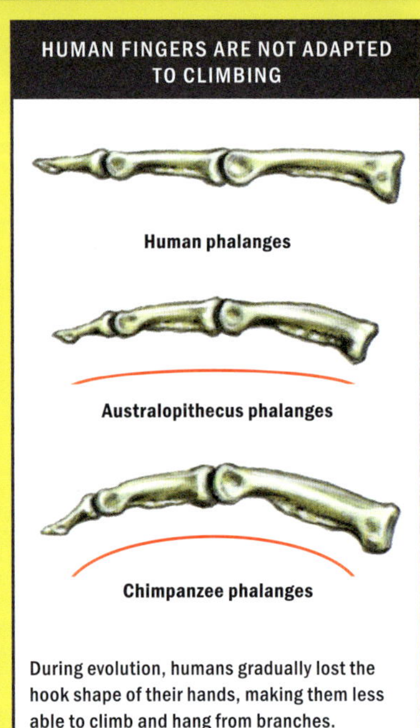

During evolution, humans gradually lost the hook shape of their hands, making them less able to climb and hang from branches.

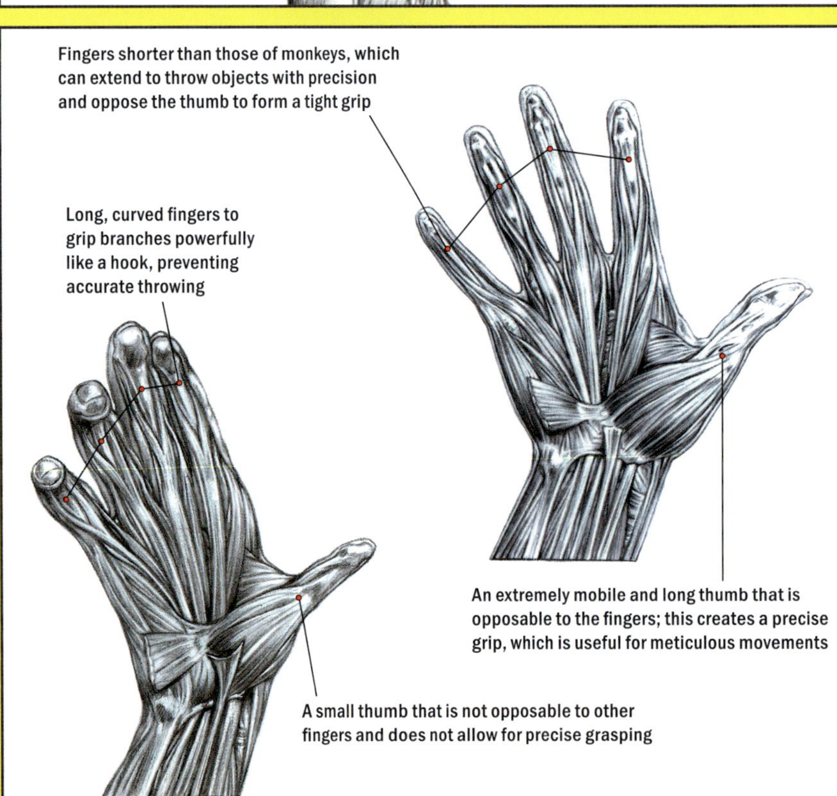

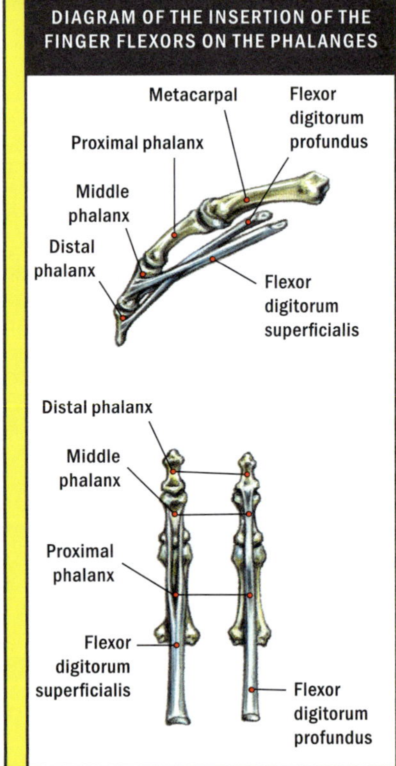

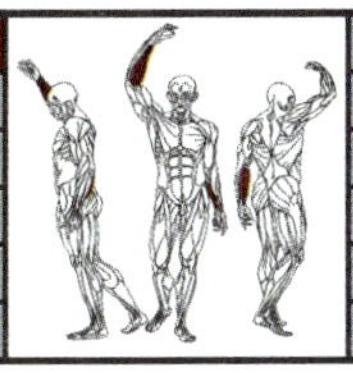

Sternocleidomastoid
Splenius capitis
Levator scapulae
4th cervical vertebra
Splenius capitis
Clavicle
Acromion
Head of humerus
Scapula
Deltoid tuberosity
Humerus

Trapezius
Upper portion
Middle portion
Lower portion

Spine of scapula
Acromion
Posterior deltoid
Infraspinatus
Teres minor
Rhomboid
Teres major

Triceps brachii
Long head
Lateral head
Medial head

Brachioradialis
Biceps brachii
Brachialis
Flexor carpi ulnaris
Flexor digitorum muscles
Anconeus
Antebrachial fascia

Latissimus dorsi

Flexor digitorum superficialis

Flexor retinaculum covering the carpal tunnel

Extensor carpi ulnaris
Flexor carpi radialis
Palmaris longus
Brachioradialis, tendon

Flexor digitorum superficialis, tendons

Flexor pollicis longus
Abductor digiti minimi
Opponens digiti minimi
Aponeurosis palmaris

Flexor digitorum profundus, tendons

Abductor pollicis brevis
Flexor pollicis brevis
Flexor retinaculum

Lumbricals

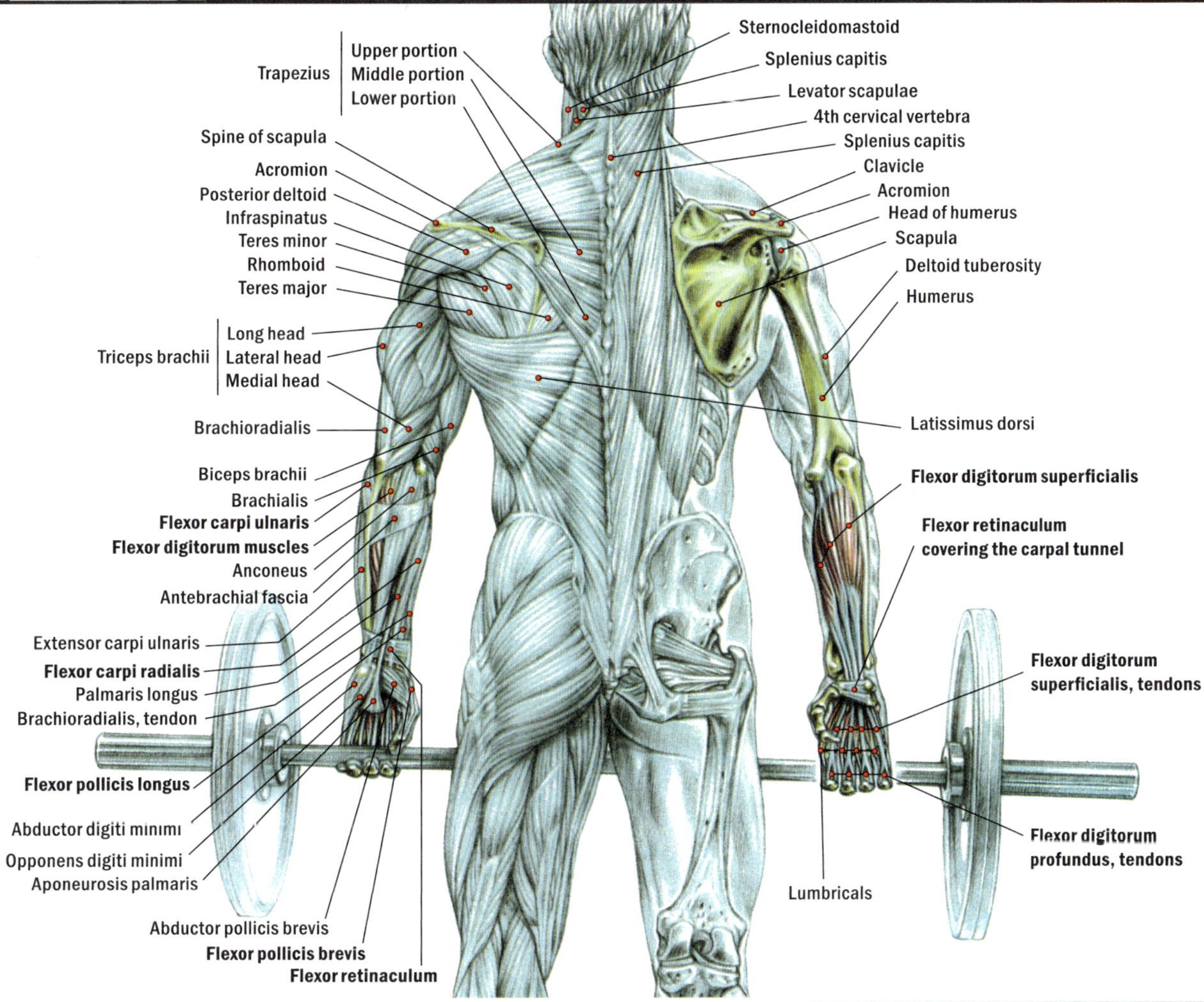

Stand and grasp the bar with an overhand grip:

- Roll the bar to the end of your fingers.
- Bend your fingers to bring the bar back into the palm of your hands.

This exercise works the deep and superficial finger flexor muscles; these muscles are used to grasp objects and to make a strong fist.

This exercise is helpful for strengthening the grip, allowing you to hold barbells and dumbbells better and, therefore, to lift heavier weights. It also helps improve your grip on the bar during pull-ups.

This is an excellent complementary exercise for combat sports such as judo and wrestling in which the power of the grip is key to grabbing and pulling an opponent. Sets of 10 to 30 reps give very good results.

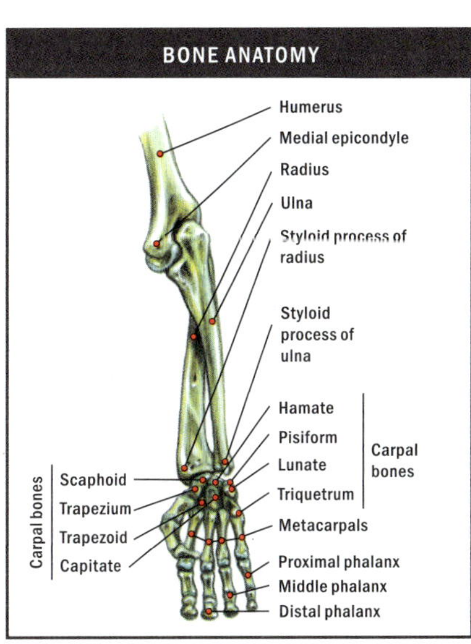

EVOLUTION OF THE HAND

DIFFERENCES IN THE ABILITY TO HANG FROM A BAR

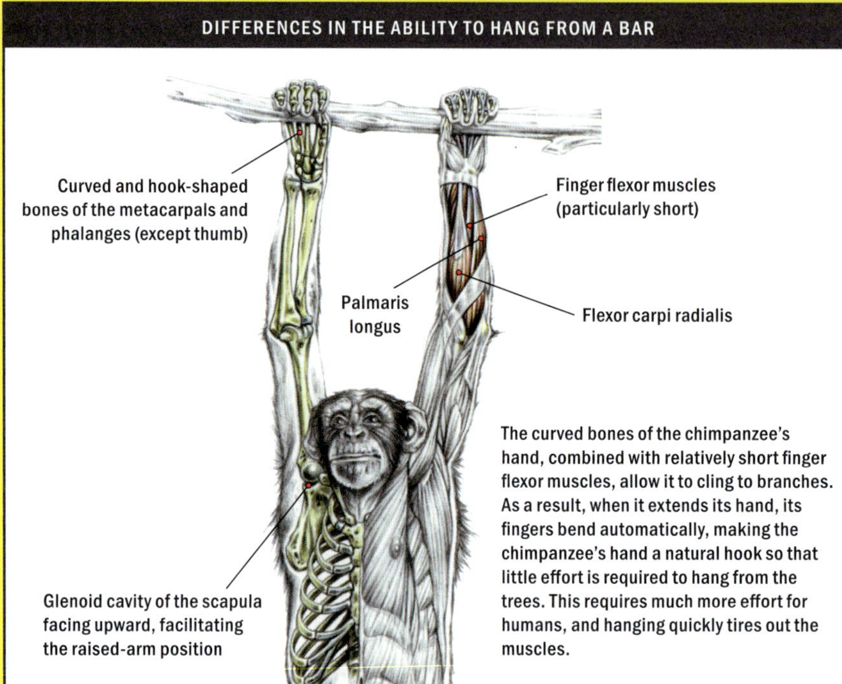

Curved and hook-shaped bones of the metacarpals and phalanges (except thumb)

Finger flexor muscles (particularly short)

Palmaris longus

Flexor carpi radialis

Glenoid cavity of the scapula facing upward, facilitating the raised-arm position

The curved bones of the chimpanzee's hand, combined with relatively short finger flexor muscles, allow it to cling to branches. As a result, when it extends its hand, its fingers bend automatically, making the chimpanzee's hand a natural hook so that little effort is required to hang from the trees. This requires much more effort for humans, and hanging quickly tires out the muscles.

HUMAN FINGERS ARE NOT ADAPTED TO CLIMBING

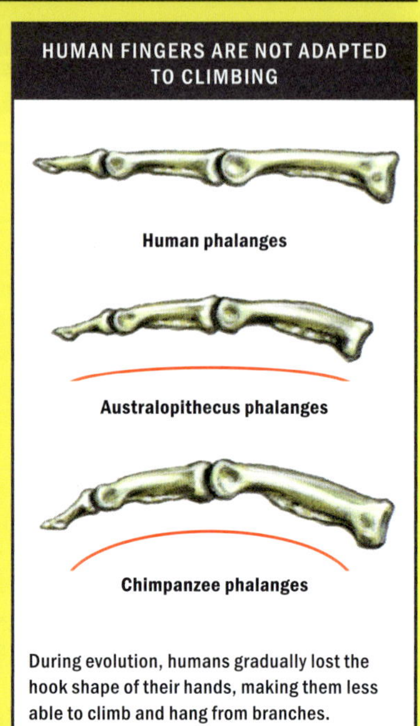

Human phalanges

Australopithecus phalanges

Chimpanzee phalanges

During evolution, humans gradually lost the hook shape of their hands, making them less able to climb and hang from branches.

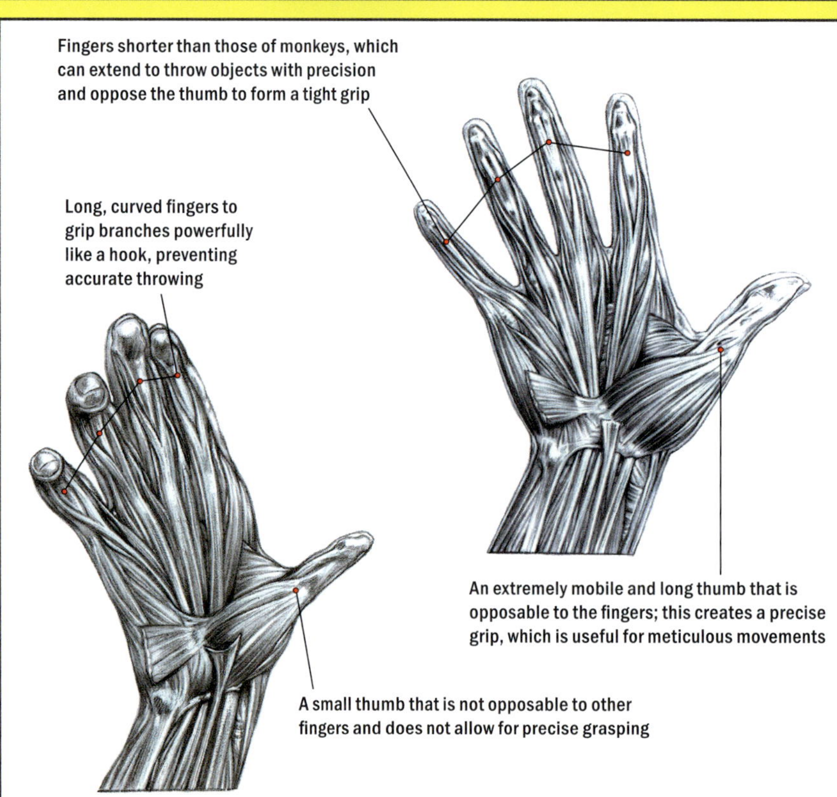

Fingers shorter than those of monkeys, which can extend to throw objects with precision and oppose the thumb to form a tight grip

Long, curved fingers to grip branches powerfully like a hook, preventing accurate throwing

An extremely mobile and long thumb that is opposable to the fingers; this creates a precise grip, which is useful for meticulous movements

A small thumb that is not opposable to other fingers and does not allow for precise grasping

DIAGRAM OF THE INSERTION OF THE FINGER FLEXORS ON THE PHALANGES

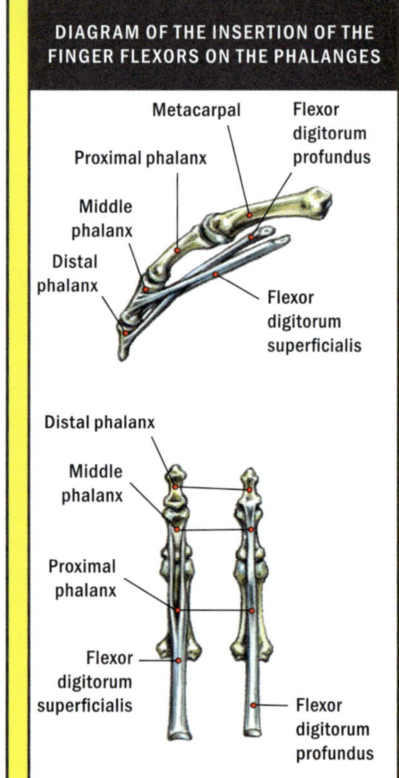

Metacarpal

Flexor digitorum profundus

Proximal phalanx

Middle phalanx

Distal phalanx

Flexor digitorum superficialis

Distal phalanx

Middle phalanx

Proximal phalanx

Flexor digitorum superficialis

Flexor digitorum profundus

COMPARISON BETWEEN THE UPPER LIMBS OF A HUMAN AND A GORILLA

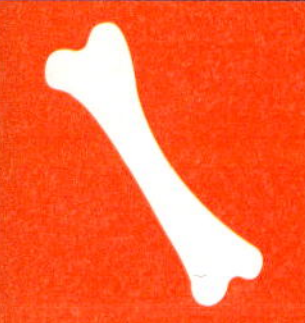

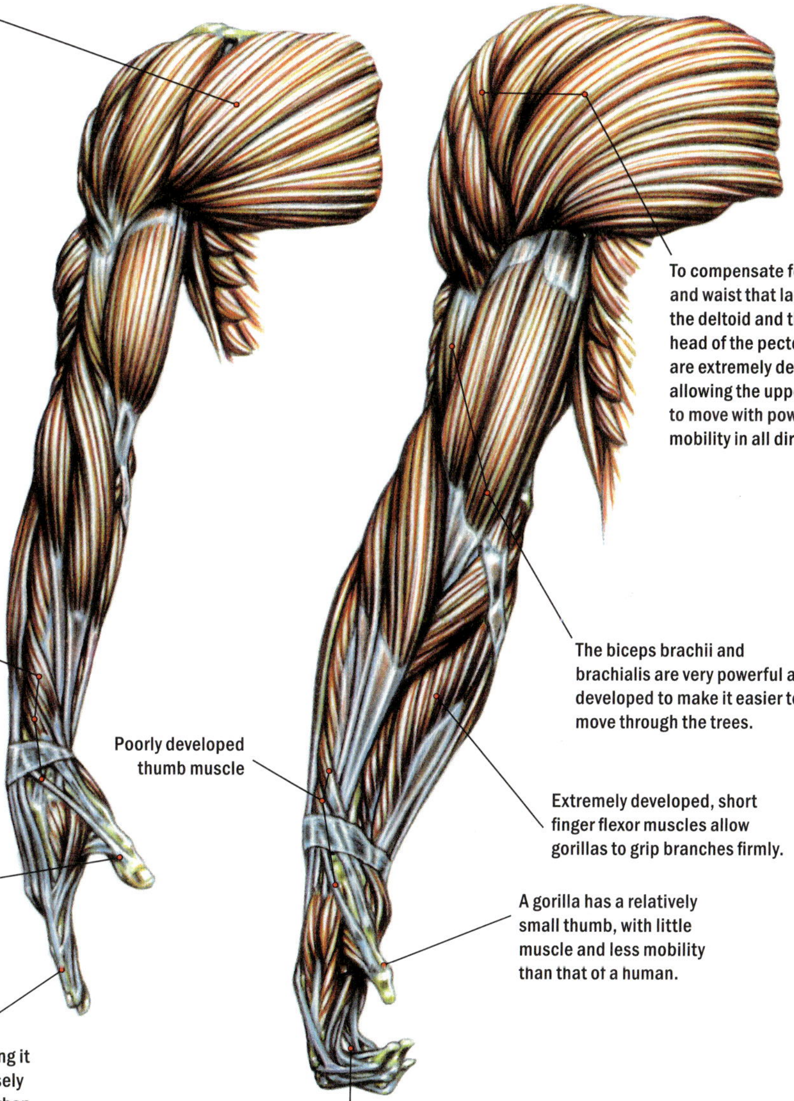
The pectoralis major is adapted more for pulling and rotating the arm toward the center of the body than for raising the arm.
To compensate for a neck and waist that lack mobility, the deltoid and the clavicular head of the pectoralis major are extremely developed, allowing the upper limb to move with power and mobility in all directions.
The abductor pollicis longus, the extensor pollicis brevis, and the extensor pollicis longus are very developed.
The biceps brachii and brachialis are very powerful and developed to make it easier to move through the trees.
Poorly developed thumb muscle
Extremely developed, short finger flexor muscles allow gorillas to grip branches firmly.
The thumb is long, very mobile, and much more muscular than that of other large primates, which allows it to be opposed to other fingers and to form a precise and relatively powerful grip.
A gorilla has a relatively small thumb, with little muscle and less mobility than that of a human.
Fingers can be extended even with the hand extended, making it easier to touch and feel precisely and allowing more precision when throwing objects, which has made man a formidable hunter.
Because the flexor digitorum muscles are very short, when the hand is extended, the fingers automatically curl into hooks; this unique feature of large arboreal primates makes it easier for them to grip the branches without tiring out the muscles.

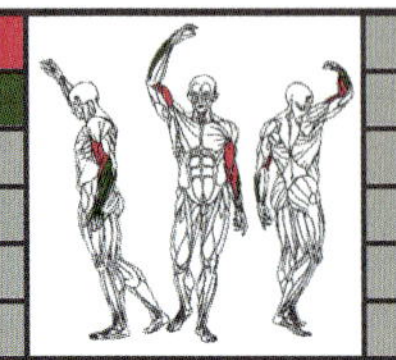

Splenius capitis
Thyrohyoid
Levator scapulae
Sternocleidomastoid
Scalene
Infraspinatus
Teres minor
Teres major
Triceps brachii | Long head
Triceps brachii | Lateral head
Brachioradialis
Extensor carpi radialis longus
Olecranon
Anconeus
Extensor carpi radialis brevis
Extensor digitorum
Extensor digiti minimi
Extensor carpi ulnaris
Flexor carpi ulnaris
Head of ulna
Extensor retinaculum

Omohyoid
Sternohyoid
Trapezius
Deltoid
Pectoralis major
Brachialis
Biceps brachii
Abductor pollicis longus
Extensor pollicis brevis

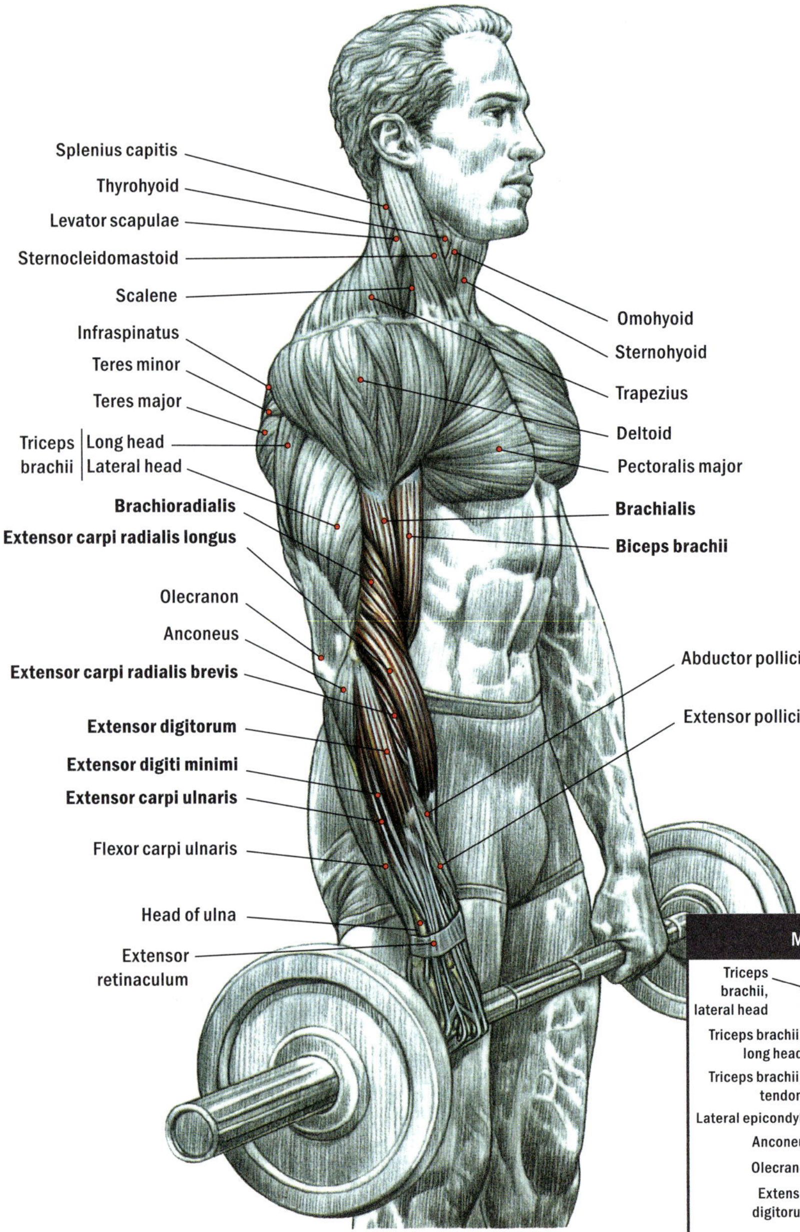

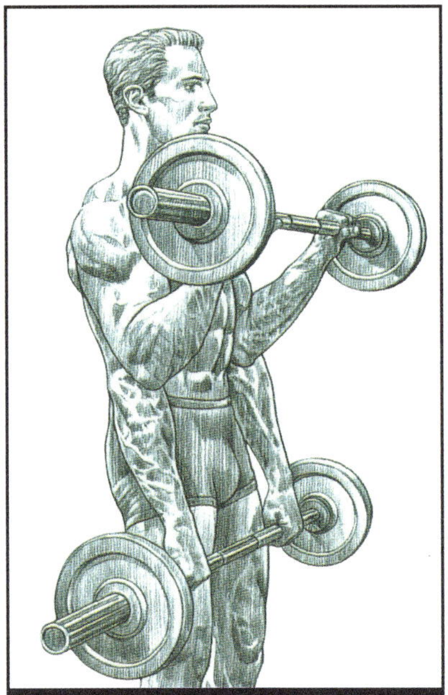

PERFORMING THE EXERCISE

MUSCLES OF THE FOREARM: FRONT VIEW

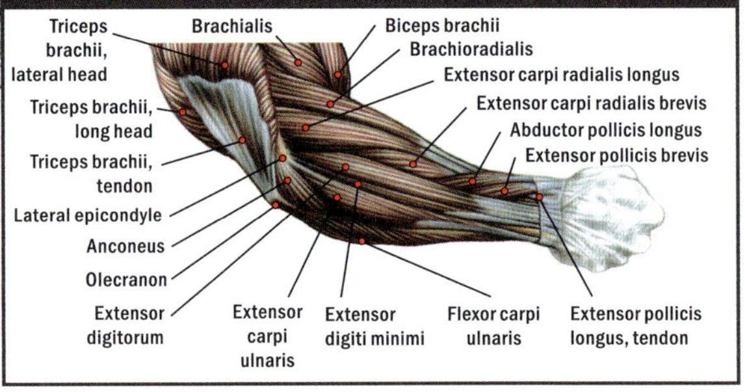

Triceps brachii, lateral head
Brachialis
Biceps brachii
Brachioradialis
Extensor carpi radialis longus
Triceps brachii, long head
Extensor carpi radialis brevis
Abductor pollicis longus
Extensor pollicis brevis
Triceps brachii, tendon
Lateral epicondyle
Anconeus
Olecranon
Extensor digitorum
Extensor carpi ulnaris
Extensor digiti minimi
Flexor carpi ulnaris
Extensor pollicis longus, tendon

Stand with your legs slightly apart and arms extended and grasp the bar with an overhand grip (with the thumbs facing each other):

- Inhale and lift your forearms, exhaling at the end of the movement.
- Return to the starting position, controlling the movement of the bar.

This exercise works the extensor muscles of the wrist (extensor carpi radialis longus, extensor carpi radialis brevis, extensor digitorum, extensor digiti minimi, and extensor carpi ulnaris). It also works the brachioradialis, brachialis, and, to a lesser degree, the biceps brachii.

This is an excellent exercise to strengthen the wrist, which is often weak because of an imbalance caused by having strong wrist flexors and weaker wrist extensors. For this reason, many boxers include the exercise in their training. Many bench press champions use it to keep their wrists from shaking when using extremely heavy weights.

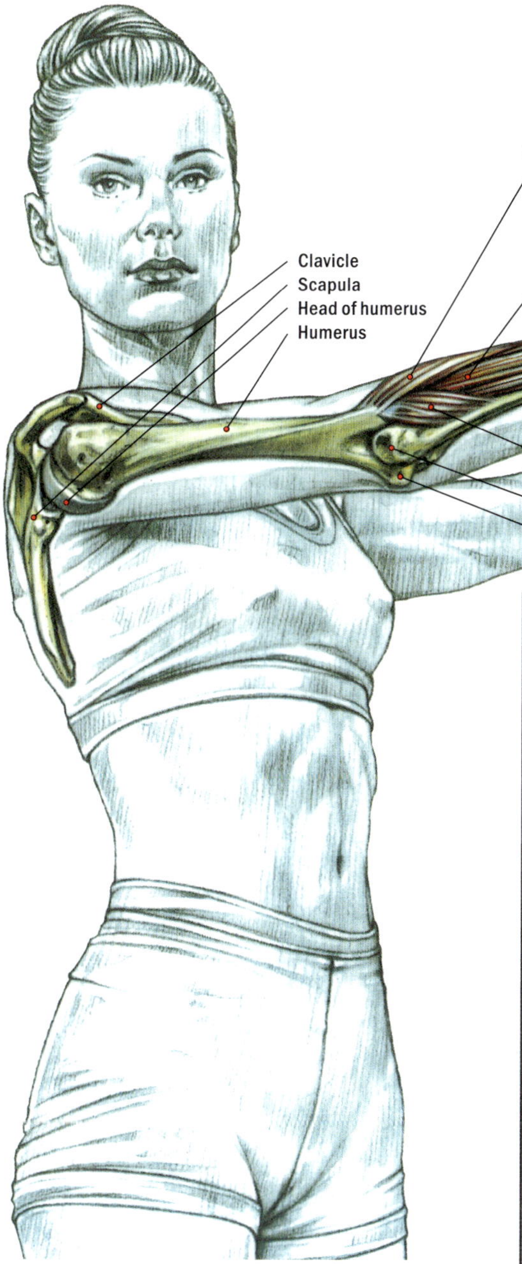

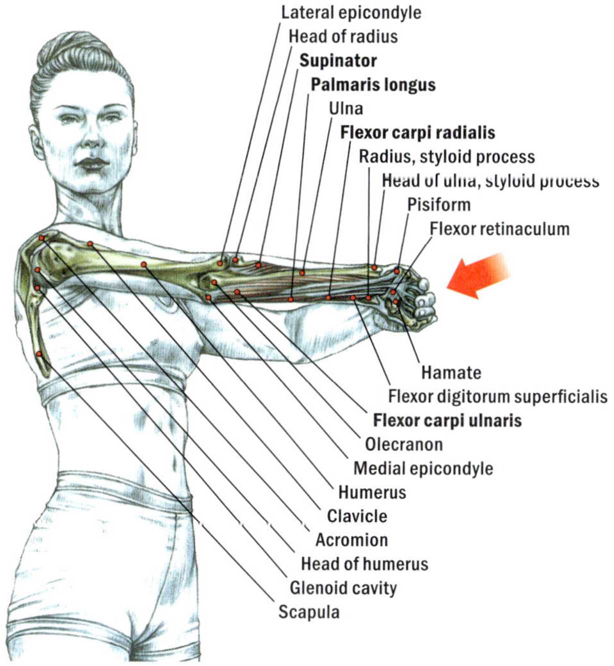

STRETCHING THE WRIST EXTENSOR MUSCLES

Extend your arm straight forward and flex your wrist. Grasp your hand with your other hand and pull slowly, as if you were trying to touch your palm to your forearm. Keep your elbow extended.

This exercise mainly stretches the extensor carpi radialis longus and brevis, extensor digitorum, extensor digiti minimi, extensor carpi ulnaris, and anconeus.

STRETCHING THE WRIST FLEXOR MUSCLES

Extend your arm in front of you with the palm of that hand facing outward. Grasp that hand with your other hand and gently pull as if you were trying to bring the top of your hand toward you while pushing the palm out. This exercise mainly stretches the palmaris longus, flexor carpi radialis, flexor carpi ulnaris, superficial and deep finger flexors, and supinator.

15 TRICEPS PUSH-DOWNS

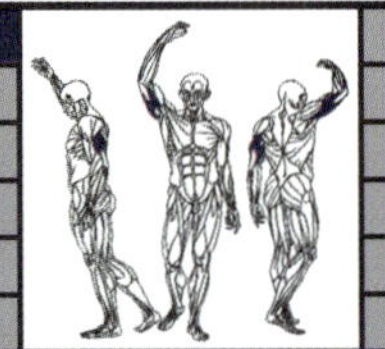

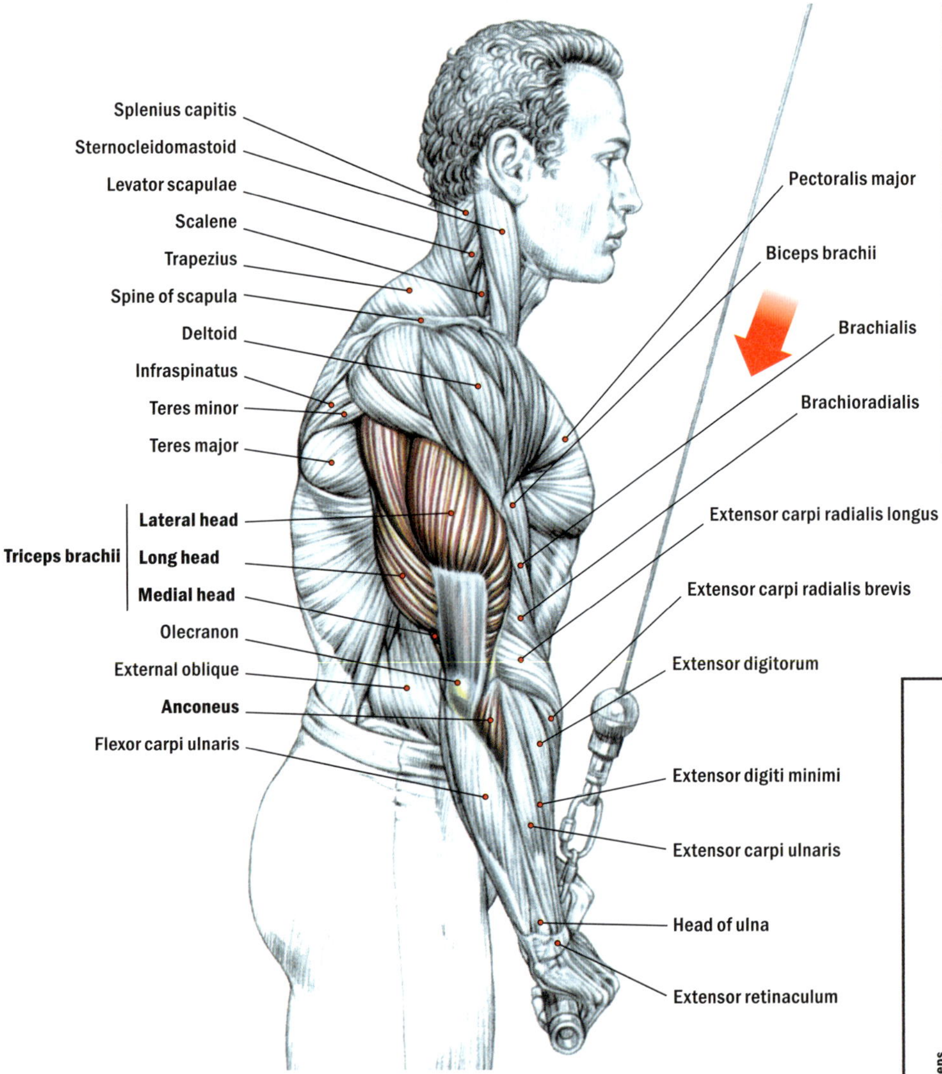

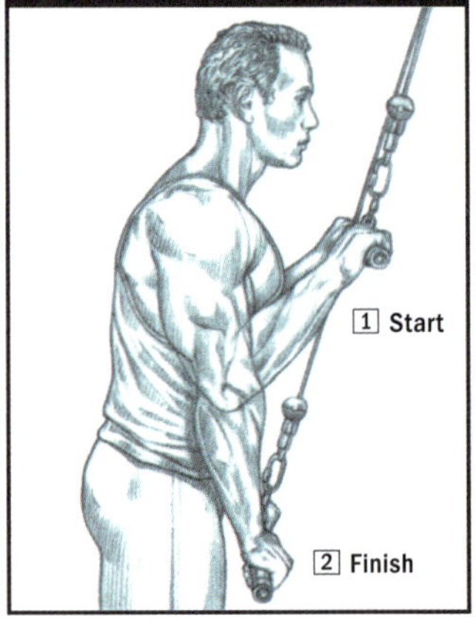

Splenius capitis
Sternocleidomastoid
Levator scapulae
Scalene
Trapezius
Spine of scapula
Deltoid
Infraspinatus
Teres minor
Teres major
Triceps brachii
Lateral head
Long head
Medial head
Olecranon
External oblique
Anconeus
Flexor carpi ulnaris
Pectoralis major
Biceps brachii
Brachialis
Brachioradialis
Extensor carpi radialis longus
Extensor carpi radialis brevis
Extensor digitorum
Extensor digiti minimi
Extensor carpi ulnaris
Head of ulna
Extensor retinaculum

PERFORMING THE EXERCISE

1 Start
2 Finish

Stand facing the machine and grasp the handle with an overhand grip, keeping your elbows tucked into your body:

- Inhale and extend your arms, keeping your elbows tucked in.
- Exhale at the end of the exercise.

This exercise isolates the triceps and the anconeus. The variation done with a rope rather than a handle (see page 35) works the lateral head of the triceps more intensely. Doing this exercise with an underhand grip will place more work on the medial head. Hold an isometric contraction for 1 or 2 seconds at the end of the exercise to feel the effort more intensely. When using heavy weights, lean forward with your torso for stability. Beginners can use this easy exercise to develop enough strength to move on to more difficult exercises.

Scapula
Humerus
Triceps
Lateral head
Long head
Medial head
Olecranon
Anconeus
Radius
Ulna
Metacarpals

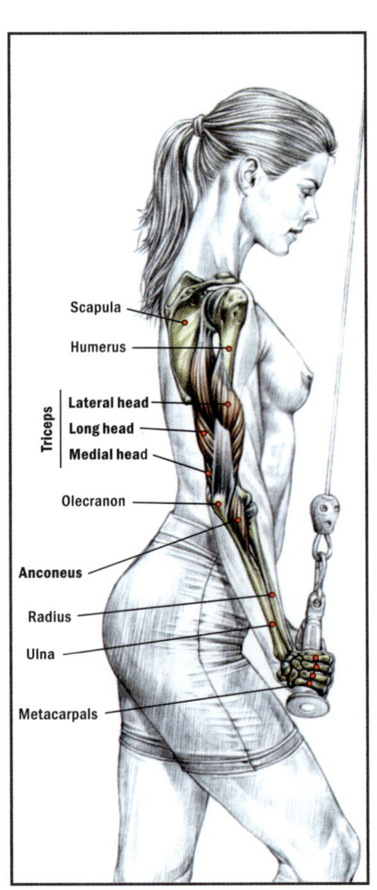

REVERSE TRICEPS PUSH-DOWNS 16

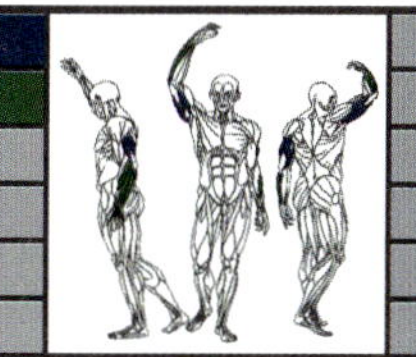

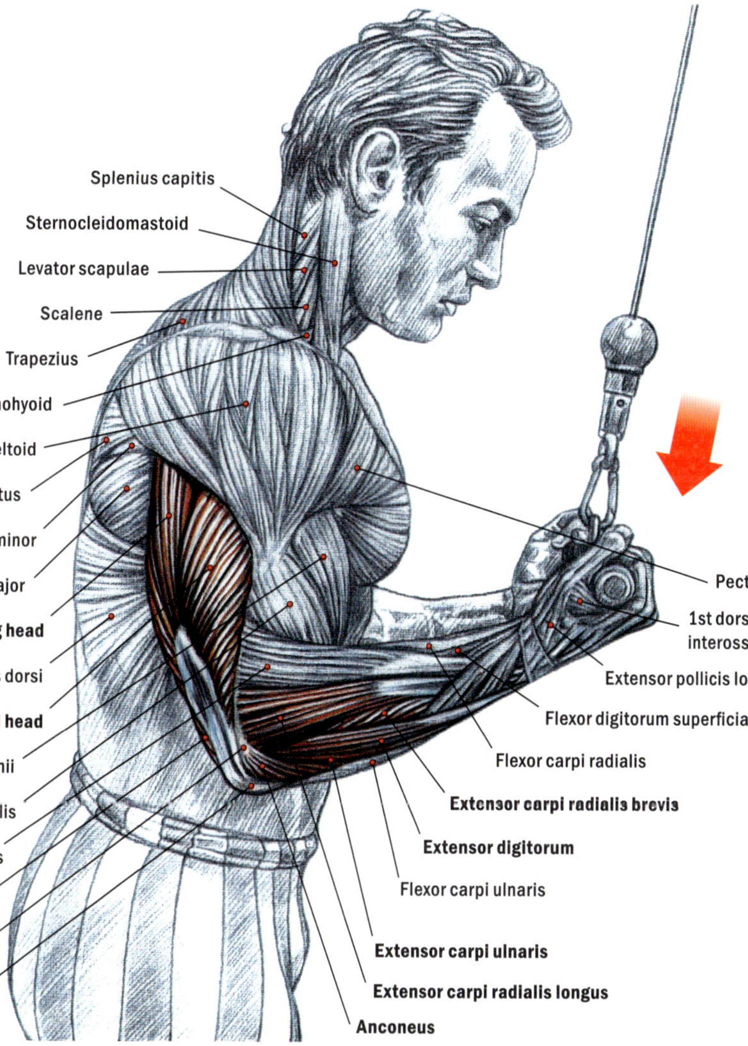

Stand facing the machine with your arms next to your body and the elbows bent. Grasp the handle:

- Inhale and straighten your arms, keeping your elbows tucked into your body.
- Exhale at the end of the exercise.

Since the underhand grip isolates the medial head of the triceps brachii, this exercise cannot be done with heavy weights.

When extending the forearms, the anconeus and wrist extensors also contract. The extensor muscles (extensor carpi ulnaris, extensor digitorum, extensor digiti minimi, and extensor carpi radialis longus and brevis) keep the wrist straight through an isometric contraction throughout the exercise.

INSERTIONS OF THE ARM MUSCLES

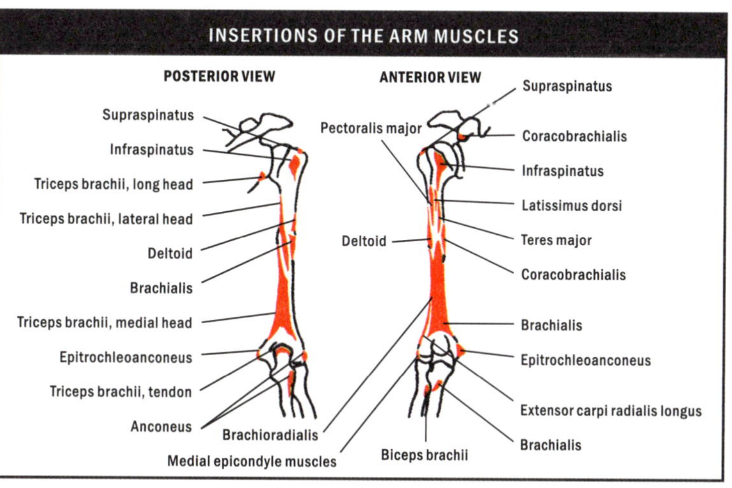

17 ONE-ARM REVERSE TRICEPS PUSH-DOWNS

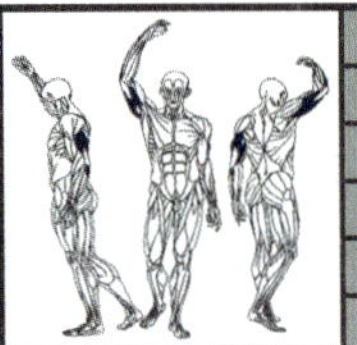

STARTING POSITION

Infraspinatus
Teres minor
Teres major
Latissimus dorsi
Triceps brachii
Lateral head
Long head
Medial head
Flexor carpi ulnaris
Extensor carpi ulnaris
Extensor digiti minimi
Extensor digitorum
Trapezius
Deltoid
Pectoralis major
Biceps brachii
Brachialis
Triceps brachii, tendon
Brachioradialis
Anconeus
Extensor carpi radialis longus
Extensor carpi radialis brevis

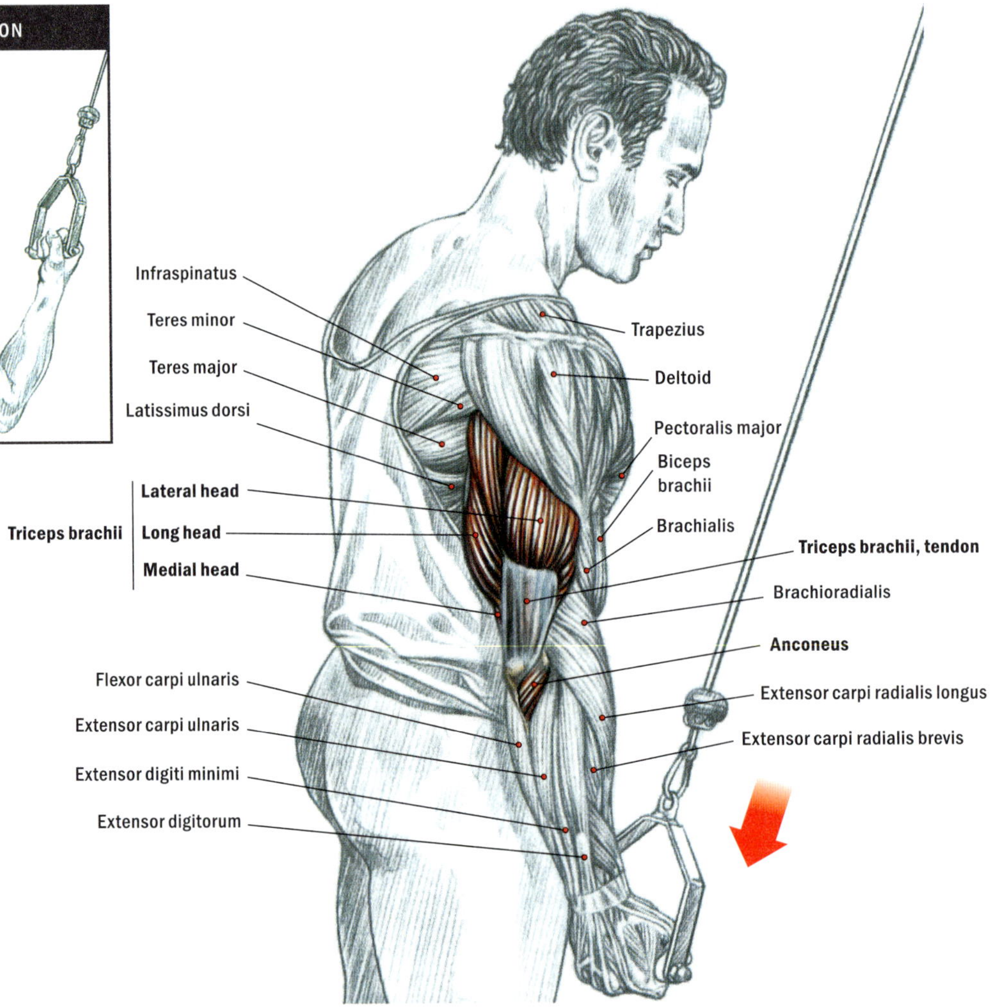

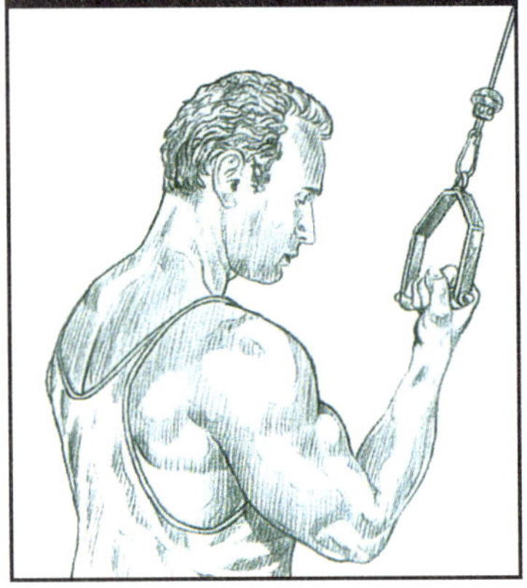

Stand facing the machine and grasp the handle with an underhand grip:

- Inhale and extend your forearm.
- Exhale at the end of the exercise.

This exercise mainly works the lateral and medial heads of the triceps.

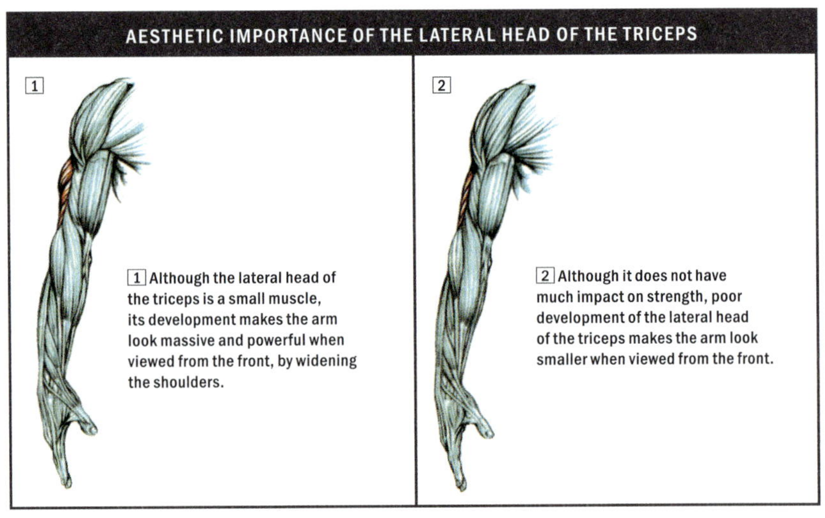

AESTHETIC IMPORTANCE OF THE LATERAL HEAD OF THE TRICEPS

1

1 Although the lateral head of the triceps is a small muscle, its development makes the arm look massive and powerful when viewed from the front, by widening the shoulders.

2

2 Although it does not have much impact on strength, poor development of the lateral head of the triceps makes the arm look smaller when viewed from the front.

TRICEPS PUSH-DOWNS WITH ROPE 18

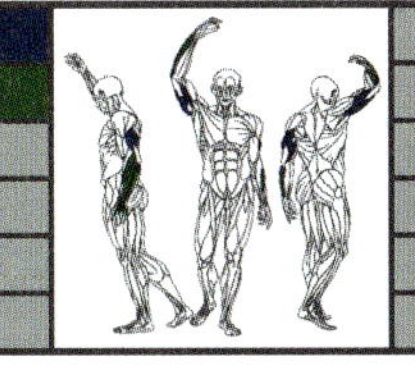

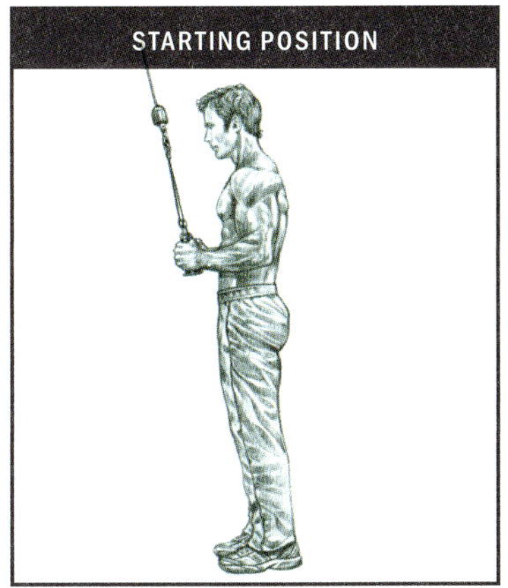

STARTING POSITION

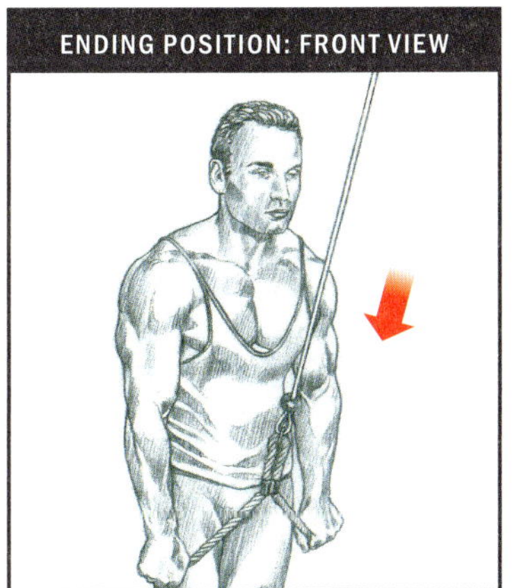

ENDING POSITION: FRONT VIEW

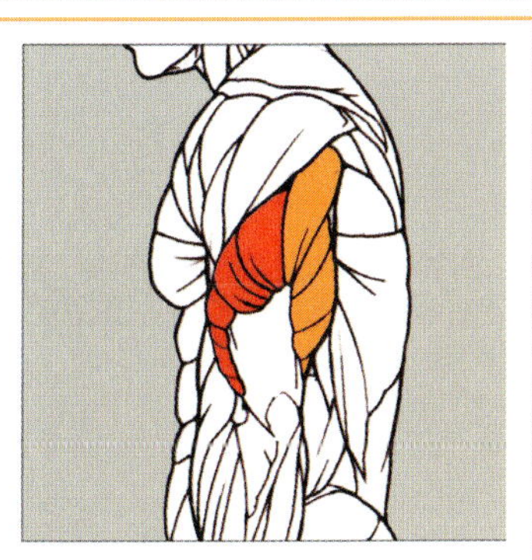

Extending the forearms using a rope or a cable works the lateral head of the triceps intensely. Using a rope is the best way to feel the muscle working. The longer the rope, the more spread out the hands will be at the end of the movement, and the more you will feel the contraction in the lateral head of the triceps.

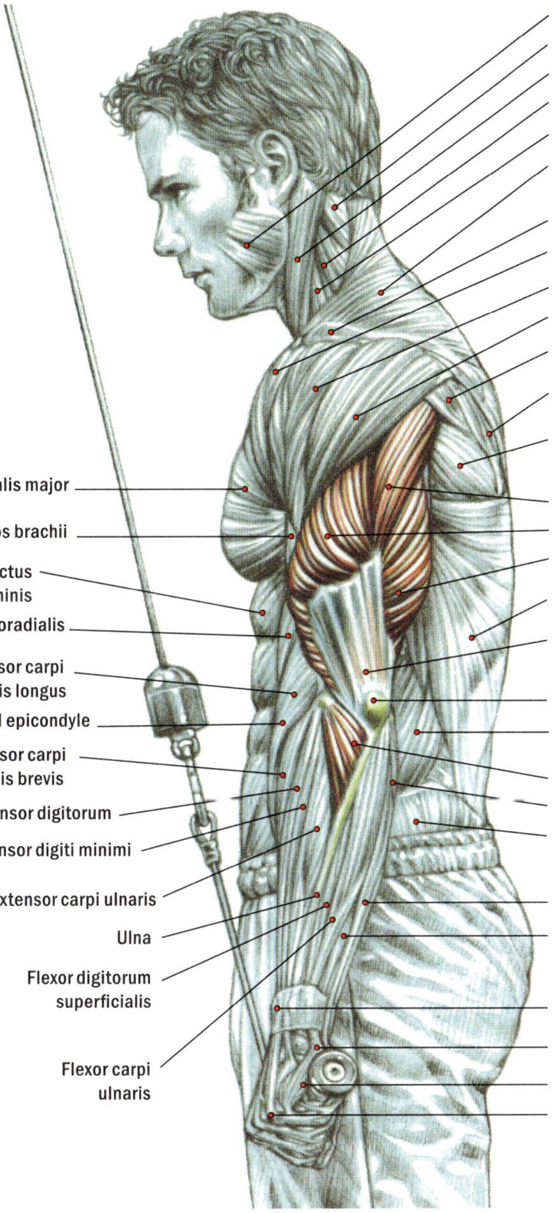

Stand facing the machine with the rope or handles in a neutral grip, keeping your elbows tucked into your body:

- Inhale and extend your forearms by trying to spread your arms outward.
- Exhale at the end of the extension and return to the starting position.

Doing this exercise with a rope or a cable contracts the lateral head of the triceps intensely.

Although it has little involvement in the arm's extension strength, the lateral head of the triceps plays an important role in the aesthetics of the upper limb when viewed from the front; it makes the arm appear broad and powerful. That is why high-pulley triceps cable extensions are an essential exercise in many bodybuilders' training routines.

To get the best results, do long sets with light weights until you start to feel a burning sensation in the muscle.

19 STANDING CABLE OVERHEAD TRICEPS EXTENSIONS

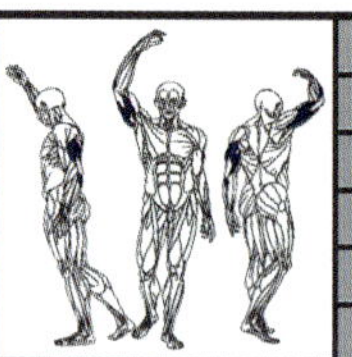

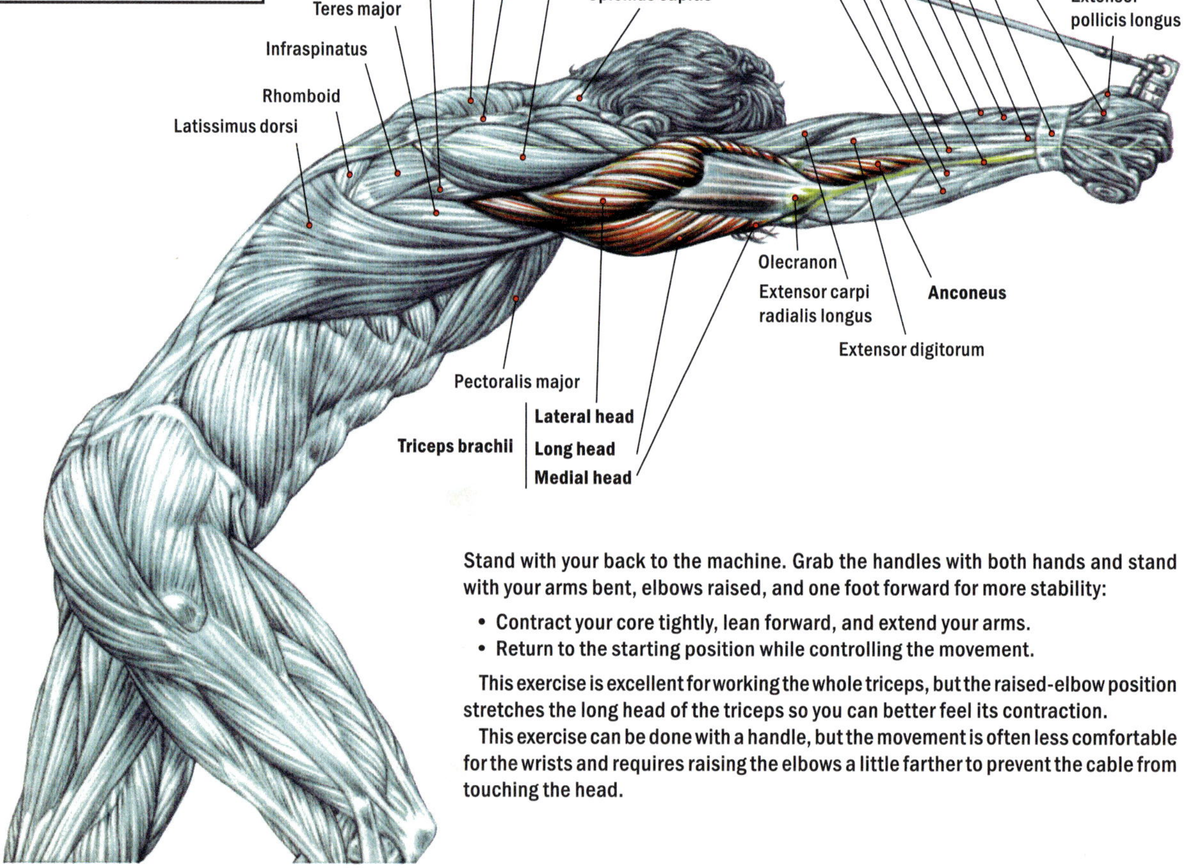

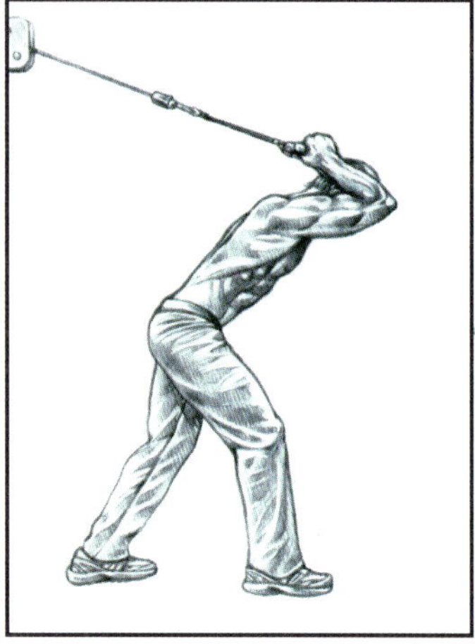

Stand with your back to the machine. Grab the handles with both hands and stand with your arms bent, elbows raised, and one foot forward for more stability:

- Contract your core tightly, lean forward, and extend your arms.
- Return to the starting position while controlling the movement.

This exercise is excellent for working the whole triceps, but the raised-elbow position stretches the long head of the triceps so you can better feel its contraction.

This exercise can be done with a handle, but the movement is often less comfortable for the wrists and requires raising the elbows a little farther to prevent the cable from touching the head.

Better recruitment of the muscle fibers of the long head of the triceps allows you to use significantly more weight than in triceps exercises in which you are facing the machine. The higher your elbows, the harder the long head of the triceps will work.

This exercise can be integrated into strength training that is tailored to throwing sports and combat sports that involve striking because its execution is similar to the upper limb movements performed in these activities.

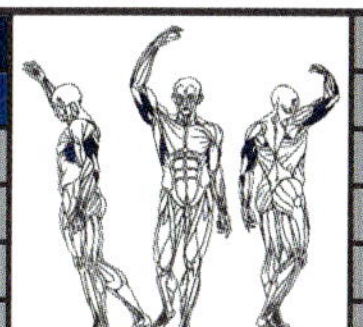

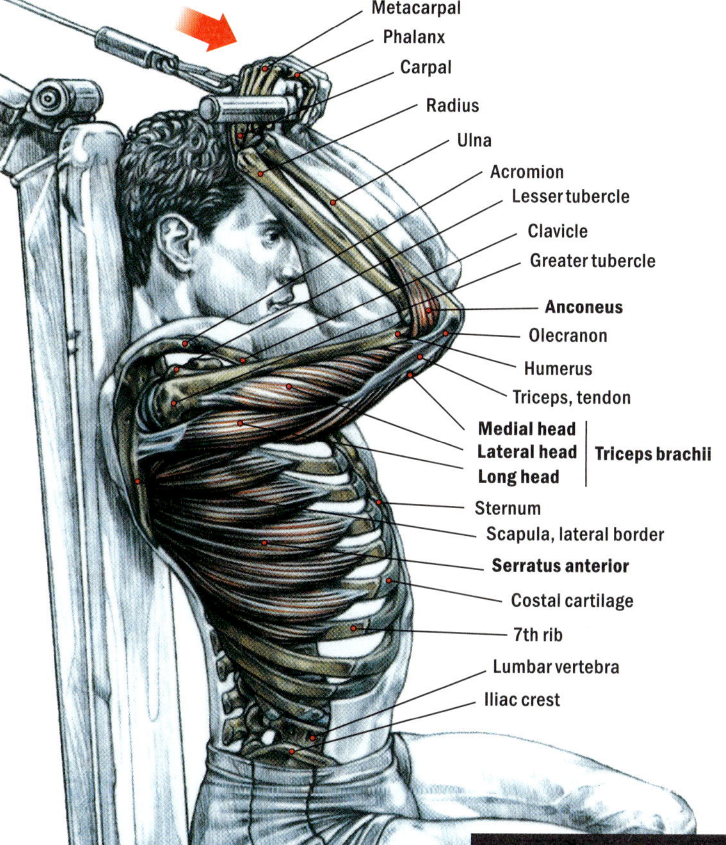

Sit with your back against a pulley machine. Grasp the pulley with an overhand grip with the arms bent and the upper arms slightly above a horizontal position:

- Inhale and extend your arms, taking care not to spread your elbows too far apart.
- Exhale at the end of the exercise.

This exercise works the triceps brachii and anconeus as well as the serratus anterior, which keeps the scapulae fixed against the rib cage throughout the exercise.

Notice that the elevated position of the elbows stretches the long heads of the triceps at the beginning of the exercise; this promotes its contraction during the effort.

Using a pulley for this exercise is an easier way to replicate the same movement as lying triceps extensions done with a bar while lying on a bench (see page 38).

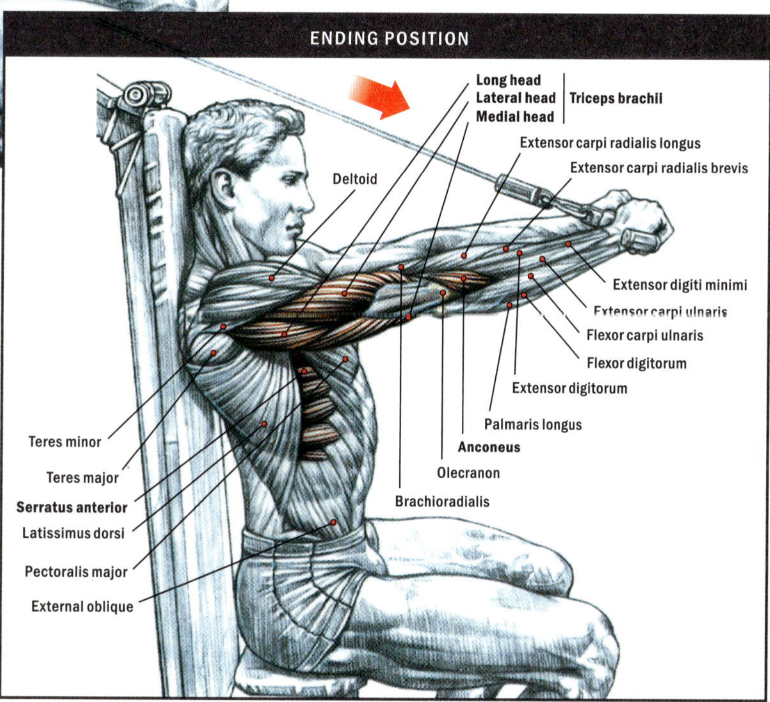

21 LYING BARBELL TRICEPS EXTENSIONS

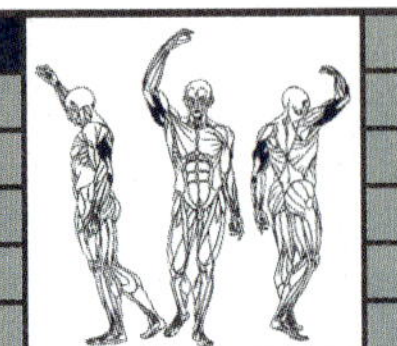

Palmaris longus
Flexor carpi radialis
Flexor digitorum superficialis
Flexor pollicis longus
Abductor pollicis longus
Extensor pollicis brevis
Flexor carpi ulnaris
Biceps brachii, aponeurotic expansion
Pronator teres
Brachialis
Olecranon
Lateral head
Medial head
Long head
Triceps brachii
Biceps brachii
Coracobrachialis
Pectoralis major
Serratus anterior
Subscapularis
Teres major
Posterior deltoid
Latissimus dorsi

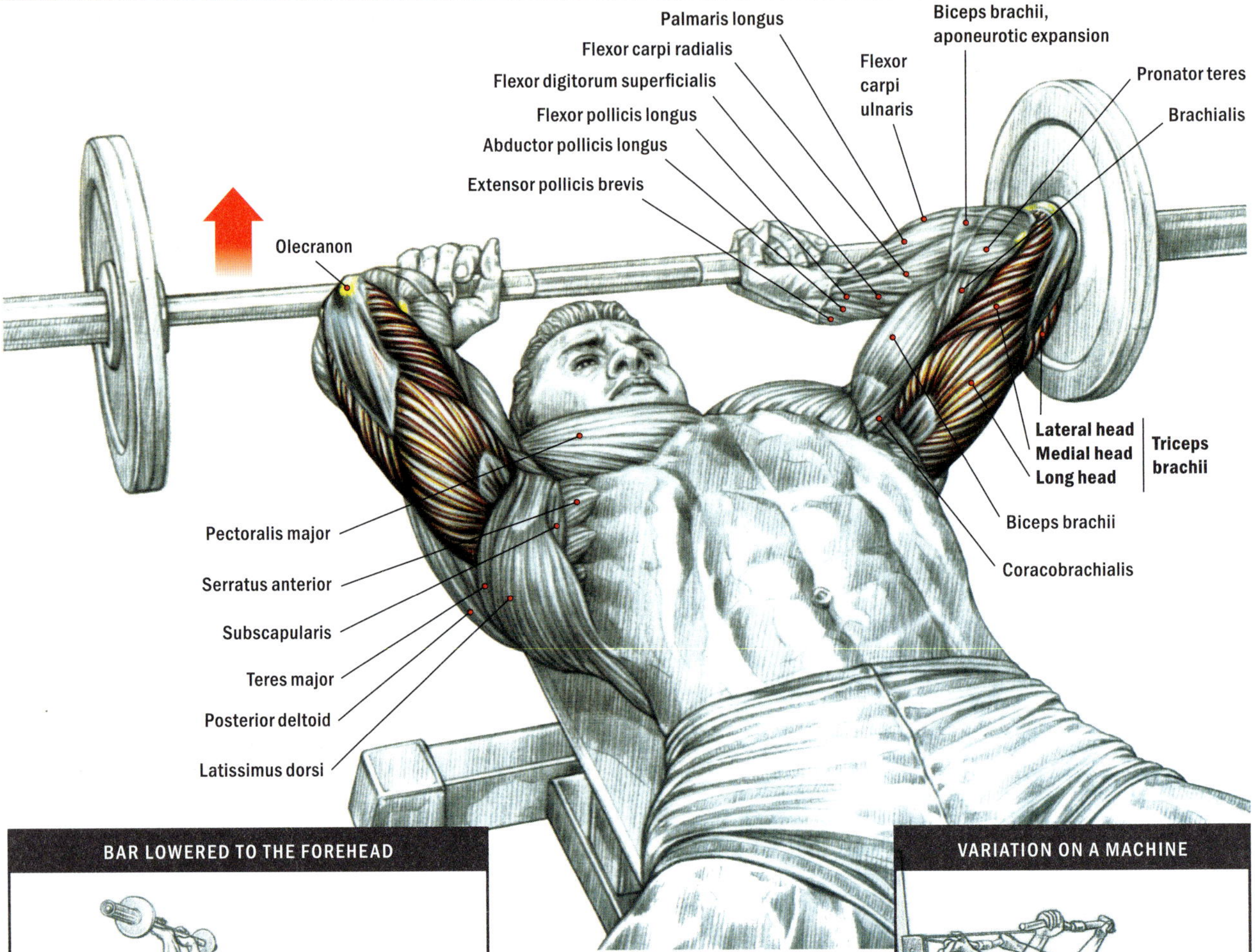

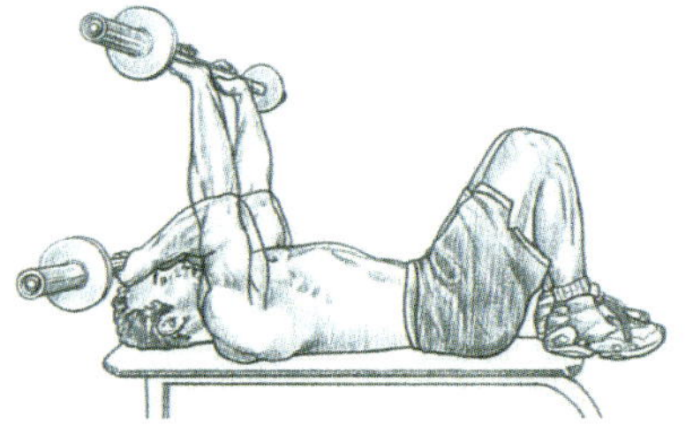

BAR LOWERED TO THE FOREHEAD

Focuses the work on the medial and lateral heads of the triceps brachii

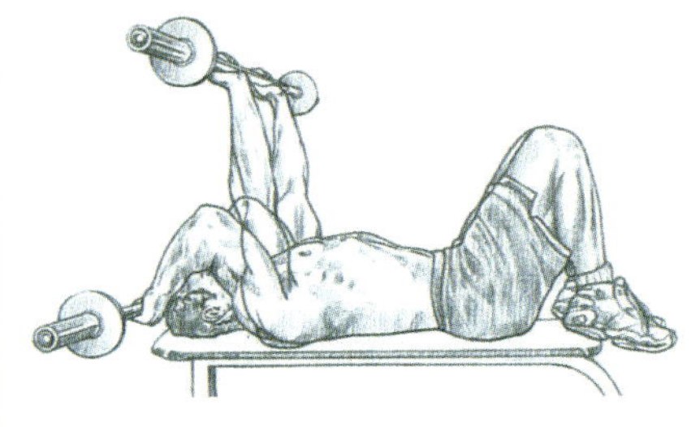

BAR LOWERED BEHIND THE HEAD

Focuses the work on the long head of the triceps brachii

Lie on a flat bench and grasp the barbell with an overhand grip and your arms vertical:

- Inhale and lower your forearms, taking care not to spread your elbows too far apart. Lower the barbell to your forehead or behind your head.
- Return to the starting position and exhale at the end of the exercise.

Because of individual variations in shoulder width, valgus angle at the elbows, and wrist flexibility, the hands can be closer or farther apart on the bar and the elbow angle more or less open during the exercise.

Using an EZ curl bar helps prevent excessive strain on the wrists during this exercise.

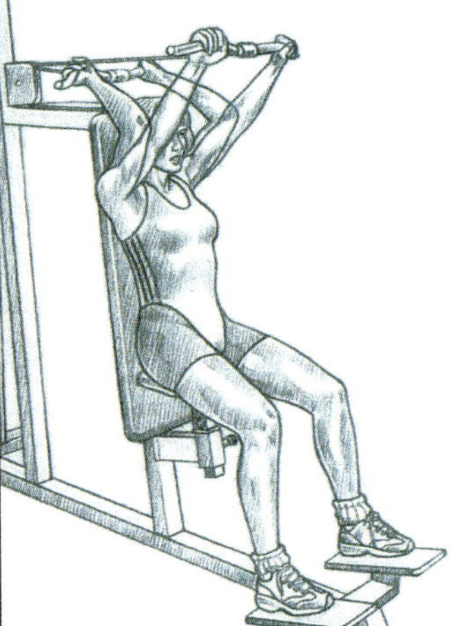

VARIATION ON A MACHINE

Doing this exercise with a pulley makes it easier to simulate the same movement done in the barbell version, and it enables you to isolate the long head of the triceps brachii.

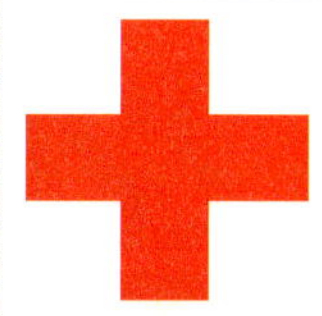

In strength training, injuries to the elbow at the insertion of the triceps are most often caused by lifting weights that are too heavy, coupled with repetitive forearm extensions, as well as a personal predisposition.

With age, lifting heavy weights repeatedly combined with individual fragility of the triceps tendon may lead to painful inflammation and calcifications or osteophytes that weaken the tendon insertion and increase the risk of tendon rupture.

At the first sign of pain, you should take a break from any activities involving the triceps for a while. Then find exercises and work angles more suited to your body structure. If you suspect a tear in the triceps tendon (this injury may not be very painful), it is important to have the injury diagnosed as soon as possible so that the tendon can be reattached to the olecranon.

When you are standing, the arm can be bent by the biceps and straightened by gravity, so a tear may not be immediately apparent. To check this, lie on your stomach with your arm resting on the bed. Bend your arm and try to straighten it. If you cannot straighten it, the triceps tendon is completely ruptured.

The biceps brachii contracts to flex the forearm while resisting gravity during our daily activities and is still able to pull the full body weight upward as it did for our arboreal ancestors. However, the triceps brachii is a muscle designed specifically to prevent the forearm from dropping down and to extend the arm explosively to hit or throw light objects like sticks or small stones.

The triceps, apart from its long head, which brings the arm powerfully toward the torso, is not designed to extend the arm with force. This muscle adapted to the predatory function of our hunter ancestors. The repetitive throwing of heavy objects weighing several pounds or the repeated extension of the arm against strong resistance (as in strength training) is not natural for it. In the long run, these actions may cause inflammation in the elbow and premature wear and tear of the insertion of the triceps tendon; this can eventually lead to total rupture.

RUPTURE OF THE DISTAL TRICEPS TENDON

INFLAMMATORY CALCIFICATION

Personal predisposition, as well as intense and repetitive triceps work, can lead to inflammation of the elbow, which, in the long run, may lead to abnormal development of the olecranon (prominent bone of the elbow).

WEAKENED TRICEPS TENDON

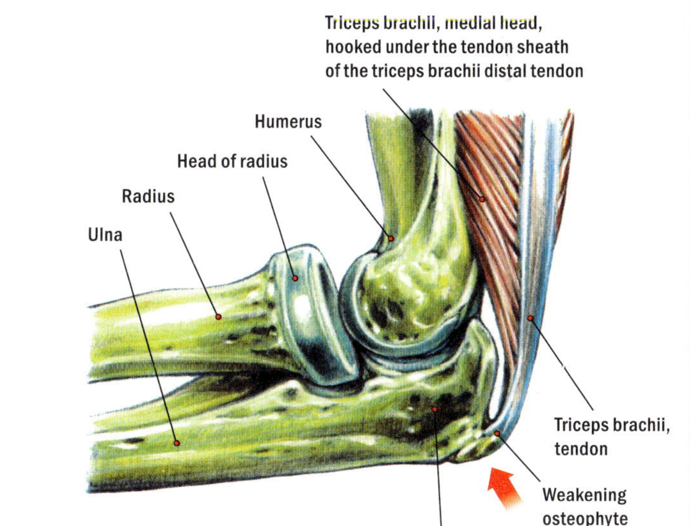

Personal predisposition, combined with intense and repetitive triceps work, can lead to inflammation with osteophyte formation (bone that grows abnormally) at the base of the triceps brachii tendon. This condition weakens the tendon, which can then tear when lifting heavy weights.

22 LYING DUMBBELL TRICEPS EXTENSIONS

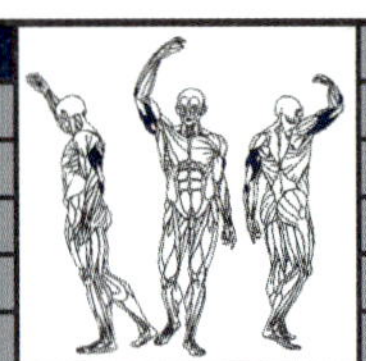

Abductor pollicis longus
Extensor pollicis brevis
Extensor pollicis longus
Flexor carpi ulnaris
Extensor carpi ulnaris
Extensor digiti minimi
Extensor digitorum
Extensor carpi radialis brevis
Anconeus
Extensor carpi radialis longus
Brachioradialis
Brachialis
Medial head
Lateral head
Long head
Triceps brachii
Serratus anterior
Latissimus dorsi
Teres major
Teres minor
Infraspinatus
Anterior deltoid
Biceps brachii
Middle deltoid
Posterior deltoid

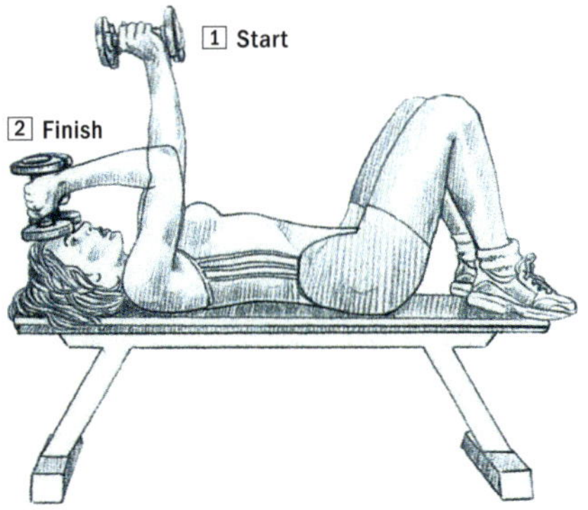

1 Start
2 Finish

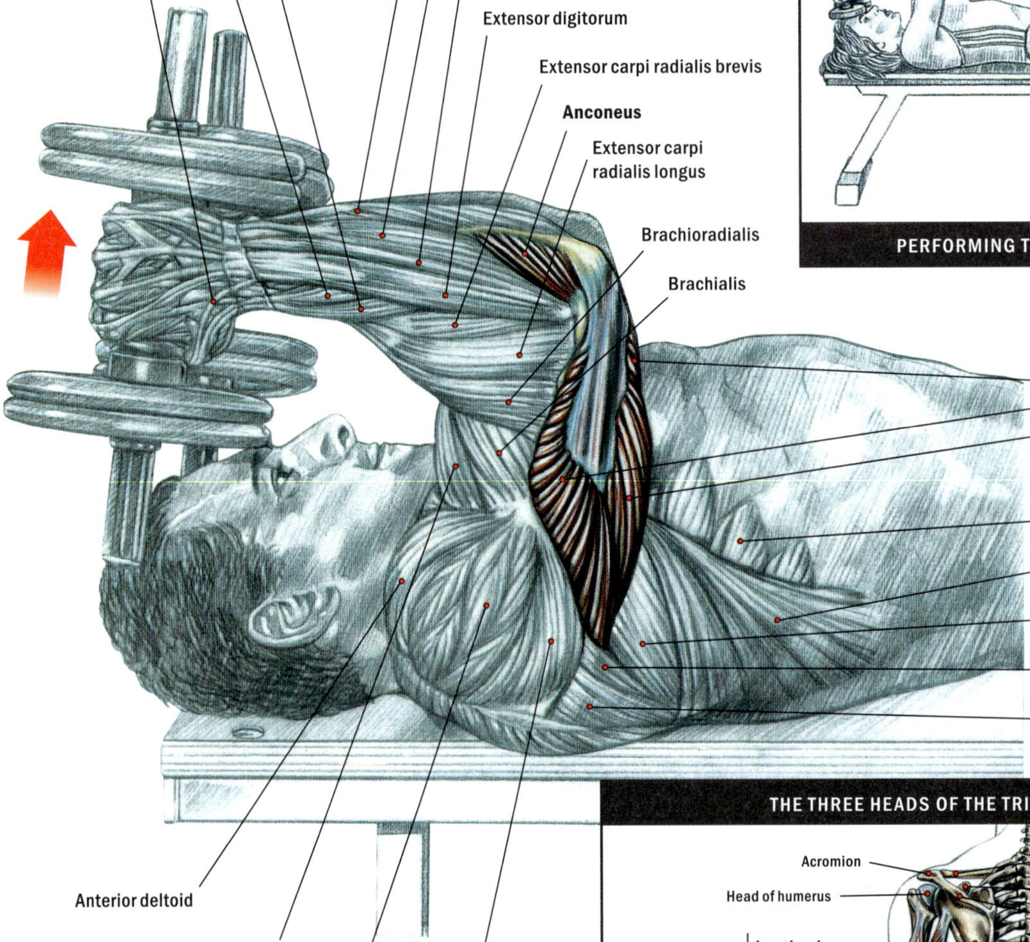

PERFORMING THE EXERCISE

THE THREE HEADS OF THE TRICEPS

Acromion
Head of humerus
Triceps brachii
Long head
Lateral head
Medial head
Triceps brachii, tendon
Radius
Ulna
Styloid process of ulna
Clavicle
Coracoid process
Spine of scapula
Scapula
Vertebra
Rib
Medial epicondyle
Olecranon
Anconeus
Carpal
Metacarpal
Proximal phalanx
Middle phalanx
Distal phalanx

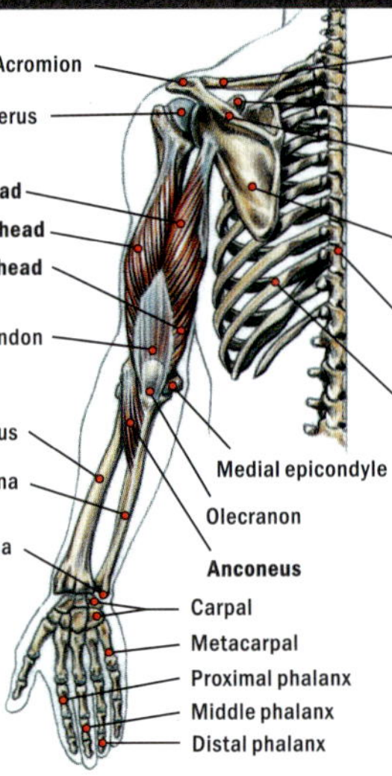

Lie on a flat bench and grasp a dumbbell in each hand with your arms vertical:

- Inhale and lower your forearms with a controlled movement.
- Return to the starting position and exhale at the end of the exercise.

This exercise works all three heads of the triceps brachii equally.

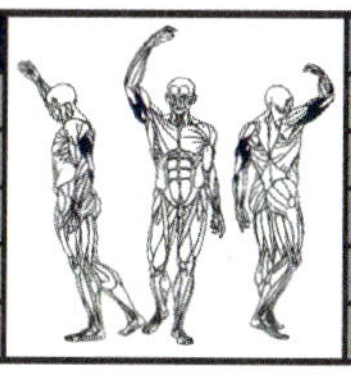

ONE-ARM OVERHEAD DUMBBELL TRICEPS EXTENSIONS 23

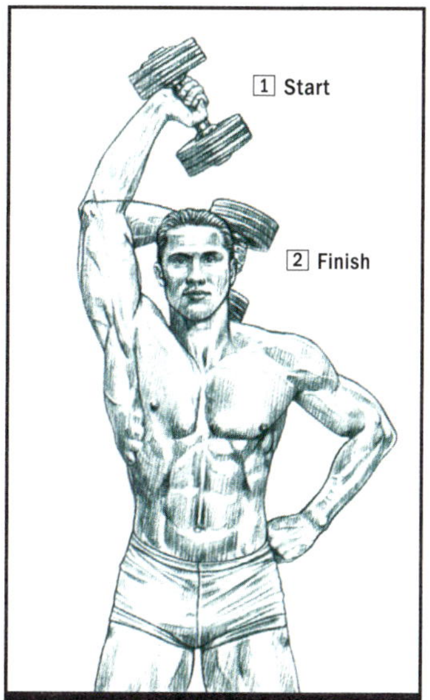

1 Start
2 Finish

PERFORMING THE EXERCISE

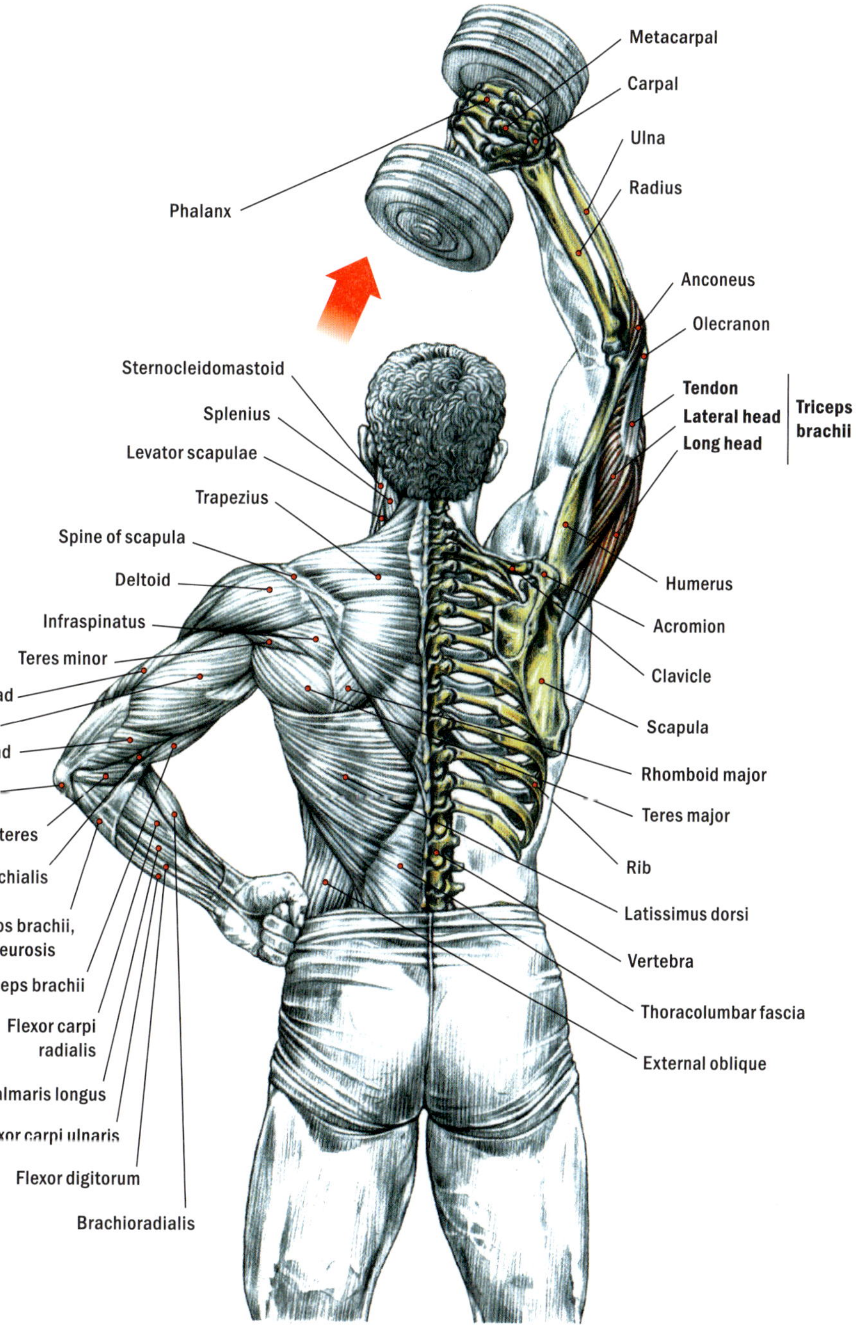
Metacarpal
Carpal
Ulna
Radius
Phalanx
Anconeus
Olecranon
Sternocleidomastoid
Splenius
Levator scapulae
Trapezius
Tendon
Lateral head
Long head
Triceps brachii
Spine of scapula
Deltoid
Humerus
Acromion
Infraspinatus
Teres minor
Clavicle
Triceps brachii
Lateral head
Long head
Medial head
Scapula
Rhomboid major
Olcranon
Teres major
Pronator teres
Rib
Brachialis
Latissimus dorsi
Biceps brachii, aponeurosis
Vertebra
Biceps brachii
Thoracolumbar fascia
Flexor carpi radialis
External oblique
Palmaris longus
Flexor carpi ulnaris
Flexor digitorum
Brachioradialis

Sit or stand and grip a dumbbell in one hand with the arm vertical:

- Inhale and bend your arm to lower the dumbbell behind your neck.
- Return to the starting position and exhale at the end of the exercise.

The vertical position of the arm stretches the long head of the triceps brachii, promoting its contraction during the exercise.

It is important to engage the core to prevent arching the lower back. If possible, use a bench with a short backrest if performing the exercise while sitting.

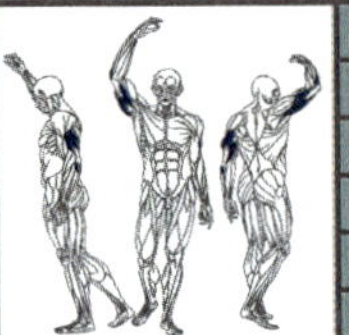

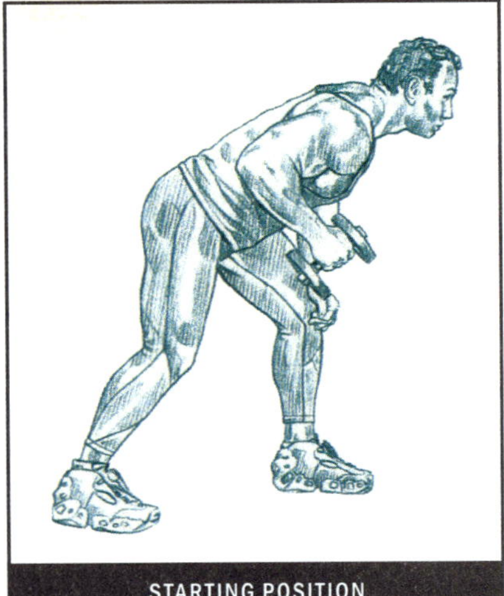

STARTING POSITION

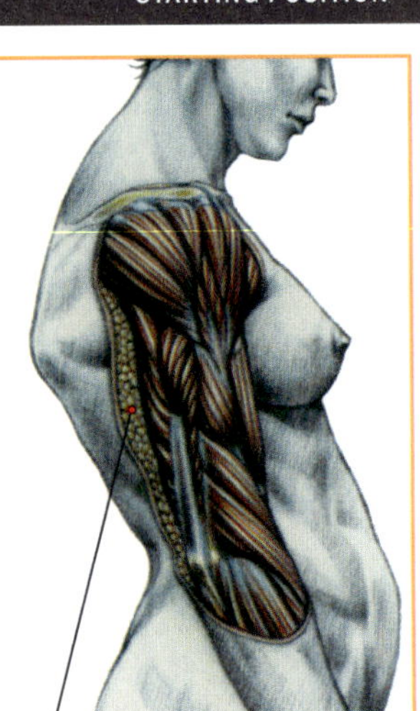

Location of fat in the arm

Triceps brachii — Lateral head / Long head

Brachioradialis

Anconeus

Flexor carpi ulnaris

Extensor digitorum

Extensor digiti minimi

Extensor carpi ulnaris

Extensor pollicis brevis

Teres major

Deltoid

Biceps brachii

Pectoralis major

Brachialis

Extensor carpi radialis longus

Extensor carpi radialis brevis

Abductor pollicis longus

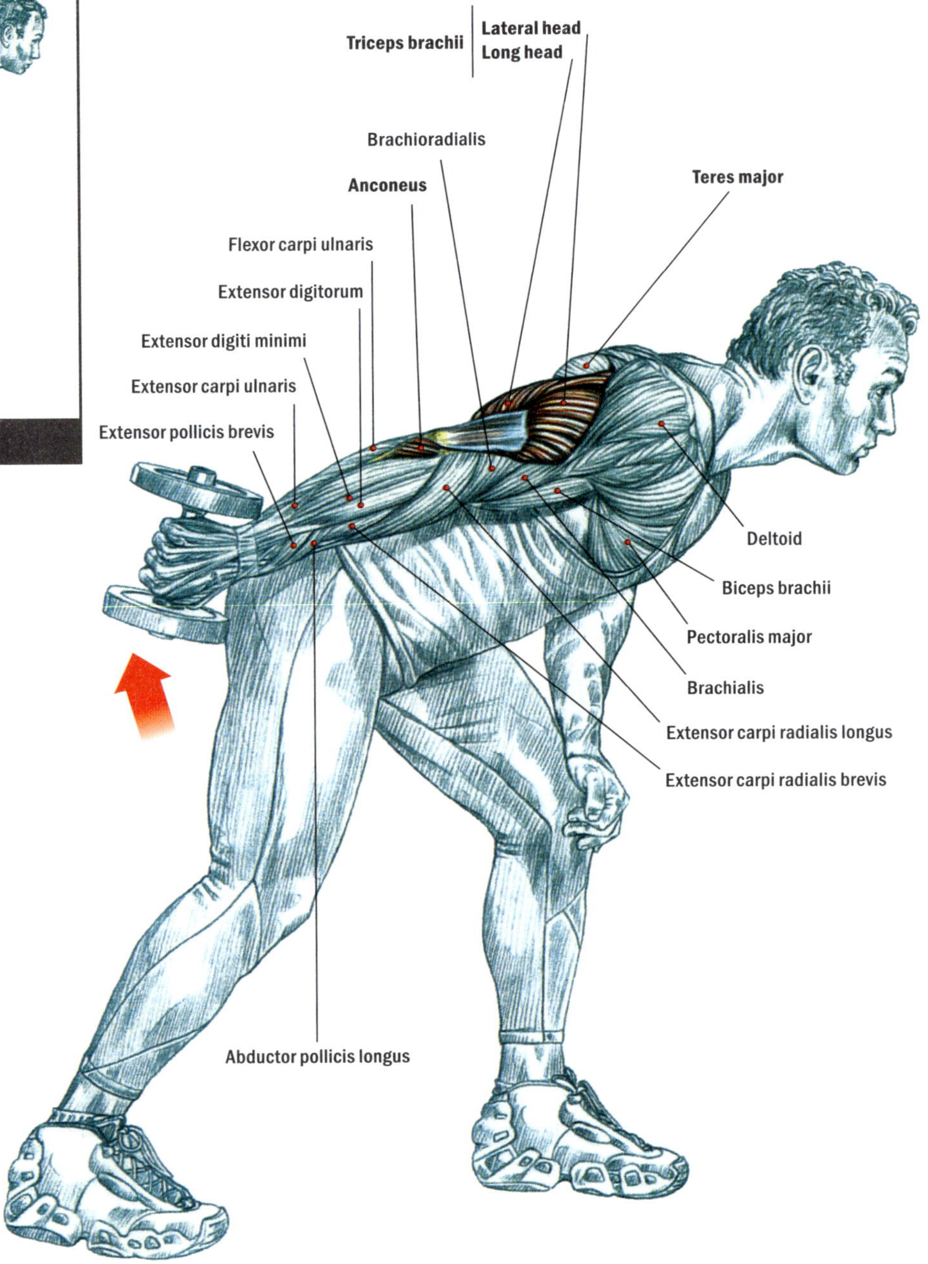

The back of the arm often contains relatively thick adipose tissue. Apart from storing energy, this fat protects the nerves and the arteries in the upper, inner region of the arm.

Although a dietary plan is the best way to lose fat, strength training exercises for the triceps (in high numbers of reps until you start to feel a burn) help target muscle growth in the back of the arm.

Stand with your knees slightly bent and lean forward at your waist, maintaining a straight back. Bend your arm and keep your upper arm parallel to your torso and alongside your body:

- Inhale and extend your forearm.
- Exhale at the end of the exercise.

This is an excellent exercise for pumping up the entire triceps muscle. For best results, do this exercise in long sets until you feel a burn.

SEATED DUMBBELL TRICEPS EXTENSIONS 25

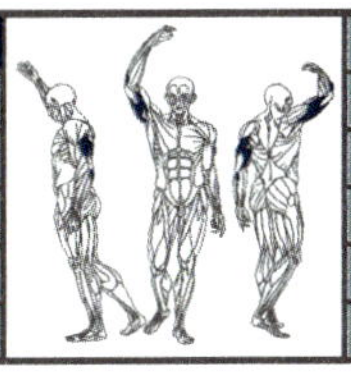

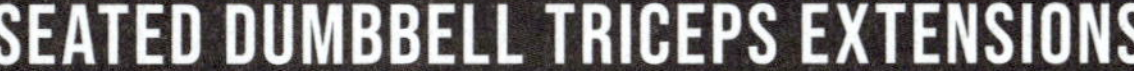

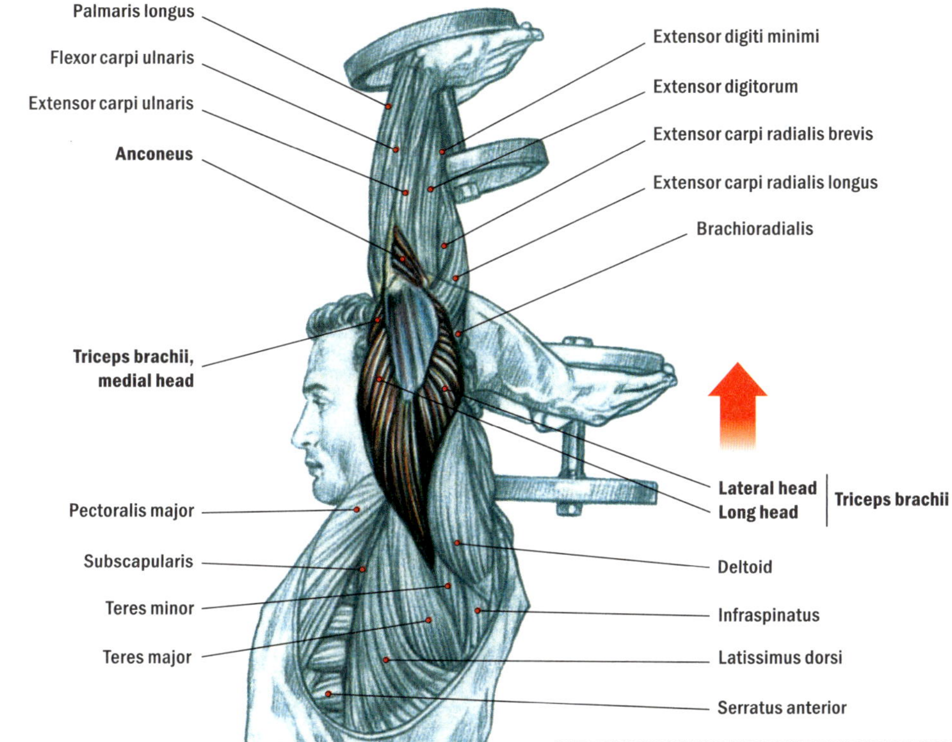

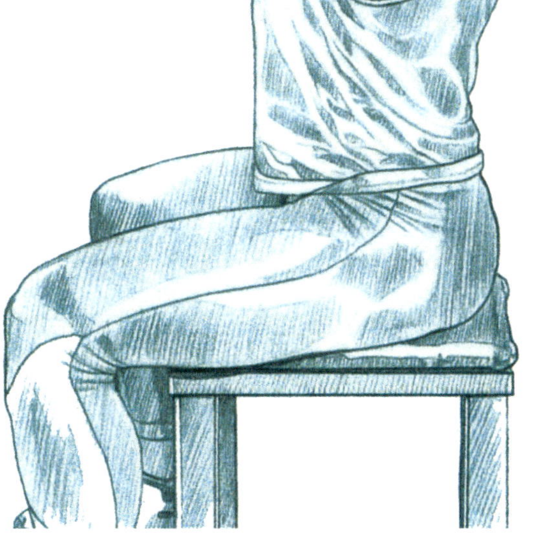

Sit and grasp a dumbbell with both hands, holding it behind your neck:

- Inhale and extend your forearms.
- Exhale at the end of the exercise.

The vertical position of the arms strongly stretches the long head of the triceps brachii, emphasizing the contraction in this area during the exercise.

It is important to engage the core to prevent arching the lower back. If possible, use a bench with a short backrest.

DIAGRAM OF THE DISTINCTIVE HORSESHOE SHAPE OF THE TRICEPS IN CONTRACTION

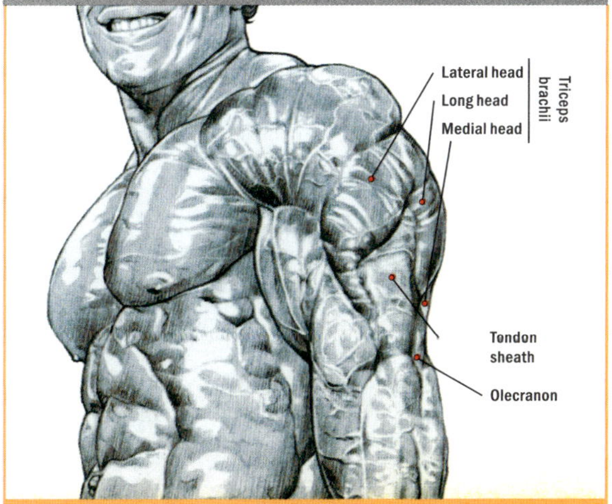

The fibers of the three heads of the triceps attach to a common tendinous plate, which in turn is attached to the olecranon by a tendon. When the triceps contracts, these tendinous fibers sink into the muscle, like a hot knife sinking into butter. The contracted muscle pushes outward, creating the characteristic horseshoe shape.

26 SEATED EZ CURL BAR TRICEPS EXTENSIONS

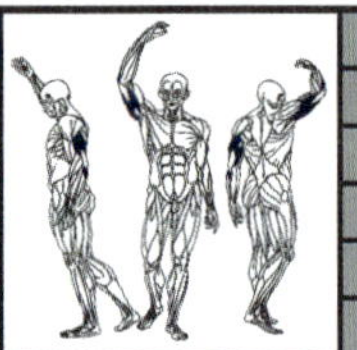

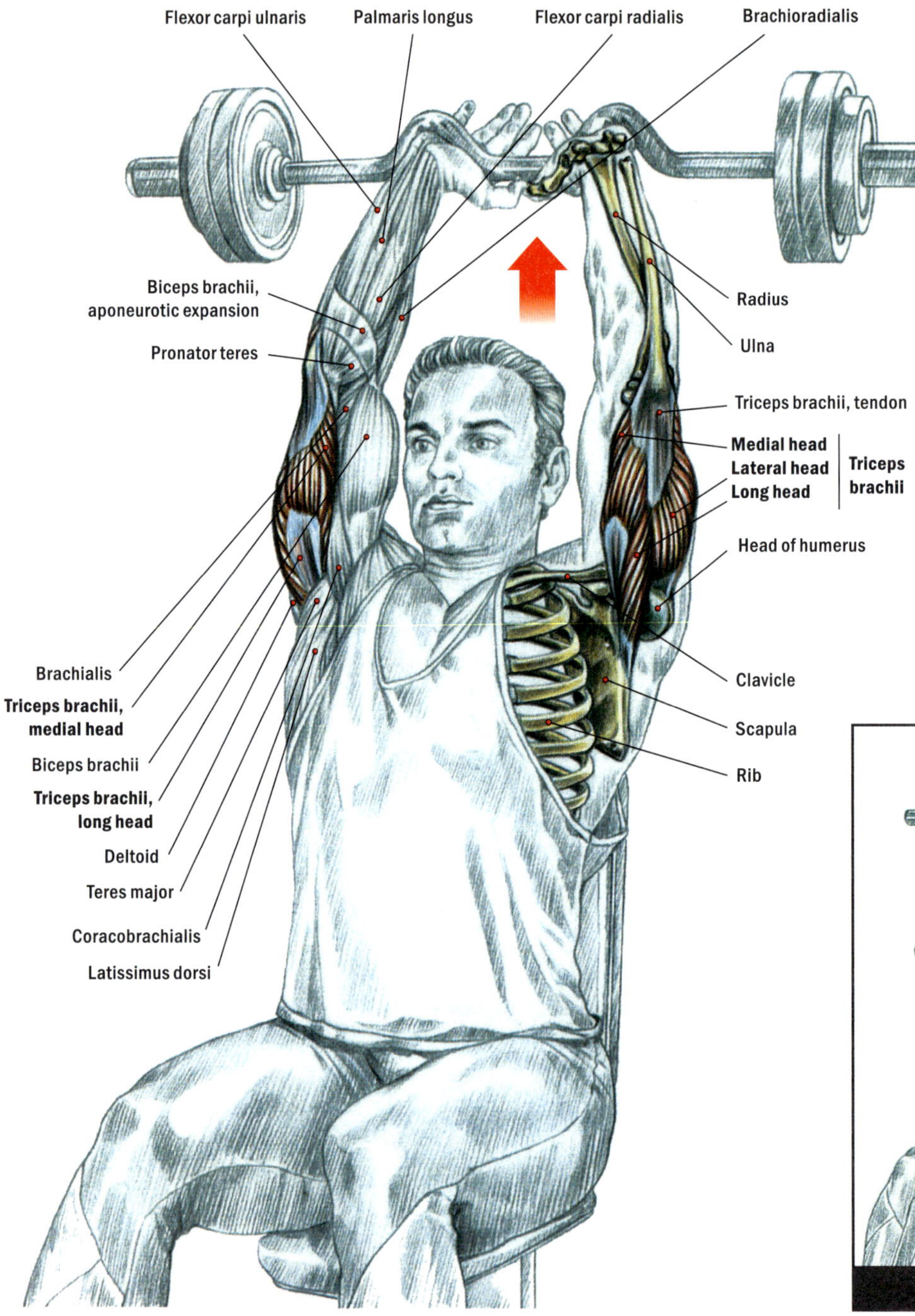

Flexor carpi ulnaris
Palmaris longus
Flexor carpi radialis
Brachioradialis
Biceps brachii, aponeurotic expansion
Pronator teres
Radius
Ulna
Triceps brachii, tendon
Medial head
Lateral head
Long head
Triceps brachii
Head of humerus
Clavicle
Scapula
Rib
Brachialis
Triceps brachii, medial head
Biceps brachii
Triceps brachii, long head
Deltoid
Teres major
Coracobrachialis
Latissimus dorsi

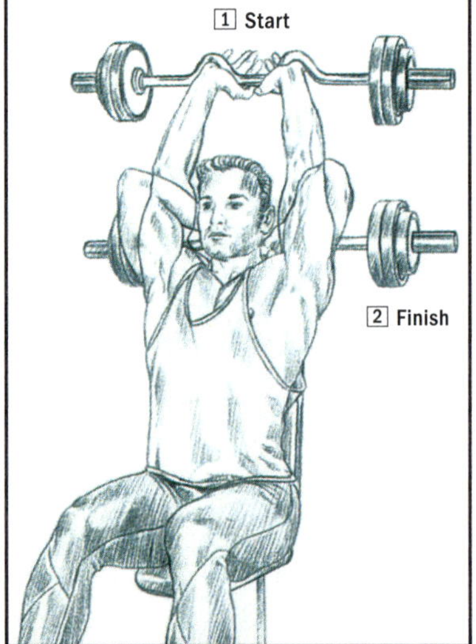

1 Start
2 Finish

PERFORMING THE EXERCISE

Sit and grasp a bar with an overhand grip and arms vertical:

- Inhale and bend your elbows to lower the bar behind your head.
- Return to the starting position and exhale at the end of the extension.

The vertical position of the arms strongly stretches the long head of the triceps brachii, emphasizing its contraction during the exercise. Additionally, the overhand grip promotes the contraction of the lateral head.

For safety reasons, you must avoid arching the lower back. If possible, use a bench with a short backrest.

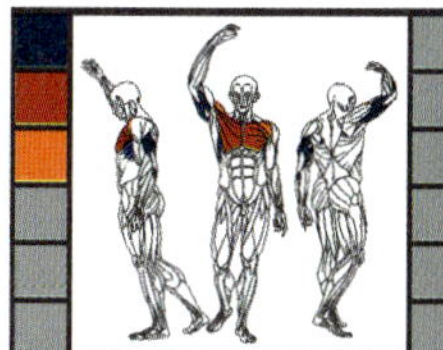

STARTING POSITION

Deltoid
Pectoralis major

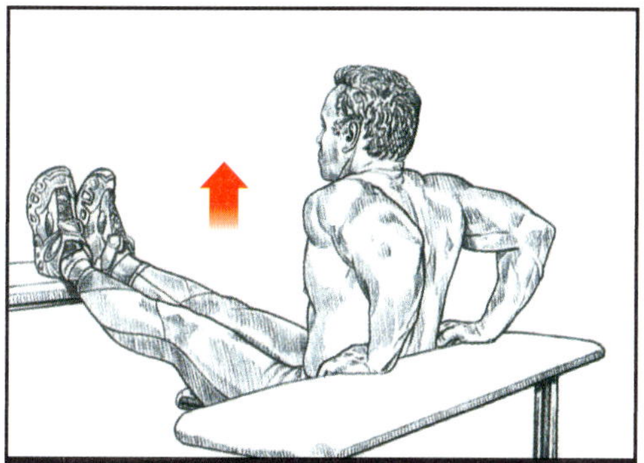

Triceps brachii
Lateral head
Long head
Medial head

Anconeus

Extensor digitorum

Extensor digiti minimi

Trapezius
Teres minor
Infraspinatus
Teres major
Rhomboid
Latissimus dorsi
Flexor carpi radialis
Palmaris longus
Extensor carpi ulnaris
Flexor carpi ulnaris

Suspend your body between two benches by placing your hands on the edge of one bench and your feet on the other bench:

- Inhale, then dip by bending your arms and rise by straightening your arms.
- Exhale at the end of the exercise.

This exercise works the triceps and pectoral muscles as well as the anterior deltoid.

You can place weights on top of the thighs to increase the difficulty and intensity of the exercise.

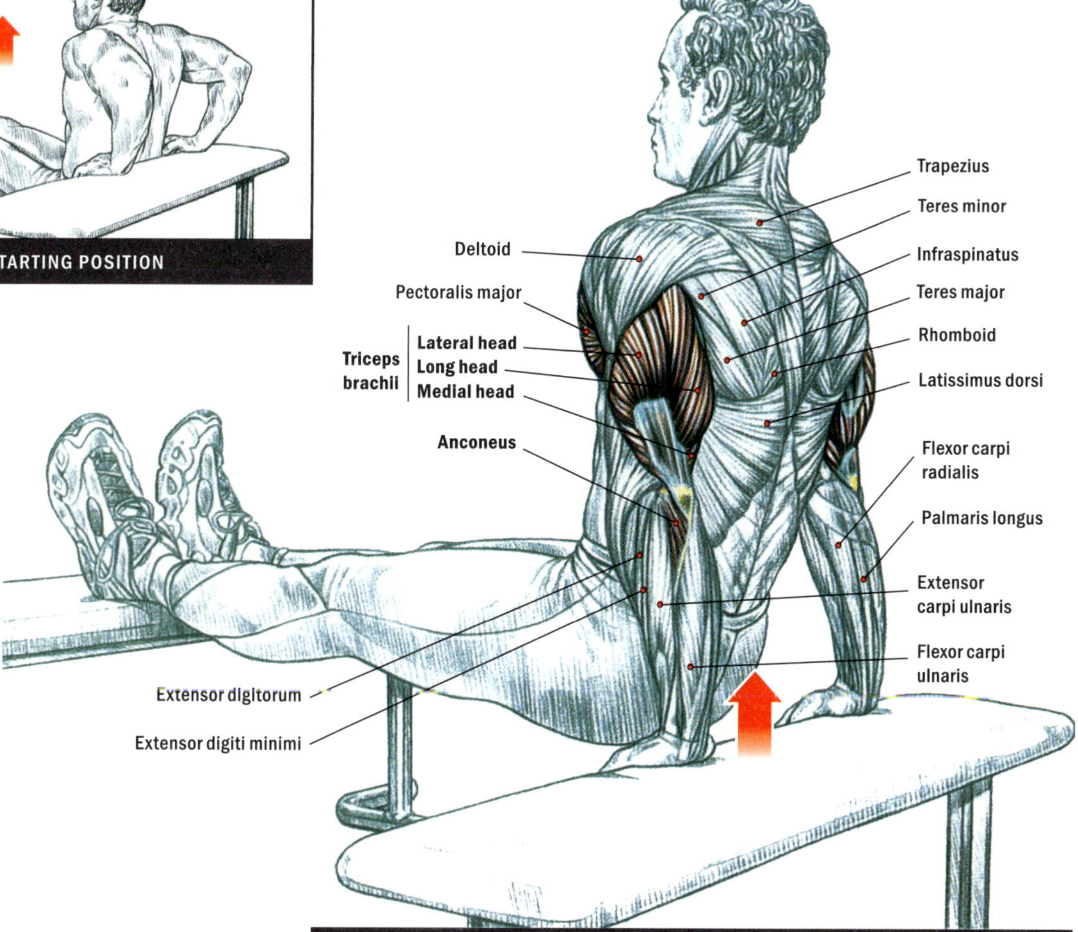

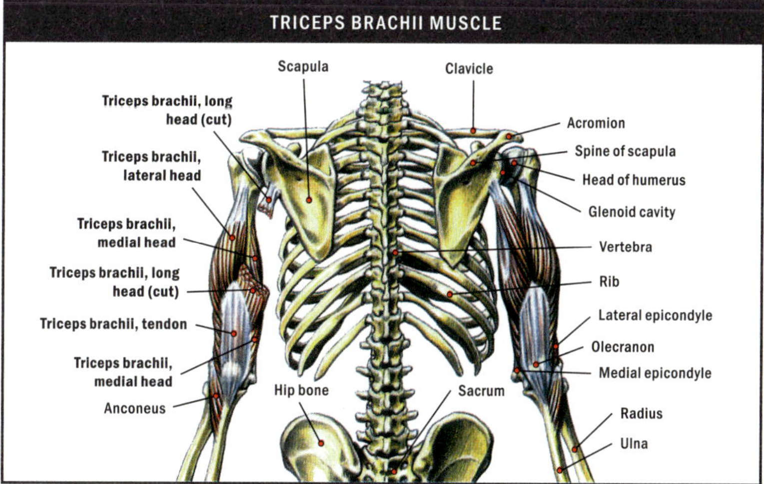

TRICEPS BRACHII MUSCLE

Triceps brachii, long head (cut)
Triceps brachii, lateral head
Triceps brachii, medial head
Triceps brachii, long head (cut)
Triceps brachii, tendon
Triceps brachii, medial head
Anconeus

Scapula
Clavicle
Acromion
Spine of scapula
Head of humerus
Glenoid cavity
Vertebra
Rib
Lateral epicondyle
Olecranon
Medial epicondyle
Radius
Ulna

Hip bone
Sacrum

STRETCHING THE TRICEPS

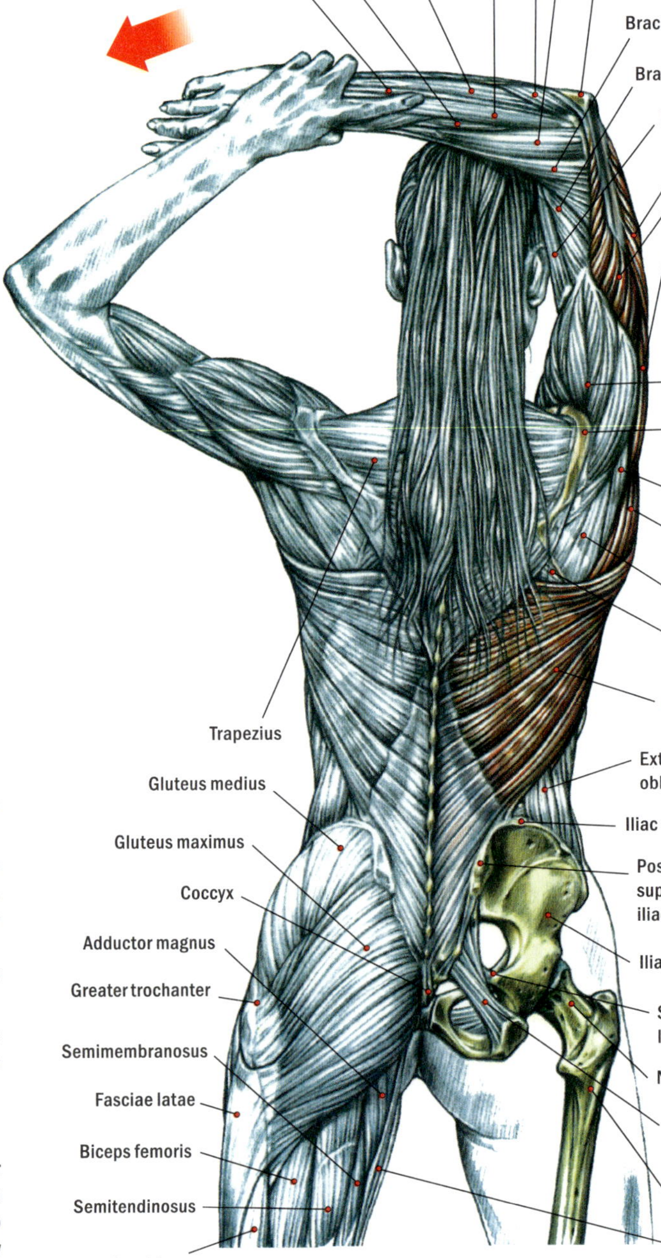

Stand or sit with a very straight back. Hold one arm straight up against the side of your head and bend your elbow to 90 degrees:

- Grab your wrist with your other hand and pull slowly, trying to bring your elbow behind your head.
- Hold the stretch for a few seconds while breathing slowly.

This exercise mainly stretches the triceps, teres major, and latissimus dorsi.

Variation

To accentuate the stretch on your triceps, do this stretch with your arm bent. Use the opposite hand to grasp your elbow and slowly pull your elbow down behind your head, as shown on the next page.

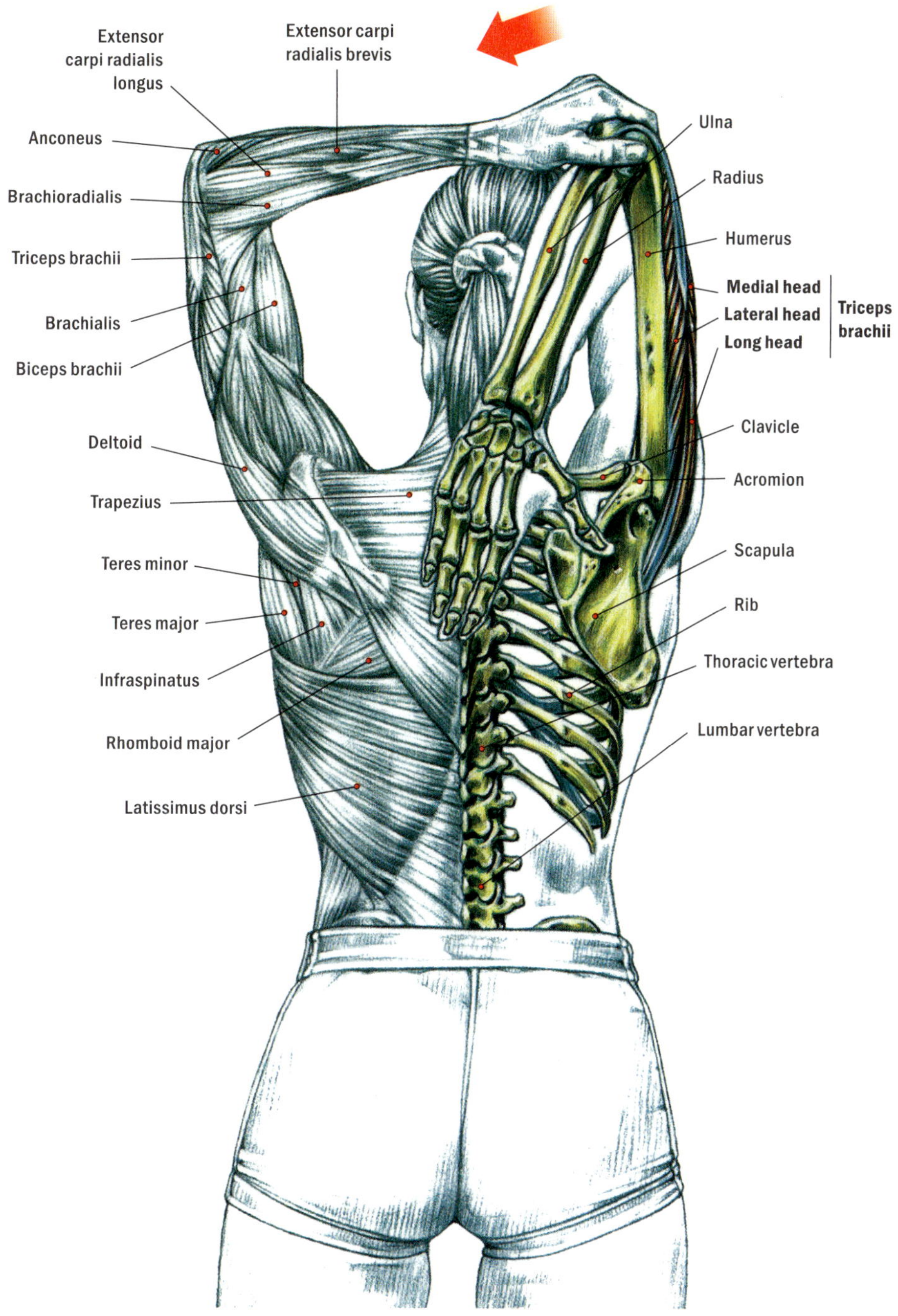

Stand or sit with your back straight and one arm raised vertically beside your head. Bend your arm at the elbow so that your hand touches your upper back:

- With your other hand, grasp your elbow and slowly try to pull it behind your head.
- Hold the stretch for a few seconds while breathing slowly.

This stretches the teres major, the long head of the triceps brachii, and, to a lesser extent, the latissimus dorsi.

Variations

- Pull the hand rather than your elbow.
- For greater intensity, place the raised arm against a wall.

These triceps stretches can help prevent tears that can happen when using heavy weights during triceps exercises but also when doing pullovers or upright rows with heavy weights. Upright rows tend to pull excessively on the long head of the triceps.

02 SHOULDERS

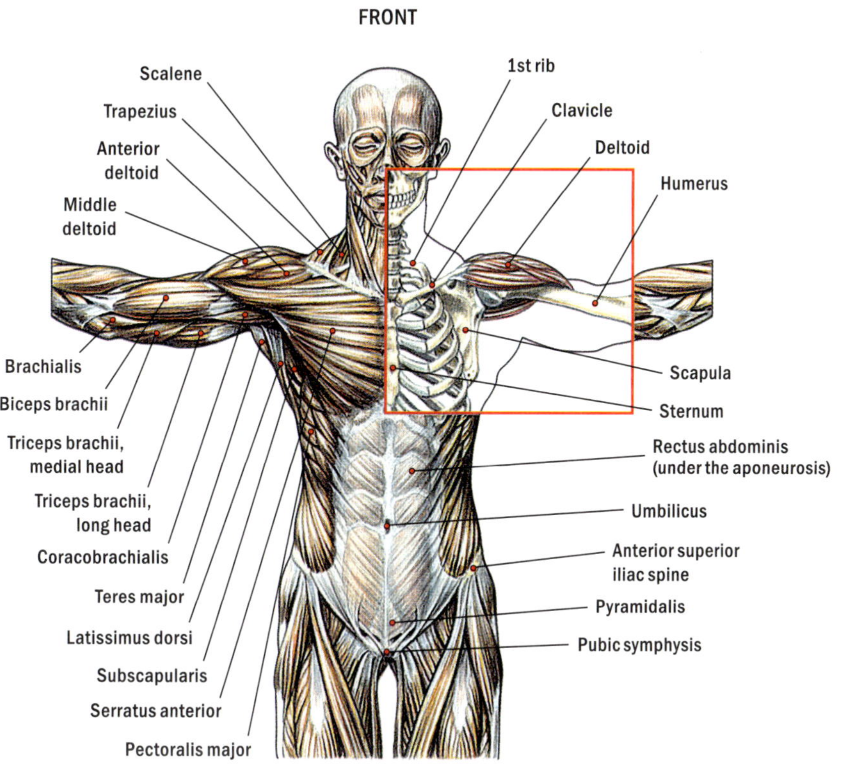

FRONT
Scalene
Trapezius
Anterior deltoid
Middle deltoid
Brachialis
Biceps brachii
Triceps brachii, medial head
Triceps brachii, long head
Coracobrachialis
Teres major
Latissimus dorsi
Subscapularis
Serratus anterior
Pectoralis major
1st rib
Clavicle
Deltoid
Humerus
Scapula
Sternum
Rectus abdominis (under the aponeurosis)
Umbilicus
Anterior superior iliac spine
Pyramidalis
Pubic symphysis

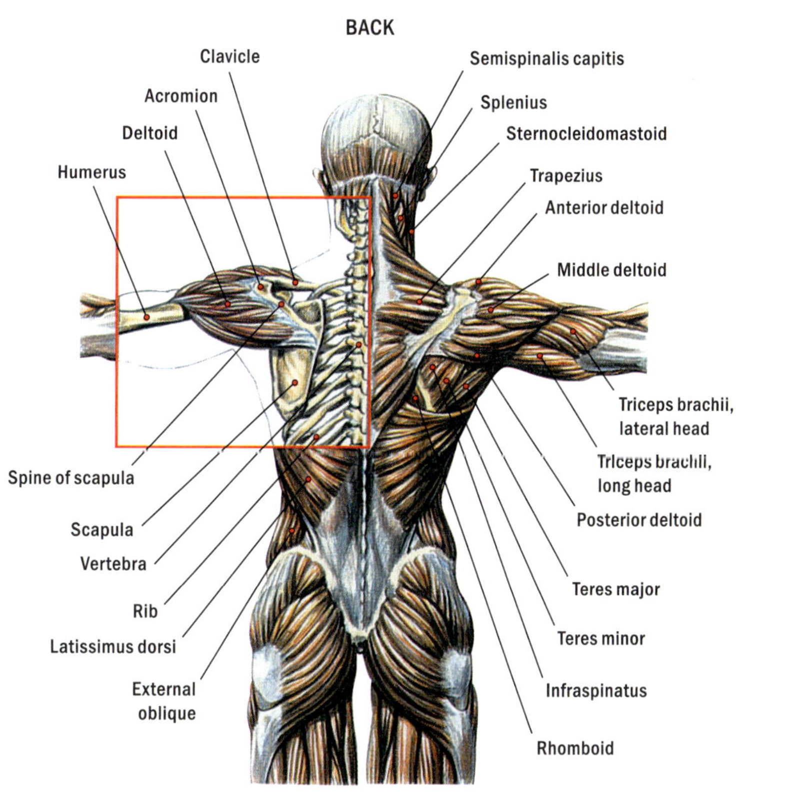

BACK
Clavicle
Acromion
Deltoid
Humerus
Spine of scapula
Scapula
Vertebra
Rib
Latissimus dorsi
External oblique
Semispinalis capitis
Splenius
Sternocleidomastoid
Trapezius
Anterior deltoid
Middle deltoid
Triceps brachii, lateral head
Triceps brachii, long head
Posterior deltoid
Teres major
Teres minor
Infraspinatus
Rhomboid

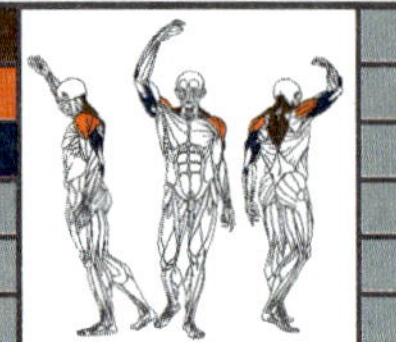

Occipitofrontalis, occipital belly

Diagram labels (clockwise):
- Deltoid: **Anterior deltoid**, **Middle deltoid**, **Posterior deltoid**
- Semispinalis capitis
- Splenius capitis
- Sternocleidomastoid
- Brachioradialis
- Extensor digitorum
- Extensor carpi radialis brevis
- Extensor carpi ulnaris
- Extensor carpi radialis longus
- Anconeus
- Triceps brachii: **Lateral head**, **Medial head**, **Long head**
- Brachialis
- Biceps brachii
- Trapezius
- Teres minor
- Teres major
- Infraspinatus
- Rhomboid major
- Latissimus dorsi
- External oblique
- Thoracolumbar fascia
- Cranium
- Mastoid process
- Cervical vertebra
- Clavicle
- **Supraspinatus**
- Acromion
- Spine of scapula
- Radius
- Ulna
- Humerus
- Scapula
- 9th rib
- Thoracic vertebra
- Lumbar vertebra

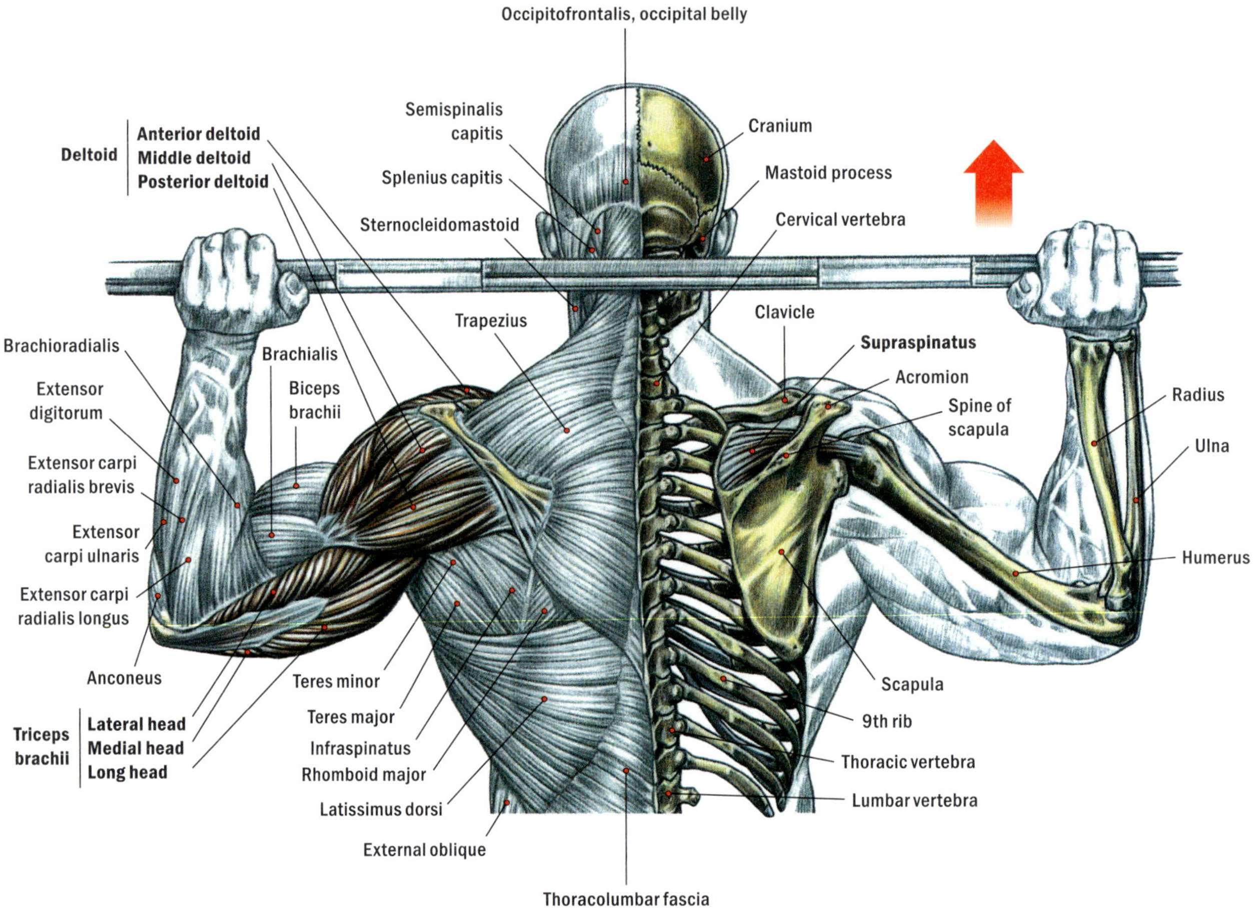

Sit with your back straight and hold the bar behind your neck with an overhand grip:

- Inhale and push the bar straight up, keeping your lower back as straight as possible.
- Exhale at the end of the exercise.

This exercise works the deltoid, mainly the middle and posterior fibers, as well as the trapezius, triceps brachii, and the serratus anterior. Although they are not worked as intensely, the rhomboids, infraspinatus, teres minor, and, deeper in, the supraspinatus also contract. You can also do this exercise while standing or using a rack. There are also many specific machines available for doing this exercise.

> ⚠ To prevent injury to the shoulder joint, which is vulnerable, lower the bar only as far as your unique shoulder structure and flexibility allow you to do comfortably (see page 56).

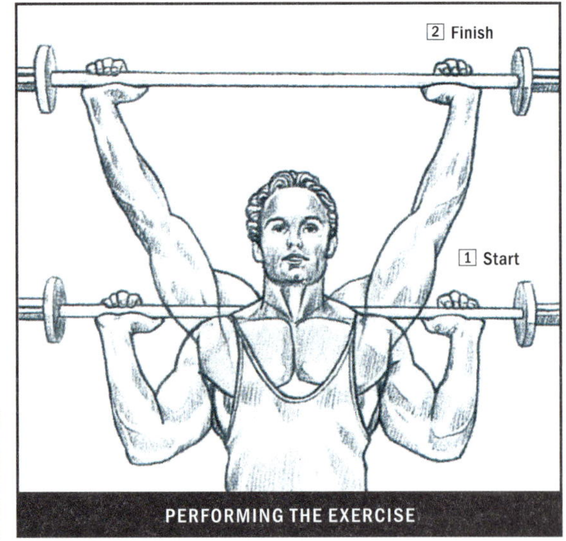

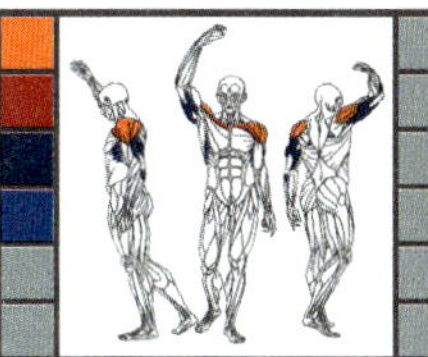

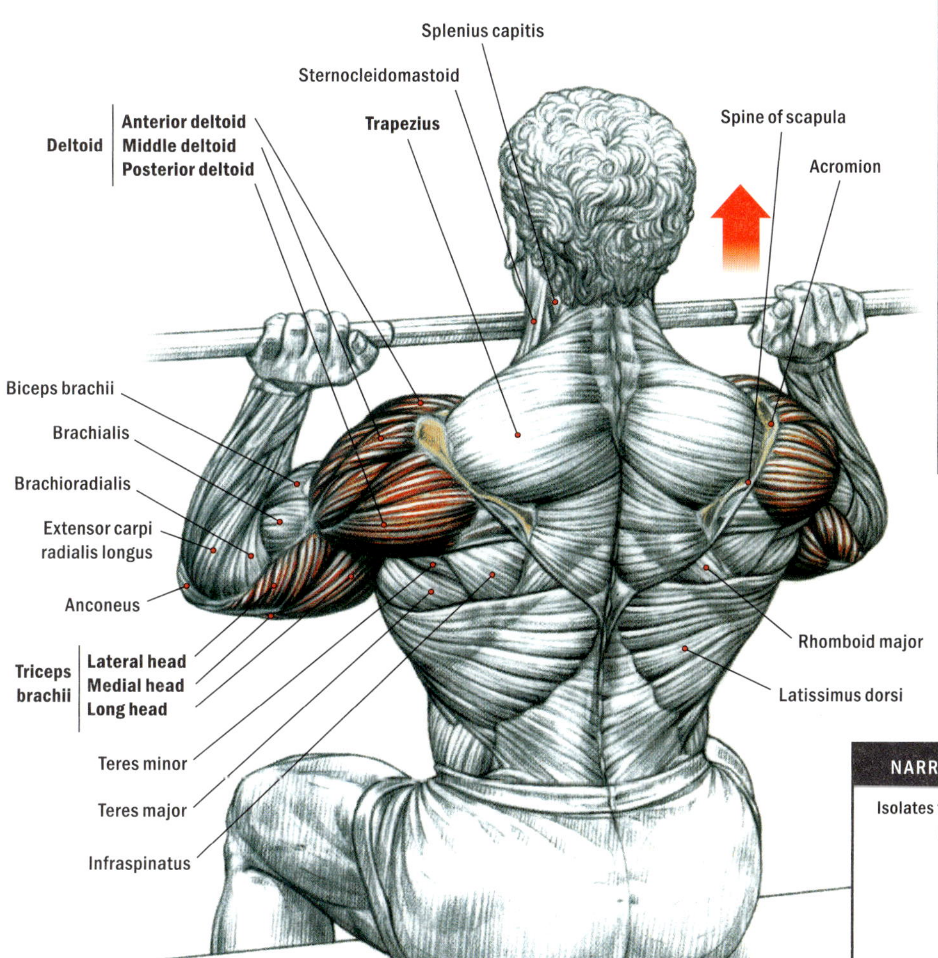

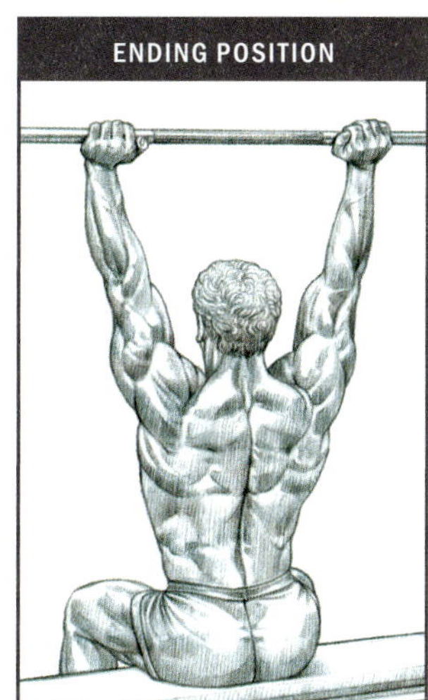
ENDING POSITION

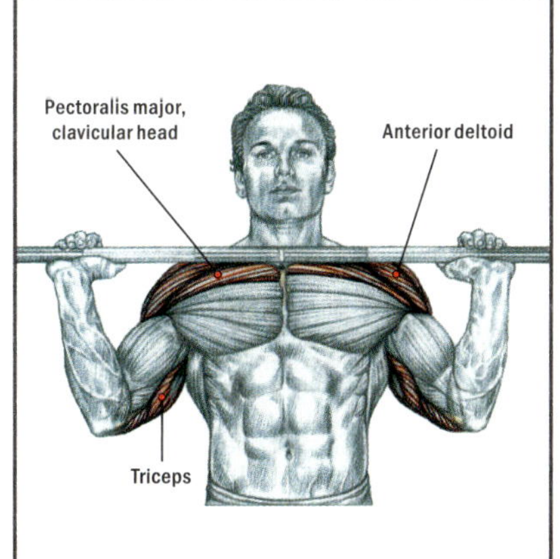
STARTING POSITION: FRONT VIEW

Sit with your back straight and hold the bar with an overhand grip, resting it across your upper chest:

- Inhale and push the bar up.
- Exhale at the end of the exercise.

This core exercise mainly uses the anterior and lateral deltoids, the clavicular head of the pectoralis major, triceps brachii, serratus anterior, trapezius, and, deeper in, the supraspinatus.

You can also perform this exercise standing, as long as you keep your back straight, avoiding any arching of your lumbar spine.

You can use various machines and racks to do this exercise; these allow you to do the exercise without worrying about positioning, and they help focus the work on the deltoid.

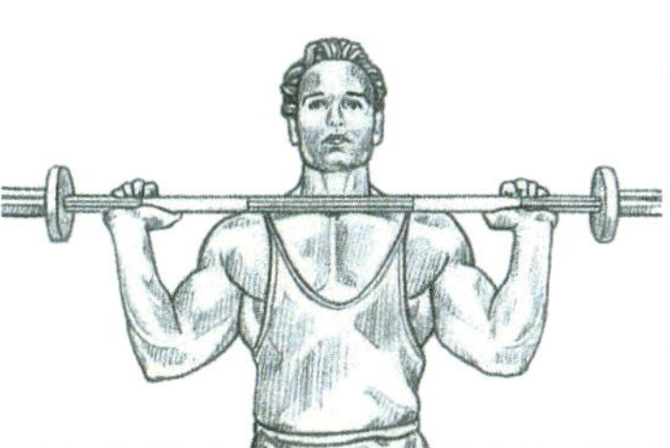
NARROW GRIP, ELBOWS FORWARD

Isolates the anterior deltoid and the clavicular head of the pectoralis major.

WIDE GRIP, ELBOWS SPREAD OUT

Isolates the anterior and middle deltoids.

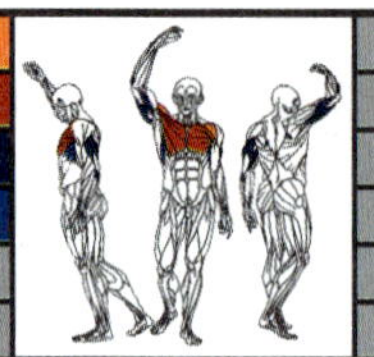

03 SEATED DUMBBELL PRESSES

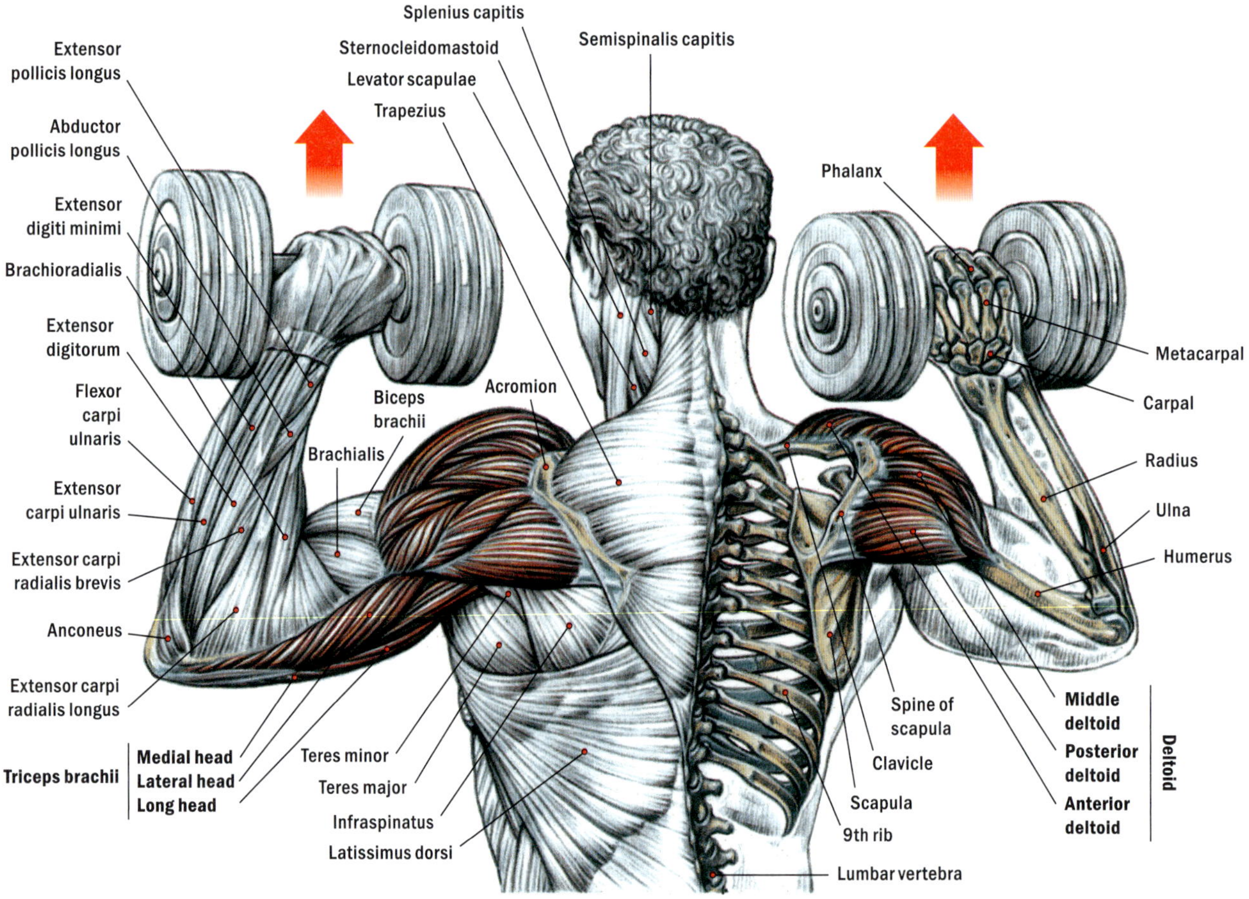

Splenius capitis
Sternocleidomastoid
Semispinalis capitis
Levator scapulae
Trapezius
Extensor pollicis longus
Abductor pollicis longus
Extensor digiti minimi
Brachioradialis
Extensor digitorum
Flexor carpi ulnaris
Extensor carpi ulnaris
Extensor carpi radialis brevis
Anconeus
Extensor carpi radialis longus
Triceps brachii
Medial head
Lateral head
Long head
Biceps brachii
Brachialis
Acromion
Teres minor
Teres major
Infraspinatus
Latissimus dorsi
Phalanx
Metacarpal
Carpal
Radius
Ulna
Humerus
Spine of scapula
Clavicle
Scapula
9th rib
Lumbar vertebra
Middle deltoid
Posterior deltoid
Anterior deltoid
Deltoid

VARIATION WITH PALMS FACING EACH OTHER

2 Finish
1 Start

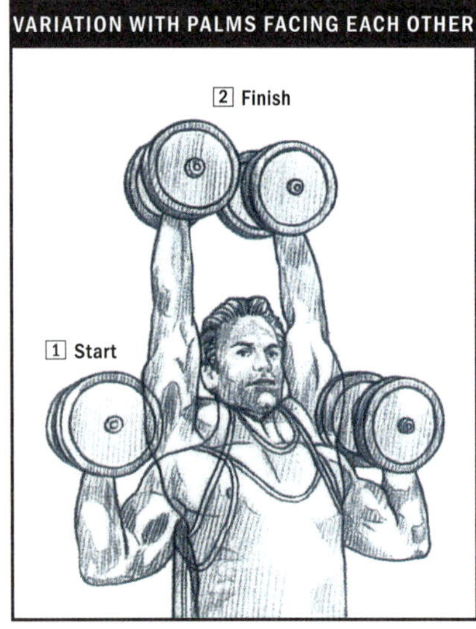

Sit on a bench, keeping your back straight, and hold the dumbbells at shoulder level with an overhand grip (thumbs pointing inward):

- Inhale and extend your arms vertically.
- Exhale at the end of the exercise.

This exercise contracts the deltoid (primarily the middle deltoid), as well as the trapezius, serratus anterior, and triceps brachii.

This exercise can also be done while standing up, and you can also alternate arms. A backrest helps prevent any arching in the back.

ENDING POSITION

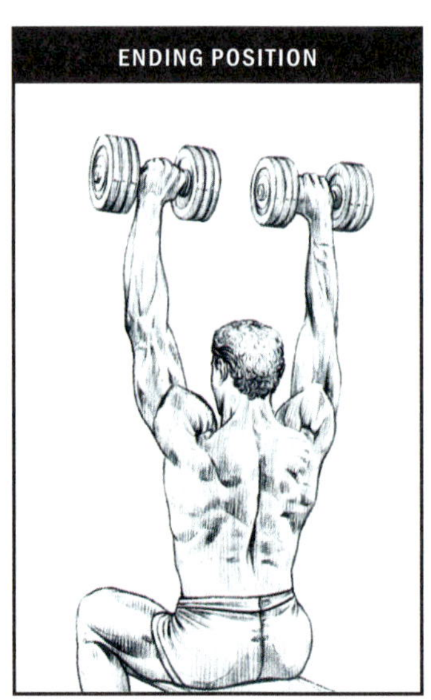

TRAINING THROUGH SHOULDER INJURIES WITH LYING DUMBBELL PRESSES

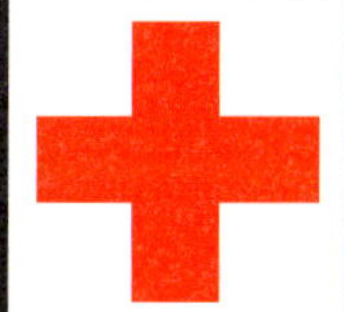

This is one of the rare exercises that can be done by those suffering from the all-too-common entrapment syndrome.

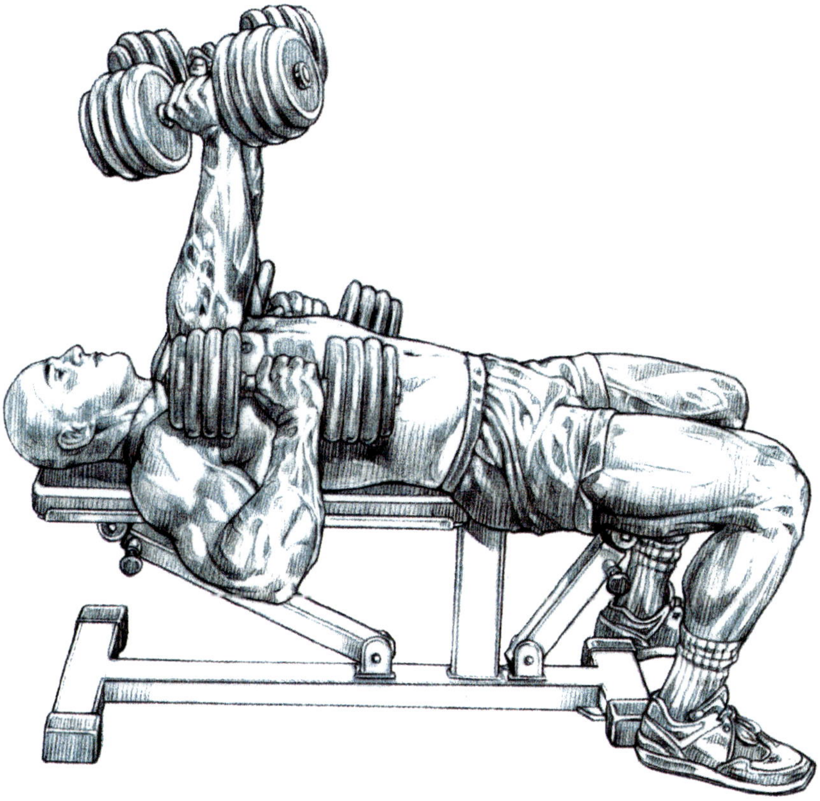

Doing dumbbell presses while lying on a bench with the elbows next to the body works the anterior deltoid intensely and, to a lesser degree, works the middle deltoid while preventing excessive rubbing at the front of the shoulder. When performed regularly, this exercise will maintain the size and tone of the deltoids despite any injuries. You can also use this exercise to reeducate the pectoralis major after a tear; pressing with the elbows against the body reduces the stretch in the pectoralis major, decreasing the risk of tearing the scarred area.

Performing the Exercise

Lie on a bench with your chest expanded, back slightly arched, feet flat on the ground, and elbows bent next to your body, holding a dumbbell in each hand.

- Inhale and extend your arms vertically.
- Exhale at the end of the exercise.
- Return to the starting position with a controlled movement.

COMPARISON OF THE HIP JOINT AND THE SHOULDER JOINT

Hip bone

Femur

1 Hip joint

Scapula

Humerus

2 Shoulder joint

Compared to the stable hip joint, the shoulder joint is less encased and is more mobile, which makes it more vulnerable to injuries.

Shoulder injuries occur frequently in strength training, especially in bodybuilding, where developing the entire deltoid group requires the athlete to perform a significant number of reps and variations in exercises, which multiplies the risk of injury.

The hip joint, where the head of the femur sits deep in the glenoid cavity of the pelvis, is very stable. On the other hand, the shoulder joint, which is very mobile to allow the arm to have a wide range of motion, is much less contained. The shoulder is a ball-and-socket joint held in place by muscles; the head of the humerus is held within the glenoid cavity of the scapula primarily by a complex musculotendinous group.

ROTATOR CUFF MUSCLES SEEN FROM THE FRONT

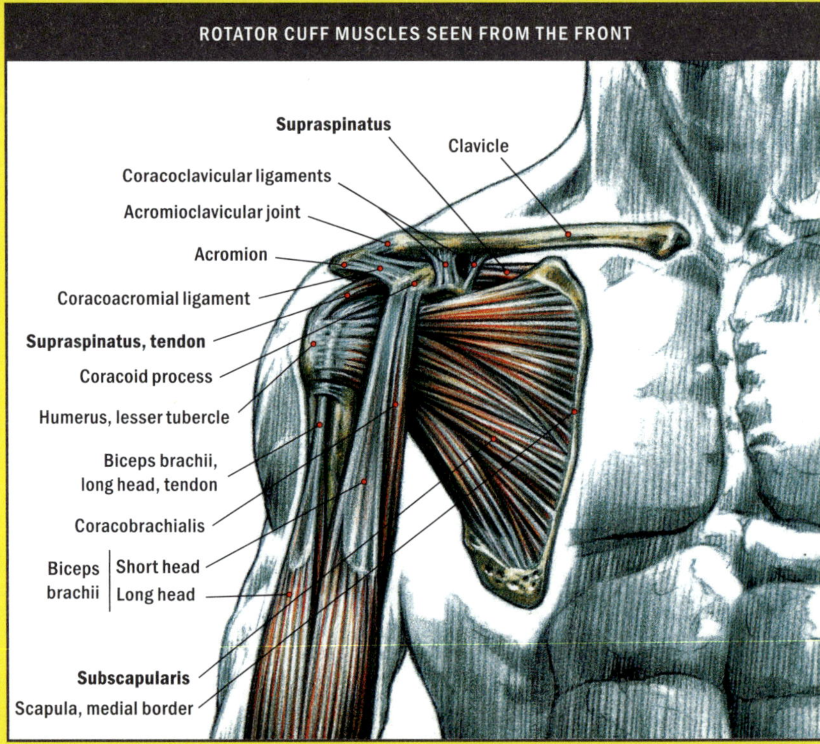

ROTATOR CUFF MUSCLES SEEN FROM BEHIND

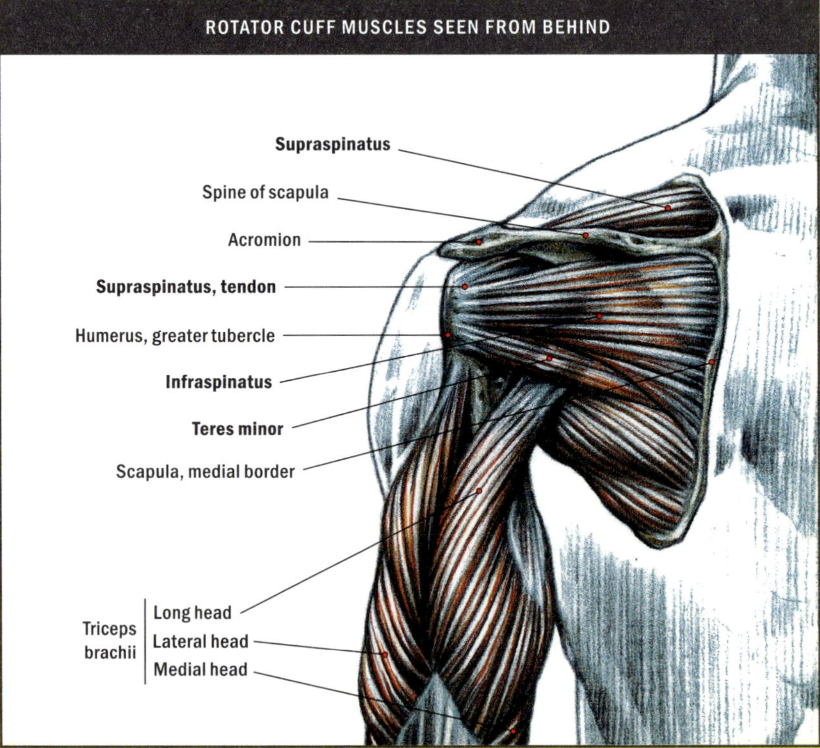

Most strength training injuries occur when training the deltoids, and they rarely result in direct injury to the muscle. Generally, these injuries are much deeper, and they appear during an odd movement or, more pernicious, after a long period of rubbing of the tendons reinforcing the articular capsule.

In contrast to violent contact sports, such as American football, or sudden arm movements, like pitching, which can create serious injuries involving dislocation or even torn tendons, the most serious injury in strength training involves entrapment, technically known as *subacromial impingement syndrome*. When certain people perform exercises in which they raise the arms, such as presses from the neck or lateral raises, the supraspinatus tendon is rubbed and compressed between the head of the humerus and the osteoligamentous arch created by the inferior surface of the acromion and the coracoacromial ligament.

Inflammation follows. This generally begins with the serous bursa, which normally protects the supraspinatus from excessive friction, and extends to the supraspinatus tendon itself, which, without treatment, ends up affecting the adjacent infraspinatus tendon posteriorly and the long head of the biceps brachii anteriorly. Raising the arm becomes extremely painful and eventually can cause irreversible deterioration of the supraspinatus tendon through calcification and even tearing; however, this usually only happens to people over 40 years of age. The space between the humerus and the coracoacromial arch varies from person to person. Some athletes cannot raise their arms laterally without excessive friction. These people should avoid all presses from the neck, lateral raises that go too high, and back presses.

All barbell presses for the shoulders must be performed to the front with the elbows slightly forward. When doing lateral dumbbell raises, you'll need to determine the proper angle to use. The correct movement is the one that does not cause any pain.

It is interesting to note that not everyone responds the same way to the same shoulder injury. Some people perform all sorts of arm raises that compress the tendon, sometimes even causing tendon degeneration, without initiating a painful inflammatory process.

This is how a torn supraspinatus tendon can be discovered during assessment without that person ever having complained of pain. Another cause of shoulder pain may be an imbalance in muscle tension around the articular capsule. Remember that the head of the humerus is solidly fixed in the glenoid cavity of the scapula by a group of muscles whose tendons adhere to or cross the joint capsule. In front is the subscapularis, a little farther to the outside is the long head of the biceps; at the top is the supraspinatus, and to the back are the infraspinatus and teres minor. Spasm, hypertonicity, or hypotonicity in one or more of these muscles can pull the shoulder joint into an incorrect position.

This incorrect position can cause friction during arm movements, resulting in inflammation.

Example: Shortening or spasm of the teres minor and the infraspinatus will externally rotate the head of the humerus, which will cause rubbing at the front of the shoulder during arm movement. Over time, this can injure the tendon of the long head of the biceps brachii. Be careful to balance the training of the shoulder muscles and avoid any exercises that feel awkward or painful.

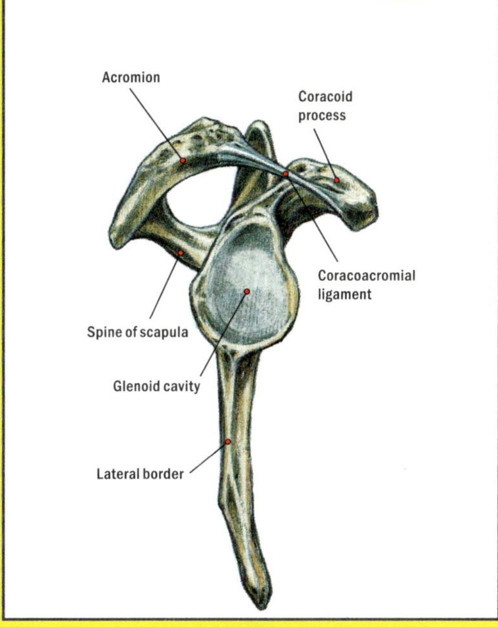

Massage, either manually or even better with an electric massager, and electrical stimulation are effective for decreasing or eliminating spasms and shortening of the teres minor and infraspinatus.

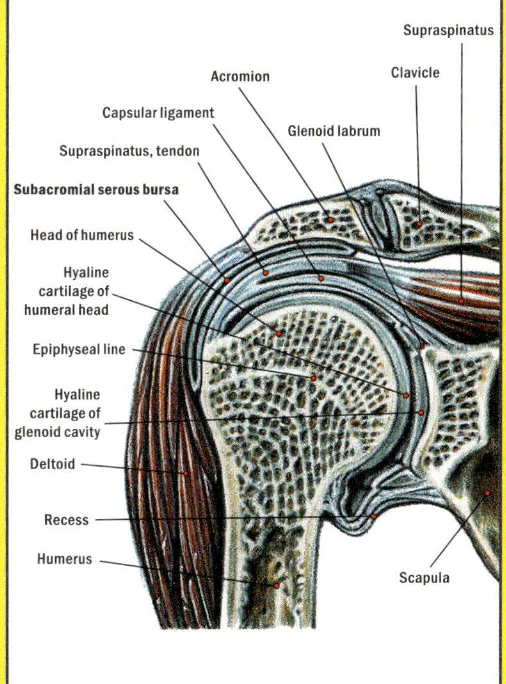

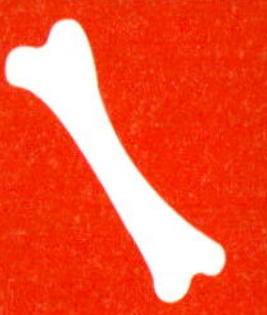

HOW BONE STRUCTURE AFFECTS THE BACK PRESS

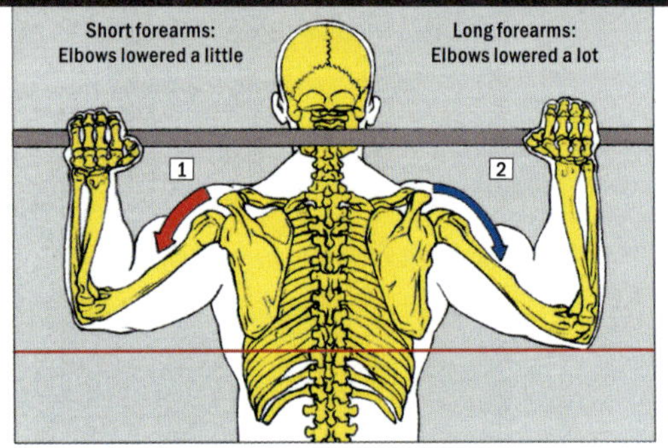

1 The deltoid is stretched optimally, allowing for recruitment of the maximum number of muscle fibers during the initiation of the movement.
2 The deltoid is overstretched, which does not allow enough muscle fibers to be recruited for a powerful initiation of the movement.

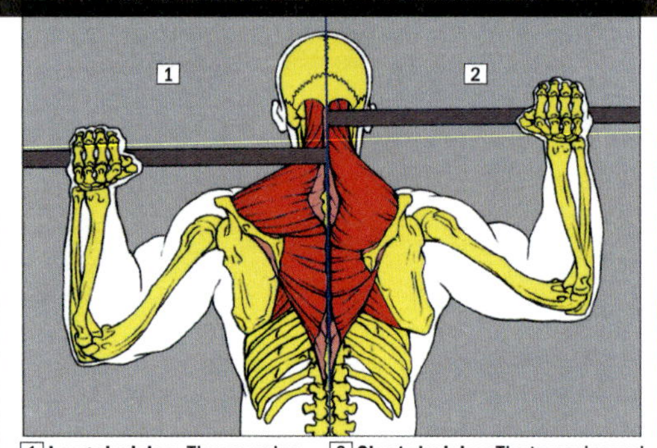

1 **Long clavicles:** The scapulae are free to rotate, and the elbows can be lowered without restriction.
2 **Short clavicles:** The trapezius and rhomboid muscles are compressed and prevent the scapulae from rotating, thereby limiting how far the elbows can be lowered.

It is important to consider individual morphological differences when training the shoulders with the back press.

The length of the arms: The length of the arms, especially the forearms, plays a fundamental role in the execution of this exercise. When lowering the bar below the ears, people with proportionately longer forearms bring their elbows down lower than people with proportionately shorter forearms. This lower placement of the elbows really stretches the deltoid, putting it in an unfavorable position by not allowing the muscle to recruit the maximum number of fibers to initiate a powerful push.

To optimize training and be able to add more weight, people with proportionately longer arms should add heavier weights and not lower the bar too much below the ears. The most important part is to be able to feel the deltoids working.

The length of the clavicles: The length of the clavicles has a considerable influence on the ability to lower the bar correctly behind the neck. Short clavicles inevitably bring the shoulder blades toward the vertebral axis. During a back press, as both shoulder blades tilt to the center of the back, their movement is significantly reduced by the compression of the trapezius and rhomboid muscles in the middle of the back. This shortened range of the shoulder blades limits the ability to correctly lower the elbows in order to feel the deltoids working.

Furthermore, the greater the development of the muscles at the center of the back, the less the shoulder blades will be able to move toward each other, and this will further limit the lowering of the bar behind the neck.

1 When the humerus rotates externally with elevation of the arm, reduced space between the glenohumeral joint and the coracoacromial arch may lead to excessive friction that, over time, can damage or even tear the supraspinatus tendon. Therefore, at the slightest sensation of unease accompanied by pain during the back press, change the movement to avoid developing degenerative tendinitis of the rotator cuff.

2 Raising the arm (as in lateral raises with dumbbells) causes the humerus to rotate internally. Too narrow a space between the glenohumeral joint and the coracoacromial arch may lead to excessive friction that risks damaging the infraspinatus tendon.

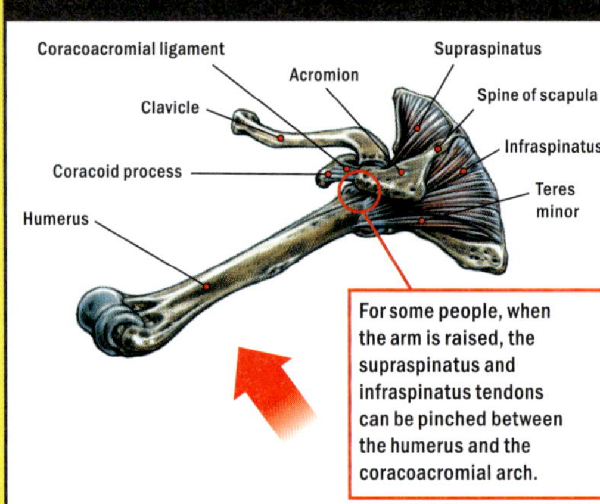

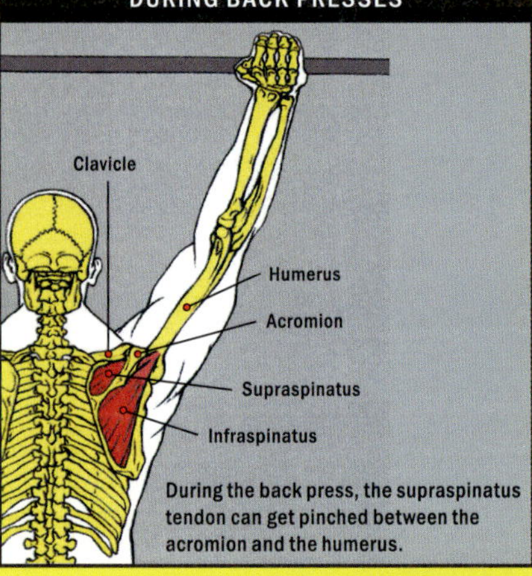

People with long forearms and short clavicles should avoid the back press to work their deltoids.

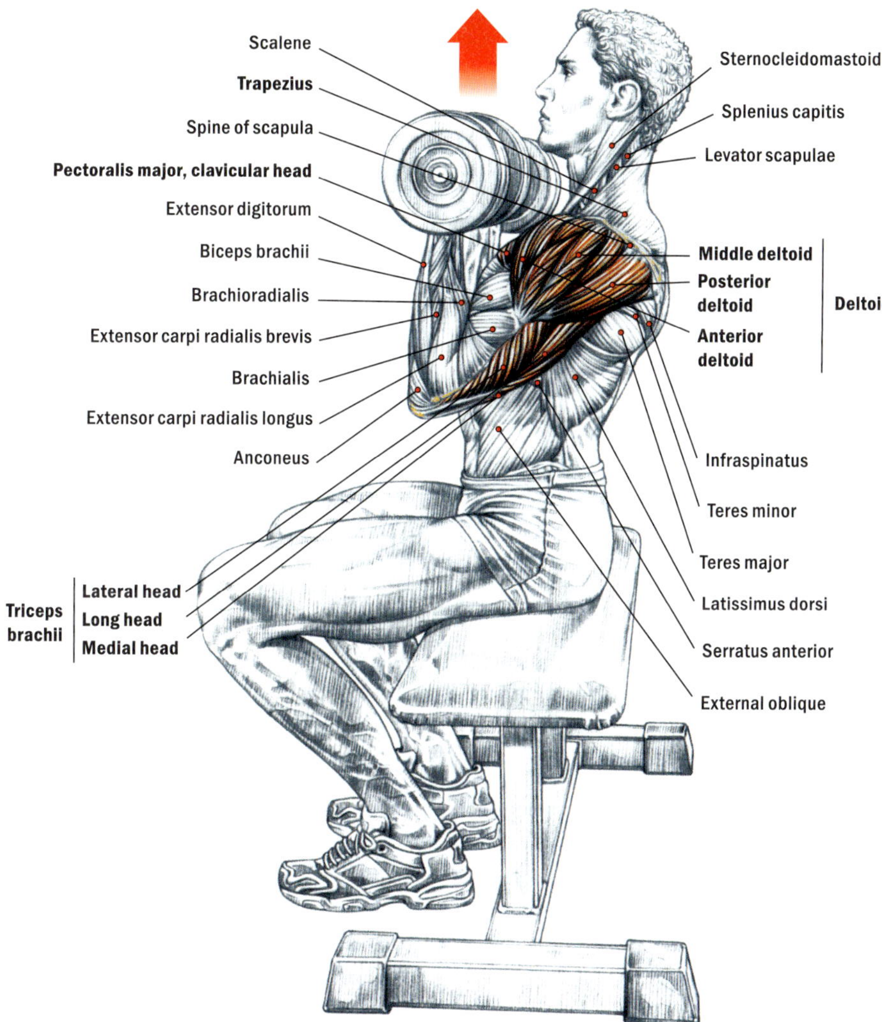

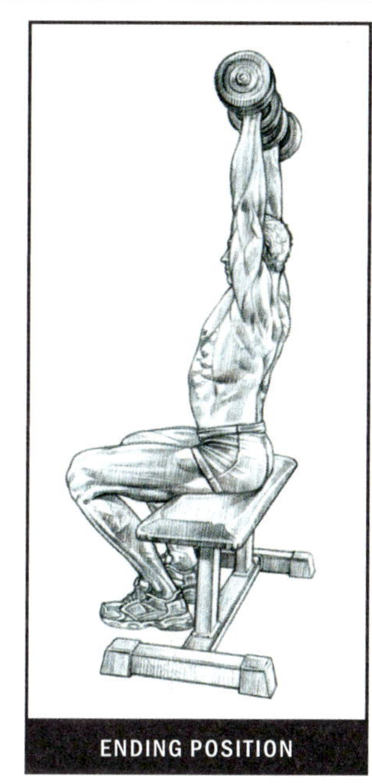

Sit on a bench, keeping your back straight. With your arms bent and your elbows pointing forward, hold the dumbbells at shoulder level with an underhand grip (thumbs pointing away from each other):

- Inhale and extend your arms overhead while rotating 90 degrees at the wrists, bringing them into an overhand grip (thumbs pointing toward each other).
- Exhale at the end of the exercise.

This exercise works the deltoid (primarily the anterior deltoid), as well as the clavicular head of the pectoralis major, triceps brachii, trapezius, and serratus anterior.

Variations
The exercise can be done

- seated against a backrest to help prevent excessive arching of the back,
- standing, or
- alternating arms.

Working with the elbows pointing forward prevents excessive friction in the shoulder joint, which can trigger inflammation that, in the long term, could results in more serious injuries. This exercise is recommended for people with weak shoulders and is meant to replace more intense exercises, such as classic dumbbell presses with the elbows pointing outward or back presses.

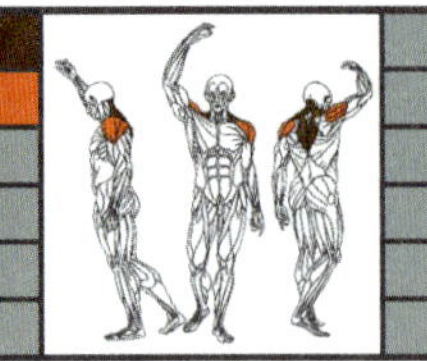

Sternocleidomastoid

Sternohyoid

Trapezius

Pectoralis major

Deltoid

Coracobrachialis

Biceps brachii

Brachialis

Brachioradialis

Pronator teres

Triceps brachii | Medial head / Long head

Teres major

Latissimus dorsi

Serratus anterior

External oblique

Rectus abdominis

Gluteus medius

Iliopsoas

Pectineus

Tensor fasciae latae

Adductor longus

Sartorius

Gracilis

1st rib

Clavicle

Anterior deltoid
Posterior deltoid | Deltoid
Middle deltoid

Ulna

Radius

Cubitus

Scapula

Sternum

Rib

Lumbar vertebra

Hip bone

Sacrum

Pubic symphysis

Femur

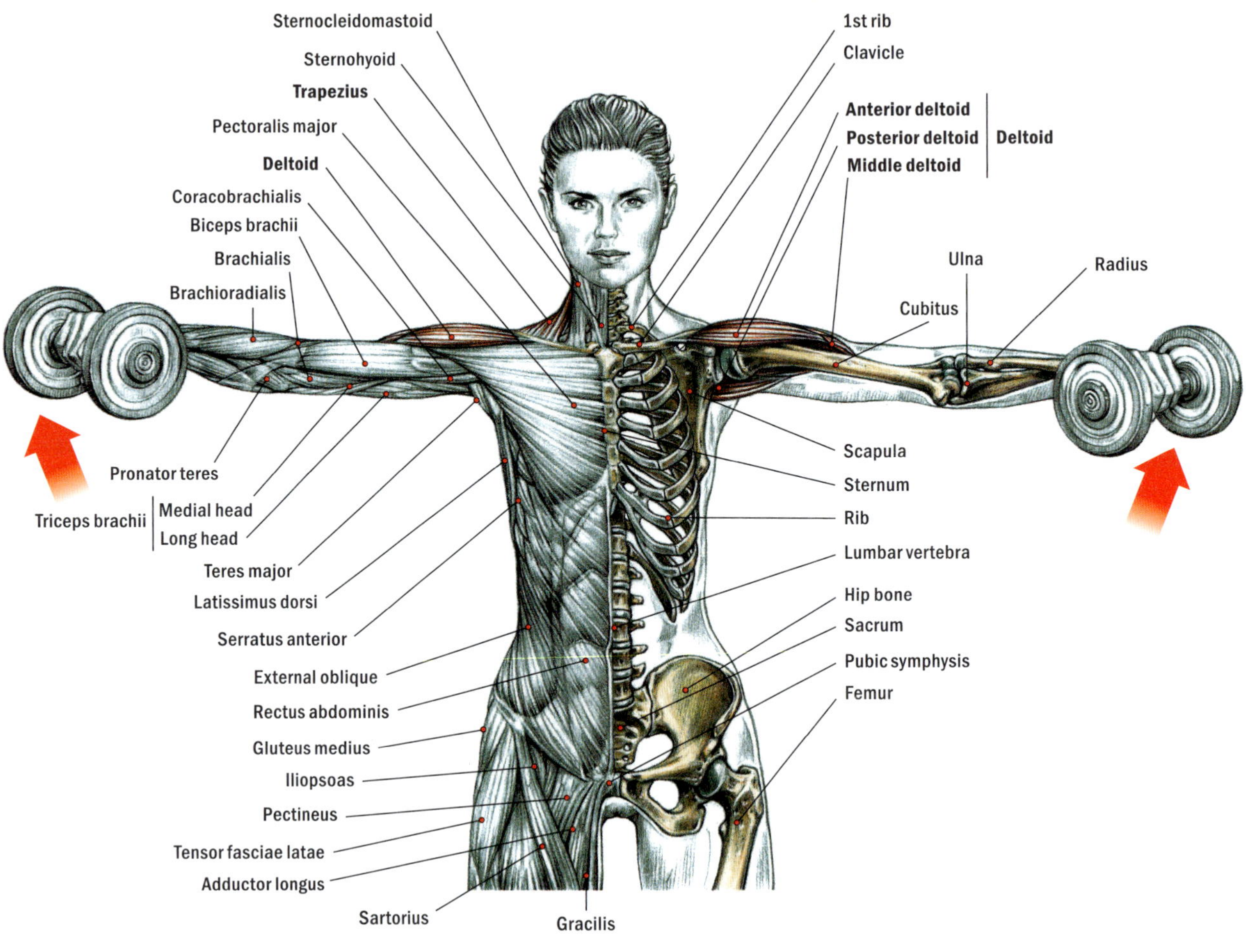

ACTION OF THE SUPRASPINATUS MUSCLE

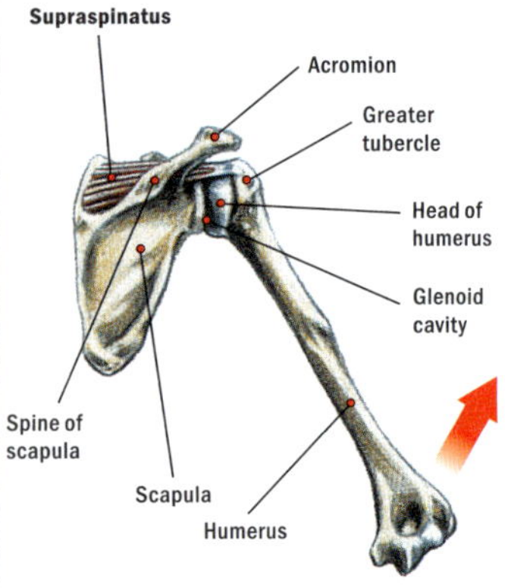

Supraspinatus

Acromion

Greater tubercle

Head of humerus

Glenoid cavity

Spine of scapula

Scapula

Humerus

The supraspinatus helps the deltoid raise the arm laterally and helps keep the head of the humerus in the glenoid cavity.

Stand with a straight back, with legs slightly apart, arms hanging next to your body, holding a dumbbell in each hand:

- Raise your arms to a horizontal position, keeping your elbows slightly bent.
- Return to the starting position.

This exercise primarily works the middle deltoid. The middle deltoid is a multipennate muscle whose different fibers converge on the humerus. Their function is to support relatively heavy weight and to move the arm precisely through its full range of motion. Therefore, it is important to adapt strength training to the specifics of this muscle by varying the starting position of the exercise (hands behind the back, at the side, or in front) to work all of the fibers of the middle deltoid. Because everyone's physical structure is different (length of the clavicle, shape of the acromion, and level of the deltoid insertion on the humerus), you must find the angle of the starting position that is most appropriate for your morphology. Lateral raises work the supraspinatus, although you cannot see the muscle because it is located deep in the supraspinatus fossa of the scapula (shoulder blade), where it attaches to the lesser tubercle of the humerus. Raising the arms higher than a horizontal position will work the upper part of the trapezius. However, many bodybuilders do not go above horizontal so that they can focus the work on the lateral part of the deltoid.

This exercise is never done with heavy weights. For the best results, do sets of 10 to 25 reps, while varying the working angle without much rest time until you feel a burn.

To increase the intensity, maintain an isometric contraction for a few seconds between each pair of repetitions while keeping the arms horizontal.

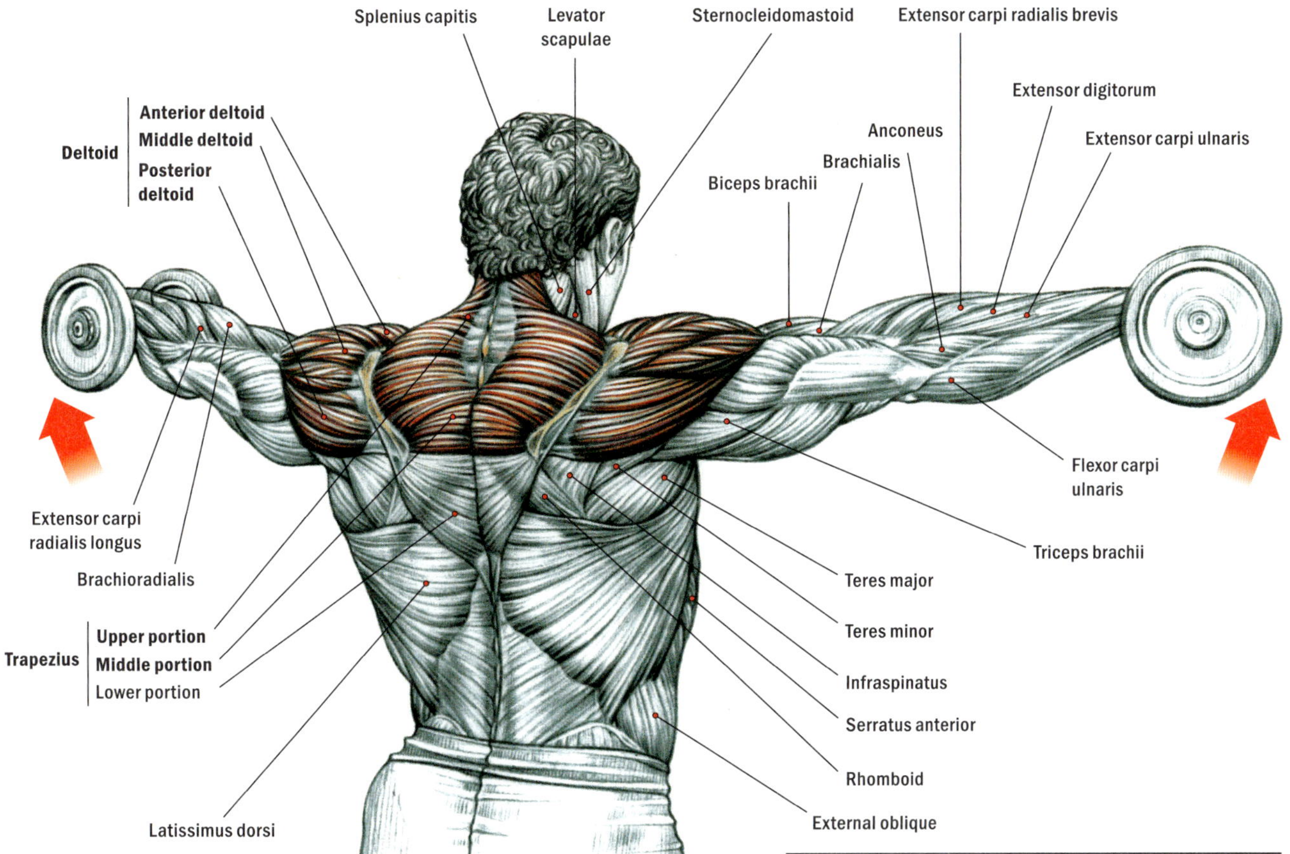

Splenius capitis
Levator scapulae
Sternocleidomastoid
Extensor carpi radialis brevis
Extensor digitorum
Anconeus
Extensor carpi ulnaris
Brachialis
Biceps brachii
Deltoid
Anterior deltoid
Middle deltoid
Posterior deltoid
Flexor carpi ulnaris
Extensor carpi radialis longus
Triceps brachii
Brachioradialis
Teres major
Trapezius
Upper portion
Middle portion
Lower portion
Teres minor
Infraspinatus
Serratus anterior
Rhomboid
External oblique
Latissimus dorsi

STARTING POSITION: VARIATIONS

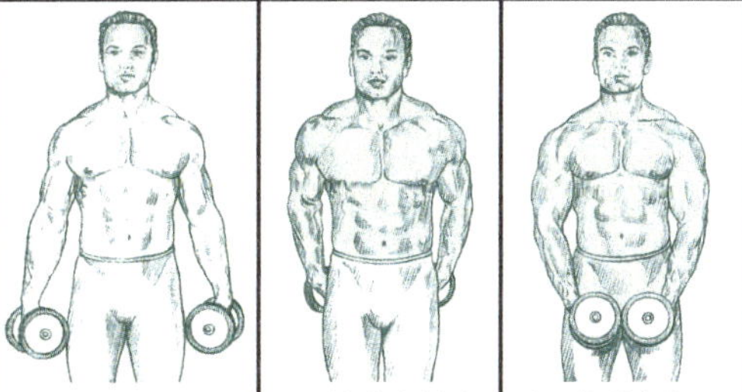

Dumbbells on the side | Dumbbells behind the back | Dumbbells in front of the thighs

ENDING POSITION: VARIATIONS

1
2

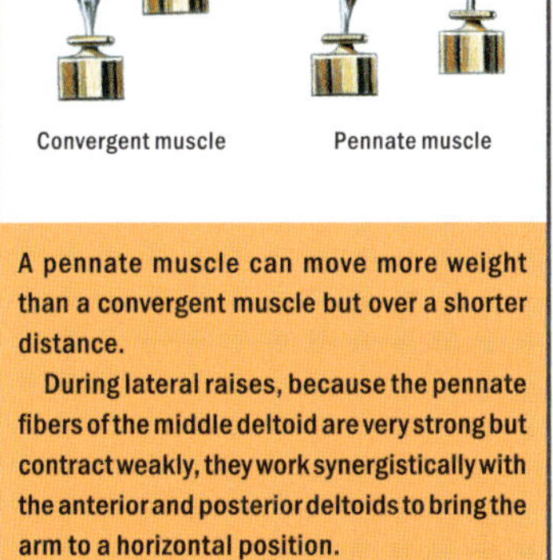

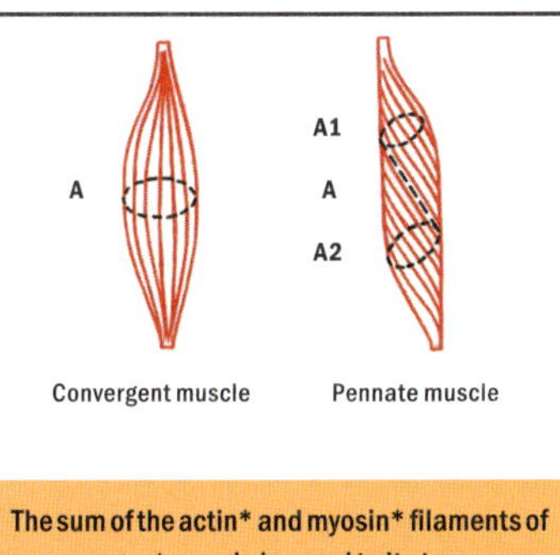

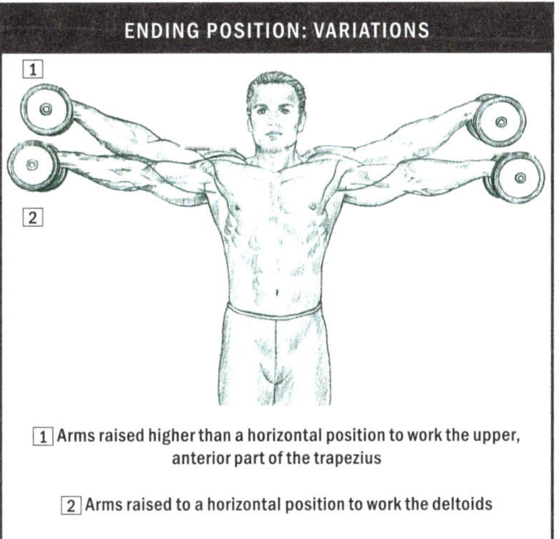

[1] Arms raised higher than a horizontal position to work the upper, anterior part of the trapezius

[2] Arms raised to a horizontal position to work the deltoids

Convergent muscle | Pennate muscle

A pennate muscle can move more weight than a convergent muscle but over a shorter distance.

During lateral raises, because the pennate fibers of the middle deltoid are very strong but contract weakly, they work synergistically with the anterior and posterior deltoids to bring the arm to a horizontal position.

A
A1
A
A2

Convergent muscle | Pennate muscle

The sum of the actin* and myosin* filaments of a convergent muscle is equal to its transverse section (A).

The sum of the actin and myosin filaments of a pennate muscle is equal to the sum (A) of its oblique sections (A1 and A2).

*The motor elements of a muscle whose maximum force of contraction is approximately five kilograms per centimeter squared (71 psi) per section.

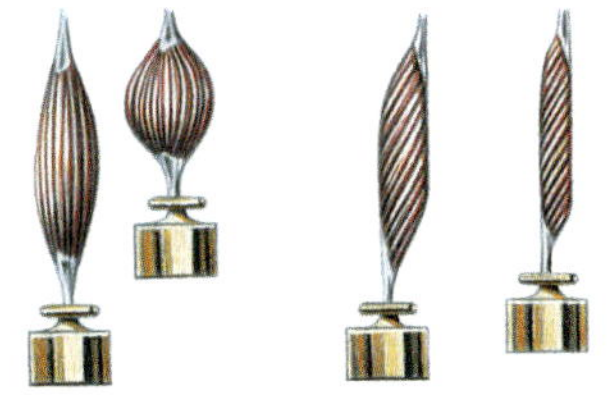

06 BENT-OVER LATERAL DUMBBELL RAISES

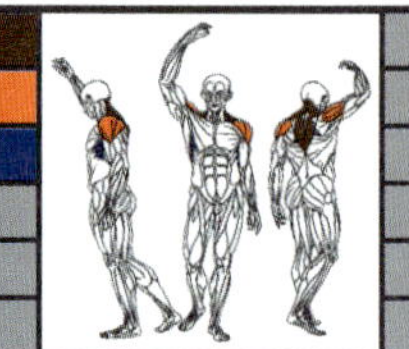

Clavicle
Trapezius
Rhomboid
Infraspinatus
Latissimus dorsi
External oblique
Teres minor
Teres major
Acromion
Deltoid
Anterior deltoid
Posterior deltoid
Middle deltoid
Triceps brachii
Brachialis
Biceps brachii
Brachioradialis
Extensor carpi radialis longus
Anconeus
Flexor carpi ulnaris
Extensor carpi radialis brevis
Extensor carpi ulnaris
Extensor digiti minimi
Sternocleidomastoid
Pectoralis major
Biceps brachii
Brachioradialis
Pronator teres
Flexor carpi radialis
Palmaris longus
Flexor digitorum superficialis
Extensor digitorum

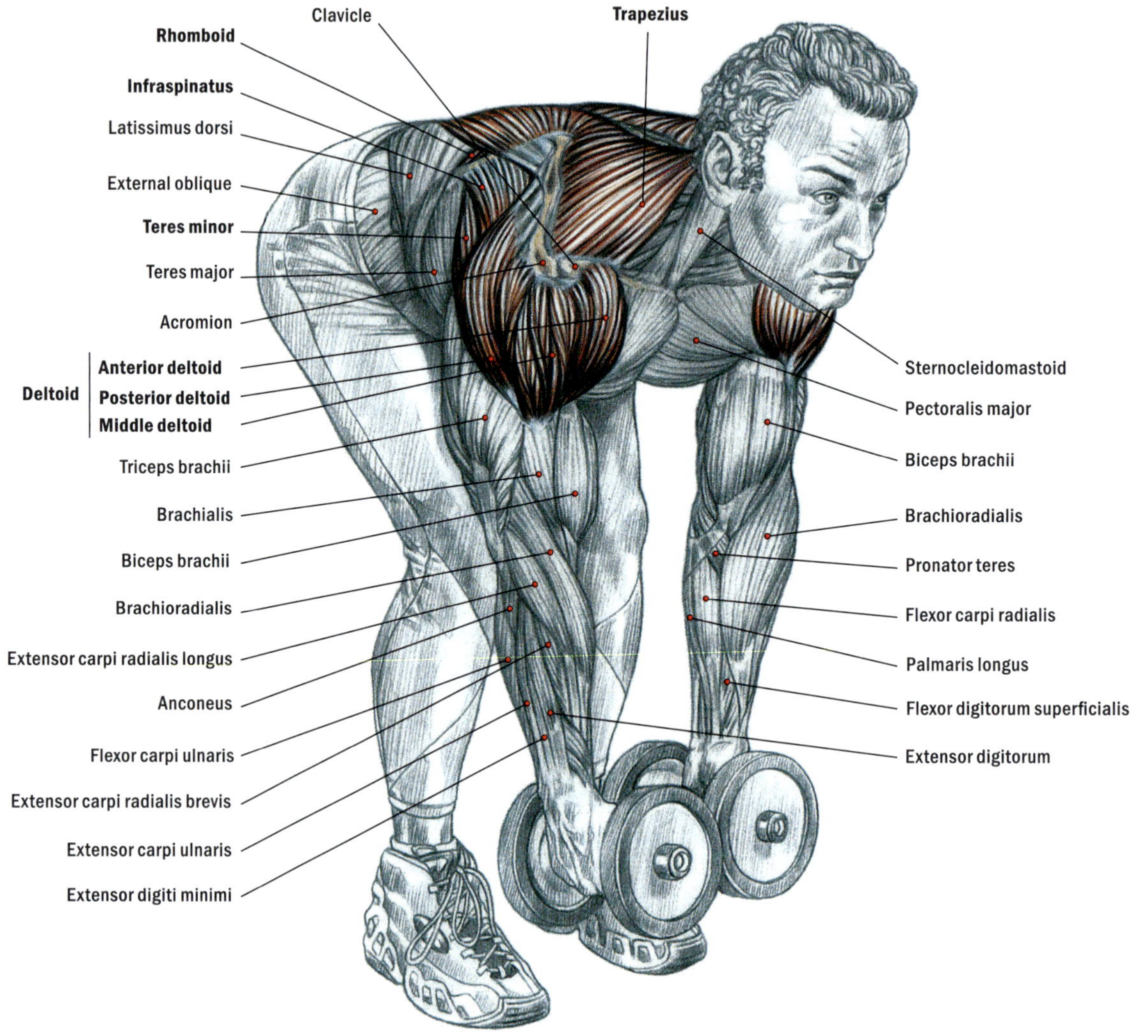

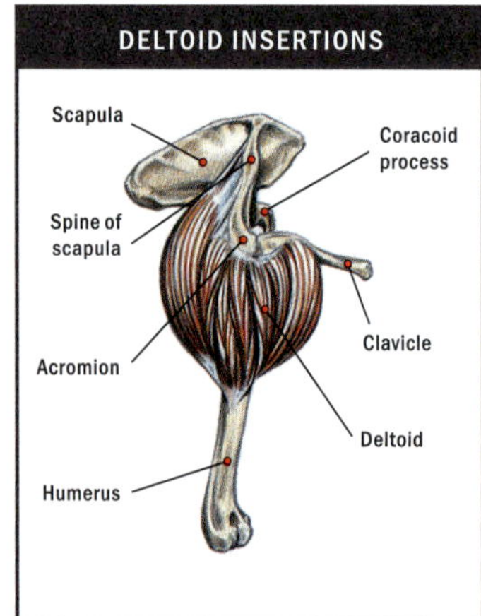

DELTOID INSERTIONS

Scapula
Coracoid process
Spine of scapula
Clavicle
Acromion
Deltoid
Humerus

Stand with your legs slightly apart and knees slightly bent. Lean forward at your waist while keeping your back straight. With your arms hanging down, grasp the dumbbells with your elbows slightly bent:

- Inhale and raise your arms to a horizontal position.
- Exhale at the end of the exercise.

This exercise works the entire shoulder, accenting the work of the posterior deltoid. Squeeze the shoulder blades together at the end of the exercise to contract the middle and lower portions of the trapezius as well as the rhomboids, teres minor, and infraspinatus.

Variation

The exercise may be done facedown on an incline bench to support the torso.

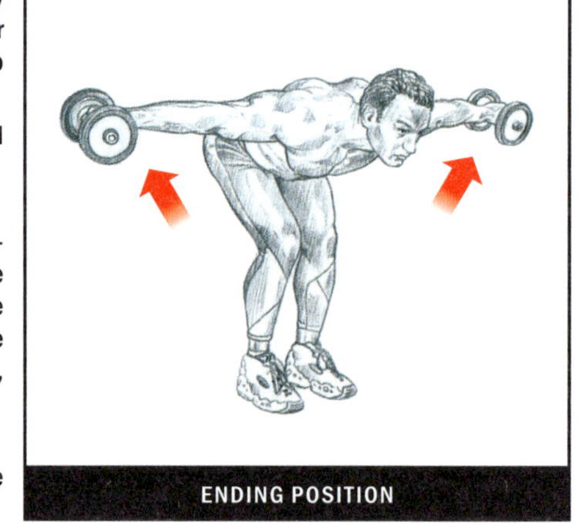

ENDING POSITION

ALTERNATING FRONT DUMBBELL RAISES 07

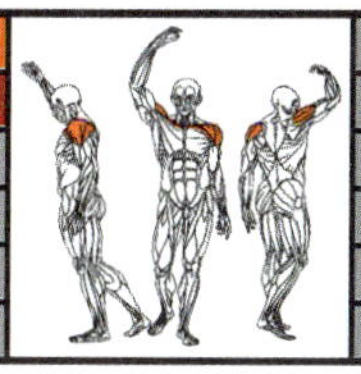

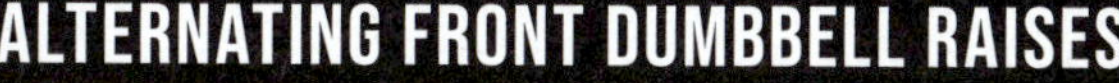

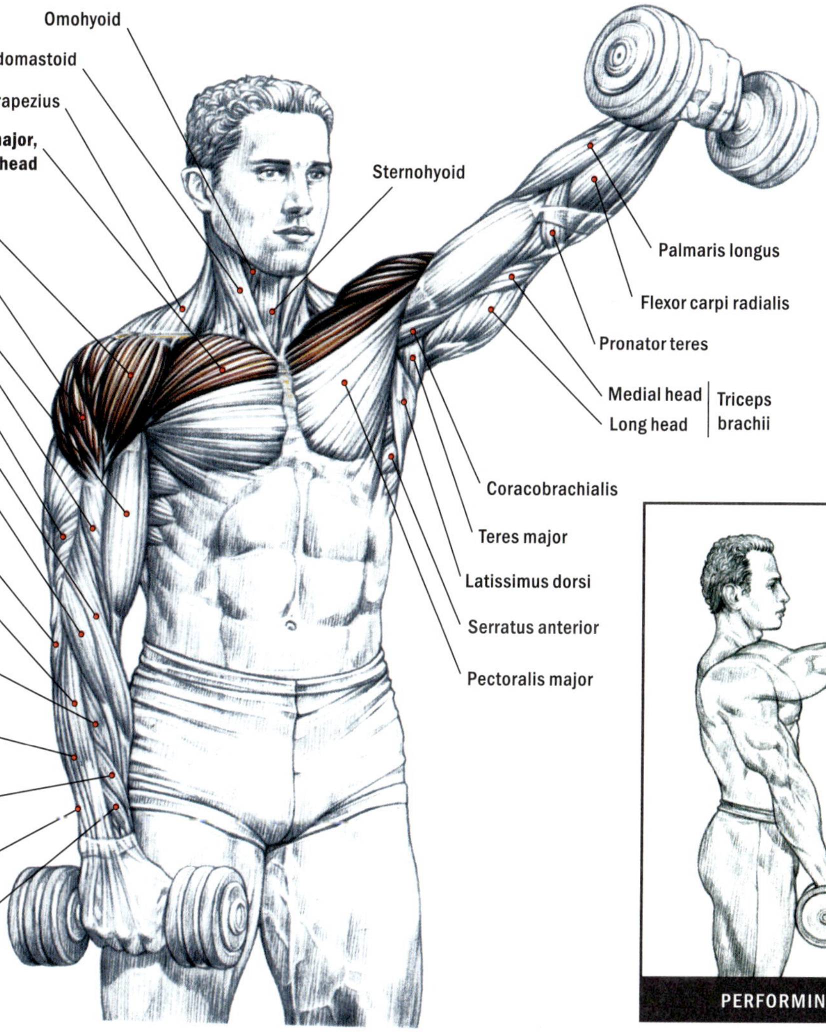

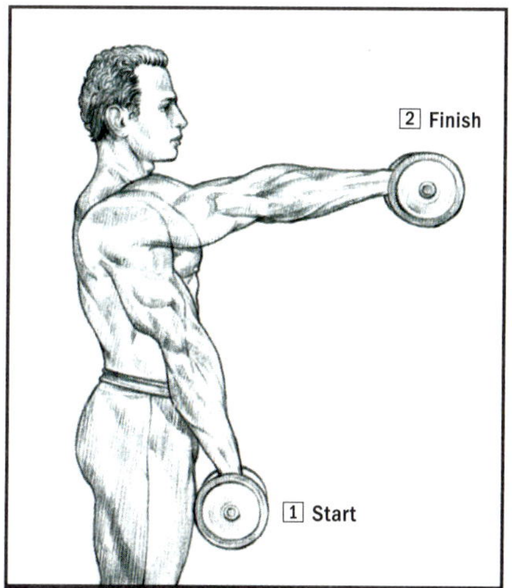

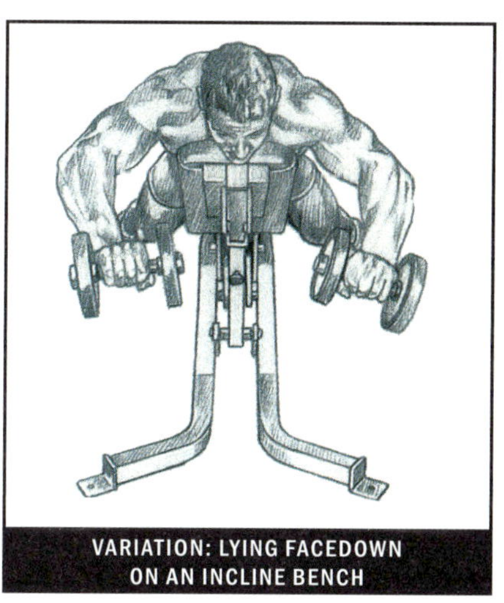

PERFORMING THE EXERCISE

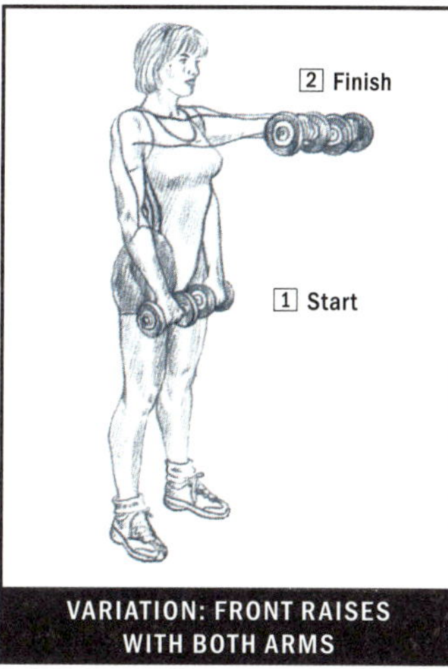

VARIATION: FRONT RAISES WITH BOTH ARMS

Stand with your feet slightly apart. Hold the dumbbells with an overhand grip as they rest against the front of your thighs or slightly to the sides:

- Inhale and alternate raising each arm to the front until it reaches eye level.
- Exhale at the end of the exercise.

This exercise mainly works the anterior deltoid, the clavicular head of the pectoralis major, and, to a lesser degree, the other parts of the deltoid. All movements that raise the arms also work the muscles that anchor the scapula to the rib cage, such as the serratus anterior and rhomboid. This allows the humerus to move from a stable base of support.

VARIATION: LYING FACEDOWN ON AN INCLINE BENCH

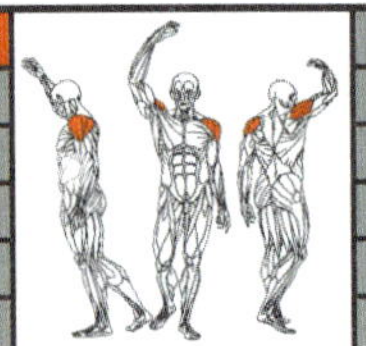

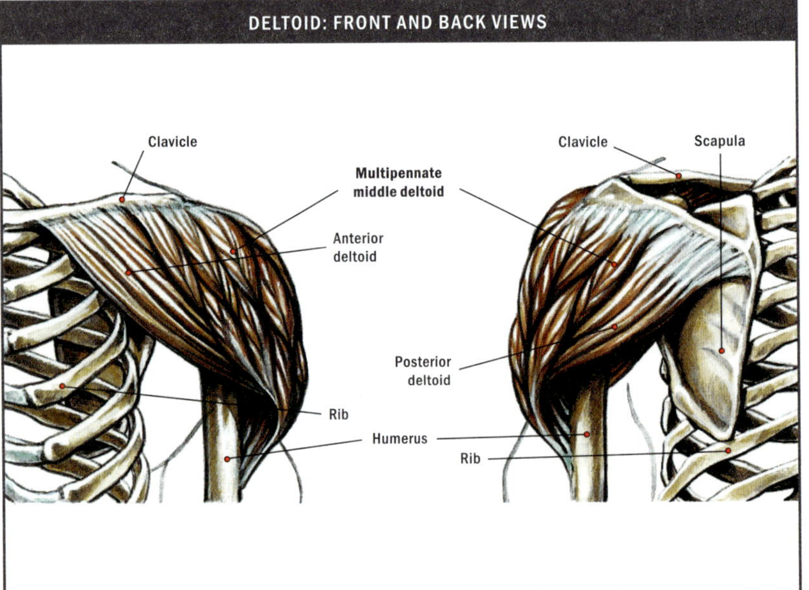

DELTOID: FRONT AND BACK VIEWS

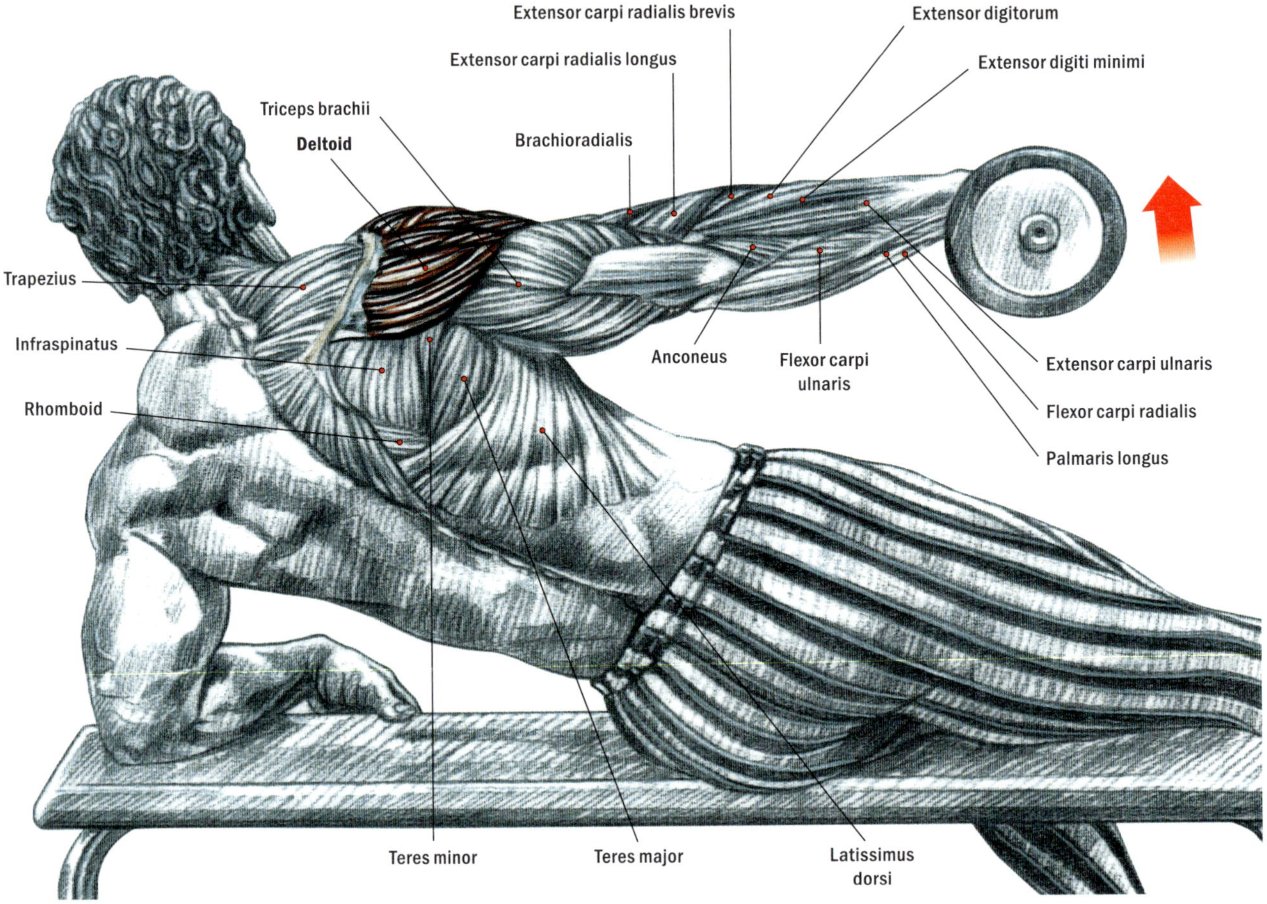

Lie on one side on the floor or on a bench while holding a dumbbell with an overhand grip:

- Inhale and raise your arm to a vertical position.
- Exhale at the end of the exercise.

Unlike standing raises, which progressively work the muscle to maximum intensity at the end of the movement (when the arm reaches a horizontal position), this exercise works the deltoid differently by focusing the effort at the beginning of the raise. Sets of 10 to 20 reps work best.

This exercise works the supraspinatus, which is the muscle mainly responsible for initiating lifting of the arm. Varying the starting position (with the dumbbell in front of the body, on the thigh, or behind the body) allows you to work all parts of the deltoid.

To increase the intensity of the movement, do this exercise under continuous tension without resting the dumbbell on the thigh.

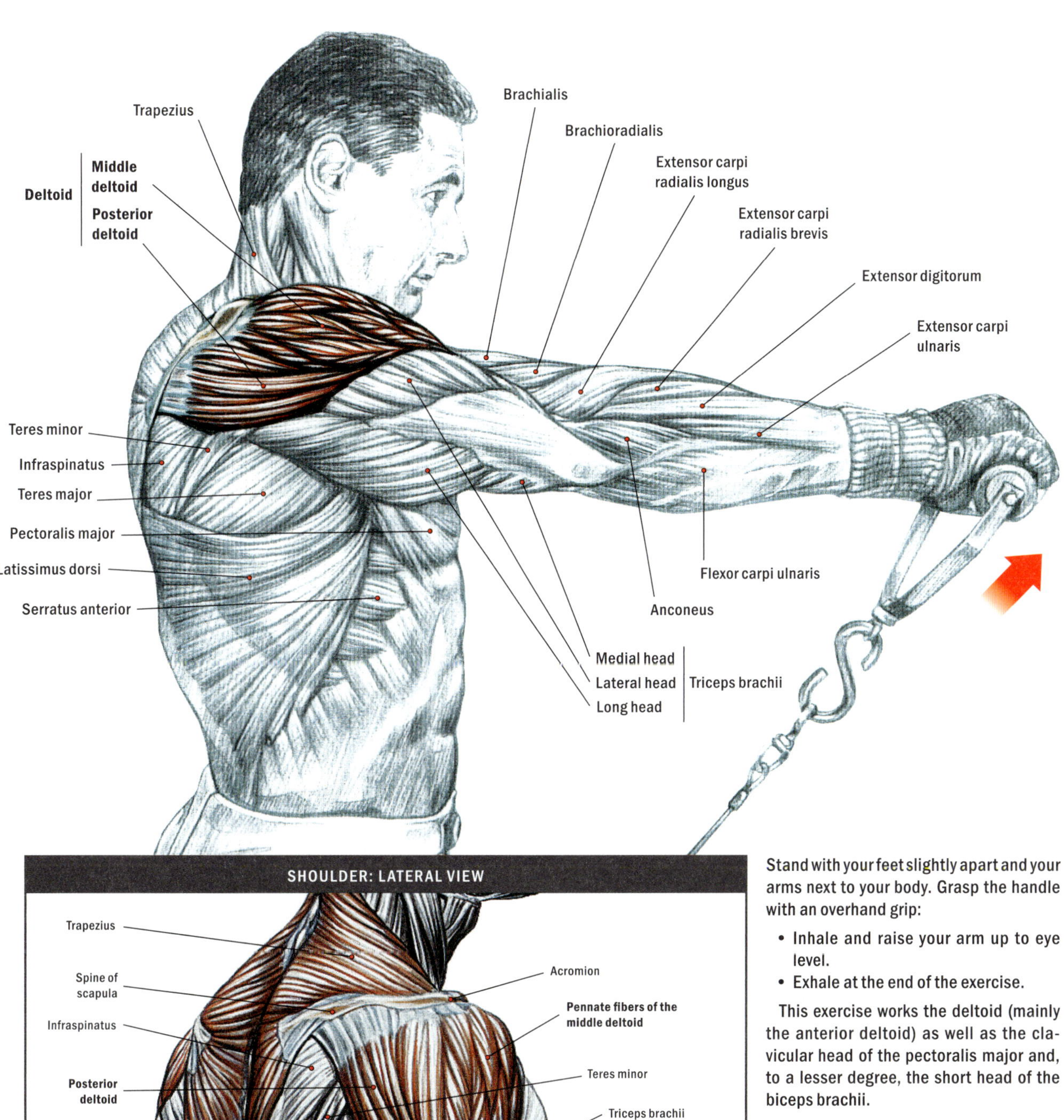

Stand with your feet slightly apart and your arms next to your body. Grasp the handle with an overhand grip:

- Inhale and raise your arm up to eye level.
- Exhale at the end of the exercise.

This exercise works the deltoid (mainly the anterior deltoid) as well as the clavicular head of the pectoralis major and, to a lesser degree, the short head of the biceps brachii.

10 LOW-PULLEY FRONT RAISES WITH A NEUTRAL GRIP

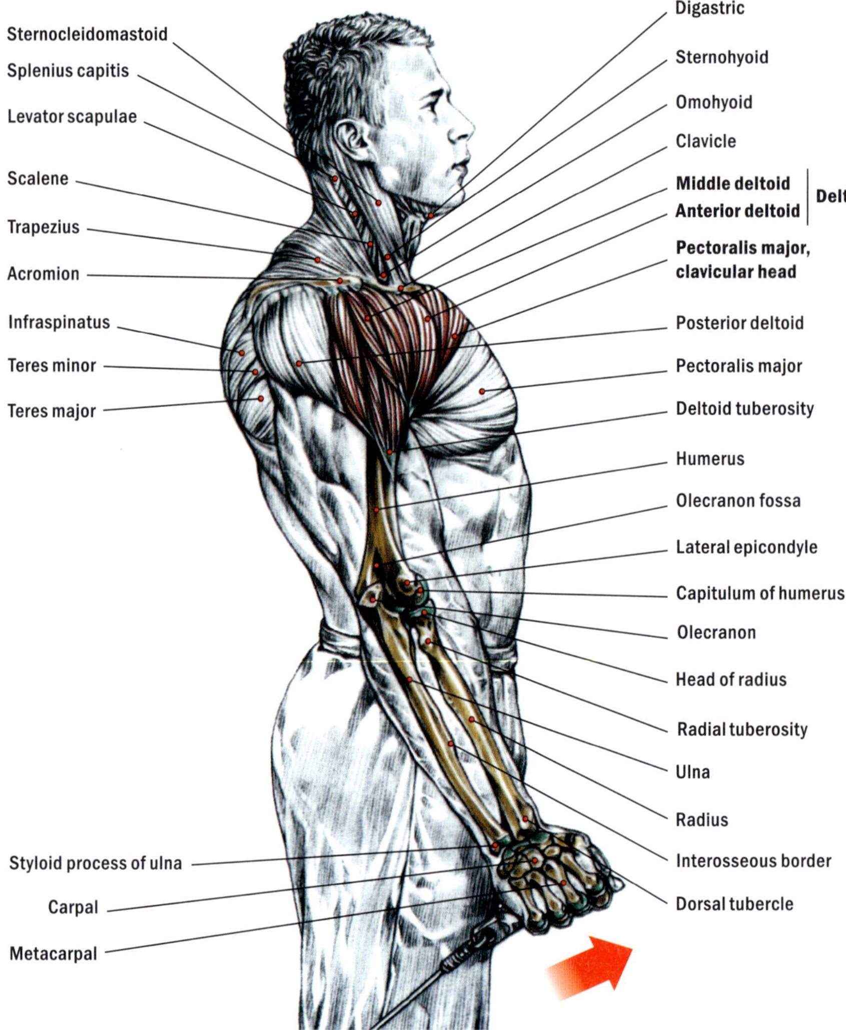

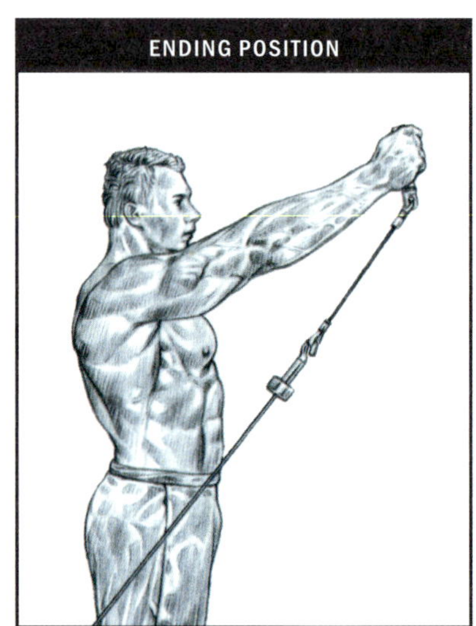

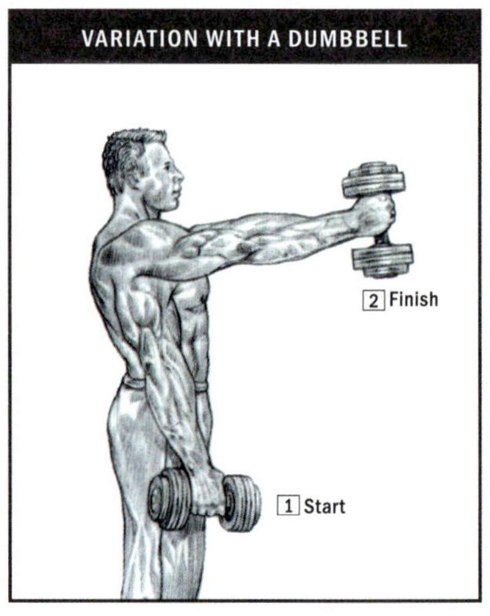

Stand with your legs slightly apart and your arm by your side holding the handle of the low pulley with a neutral (semipronated) grip (this exercise uses a handle designed for this grip):

- Inhale and raise your arm to eye level, exhaling at the end.
- Slowly return to the starting position and repeat.

This exercise mainly works the anterior deltoid as well as the clavicular part of the pectoralis major and, to a lesser degree, the middle deltoid and the short head of the biceps.

It is preferable to do this exercise in long sets.

Variation

You can also do this exercise with dumbbells.

This exercise is excellent for people who have difficulty developing the anterior deltoid. The semipronated grip externally rotates the humerus, which, at the beginning of the exercise, stretches the anterior fibers of the deltoid, allowing you to feel them working.

STRETCHING THE ANTERIOR DELTOIDS

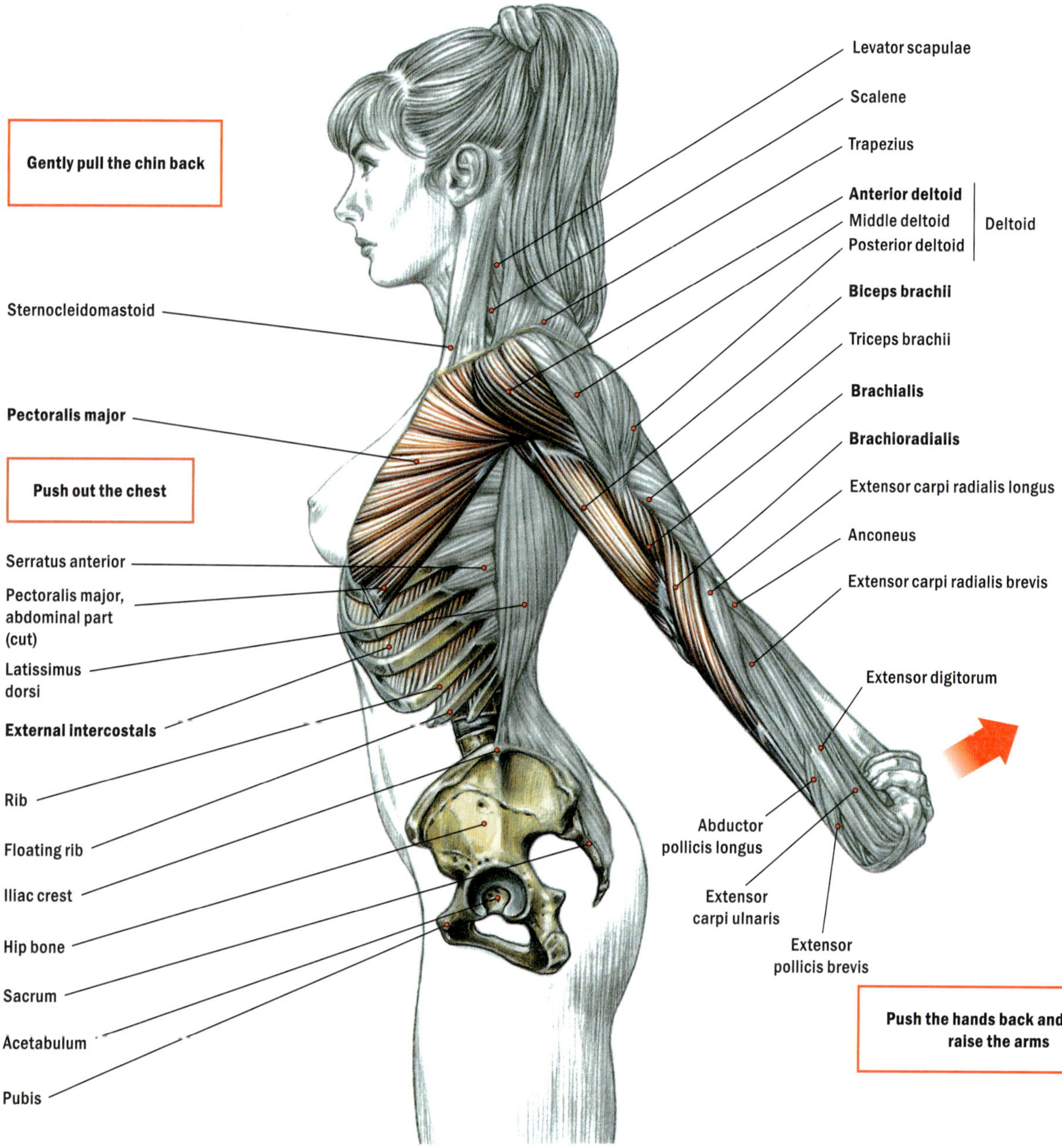

Stand with your legs shoulder-width apart and arms extended behind your back with one hand grasping the other:

- Push your arms as far back as possible, then slowly raise them while pushing out your chest and pulling your chin in.
- Hold this position for 10 seconds.

This exercise mainly stretches the anterior deltoid as well as the pectoralis major and biceps brachii. The brachialis, brachioradialis, and all of the wrist extensor muscles are also stretched.

HIGH-PULLEY LATERAL EXTENSIONS

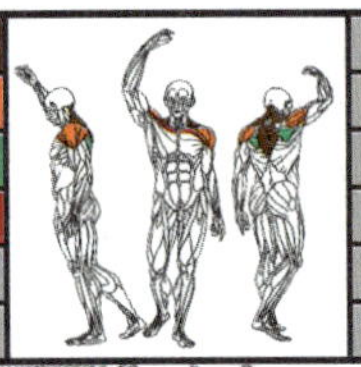

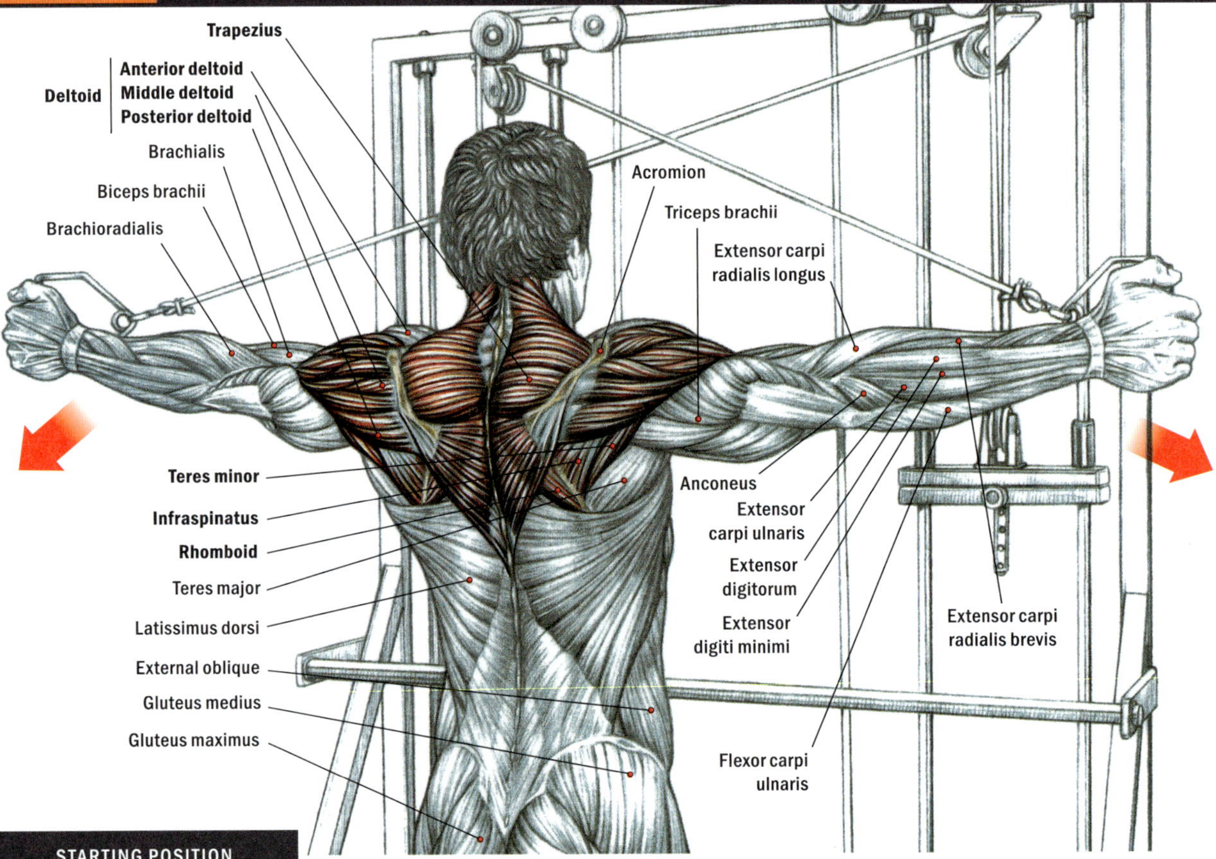

Trapezius

Deltoid — Anterior deltoid / Middle deltoid / Posterior deltoid

Brachialis

Biceps brachii

Brachioradialis

Acromion

Triceps brachii

Extensor carpi radialis longus

Teres minor

Infraspinatus

Rhomboid

Teres major

Latissimus dorsi

External oblique

Gluteus medius

Gluteus maximus

Anconeus

Extensor carpi ulnaris

Extensor digitorum

Extensor digiti minimi

Extensor carpi radialis brevis

Flexor carpi ulnaris

STARTING POSITION

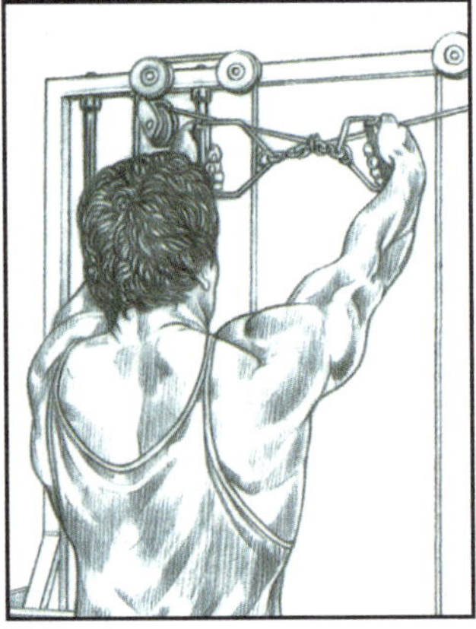

People who carry their shoulders forward because of overdevelopment of the chest muscles can do this exercise in addition to posterior shoulder work on machines to help rebalance their posture. To realign the shoulders where they belong, work with moderate weights and squeeze the shoulder blades together at the end of each repetition.

RHOMBOID MAJOR AND MINOR MUSCLES

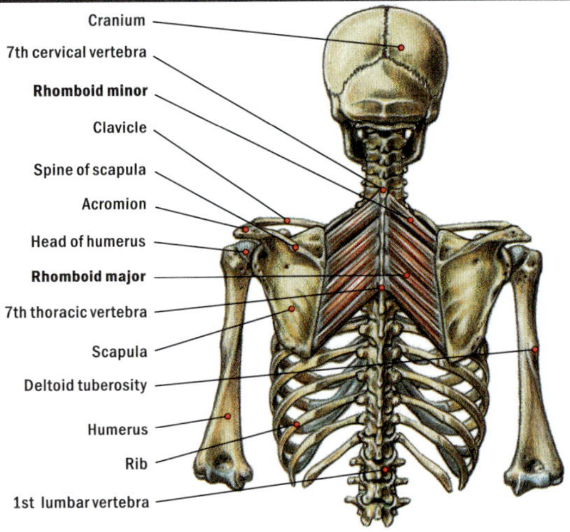

Cranium

7th cervical vertebra

Rhomboid minor

Clavicle

Spine of scapula

Acromion

Head of humerus

Rhomboid major

7th thoracic vertebra

Scapula

Deltoid tuberosity

Humerus

Rib

1st lumbar vertebra

Stand facing the pulleys with your arms extended to the front. Grip the right handle with your left hand and the left handle with your right hand:

- Inhale and extend your arms to the side and back, exhaling at the end of the movement.
- Return to the starting position with control and repeat.

This exercise mainly contracts the posterior deltoid, infraspinatus, and teres minor. At the end of the exercise as the shoulder blades come together, it contracts the trapezius and, deeper in, the rhomboids.

Located deep under the trapezius, the rhomboids pull the shoulder blades together toward the spine and press them against the rib cage.

In some people, the major and minor rhomboids are fused into one muscle.

PULLEY EXTERNAL ARM ROTATIONS 12

PERFORMING THE EXERCISE

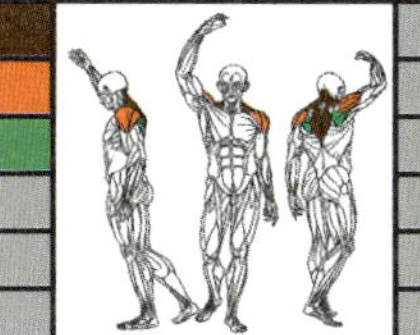

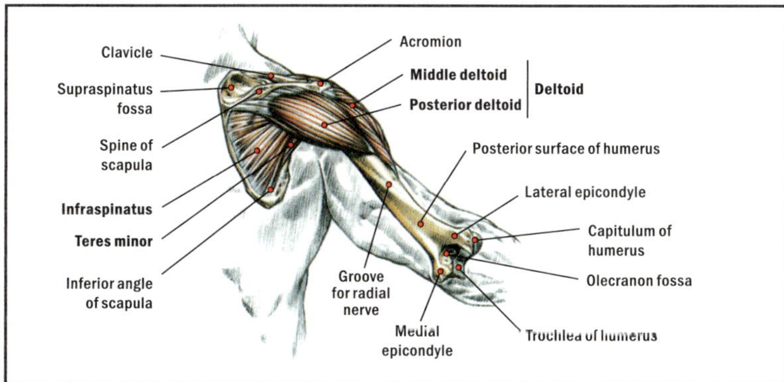

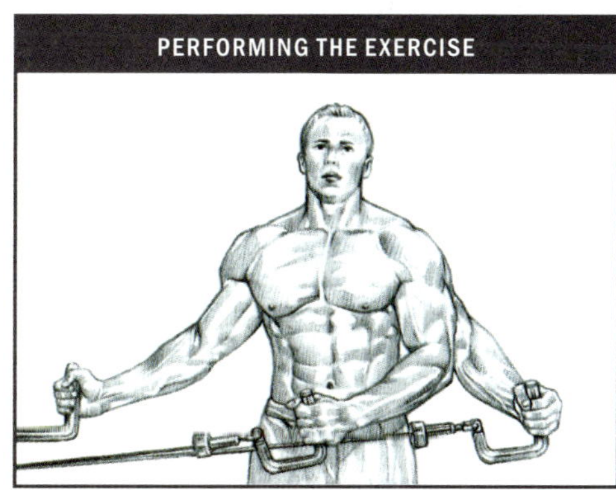

Set the pulley at waist level and position your body in line with the machine. Grip the handle with your forearm in front of your body, your elbow bent, and your upper arm against your body:

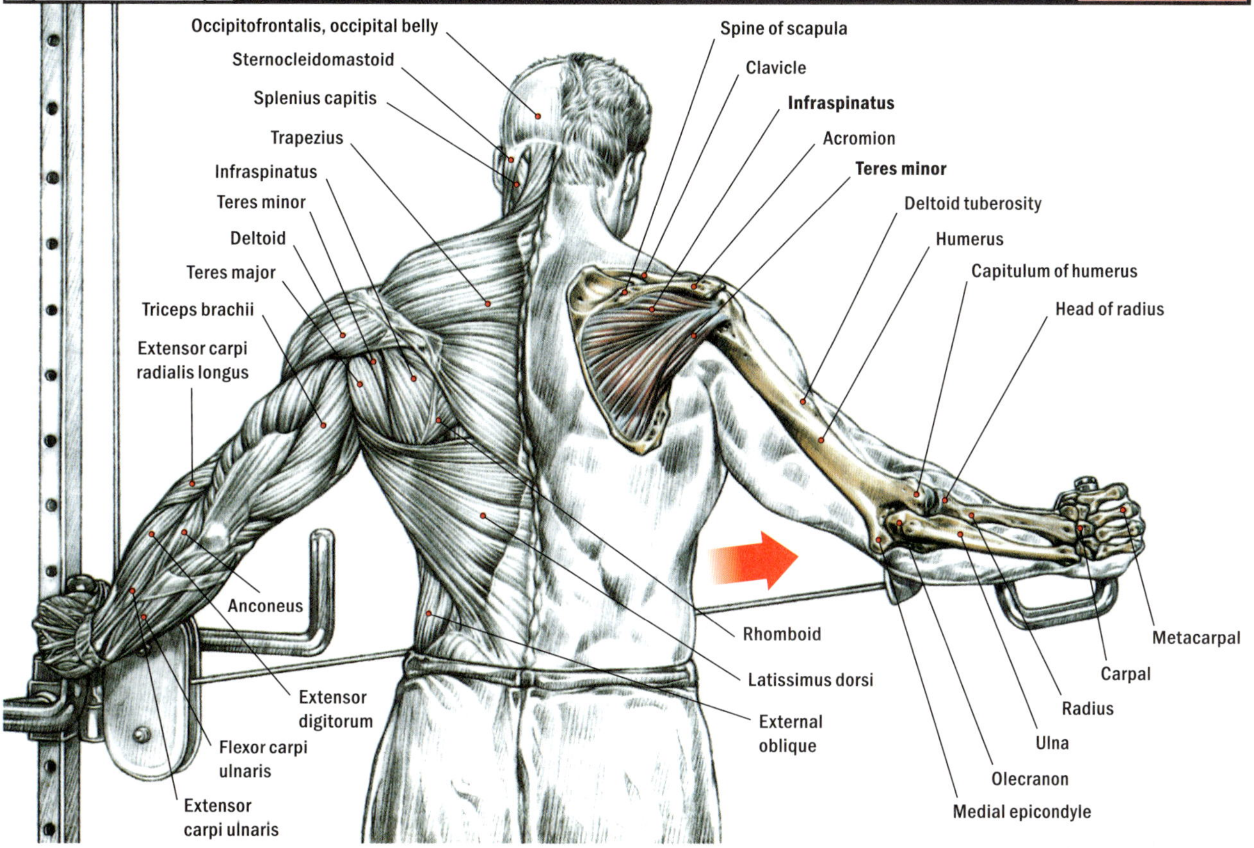

- Externally rotate your arm, trying to keep your upper arm against your body with your elbow bent.

This exercise mainly works the infraspinatus, the teres minor, and the posterior deltoid. If you bring the scapula toward the center of the body at the end of the movement, you will also work the rhomboids and the middle and inferior portions of the trapezius.

This exercise is mainly used to strengthen the infraspinatus and prevent painful cramps and injuries that are frequent with this muscle. External arm rotations with a pulley are often recommended as a reeducation exercise during recovery from a tear or partial tear of the infraspinatus. Use very light weights initially.

This exercise can be done with the goal of working the posterior deltoid, which is often difficult to recruit. In this case, move your arm slightly away from the body and extend the elbow at the end of the movement.

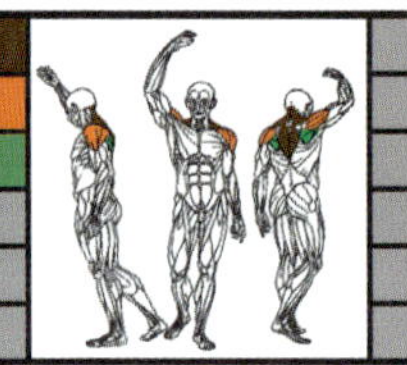

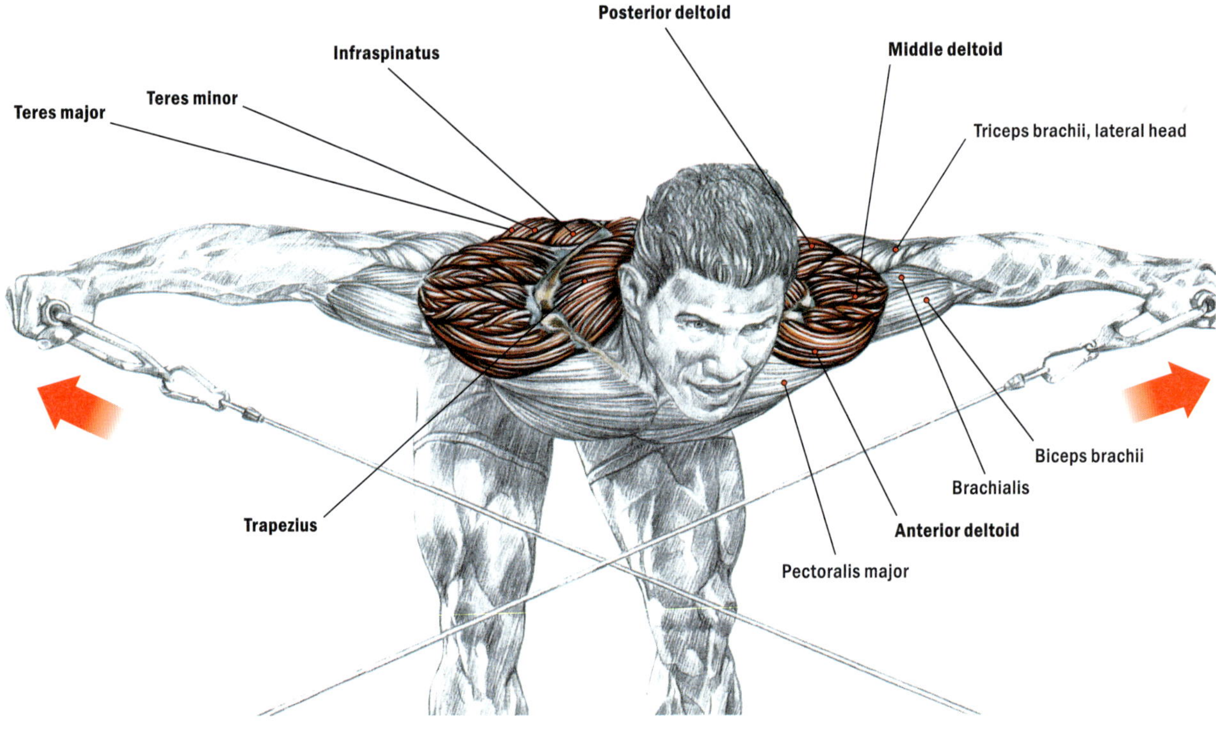

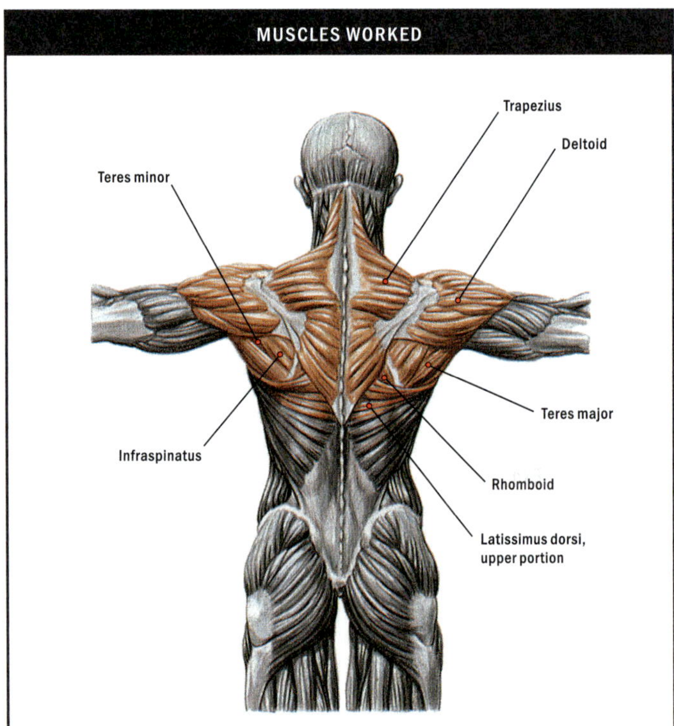

Stand with your feet apart and legs slightly bent. Lean forward from your waist, keeping a flat back, and let your arms hang down. Grip a handle in each hand with the cables crossed:

- Inhale and raise your arms to a horizontal position.
- Exhale at the end of the exercise.

This exercise mainly works the posterior deltoid. At the end of the exercise, as the shoulder blades squeeze together, the rhomboids and the middle and lower portions of the trapezius contract.

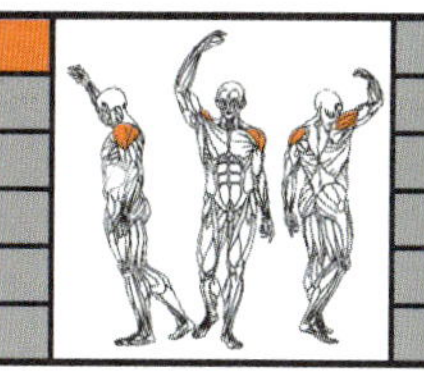

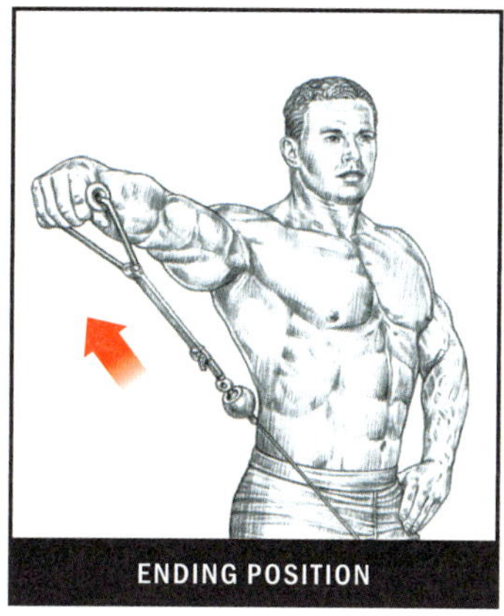

ENDING POSITION

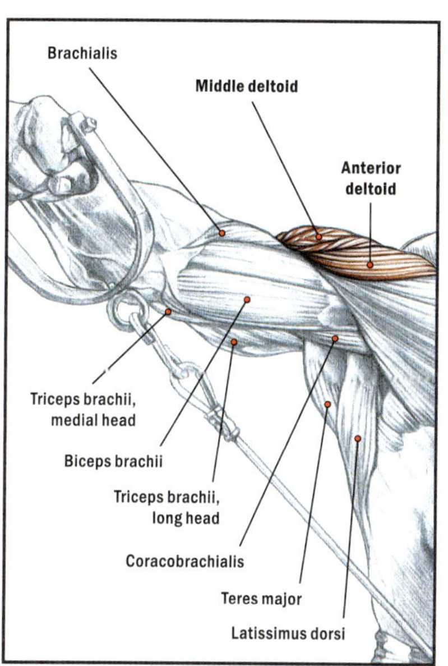

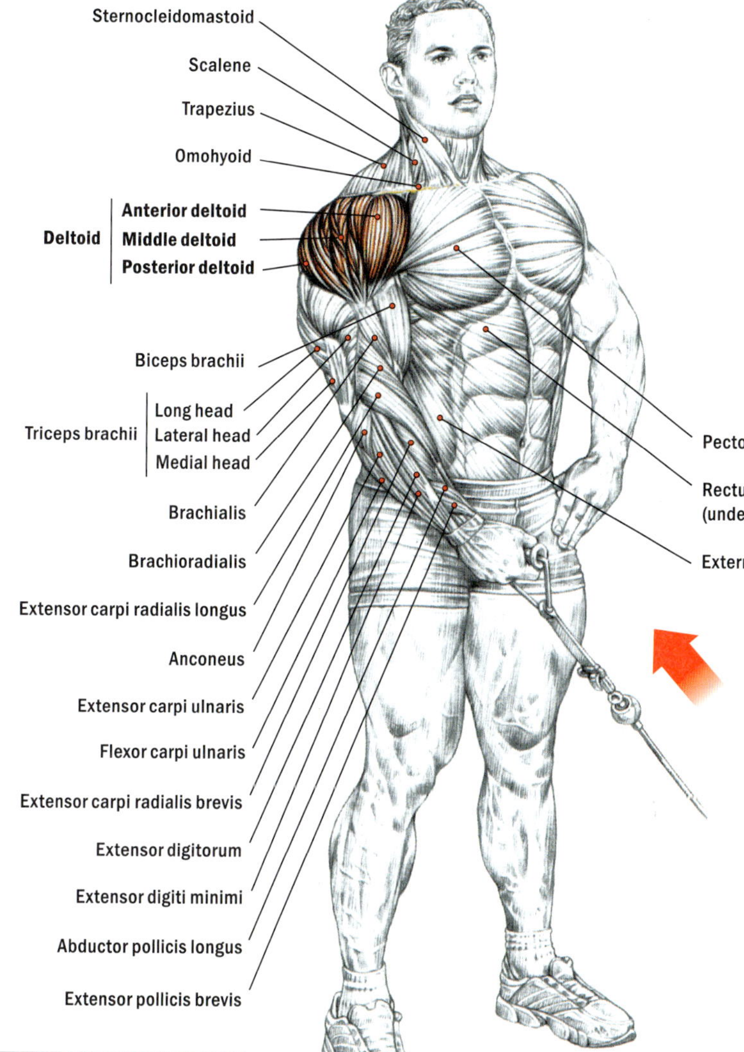

DELTOID MUSCLE ACTION

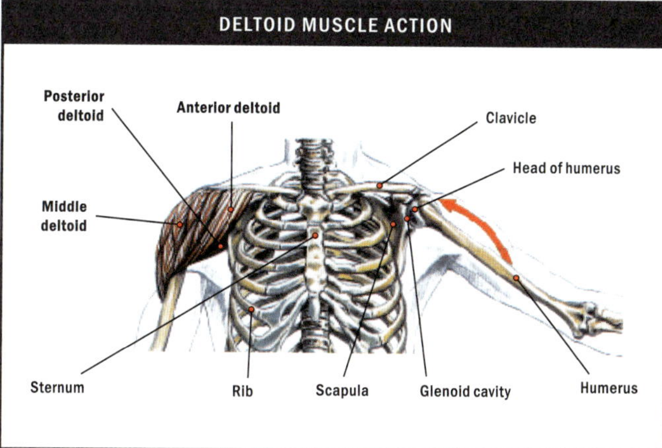

Grasp the handle with your arm next to your body:

- Inhale and raise your arm to a horizontal position.
- Exhale at the end of the exercise.

This exercise mainly develops the middle deltoid. Because the muscle is multipennate, composed of many fibers in the shape of a feather, it is best to vary the working angles to work all the fibers.

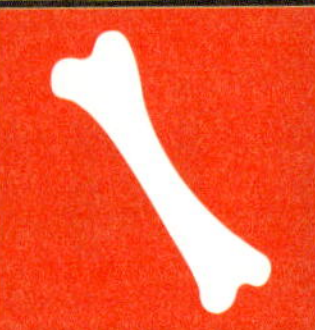

THE IMPORTANCE OF PULLING THE SHOULDERS BACK

MUSCLES ENGAGED WHEN PULLING THE SHOULDERS BACK

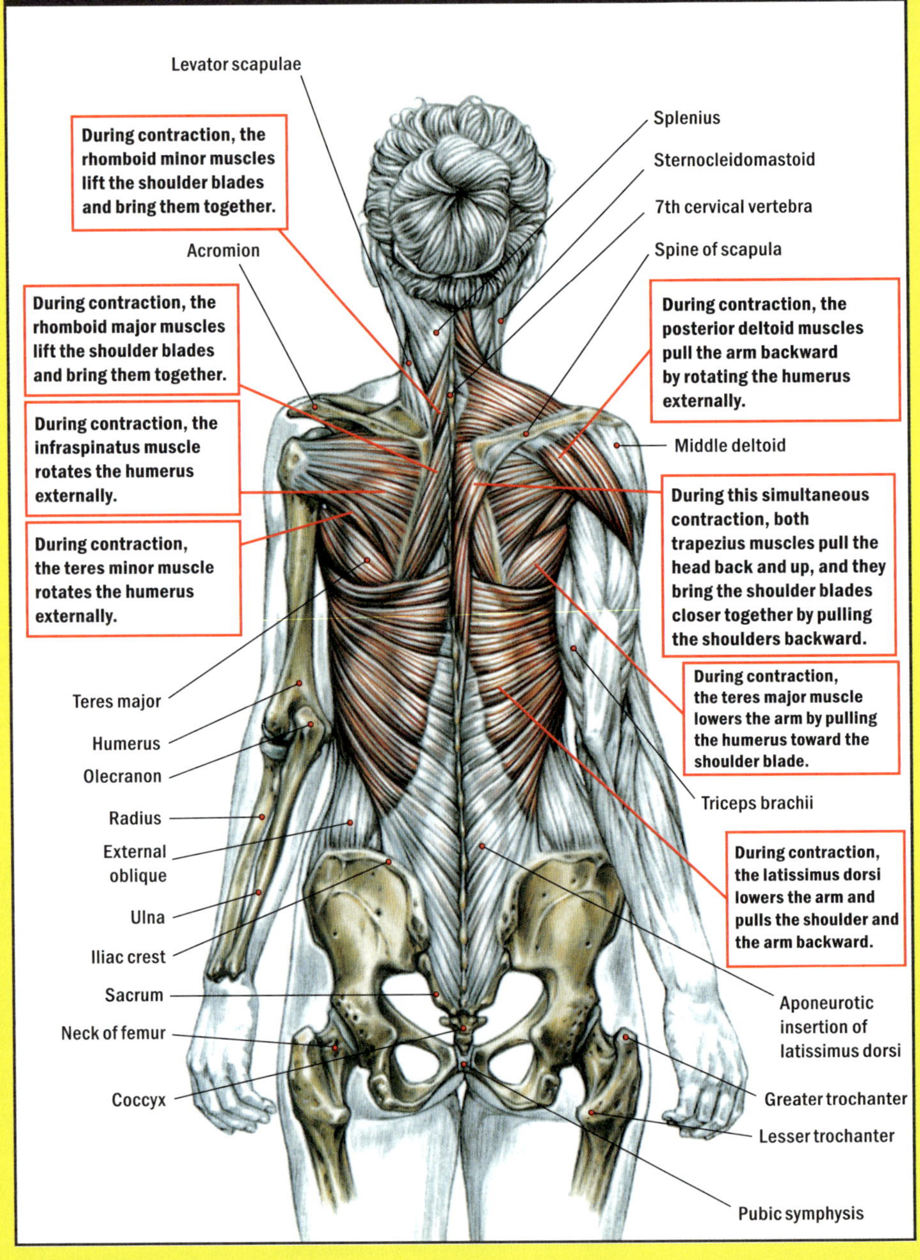

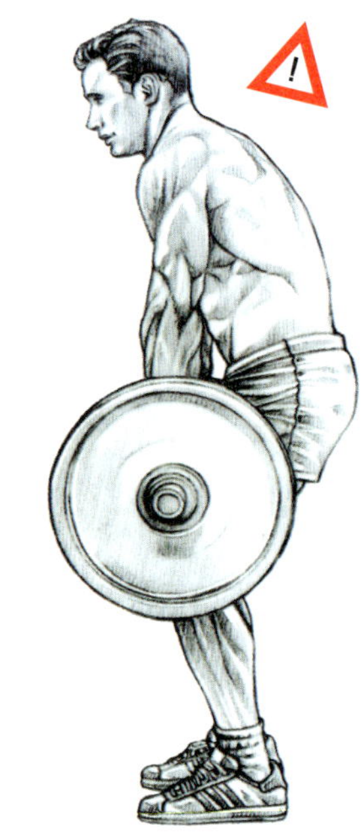

Rounding the upper back during deadlifts limits the power of the lift. To avoid rounding the back, do specific exercises to strengthen the muscles responsible for straightening the shoulders.

In powerlifting, with heavy deadlifts, it is essential to avoid rounding the shoulders forward and tipping forward at the hips, which can restrict the power of the lift. Always pull the shoulders back during the exercise. To achieve this, you should do specific exercises to prepare the shoulders.

One of the major postural defects encountered frequently in modern society, where we spend inordinate amounts of time sitting, is kyphosis (rounding of the upper thoracic spine).

This poor upper body position is usually due to the hypotonicity of the muscles close to the shoulder blades and the external rotator muscles of the arms; in men, it is often due to hypertonicity and overdevelopment of the chest muscles.

In strength training, focusing extensively on the pectorals or doing too many bench presses can also contribute to this postural issue. In any case, it is important to rebalance the posture through specific exercises to straighten the shoulders, such as the pec deck rear-delt laterals (page 77), high-pulley lateral extensions (page 66), or bent-over lateral dumbbell raises (page 60).

ONE-DUMBBELL FRONT RAISES 15

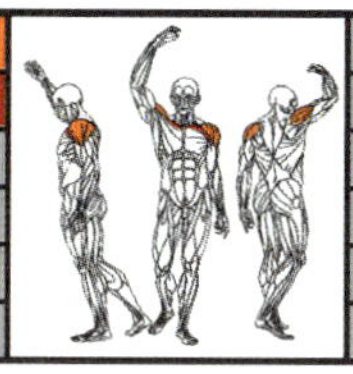

Sternocleidomastoid
Splenius
Levator scapulae
Scalene
Omohyoid
Trapezius
Pectoralis major, clavicular head
Deltoid
Middle deltoid
Posterior deltoid
Anterior deltoid
Triceps brachii, long head
Triceps brachii, lateral head
Brachioradialis
Anconeus
Extensor digitorum
Extensor carpi radialis brevis
Flexor carpi ulnaris
Extensor carpi ulnaris
Extensor digiti minimi
Pectoralis major
Extensor carpi radialis longus
Biceps brachii
Brachialis

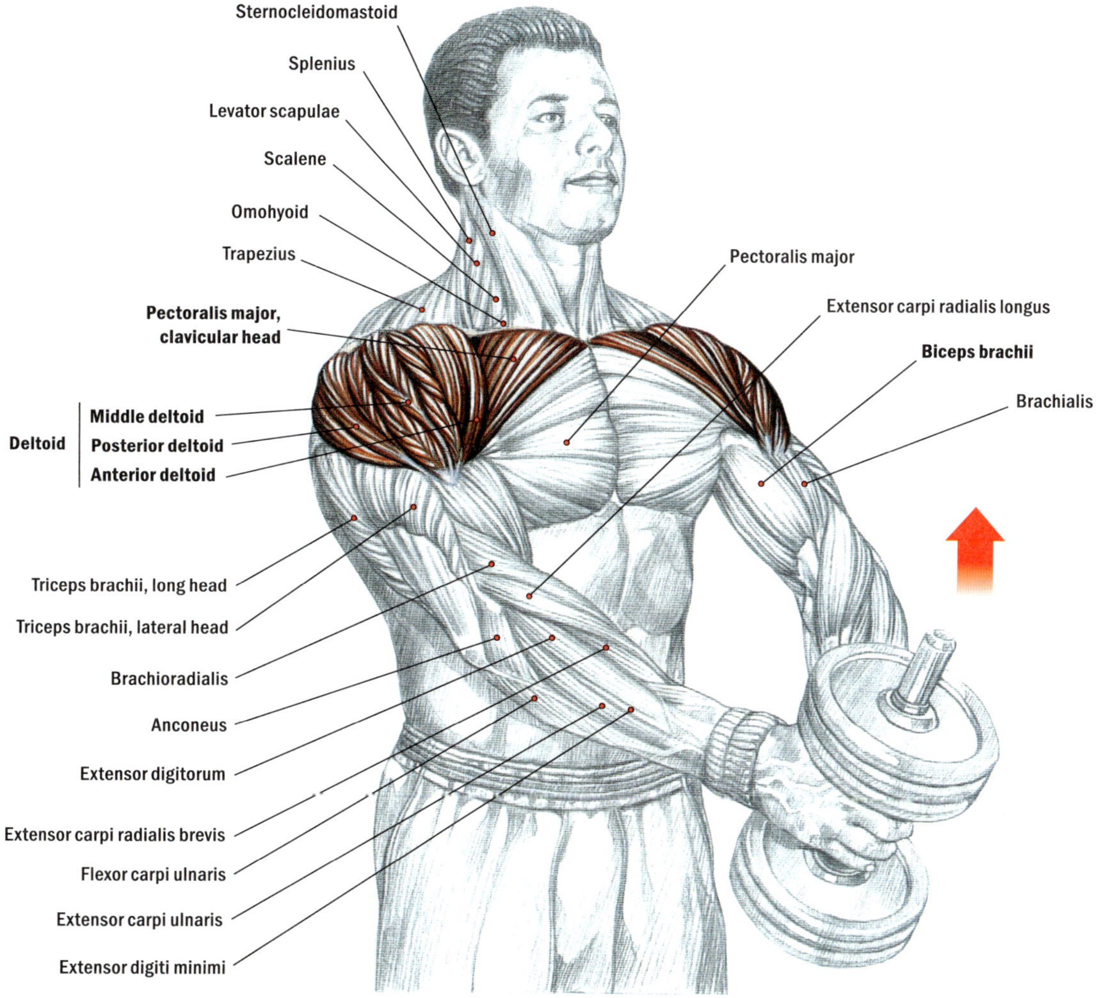

Stand with your legs slightly apart, your back straight, and your abdominal muscles engaged. With your arms extended, grasp a dumbbell in both hands with fingers crossed over each other and rest the dumbbell against your thighs:

- Inhale and raise the dumbbell to eye level.
- Lower gently, avoiding any abrupt movement.
- Exhale at the end of the exercise.

This exercise primarily works the anterior deltoid, the clavicular head of the pectoralis major, and the short head of the biceps.

Note that all the fixators of the scapula (shoulder blade) are used during the isometric contraction, which allows the humerus to move on a stable support.

Rib
Sternal manubrium
Clavicle
Acromion
Pectoralis major, clavicular head
Coracoid process
Sternum
Humerus
Costal cartilage
Xiphoid process

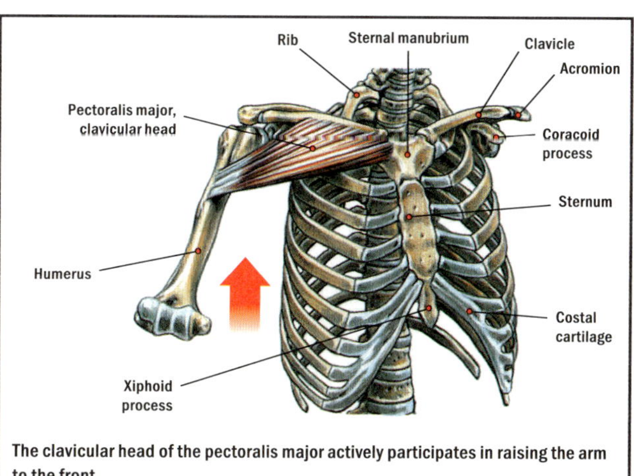

The clavicular head of the pectoralis major actively participates in raising the arm to the front.

16 BARBELL FRONT RAISES

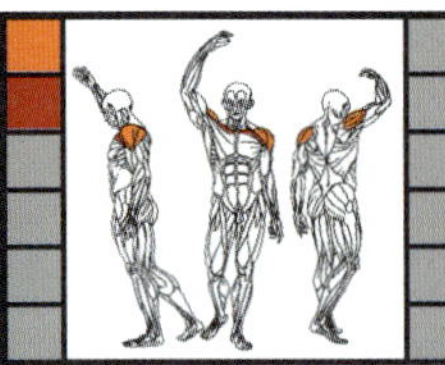

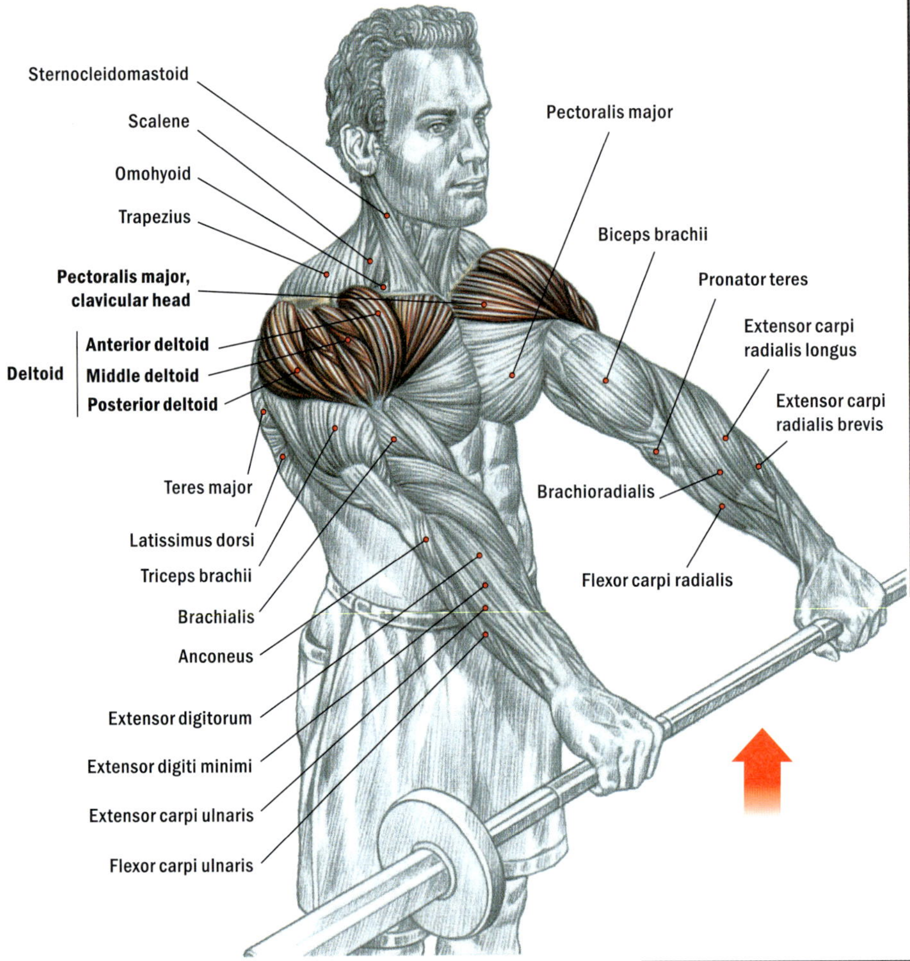

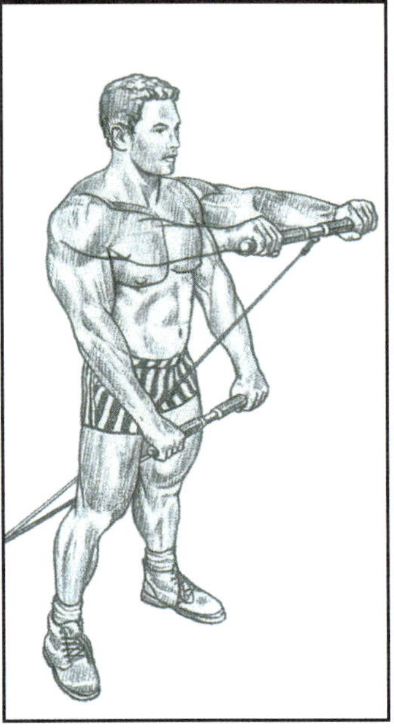

Sternocleidomastoid
Scalene
Omohyoid
Trapezius
Pectoralis major, clavicular head
Deltoid
Anterior deltoid
Middle deltoid
Posterior deltoid
Teres major
Latissimus dorsi
Triceps brachii
Brachialis
Anconeus
Extensor digitorum
Extensor digiti minimi
Extensor carpi ulnaris
Flexor carpi ulnaris
Pectoralis major
Biceps brachii
Pronator teres
Extensor carpi radialis longus
Extensor carpi radialis brevis
Brachioradialis
Flexor carpi radialis

VARIATION: USING A LOW PULLEY

Stand with your legs slightly apart and your back straight, contracting your abdominal muscles. Hold the barbell with an overhand grip and rest it against your thighs:

- Inhale and raise the barbell with extended arms to eye level.
- Exhale at the end of the exercise.

This exercise contracts the anterior deltoid, the clavicular head of the pectoralis major, the infraspinatus, and, to a lesser degree, the trapezius, serratus anterior, and short head of the biceps.

If you continue raising your arms above eye level, the posterior deltoids will contract, supporting the work of the other muscles and allowing you to raise your arms to a vertical position.

The exercise can also be done using a low pulley, with your back to the machine and the cable passing between your legs.

The biceps brachii participates, although to a lesser degree, in all front arm raises.

PERFORMING THE EXERCISE

1 Start
2 Finish

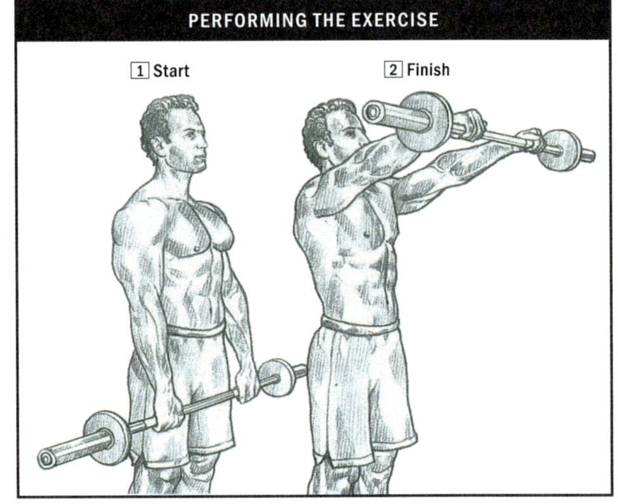

TEARS AND RUPTURES IN THE UPPER PART OF THE SHORT HEAD OF THE BICEPS BRACHII

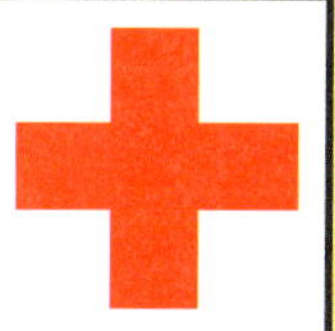

DIAGRAM OF A RUPTURE IN THE TENDON OF THE SHORT HEAD OF THE BICEPS BRACHII

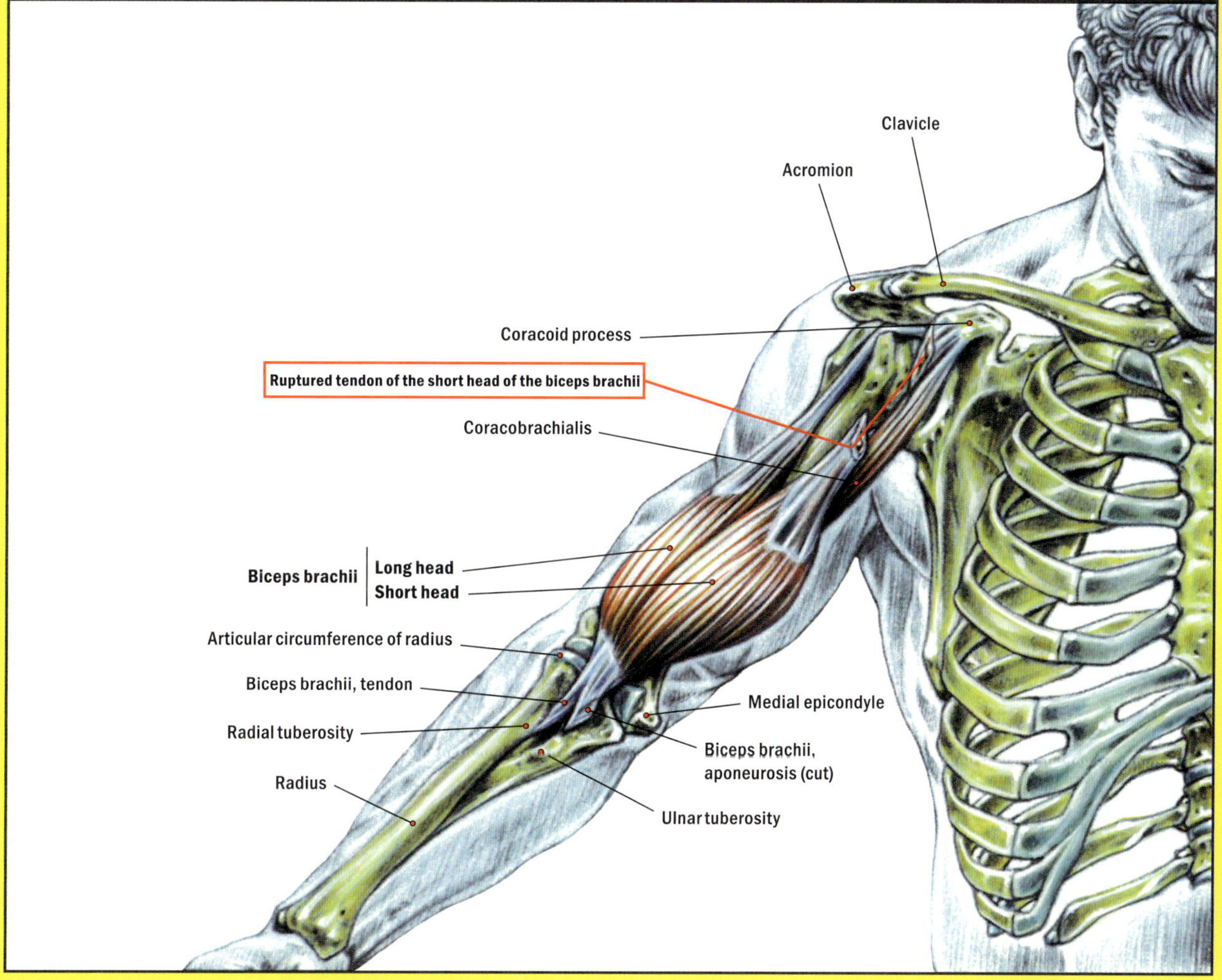

Tears and ruptures in the upper part of the short head of the biceps are incredibly rare, even rarer than injuries to the long head of the biceps brachii or distal biceps tendon. They seem to occur more frequently in two types of movements: the snatch and upright rows. When performing upright rows, the heavier the weight, the greater the distance between the hands, and the more the elbows extend outward, the greater the strain on the inner part of the biceps.

Apart from these two types of movements, injuries to this area are relatively rare. However, these injuries are sometimes found in strength sports such as Atlas stones lifting.

If you start to feel any strain in the upper and inner part of the biceps when doing upright rows, stop the exercise and move your hands closer together on the bar.

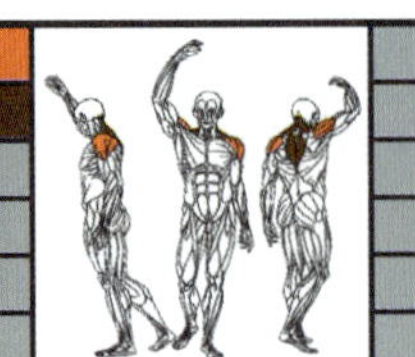

17 UPRIGHT ROWS

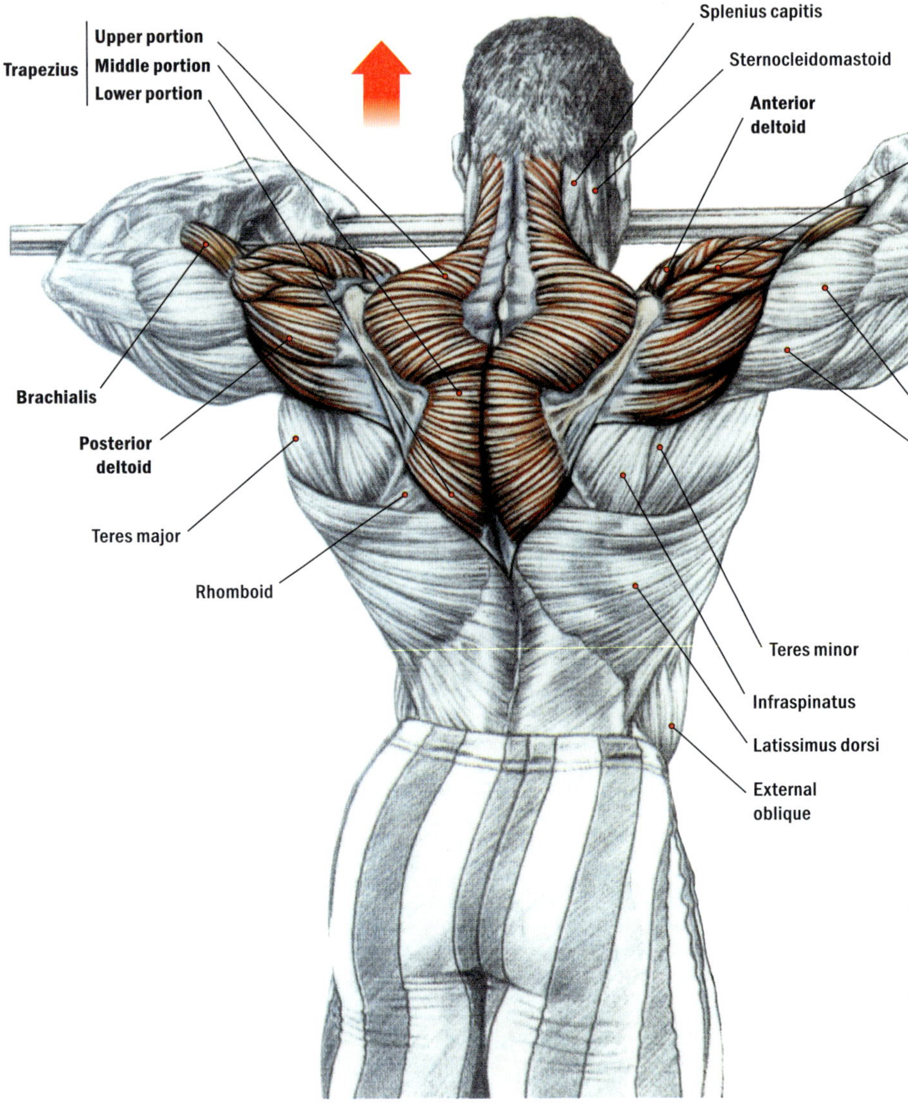

Trapezius
Upper portion
Middle portion
Lower portion
Splenius capitis
Sternocleidomastoid
Anterior deltoid
Middle deltoid
Brachialis
Posterior deltoid
Teres major
Rhomboid
Medial head
Lateral head
Long head
Triceps
Teres minor
Infraspinatus
Latissimus dorsi
External oblique

2 Finish
1 Start

PERFORMING THE EXERCISE

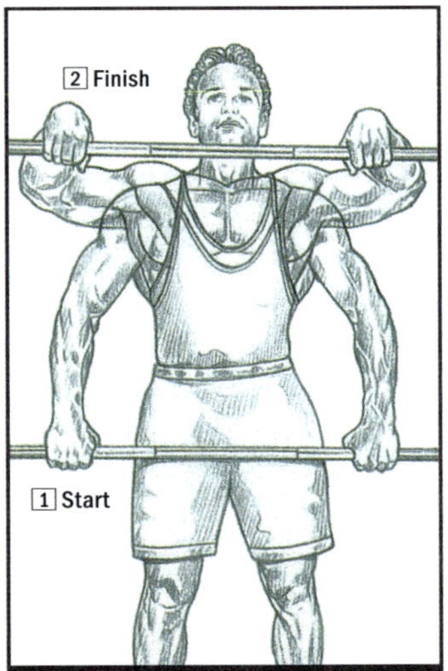

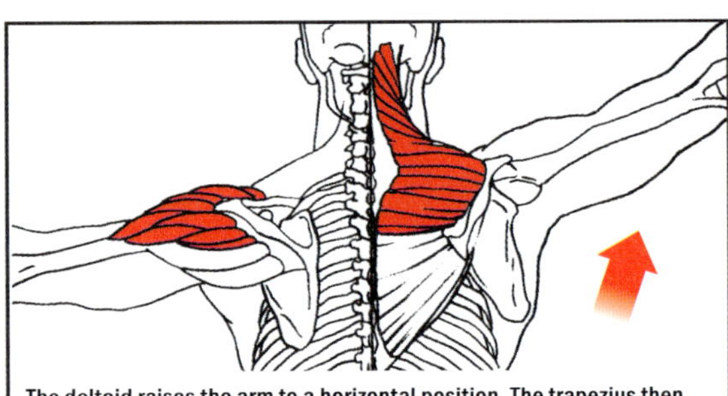

Stand with your legs slightly apart and your back straight. Grasp the barbell with an overhand grip slightly wider than shoulder width and rest it against your thighs:

- Inhale and pull the barbell up along your body to your chin, keeping your elbows as high as possible.
- Lower the bar with control, avoiding any abrupt movements.
- Exhale at the end of the exercise.

This exercise mainly uses the deltoid, trapezius, and biceps muscles, as well as the muscles in the forearms, the lumbosacral region, the gluteus muscles, and the abdominal muscles.

This is a fundamental exercise that is comprehensive and helps develop a Herculean physique.

The deltoid raises the arm to a horizontal position. The trapezius then takes over to rotate the scapula (shoulder blade), allowing the arm to continue its upward course.

HOW MORPHOLOGY AFFECTS UPRIGHT ROWS

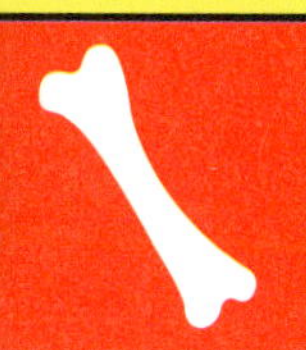

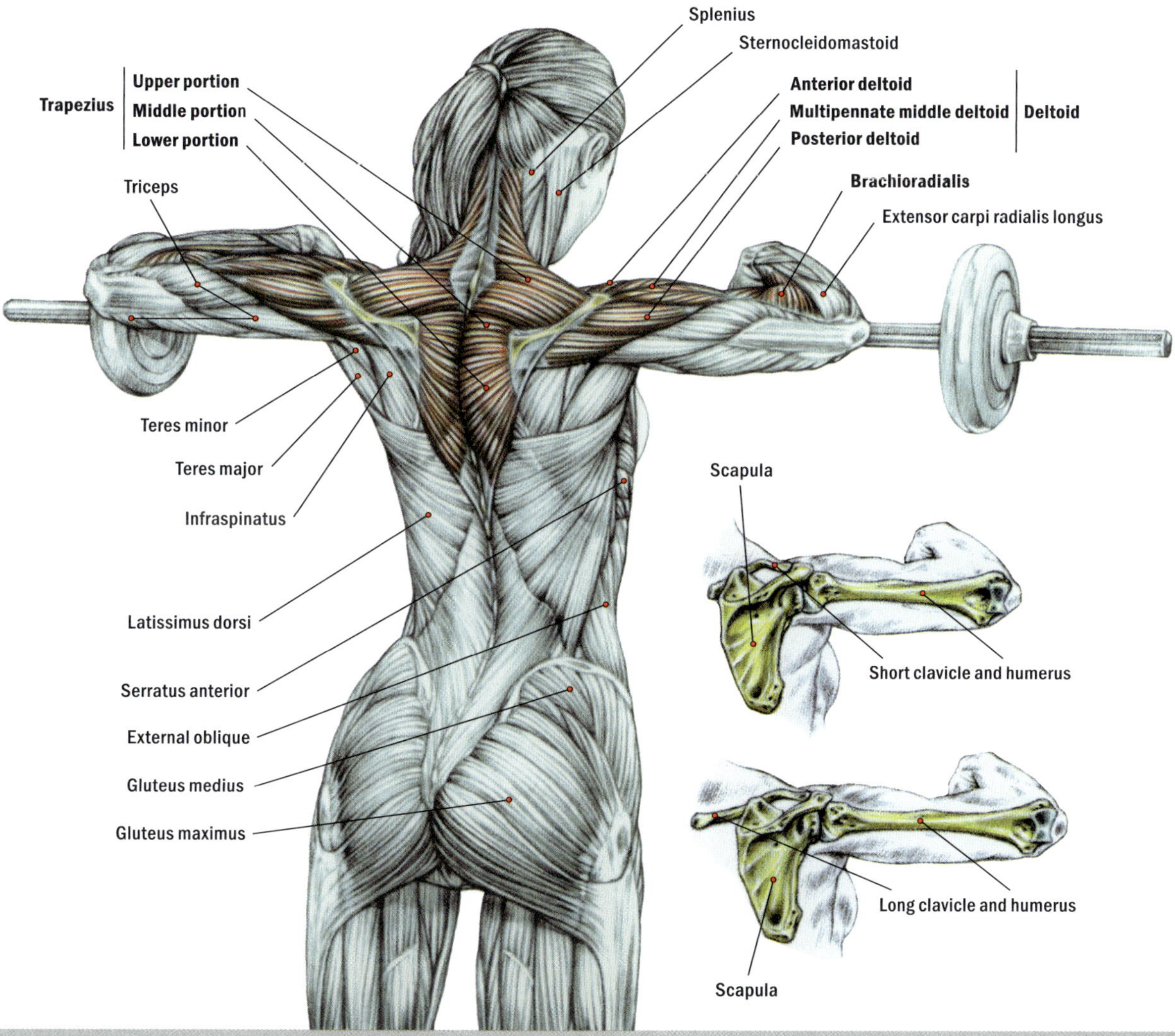

In strength training, the shape and size of the levers play a huge role in determining a person's ability to lift heavy weights. In upright rows, the longer the humerus and clavicle bones are, the harder it is to lift heavier weights. The best morphology for doing upright rows with heavy vertical pulls is to have short clavicle and humerus bones.

18 MACHINE LATERAL RAISES

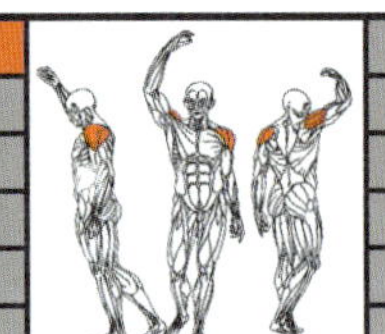

Sternohyoid
Pectoralis major, clavicular head
Pectoralis major
Clavicle
Sternum
Deltoid
Biceps brachii
Triceps
Long head
Medial head
Brachialis
Pronator teres
Brachioradialis
Flexor digitorum superficialis
Flexor carpi ulnaris
Extensor carpi radialis longus
Palmaris longus
Flexor carpi radialis
Sternocleidomastoid
Levator scapulae
Omohyoid
Trapezius
Scalene
Middle deltoid
Anterior deltoid
Deltoid
Triceps brachii, lateral head

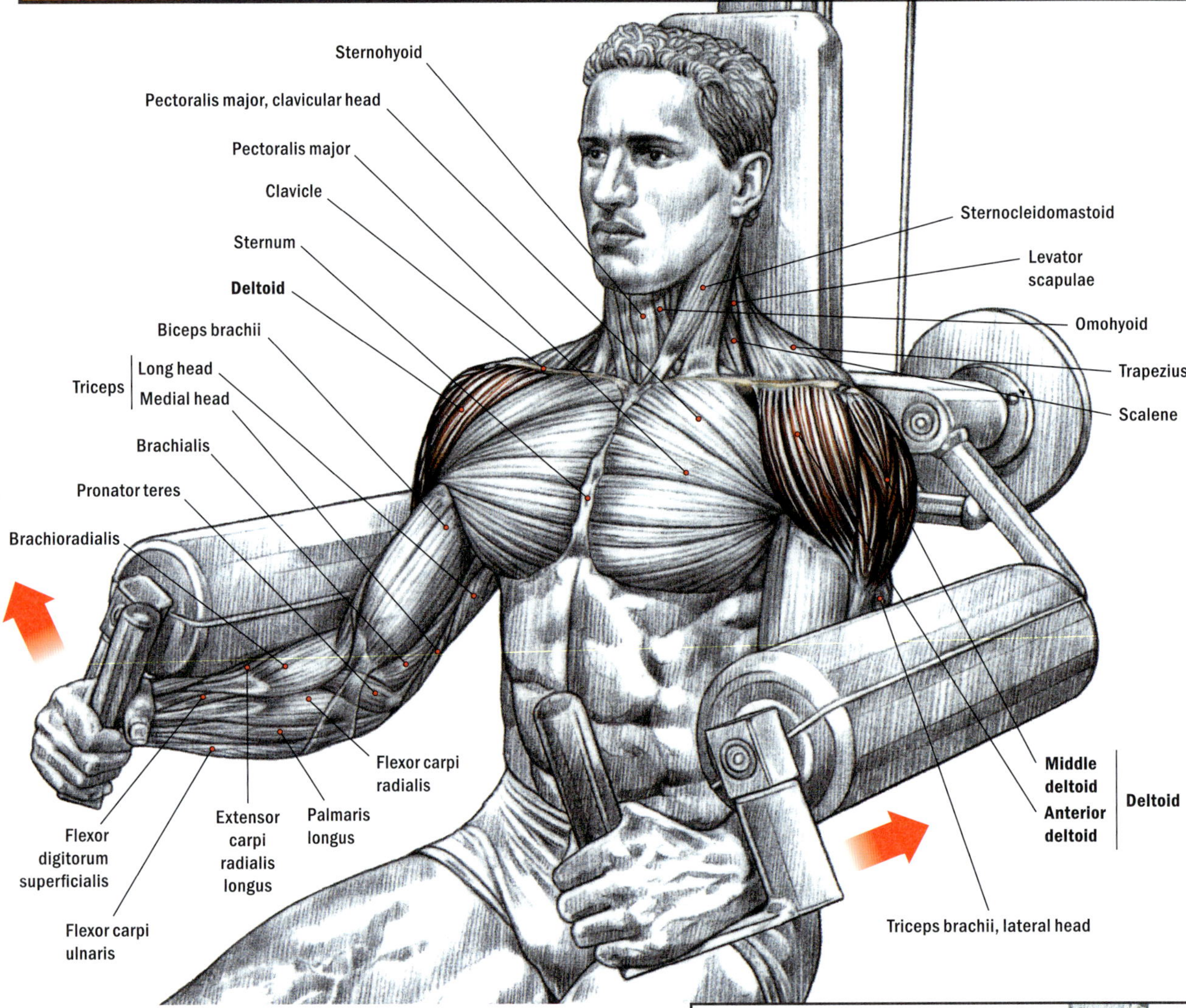

Sit at a machine and grasp the handles:

- Inhale and raise your elbows so the arms are in a horizontal position.
- Exhale at the end of the exercise.

This exercise uses the deltoid (focusing most of the effort on the middle deltoid) and the supraspinatus, located under the deltoid. If you raise your arm higher than a horizontal position, the upper portion of the trapezius is also engaged.

This is an excellent exercise for beginners, because you do not have to worry about your positioning, and you can do long sets.

2 Finish
1 Start

PERFORMING THE EXERCISE

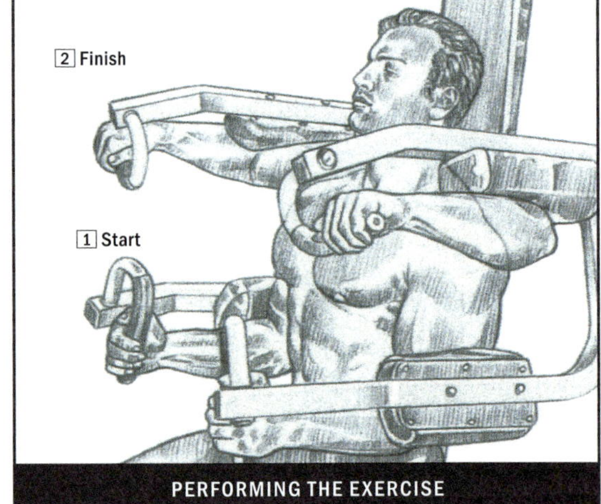

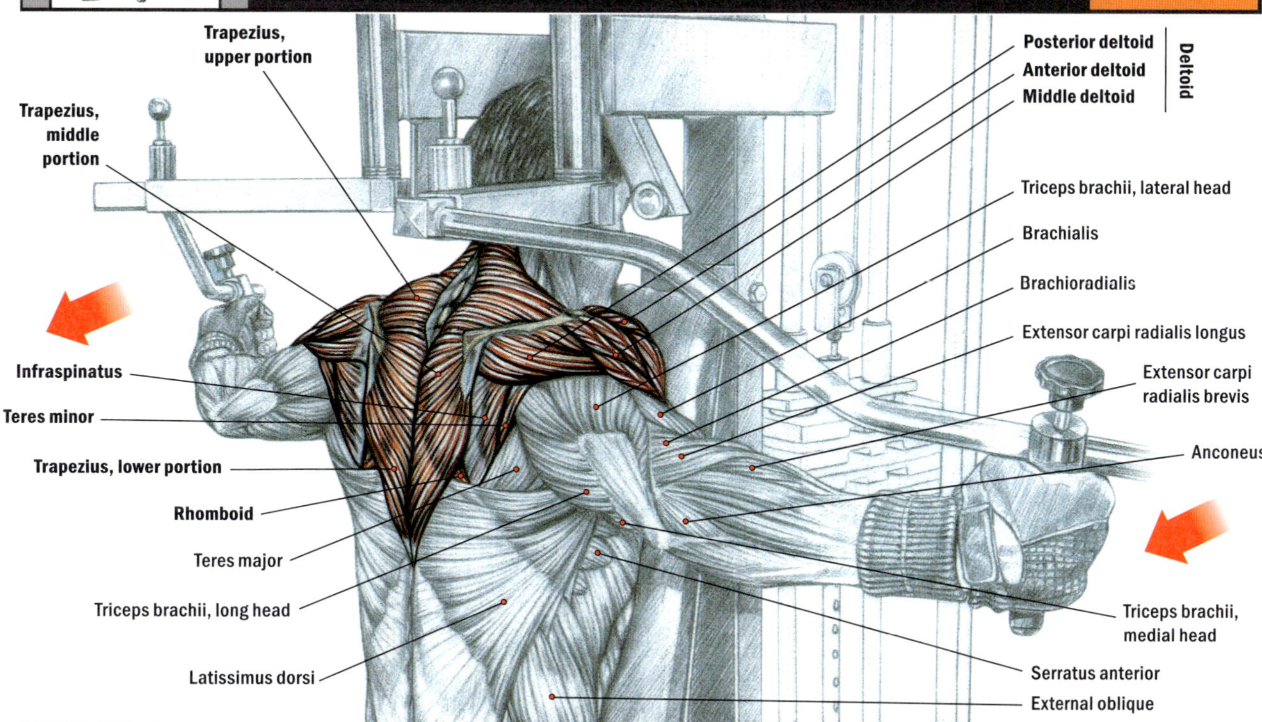

INFRASPINATUS AND TERES MINOR

Both of these muscles arise from the posterior surface of the scapula (shoulder blade), pass over the scapulohumeral joint (adhering to its articular capsule), and insert on the greater tubercle of the humerus. They play an important role in external rotation of the arm and reinforce the action of the shoulder ligaments by actively reinforcing the attachment of the arm to the chest.

In some people, the teres minor and infraspinatus are fused, forming one muscle.

PERFORMING THE EXERCISE

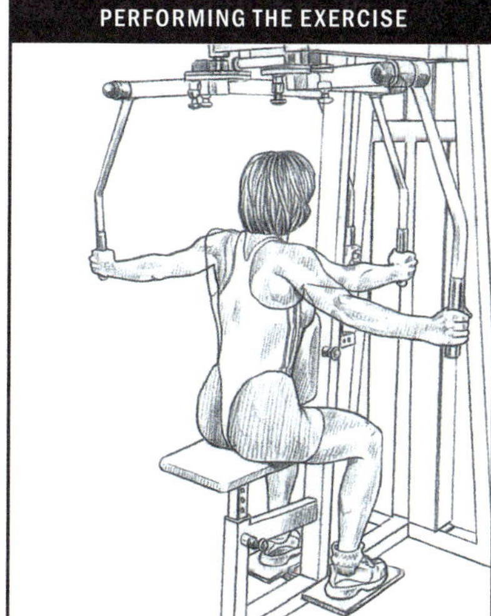

Sit facing the machine, with your torso against the back pad and your arms forward, gripping the handles:

- Inhale and separate your arms, squeezing your shoulder blades together at the end of the movement.
- Exhale.

This exercise mainly works the posterior deltoid, infraspinatus, and teres minor and, at the end of the movement when the shoulder blades come together, the trapezius and rhomboids.

STRETCHING THE POSTERIOR ROTATOR CUFF MUSCLES

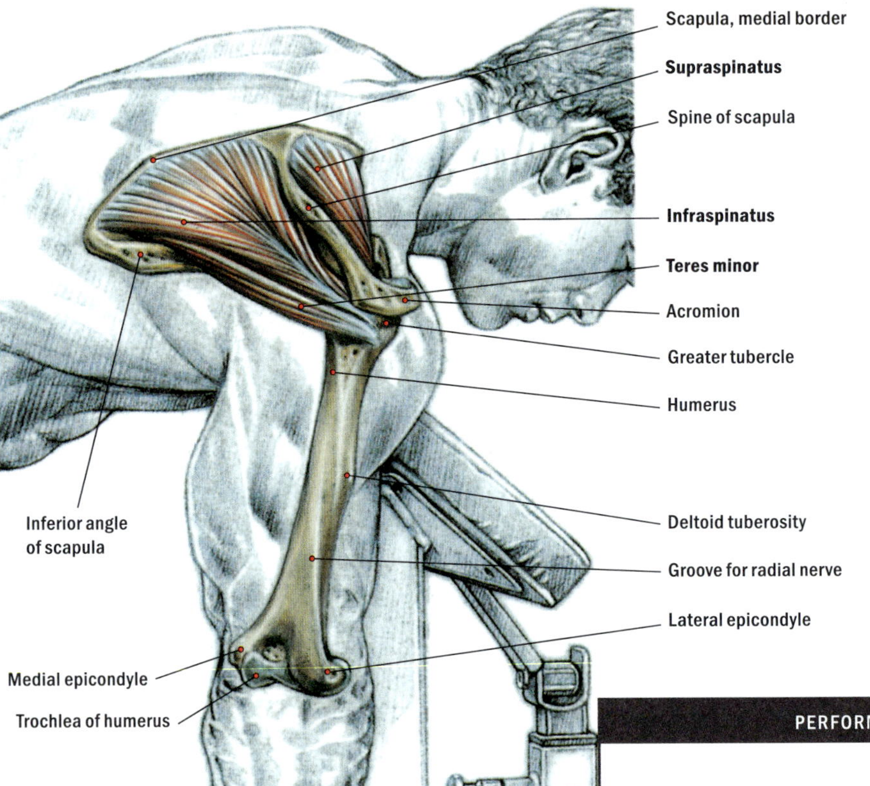

Stand with a dumbbell in your hand, lean your torso forward and rest it on a machine (for example, on a 45-degree back extension machine):

- With your arm relaxed, let the dumbbell hang for a minute while trying to relax the shoulder.

This exercise allows you to stretch the infraspinatus, teres minor, and, to a lesser extent, the supraspinatus; these muscles attach to the posterior surface of the scapula.

In strength training, these muscles are often the site of cramps and spasms that can pull the shoulder into a bad position. Over time, this can lead to overuse injuries in the tendon that are particularly incapacitating.

Cramps or spasms of the teres minor and infraspinatus will engage the humerus in external rotation. This creates excessive friction on the tendon of the long head of the biceps at the front of the arm (in the bicipital groove). If not treated, this can lead to inflammation and tearing of the tendon. Therefore, at the slightest suspicion of a cramp, it is important to do this specific stretch to relax these muscles.

PERFORMING THE EXERCISE

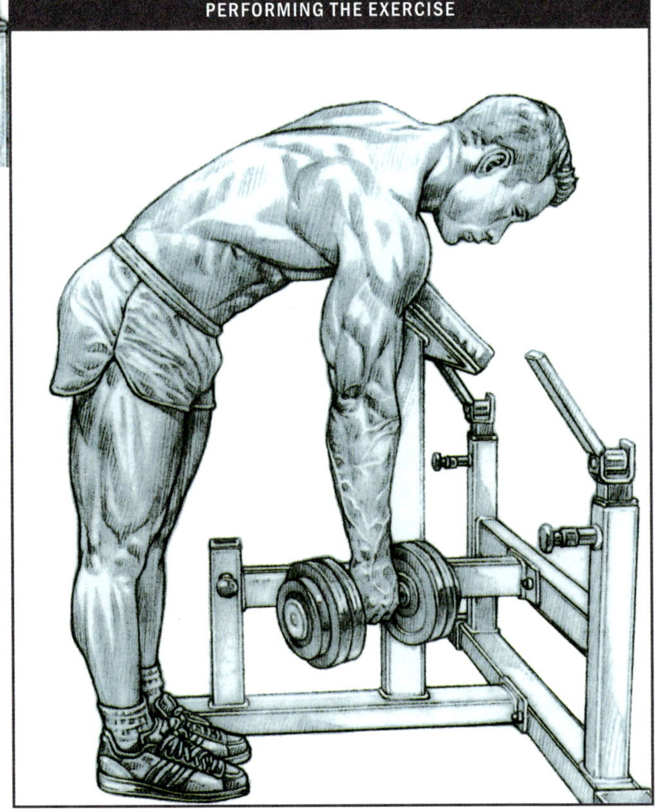

STRETCHING THE SHOULDER

TWO WAYS TO PULL ON THE ELBOW

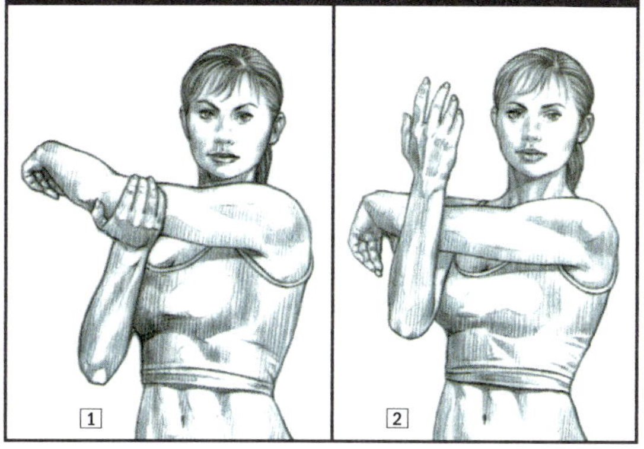

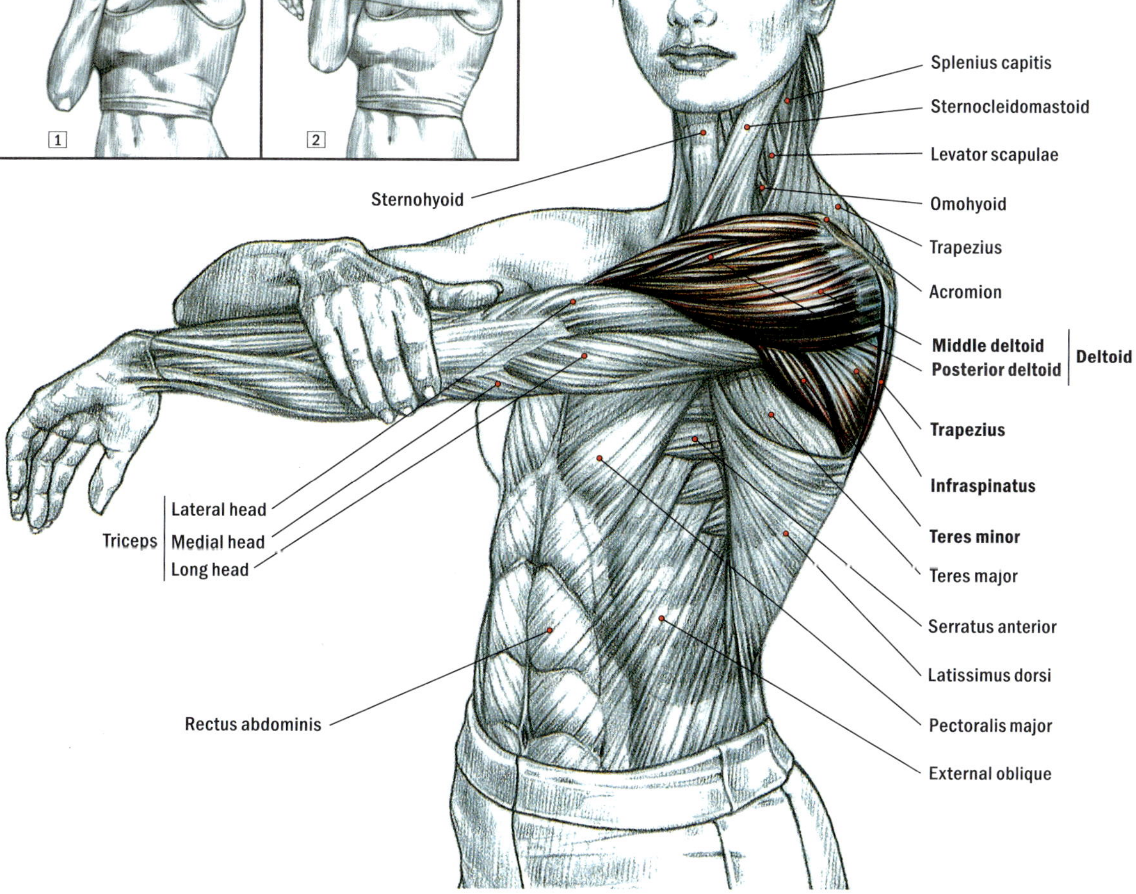

Stand with your head level and one arm horizontal:

- Grasp your elbow with the opposite hand and pull on your arm to slowly bring your elbow toward the opposite shoulder.
- Hold the stretch for 10 to 20 seconds—the time it takes to feel the stretch.

This stretch is for the both the posterior and middle deltoid and—especially important—for the teres minor and infraspinatus. These small muscles externally rotate the humerus and are often the site of cramps. These cramps can cause functional imbalances in the shoulder (such as excessive friction of the tendon of the long head of the biceps in the bicipital groove of the humerus) and may result in inflammation and injury.

The middle and inferior portions of the trapezius muscle and the rhomboid major are also stretched.

Variation

Place the other arm in front and use it to pull your elbow.

For some people with very well-developed muscles, adduction of the arm can be hindered by compression of the biceps brachii against the pectoralis major. This can limit the proper stretching of the back of the shoulder.

03 CHEST

THE IMPORTANCE OF THE PECTORALIS MAJOR MUSCLE WHEN THROWING

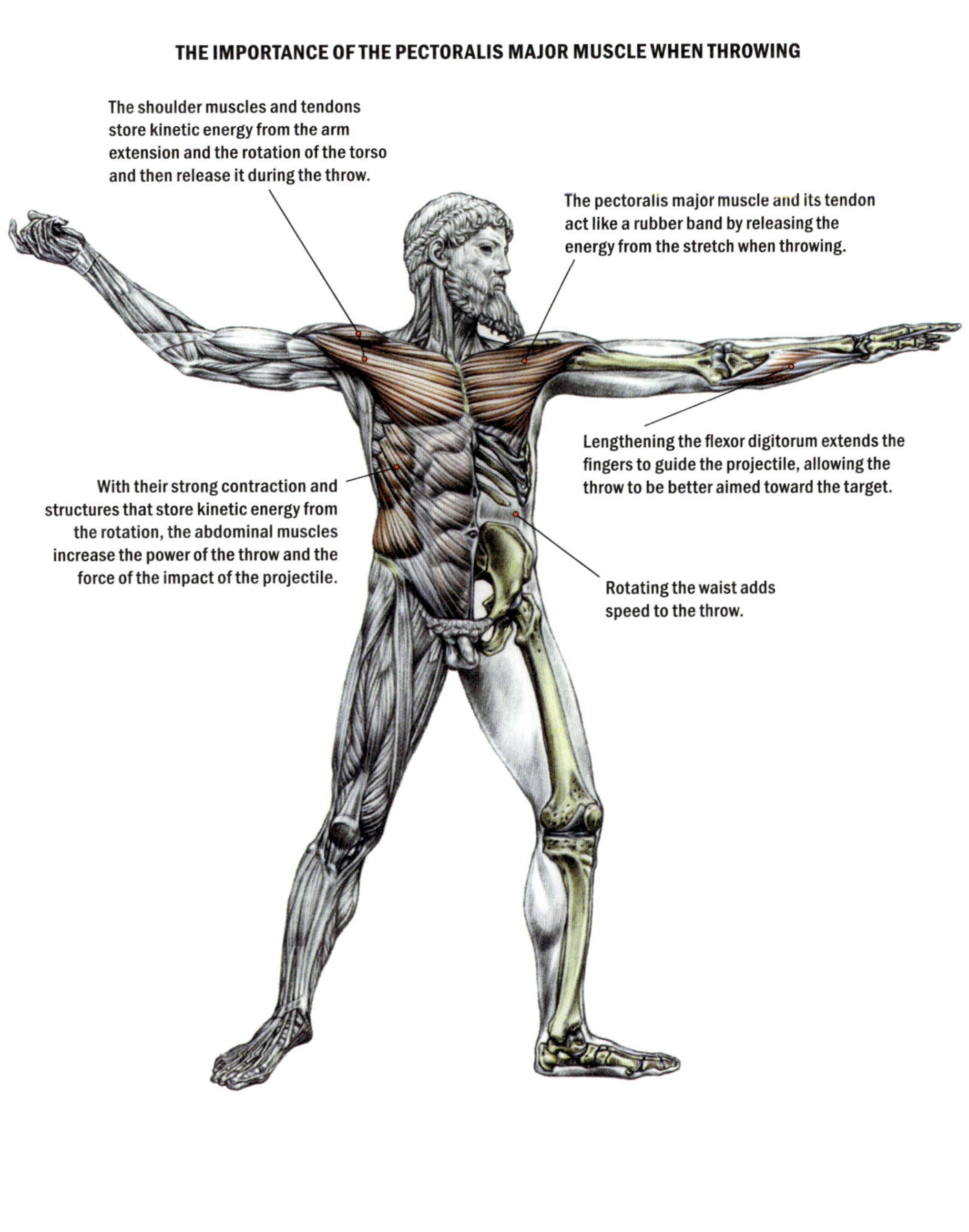

01 INCLINE BENCH PRESSES

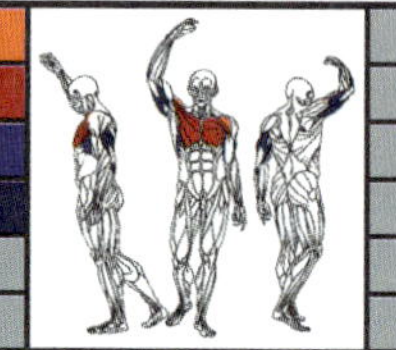

Pectoralis major
Brachioradialis
Rectus abdominis (under the aponeurosis)
Linea alba
External oblique
Teres major
Latissimus dorsi
Subscapularis
Serratus anterior
Flexor digitorum superficialis
Anterior deltoid
Coracobrachialis
Biceps brachii
Flexor carpi radialis
Palmaris longus
Flexor carpi ulnaris
Extensor carpi ulnaris
Anconeus
Triceps brachii, long head
Brachialis
Triceps brachii, medial head

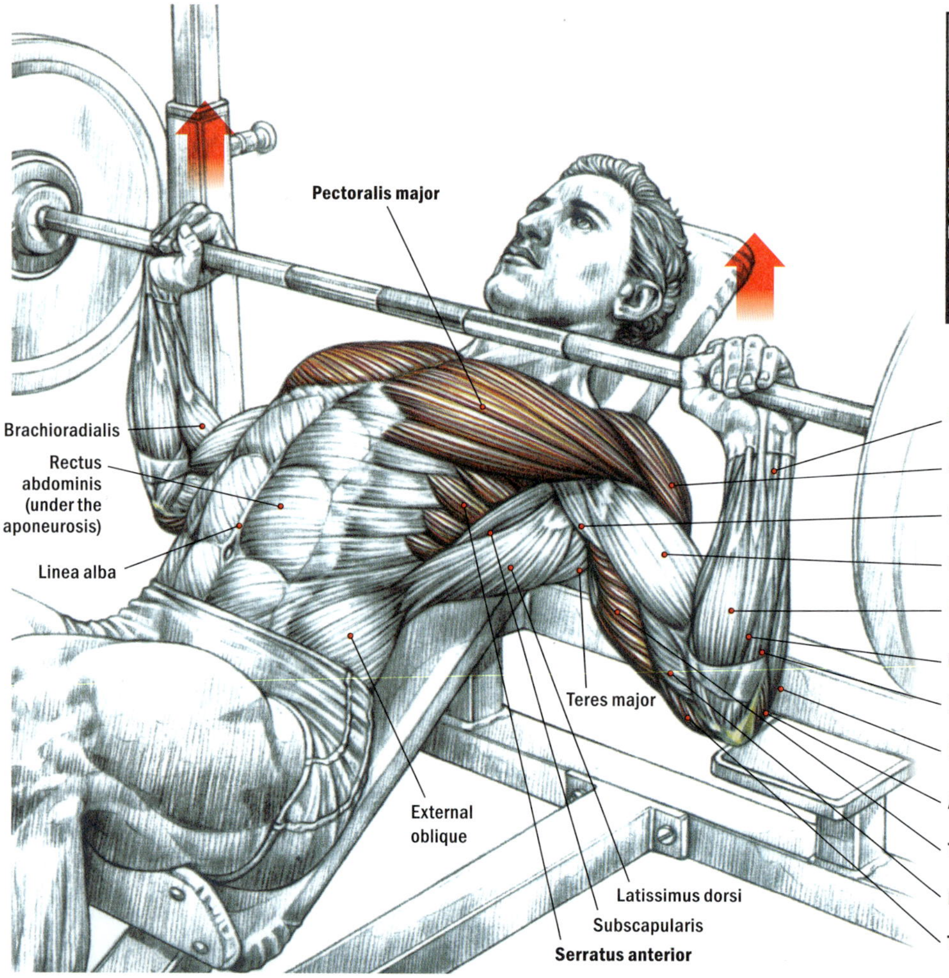

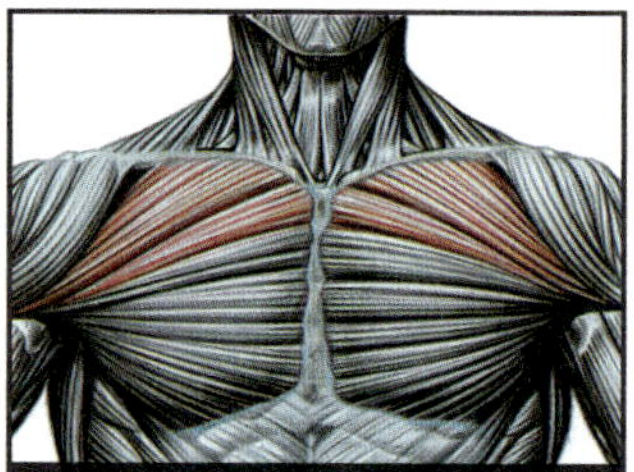

PART OF THE PECTORAL MUSCLES PRIMARILY WORKED DURING THE EXERCISE

INFLUENCE OF THE INCLINE BENCH PRESS ON THE CHEST

Clavicle
Trapezius
Deltoid
Pectoralis major
Body of the breast, mammary gland lobe
Infraspinatus
Teres minor
Teres major
Mammary papilla
Latissimus dorsi
Triceps brachii
Serratus anterior
Brachialis
Biceps brachii

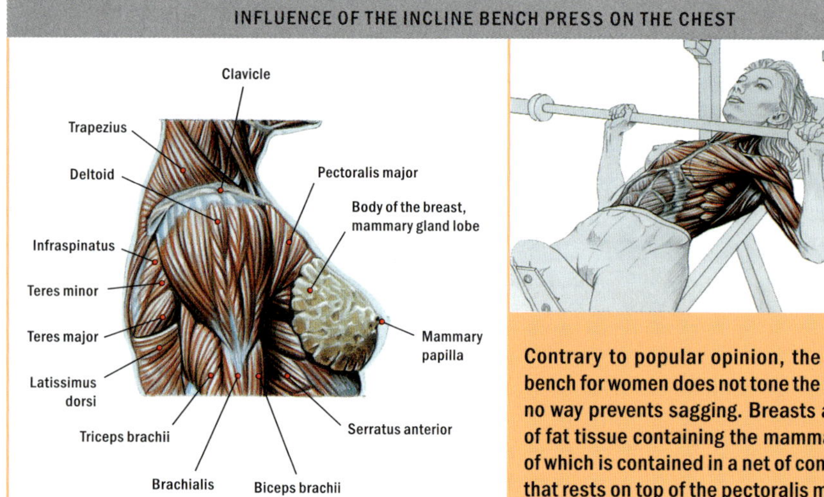

Contrary to popular opinion, the incline press bench for women does not tone the breasts and in no way prevents sagging. Breasts are composed of fat tissue containing the mammary glands, all of which is contained in a net of connective tissue that rests on top of the pectoralis major muscles.

Sit on an incline bench set at 45 to 60 degrees and grasp the barbell with an overhand grip wider than shoulder width:

- Inhale and lower the barbell to your sternal notch.
- Extend your arms.
- Exhale at the end of the exercise.

This exercise mainly works the clavicular head of the pectoralis major, anterior deltoid, triceps brachii, serratus anterior, and pectoralis minor. This exercise may be done using a rack.

STRETCHING THE PECTORALIS MAJOR

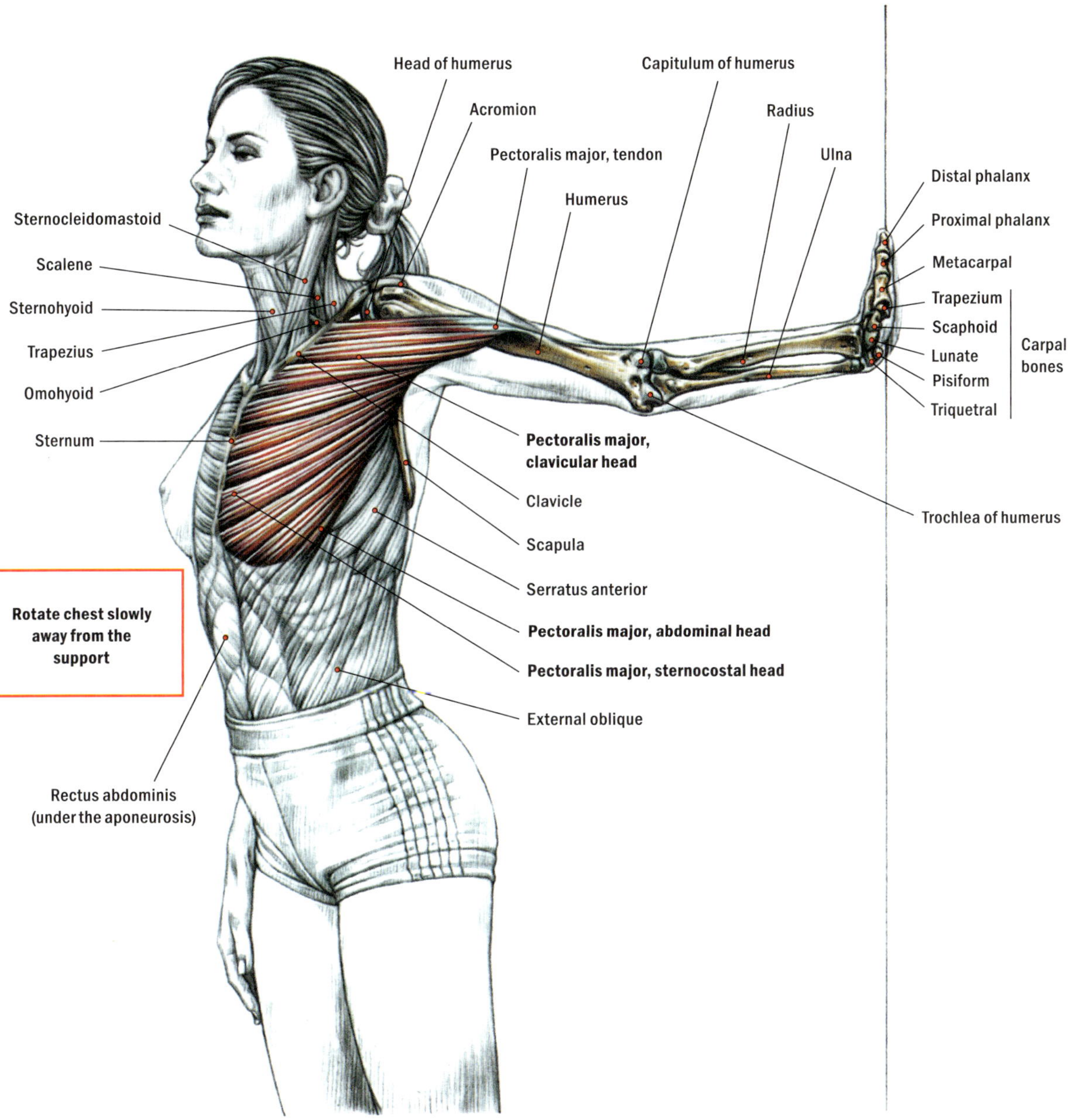

Stand with your arm extended. Grip a support with your hand and slowly rotate your chest away from the support. This exercise mainly stretches the pectoralis major, anterior deltoid, and biceps brachii.

Variation

Position your hand at various levels in order to stretch all the fibers of the pectoralis major.

This is an excellent stretch for the bench press in weightlifting, all throwing sports, and sports with a large amount of overhand motion, including baseball, softball, tennis, volleyball, and handball.

02 BENCH PRESSES

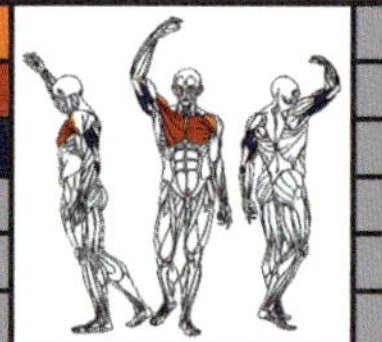

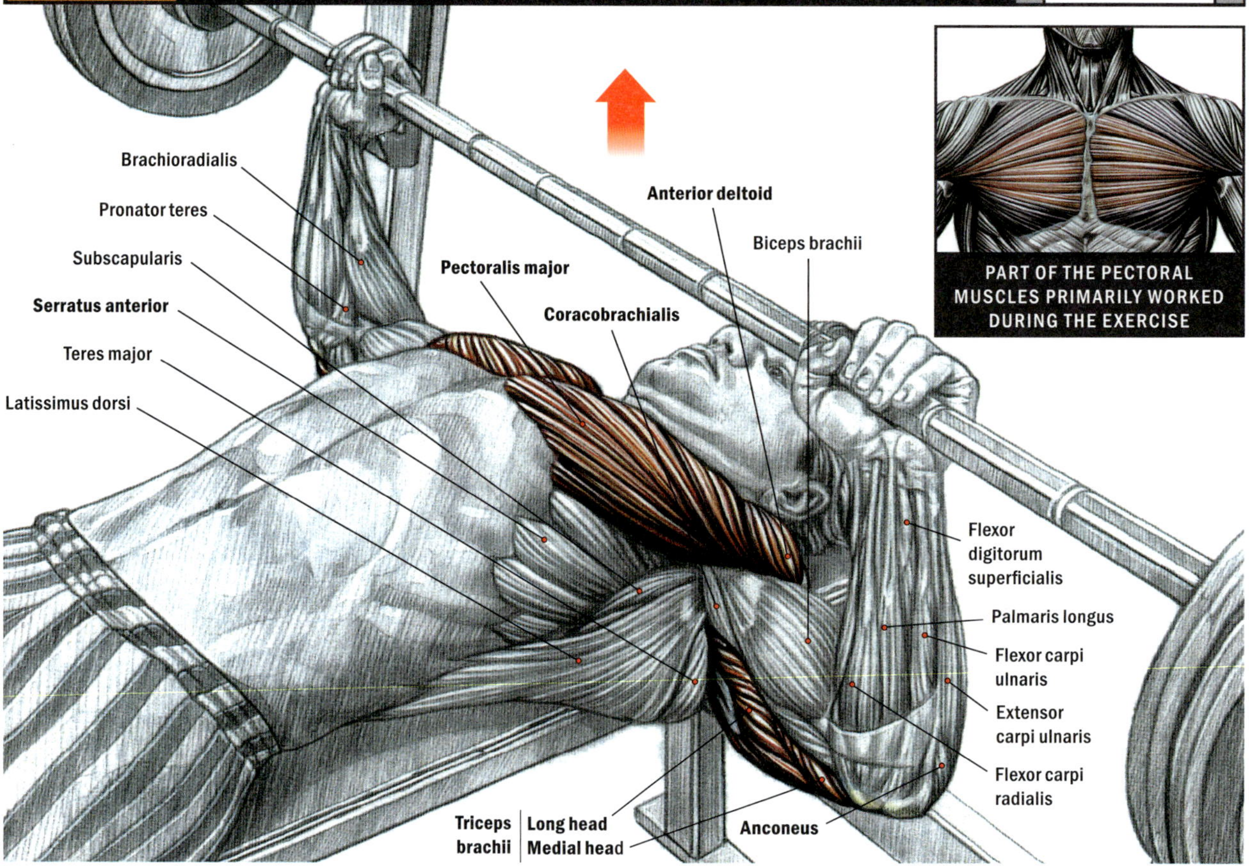

Brachioradialis
Pronator teres
Subscapularis
Serratus anterior
Teres major
Latissimus dorsi
Pectoralis major
Coracobrachialis
Anterior deltoid
Biceps brachii
Flexor digitorum superficialis
Palmaris longus
Flexor carpi ulnaris
Extensor carpi ulnaris
Flexor carpi radialis
Anconeus
Triceps brachii
Long head
Medial head

PART OF THE PECTORAL MUSCLES PRIMARILY WORKED DURING THE EXERCISE

2 Finish
1 Start

PERFORMING THE EXERCISE

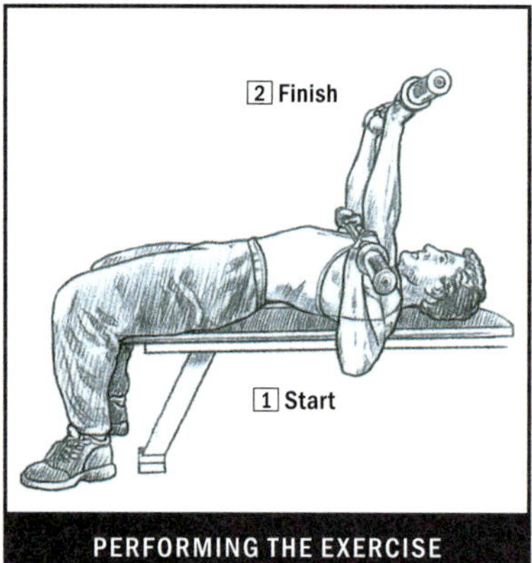

Lie on a horizontal bench, with your buttocks on the bench and your feet flat on the ground:

- Grasp the barbell with an overhand grip wider than shoulder width.
- Inhale and lower the bar to your chest with a controlled movement.
- Straighten your arms and exhale at the end of the exercise.

This exercise engages the entire pectoralis major muscle as well as the pectoralis minor, anterior deltoid, serratus anterior, triceps, and coracobrachialis.

Variations

- This exercise can be done while arching the back in powerlifter style. This position brings the more powerful lower part of the pectoral muscles into play, allowing you to press heavier weights. However, this variation should be done carefully to protect your back and avoid injury.
- Doing the press with your elbows next to your body focuses the work on the anterior deltoid.
- Varying the width of your hands works different parts of the muscle:
  - Hands close together works the central part of your pectorals.
  - Hands farther apart works the lateral part of your pectorals.
- Varying the angle of the barbell also works different parts of your muscle:
  - Lowering the bar to the costochondral border of the rib cage isolates the lower part of your pectorals.
  - Lowering the barbell to the middle part of the pectorals isolates the midline fibers.
  - Lowering the bar onto your sternal notch works the clavicular head of the muscle.
- If you have back problems or you want to isolate your pectorals, you can do the extension with your legs raised.
- Bench presses can be done in a rack.

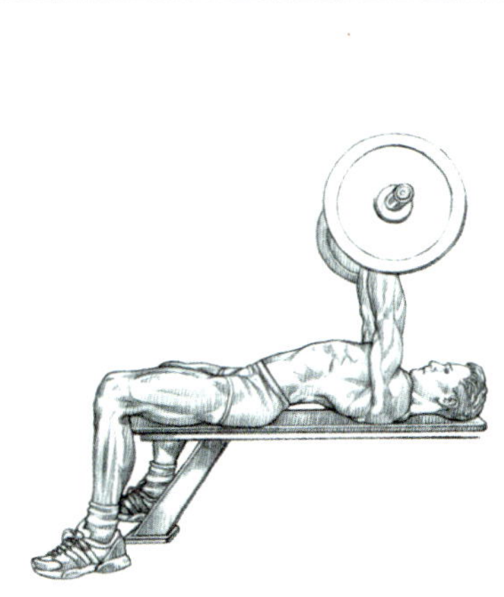

Doing the bench press with an arched back, powerlifter style, limits the range of the movement and allows you to lift significantly heavier weights because it uses mainly the lower part of the pectorals, which are very strong.

In competitions, the feet and the head should not move, and the buttocks should remain in contact with the bench. People with back problems should not do this variation.

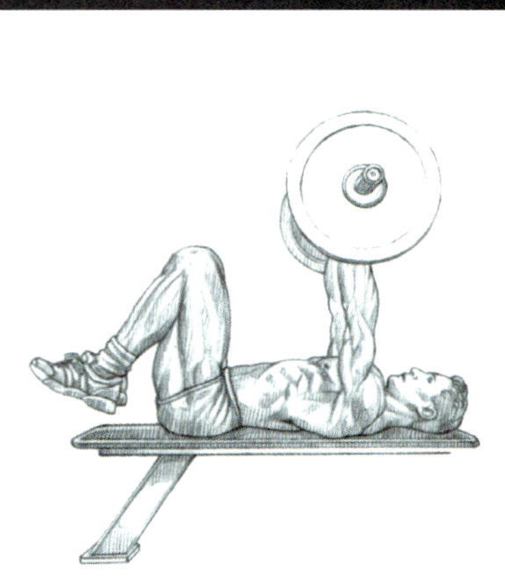

Doing the movement with raised legs helps prevent excessive arching, which can cause lower back pain. This variation can also decrease the work done by the lower pectorals by transferring the work to the middle and clavicular fibers.

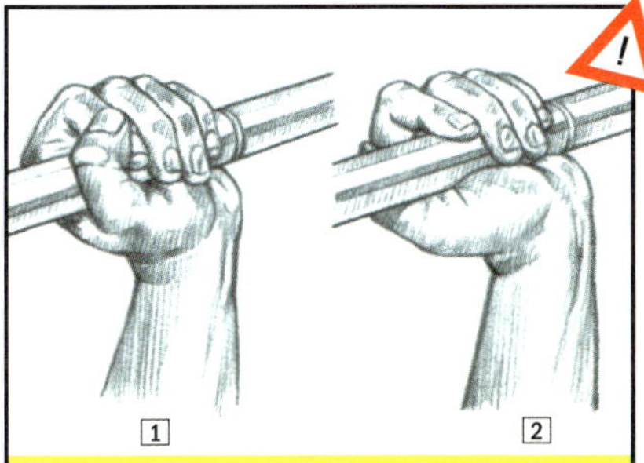

1 For maximum safety, grip the bar with the thumb and fingers opposite each other.

2 If your grip on the bar is not locked in using your thumbs, the bar could slip out of your hands at any moment and cause serious injuries by falling on the jaw or, even worse, your neck.

THE ROLE OF THE LATISSIMUS DORSI IN HEAVY BENCH PRESSES

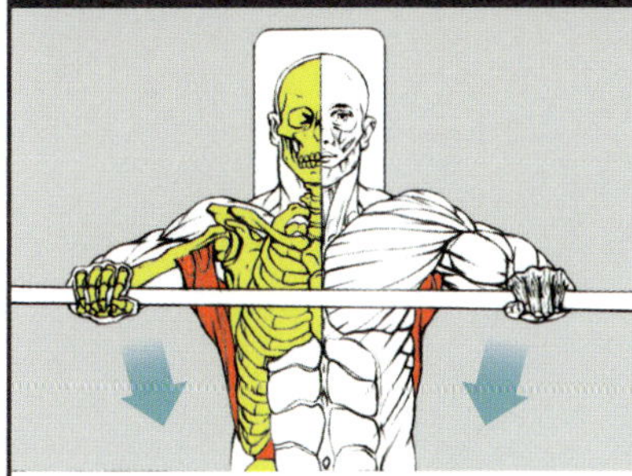

The latissimus dorsi muscle has a fundamental role in heavy bench presses. It prevents the arms from moving away from the body too much, which limits the risk of tearing the pectoralis major while making the press more stable and powerful.

HOW TO POSITION YOURSELF FOR A POWERFUL BENCH PRESS

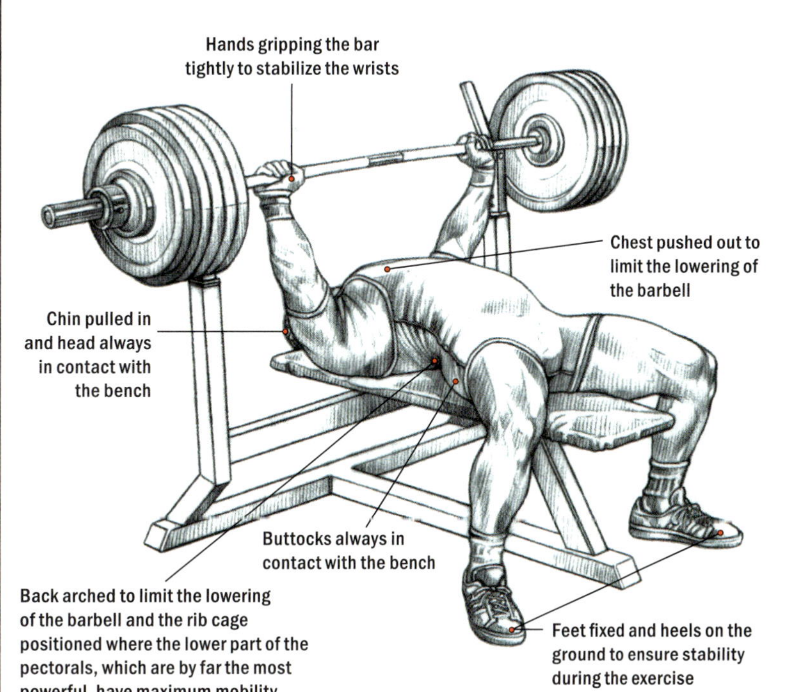

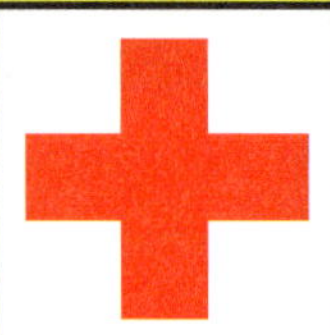

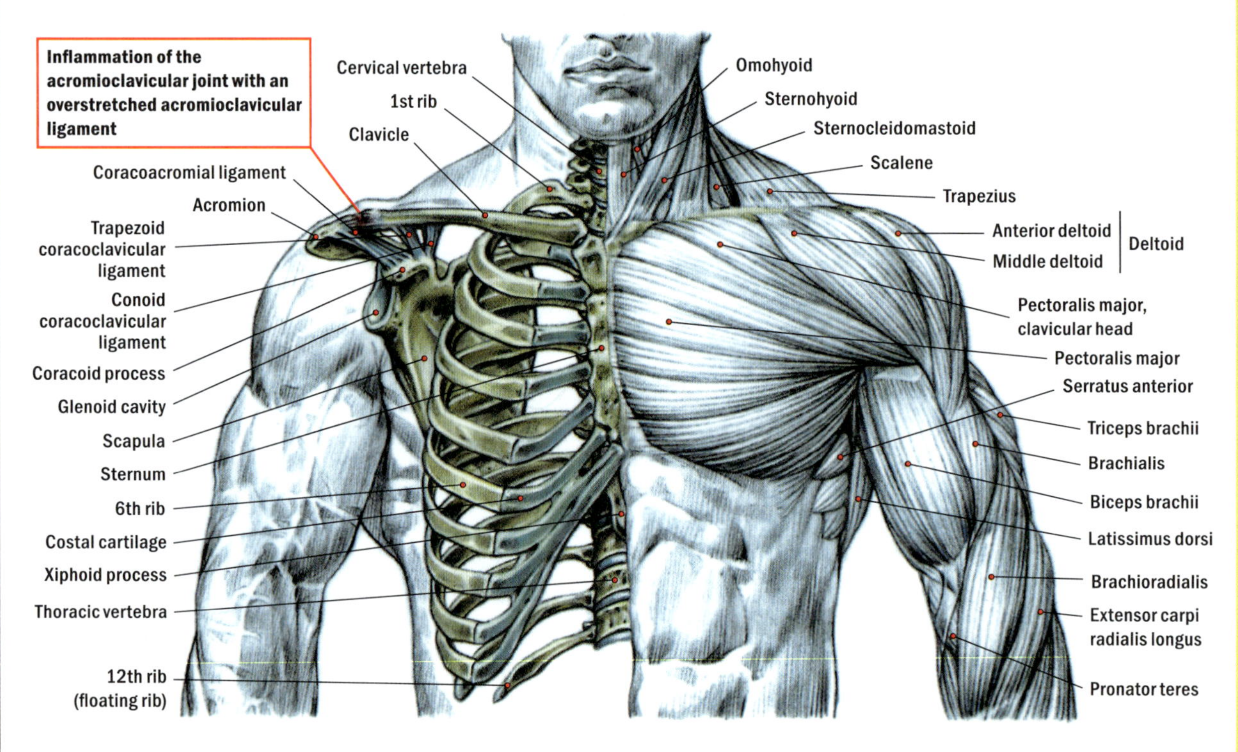

Acromioclavicular injuries are common, and most dedicated weightlifters encounter such an injury sooner or later. Unlike other sports (such as rugby, football, and equestrian), including combat sports with throws (wrestling and judo), where the shoulder joint can be seriously injured from violent contact or a fall involving acromioclavicular dislocation with ligament tearing, in weightlifting, acromioclavicular injuries are mainly due to microtraumas resulting from excessive and repetitive stress along with poor control of the shoulder joint.

The pain develops gradually. Although easily tolerated at first, the pain gradually disturbs the practice of weightlifting until it finally hinders the ability to perform many exercises such as bench presses and dips. All downward movements become painful, and supporting oneself on the elbows can also be painful.

Examination of the acromioclavicular joint usually reveals slight swelling and pain on palpation. Although not serious, this type of injury takes a long time to heal since it takes time for the inflammation to subside and for the joint capsule and the overstretched acromioclavicular ligaments, which are responsible for joint motion, to return to their normal size. If this injury occurs, you must stop all upper body training for two weeks.

CROSS SECTION OF THE ACROMIOCLAVICULAR JOINT

*The acromioclavicular ligament is a thickening of the superior part of the acromioclavicular joint capsule.

At the skeletal level, the upper extremity is attached to the chest by the clavicle, which extends from the sternum to the shoulder blade. Although not very mobile, the clavicular articulations are often overused and subject to inflammatory wear pathologies.

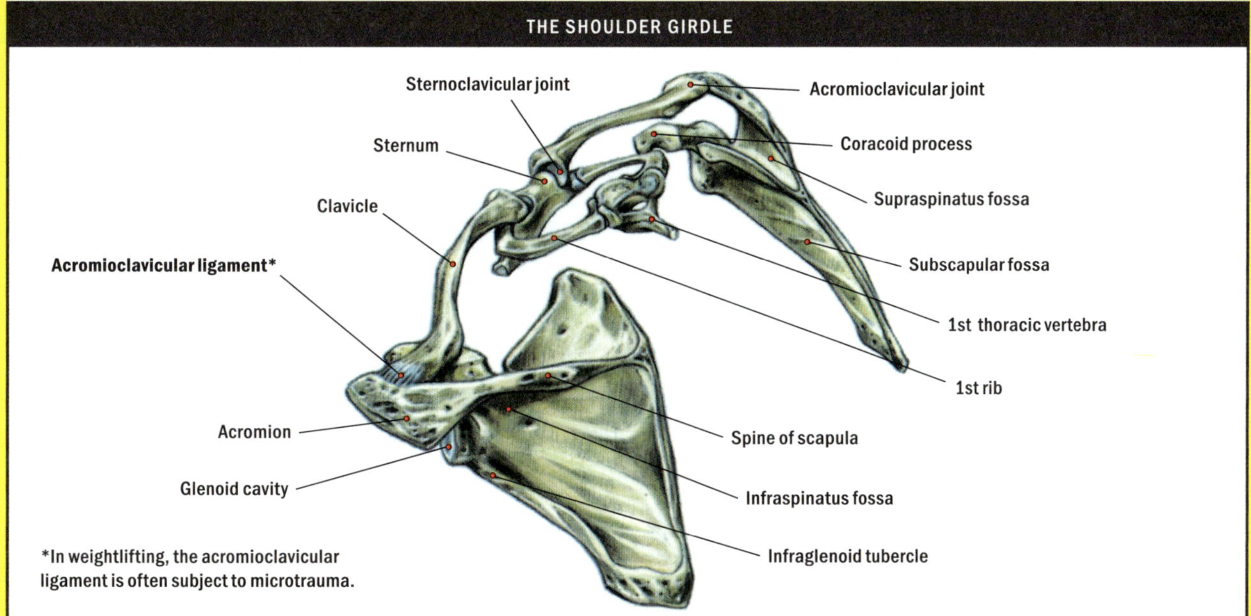

*In weightlifting, the acromioclavicular ligament is often subject to microtrauma.

On resuming training of the upper body, you should avoid the bench press and all exercises that involve pushing down, such as decline presses and dips, for at least two months because they risk stretching the acromioclavicular ligaments all over again. On the other hand, all exercises that involve pushing up, such as incline bench presses or shoulder presses with barbells and dumbbells, can be done without risk because they tend to stabilize the acromioclavicular articulation, which limits the risk of stretching the ligaments.

Disregarding this advice may cause the joint inflammation to continue, which could lead to intra-articular calcifications that could seriously compromise an athletic career.

PREVENTION

In strength training, acromioclavicular inflammation most often occurs because of overtraining in the bench press with sets that are too long or poorly controlled (rapid lowering, jerking, and bouncing off the chest). Powerlifters who bench press with an arched back are also susceptible to inflammatory pathologies from the tension placed on the acromioclavicular ligaments.

As soon as you feel any pain, stop these traumatizing techniques for some time and replace them with exercises for the pectoral muscles, such as cable crossover flys (page 109) and dumbbell exercises. Always work with an incline on the bench.

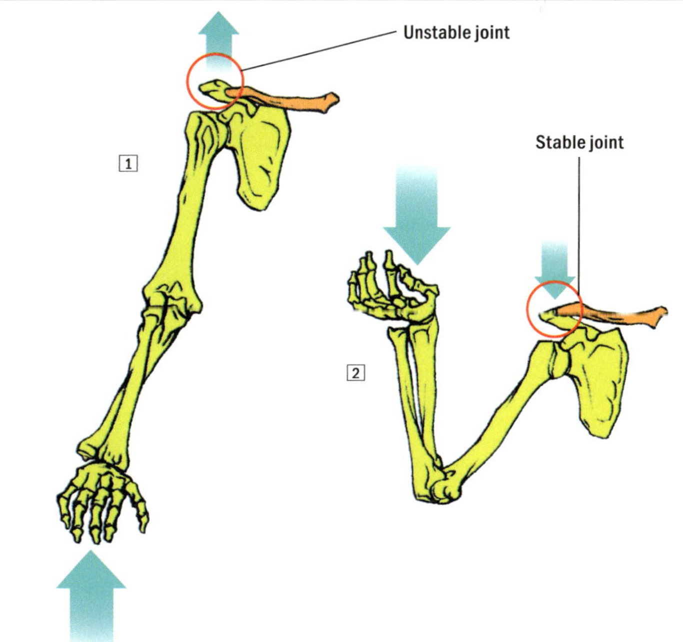

1 When pushing down (as in dips) or doing bench presses with an arched back (like powerlifters), the acromion is pushed up. If the acromioclavicular joint is injured because of an overstretched ligament, the joint will be hypermobile and will be pushed painfully upward.

2 When pushing up, such as in the incline bench presses or front presses with a bar, the acromioclavicular articulation is pressed down and stabilized.

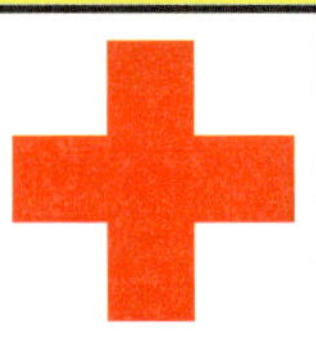

THE COMPLEXITY OF THE STERNOCLAVICULAR ZONE

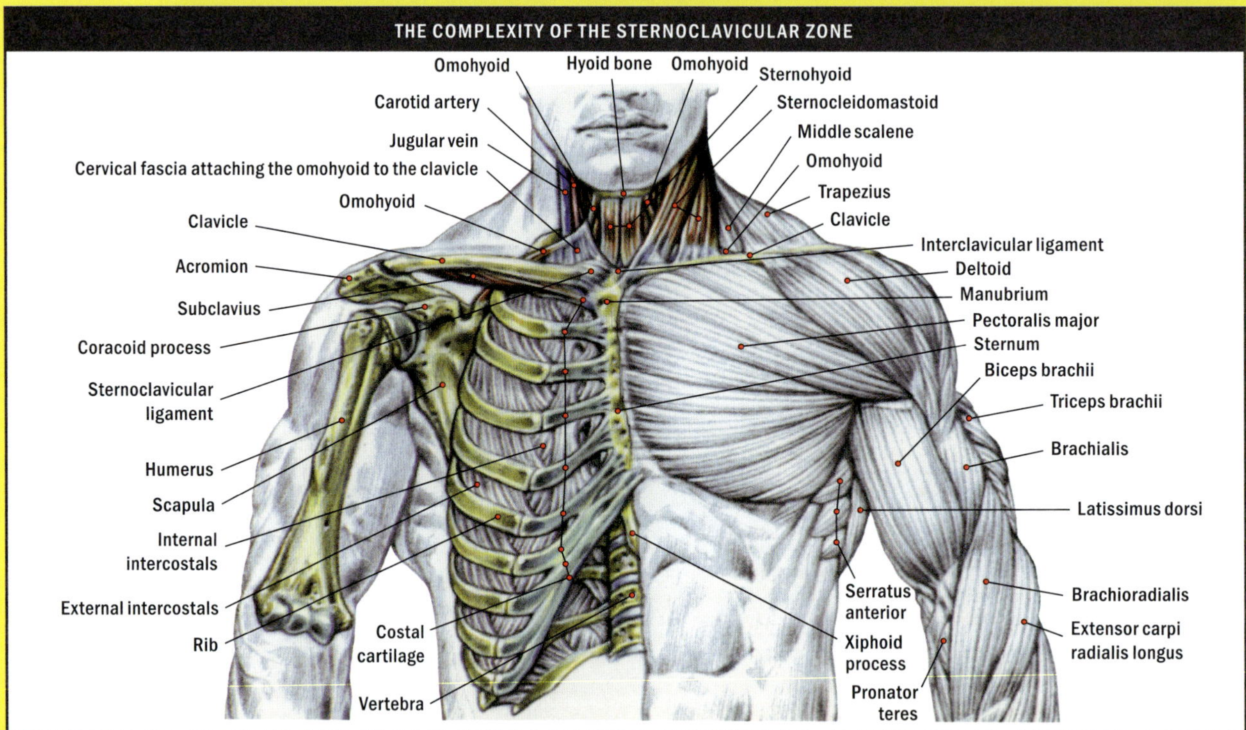

PARTIAL CROSS SECTION OF THE STERNOCLAVICULAR JOINT

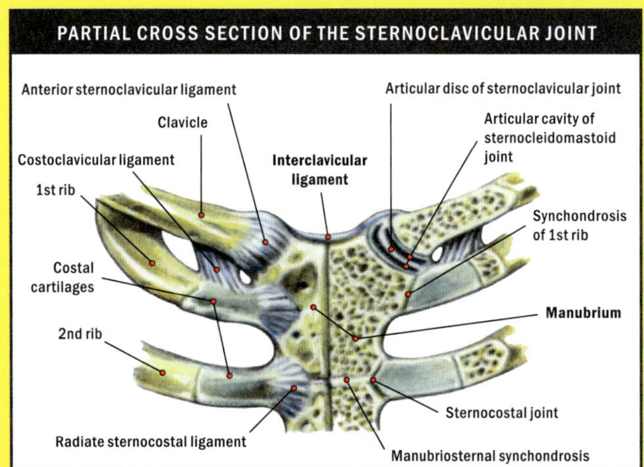

In strength training, sternoclavicular pathologies are less common than acromioclavicular pathologies, but they still affect many people. This type of injury mainly affects those who do weighted dips, decline bench presses, bench presses with an arched back (powerlifter style), or barbell bench presses with resistance bands.

These exercises tend to put a lot of stress on the sternoclavicular joint. If there is an individual predisposition (for example, a lack of resistance or ligaments that are too lax), this stress will end up stretching the sternoclavicular ligaments and deforming the joint capsule. The sternoclavicular joint slowly begins to loosen. It becomes hypermobile, painful, and swollen, which prevents you from being able to do many exercises.

This progressive sternoclavicular subluxation is typical in strength training. It is much less severe than traumatic sternoclavicular dislocation following a fall or violent contact (there is a risk of complications in the event of a clavicle dislocation, which may compress the carotid artery or the jugular vein). However, it is quite painful because excessive mobility of the clavicle stretches the subclavius muscle. The sternohyoid, omohyoid, and sternocleidomastoid muscles all attach to the sternoclavicular joint, so turning or tilting the head and swallowing can be difficult. Swelling may also occur at the base of the neck.

However, it most often heals as long as you avoid all exercises involving horizontal or downward pushes such as dips, bench presses, and decline bench presses, which put too much stress on the joint. On the other hand, because of the pressure they create, exercises that involve pushing up, such as incline or front presses, tend to press the clavicle to the sternum. Therefore, you can continue to do these exercises without risk.

> The sternoclavicular joint is the only bony connection linking the upper limb to the chest.

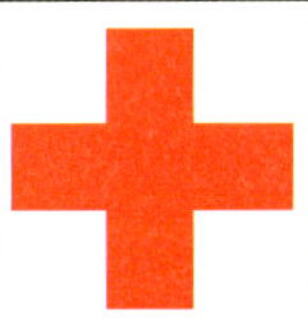

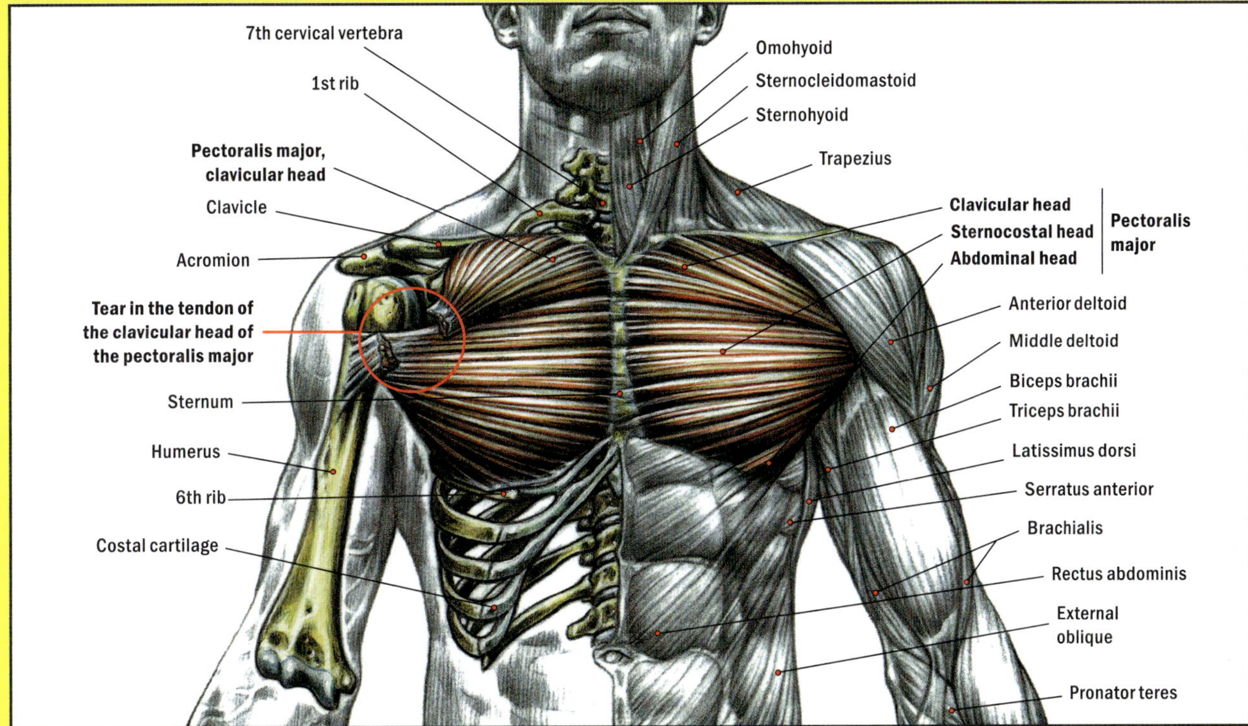

The pectoralis major originates on the anterior surface of the rib cage and inserts on the anterior surface of the upper end of the humerus. It is a powerful muscle whose main function is to bring the arms together in front of the rib cage (it is the hugging muscle).

Unlike most sports, where pectoralis major injuries are rare, weight-lifting, especially the bench press, can cause small tears in the pectoralis major and even partial rupture of its tendon. Partial ruptures are seen only in relatively powerful athletes using abnormally rapid force before the tendon has had time to strengthen. Sometimes it is associated with a low-calorie diet aimed at increased muscle definition. These diets tend to weaken the muscles, tendons, and joints.

The injury, which occurs during heavy bench pressing, generally affects only the tendon of the clavicular head of the pectoralis major. A torn tendon is extremely painful, and the athlete may faint. Swelling and bruising often appear on the front of the arm, and retraction of the clavicular head leads to a hollow underneath the anterior deltoid.

The problem with this injury is that doctors often misdiagnose it. This mistake is unfortunately common but is understandable, because, during the posttraumatic examination, the injured party is able to perform all the movements that indicate full motor function of the pectoralis major. For example, despite a tear of the clavicular head of the pectoralis major, anterior elevation of the arm, which is part of its function, is compensated for by the anterior deltoid, and abduction is performed by the sternal and abdominal heads of the pectoralis major.

If the tendon of the clavicular head of the pectoralis major is torn, it must be surgically reinserted onto the humerus as soon as possible. If this is not done promptly, retraction and fibrosis of the muscle occurs, and the operation will no longer be possible. Although the injured person can move the arm through its full range of motion without the superior head of the pectoralis major, he or she will never recover original strength and will be at a serious disadvantage in continuing heavy strength training.

INSERTION OF THE PECTORALIS MAJOR ON THE HUMERUS DEMONSTRATING HOW THE TENDON TWISTS ON ITSELF TO CREATE A *U* SHAPE

During bench presses or flys, the most lateral part of the pectoralis major tendon, which corresponds to the clavicular head, is put under the most stress. Therefore, when lifting heavy weights, this is the tendon that tears or pulls away from its insertion.

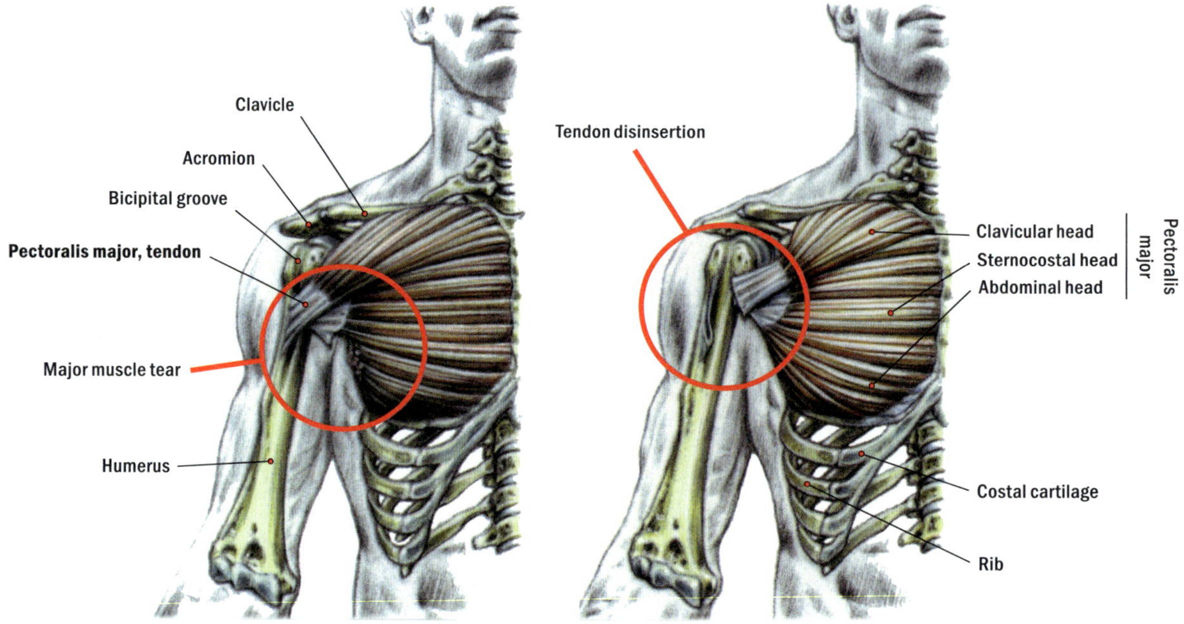

In strength training, since the goal is to gain muscle size and strength by gradually increasing the number of repetitions and the weight of the dumbbells, barbells, or weight plates used, muscle injuries are sooner or later inevitable.

Though some muscles, such as the pectorals, biceps, triceps, quadriceps, hip adductors, and hamstrings, are affected more than others, any muscle can be affected. To deal with these pathologies as pragmatically as possible, it is important to understand the difference between a major muscle tear and a tendon disinsertion.

In strength training, muscle injuries most often occur when the muscle is overstretched, the weight used is too heavy or poorly controlled, and the muscles and tendons are already slightly damaged, poorly healed, or are simply tired and stiff. Under these circumstances, not all the muscle fibers put into action during the effort are subject to the same stress. The most strained fibers will bear the load on their own and tear or, as a result, will cause uneven stress on the tendon, which will cause the tendon to partially or completely pull away from its insertion. Tendon disinsertion is more shocking because the muscle retracts into a ball and can no longer perform its motor function.

Generally, a tendon can be reinserted with screws at the exact point of its original insertion. This is why it is important to seek medical advice as soon as possible. If the injury is caught in time, healing a tendon that has pulled away from its insertion will sometimes allow full recovery of muscle motor function. However, if it is not diagnosed and operated on in time, muscle atrophy with fibrosis will prevent any possibility of later recovery.

However, it is almost impossible to reinsert a torn muscle fiber, which ends up retracting, atrophying into a fibrous mass, and leaving only a hole where the muscle once was. Note that major muscle tears generally correspond to massive disinsertions of the muscle fibers that are attached to a tendon sheath. This sheath becomes the insertion of a tendon on a bone. This type of major muscle tear is common in the tendon of the pectoralis major, under the tendon sheath of the distal tendon of the triceps brachii, under the tendon sheath of the short head of the biceps brachii, and under the tendon sheath that becomes the Achilles tendon.

To reduce the risk of tearing and tendon disinsertion, it is important to never lift heavy weights if your muscles are tired, stiff, or painful. At the beginning of a workout, do some stretching exercises to loosen any stiffness.

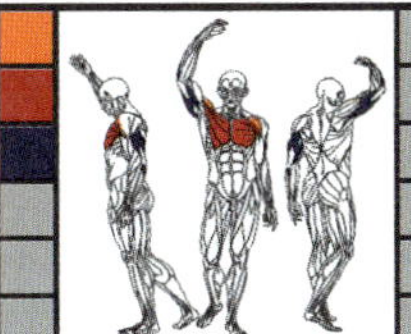

Flexor digitorum superficialis
Flexor carpi ulnaris
Biceps brachii
Anconeus

Triceps brachii
Medial head
Lateral head
Long head

Teres major
Posterior deltoid
Serratus anterior
Latissimus dorsi
Subscapularis

Palmaris longus
Brachioradialis
Flexor carpi radialis
Pronator teres
Brachialis
Pectoralis major

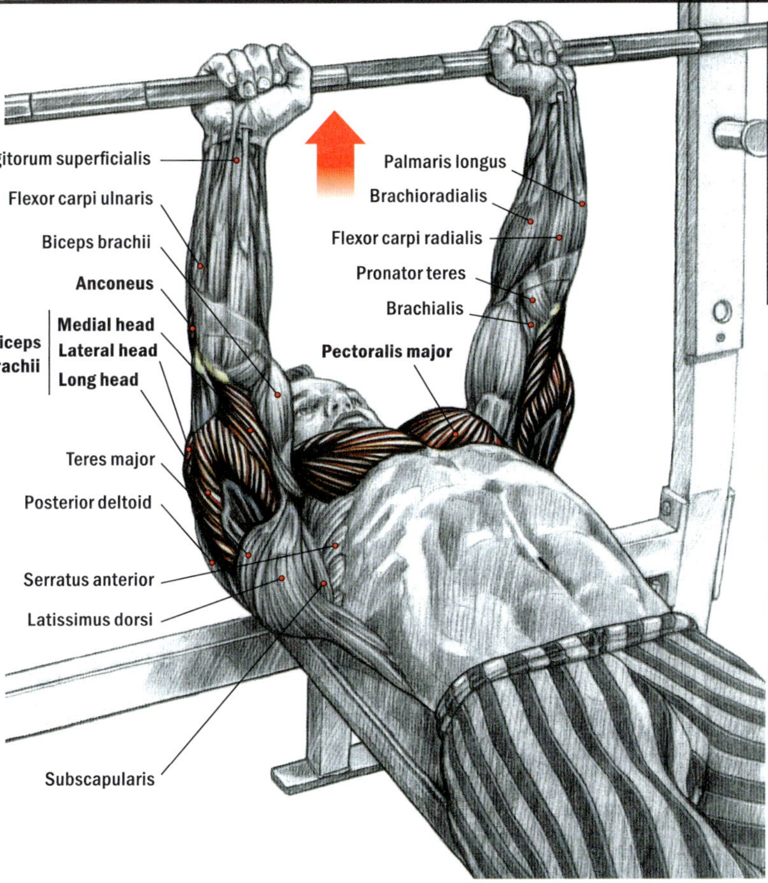

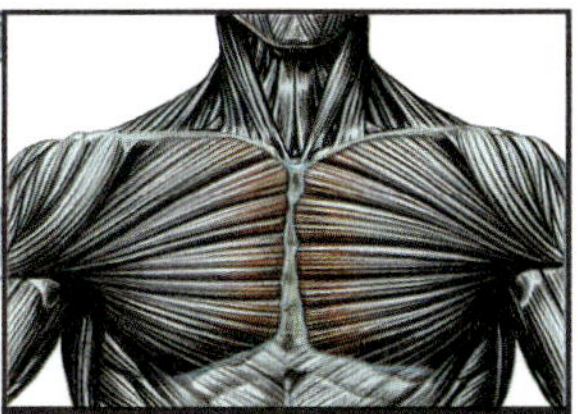

PART OF THE PECTORAL MUSCLES PRIMARILY WORKED DURING THE EXERCISE

Depending on your physical structure, the narrow grip may cause wrist pain. In this case, use a slightly wider grip.

VARIATION WITH ELBOWS OPEN

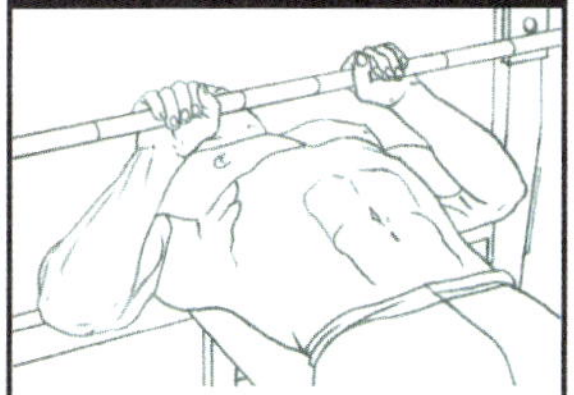

This position better isolates the triceps brachii.

Lie on a horizontal bench with your buttocks on the bench and your feet on the ground. Grip the barbell with an overhand grip and wrists 4 to 16 inches (10-40 cm) apart, depending on the flexibility of your wrists:

- Inhale and lower the bar to your chest with control, with your elbows out to your sides.
- Straighten your arms and exhale at the end of the exercise.

This exercise develops the pectoral muscles at the sternal notch and the triceps brachii. With this in mind, it may be included in a program for the arms.

By keeping your elbows next to the body as you straighten the arms, more of the work is performed by the anterior deltoid. This exercise can be done in a rack.

BENCH PRESSES AND ELBOW PAIN

Elbow pain most often develops after bench pressing. This overuse injury is generally related to overtraining with long sets.

In bench pressing, locking the straight arms at the end of the movement subjects the elbow to rubbing and microtraumas that can eventually cause inflammation. This bench press injury can rarely lead to intra-articular calcifications that are particularly crippling. In this case, surgery is often the only solution for regaining complete arm extension.

At the first sign of elbow pain, it is important to avoid exercises that involve straightening the arms. Avoiding these exercises for several days can prevent complications. When you eventually resume exercises that include arm extensions, do not completely straighten the arms at the end of the movement until the pain has completely disappeared.

CROSS SECTION OF THE ELBOW JOINT

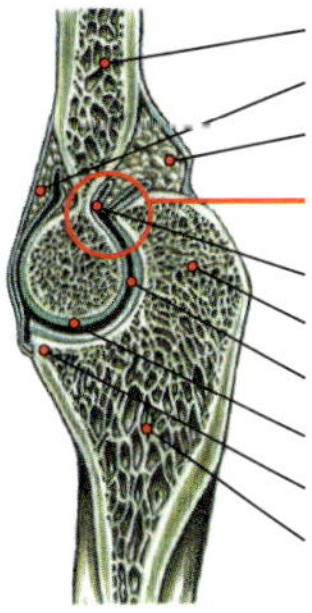

Humerus
Fat mass
Fat mass
Main zone of friction prone to inflammatory injuries
Olecranon fossa
Olecranon
Articular cavity
Trochlea, cartilage
Coronoid process
Ulna

With repeated extension of the forearm, the olecranon butts up against the olecranon fossa of the humerus. The joint then suffers from microtraumas that, over time, can cause painful inflammation on the dorsal surface of the elbow.

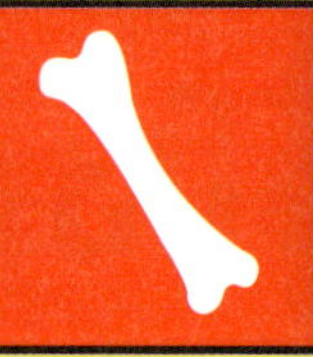

BENCH PRESSES AND MORPHOLOGY

The bench press is by far the most used exercise in strength training. It is also the exercise that causes the most injuries each year. Therefore, to do this exercise correctly and to reduce the risk of injury, you must learn the basics of individual morphological differences.

ARM LENGTH

Besides wear-and-tear pathologies, most injuries are muscle tears or tendon tears of the pectoralis major. These occur most often during the negative phase of the movement (while lowering the barbell).

As you lower the barbell to the chest, the pectoralis major, which inserts onto the humerus, becomes increasingly stretched and vulnerable as the arms are lowered. But the lowering of the arm and the stretch of the pectoralis major vary significantly depending on the individual. The longer the arms—especially the forearms—are, the lower the humerus will go down, and the more the pectoralis major will be dangerously stretched. Therefore, it is not surprising that most injuries occur in people with relatively longer arms.

THICKNESS OF THE RIB CAGE

The thicker the rib cage, the more the lowering of the barbell and, by extension, the stretching of the pectoralis major will be restricted. People with a thick rib cage can, in theory, do the bench press without much risk of injury to the pectoralis major.

It is not surprising that most of the great bench press champions are people with proportionately shorter extremities and thick chests. These two details allow them to achieve their records in relative safety by reducing the risk of tears and disinsertions of the pectoralis major.

Remember that injuries are often what limits athletes' progress. In addition to training methods, nutrition, and a good mental state, individual morphology plays a fundamental role in success in sport. It is essential to adapt your training to your morphology and to understand that what is good for one person may not be good for another.

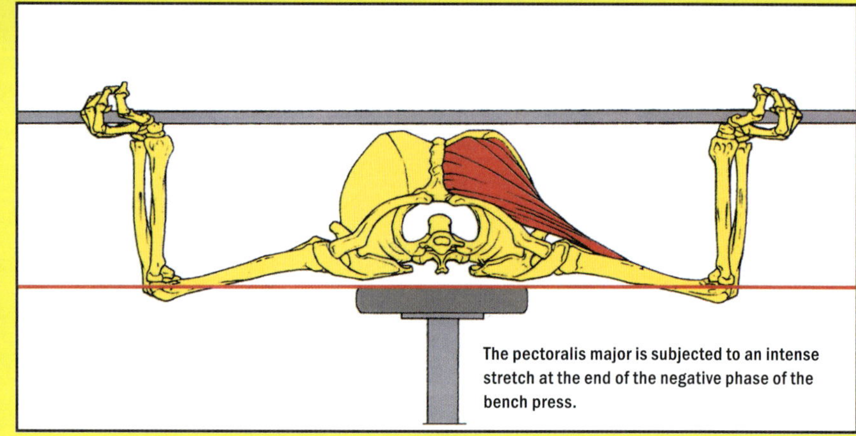

The pectoralis major is subjected to an intense stretch at the end of the negative phase of the bench press.

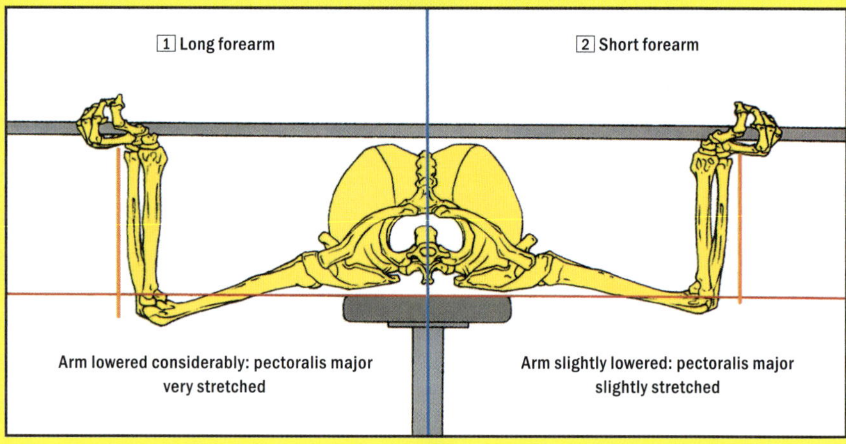

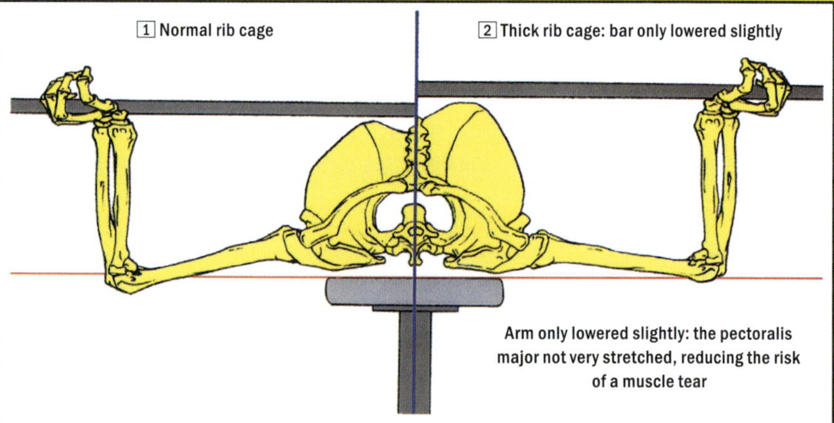

LIMITING THE RISK OF INJURY

It is possible to do the bench press by bringing the hands close together. Because this variation limits the lowering of the arms, it reduces the stretch of the pectoralis major and limits the risk of injury.

Although the range of the movement is greater, the work on the triceps is more intense, and the performance is reduced, this low-risk variation is sometimes used by certain long-limbed bench press champions.

To avoid excessive stretching of the pectoral muscles, it is possible to do a partial bench press by decreasing the descent of the bar so that it does not touch the chest.

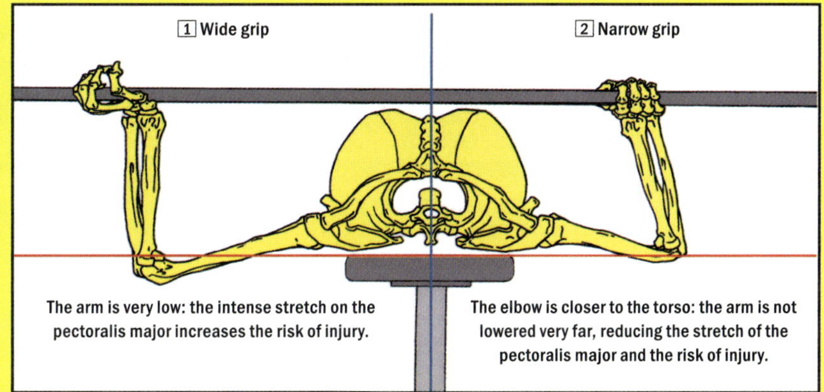

The arm is very low: the intense stretch on the pectoralis major increases the risk of injury.

The elbow is closer to the torso: the arm is not lowered very far, reducing the stretch of the pectoralis major and the risk of injury.

> ! Note that bench presses with resistance bands pose a low risk to the muscles and tendons since the stress is minimal when the muscles are stretched. However, the stress on the joints is very strong, which can cause severe damage to the joints and ligaments over time.

MUSCLE PREDOMINENCE

There are two ways of bench pressing, and these directly depend on the individual's muscle strengths.

1. The bench press can be done with the elbows apart. This technique directs most of the effort onto the pectoralis major.

2. The bench press can also be done with the elbows close together, closing the angle between the arm and chest. People who have deltoids that are stronger than their pectoralis major muscles will instinctively use this technique.

Aside from the morphology, both of these bench press types can be used to focus the work on the pectoralis major (elbows spread apart) or onto the deltoids (elbows close together).

! In the bench press, it is important to consider an individual's morphology.

A A small rib cage combined with long arms increases the trajectory of the bar, making the movement difficult while at the same time limiting the strength developed. Furthermore, when the bar approaches the chest, the pectoralis major is dangerously stretched, which increases the risk of muscle tears and tendon ruptures when heavy weights are used.

B A thick chest coupled with short arms allows one to do a bench press in complete safety by limiting the range of the movement and the stretch of the pectoralis major at the end of the descent of the bar (when the bar touches the chest). It is not surprising that the greatest bench press champions have this morphology.

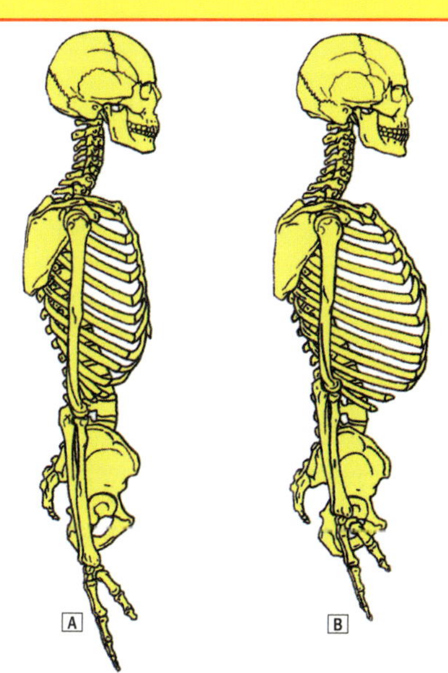

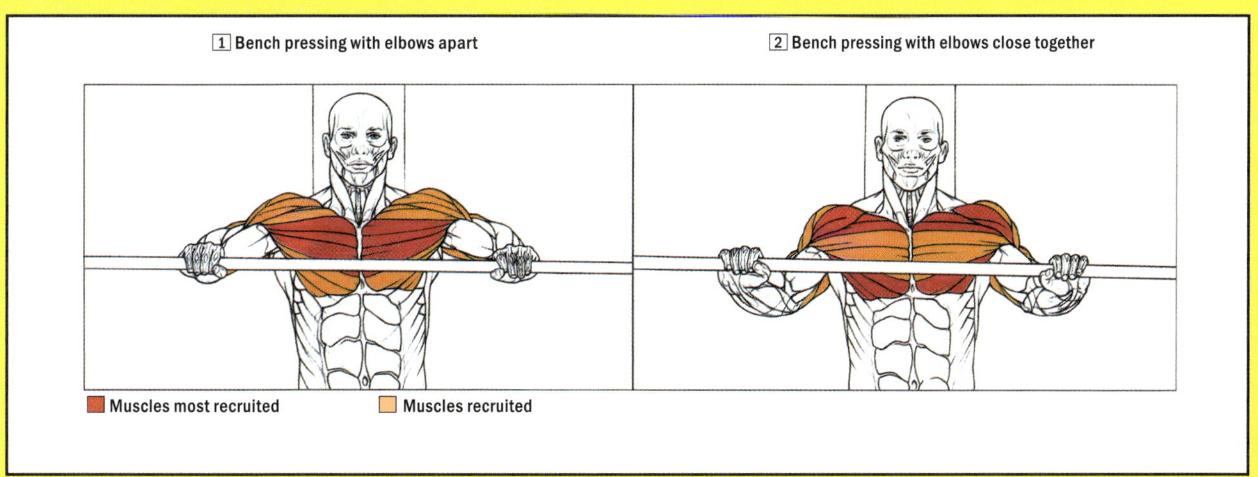

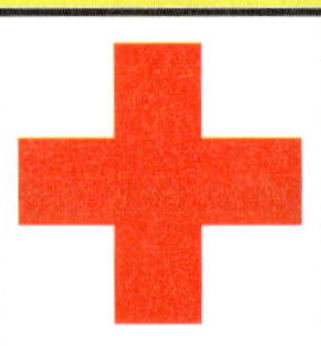

RISK OF INJURY DURING BENCH PRESSES

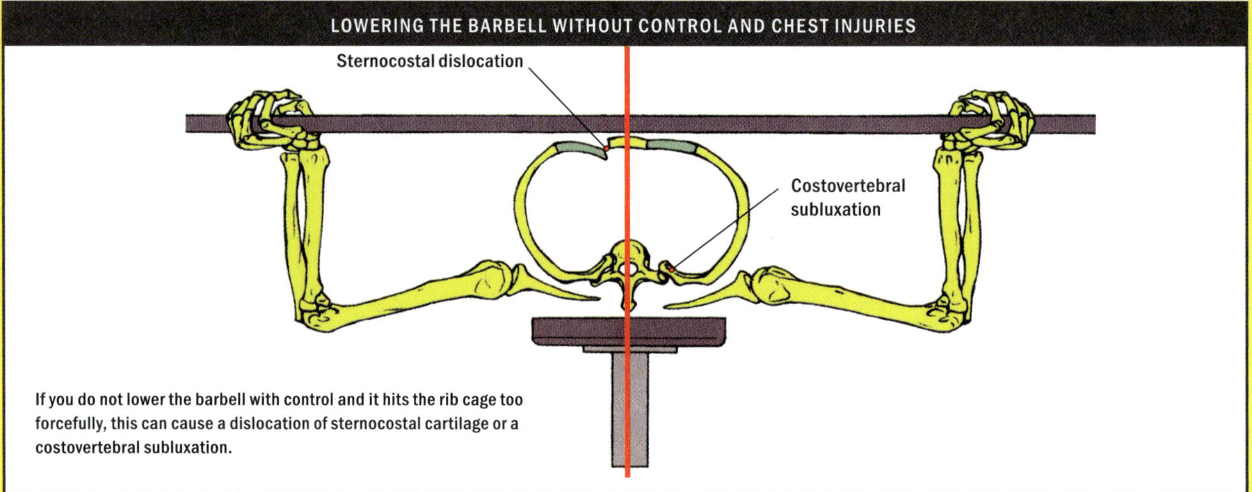

If you do not lower the barbell with control and it hits the rib cage too forcefully, this can cause a dislocation of sternocostal cartilage or a costovertebral subluxation.

Although the bench press is excellent for developing the upper body—mainly the pectorals, triceps, and anterior deltoid—it still poses some risks. Its execution requires good control and constant awareness so you can change positioning if you feel any pain to avoid severe injuries.

When doing a wide-grip bench press, the pectoralis major is particularly stretched at the end of the descent of the barbell (when it touches the chest). This is when you are at highest risk of tearing a muscle or rupturing a tendon.

To reduce the risk, it is important to warm up the muscle at the beginning of the workout with a few long and light series of bench presses and to do some specific stretching movements to equalize the stress in the muscle fibers of the pectoralis major.

If you feel that your pectoralis major is dangerously stretched when you lower the barbell, then you must, as soon as the weight becomes heavy, bring the hands a little closer together on the bar to reduce the stress on the muscles and decrease the risk of injury.

Morphologically, the longer your forearms are, the less thick your rib cage will be, the shorter your clavicles will be, and the greater the risk of injury to the pectoralis major. Although the small stretch of the pectoralis major during the narrow-grip bench press limits the risk of tears as well as tendon ruptures, the position of the glenohumeral joint at the beginning of the exercise (when the arms are straightened) creates joint instability. Subsequently, there is a risk of the humeral head slipping out of the glenoid cavity, which may cause the joint capsule to stretch backward, resulting in painful anteroposterior instability of the shoulder joint.

If you feel any shooting pain at the back of your shoulder during a narrow-grip bench press, it is a good idea to stop doing these exercises for a few weeks to allow the ligaments of the shoulder joint to tighten up so as to prevent an anteroposterior glenohumeral subluxation from developing.

It is also important to control the descent of the barbell to avoid dropping it and bouncing it off of the rib cage. At its point of impact, the force of the barbell on the chest can cause a crushing dislocation of the costal cartilage on the sternum (sternocostal dislocation) or a costovertebral subluxation.

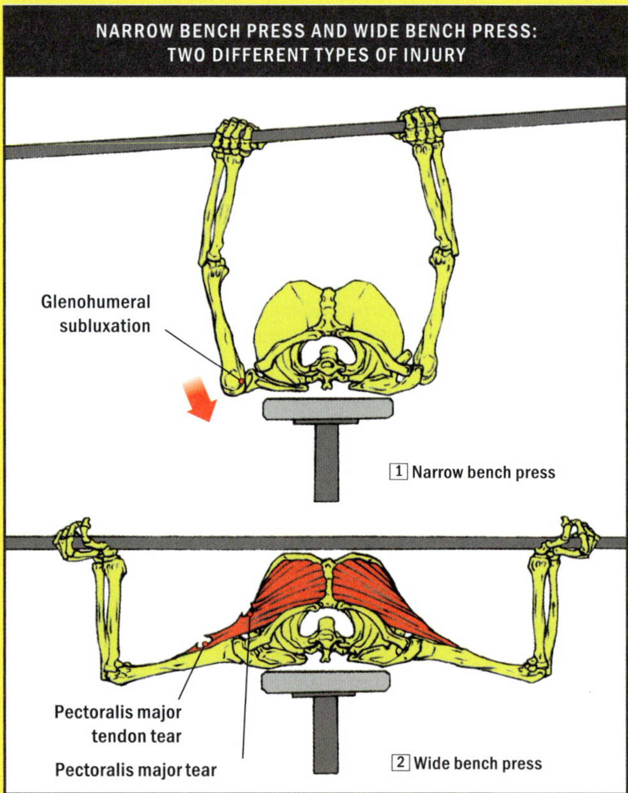

To avoid these two types of traumatic injury, do bench presses on special benches equipped with safety guards that will prevent the barbell from coming into abrupt contact with the rib cage.

ABNORMALITY OF THE BICIPITAL GROOVE OF THE HUMERUS AND DISTENSION OF THE INTERTUBERCULAR SHEATH

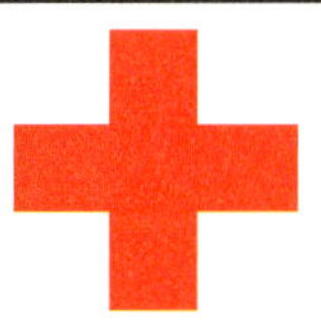

During bench presses, chest presses, shoulder presses, or incline bench presses or incline presses for the shoulders, you may a feel slight pain in the front of the shoulder as well as a feeling of a dislocation, which occurs with a small noise like a slight pop. This pain and noise are not related to the powerful deltoid muscle that covers the shoulder but are linked to two causes: Either the bicipital groove is not deep enough or there is a distension of the intertubercular sheath covering the groove—the first often causes the second.

At birth, the bicipital groove does not exist. During growth, it is the repeated friction of the long head of the biceps brachii tendon that gradually deepens the bone to form the bicipital groove.

However, in an adult, this groove may be shallow, and during arm movements, the biceps brachii tendon may pop out of its groove, deforming and excessively stretching the fibrous sheath covering the top of the groove. As a result, the long head of the biceps brachii tendon can be worn down from too much movement, causing painful tendinitis. Over time, this can even cause degeneration leading to a ruptured tendon.

So, if you feel any pain at the front of the shoulder along with hearing a small popping noise, you should avoid for some time any movements that may be causing this or slightly change the angle, range of motion, and position of the hands to prevent this pain. This allows the intertubercular sheath to tighten in order to regain its function of keeping the long head of the biceps brachii in its groove.

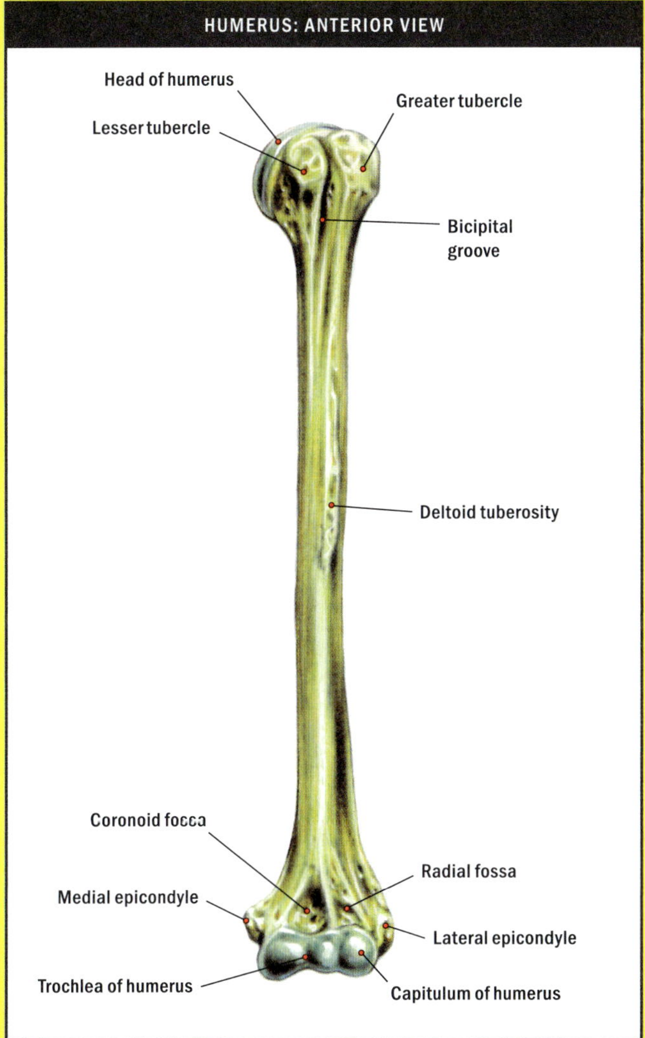

HUMERUS: ANTERIOR VIEW

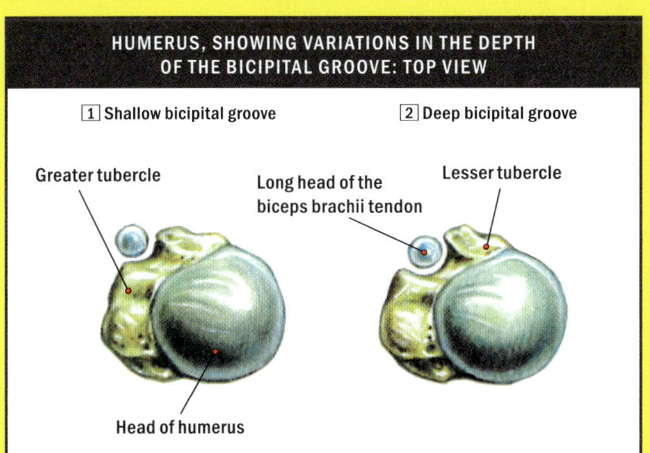

HUMERUS, SHOWING VARIATIONS IN THE DEPTH OF THE BICIPITAL GROOVE: TOP VIEW

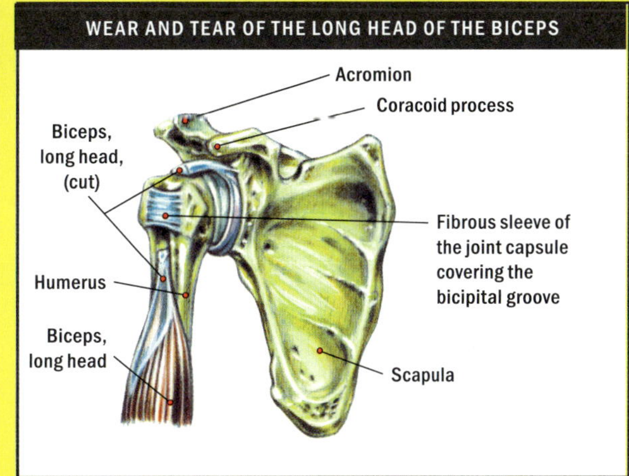

WEAR AND TEAR OF THE LONG HEAD OF THE BICEPS

INFLUENCE OF THE LENGTH OF THE CLAVICLES IN BENCH PRESSES

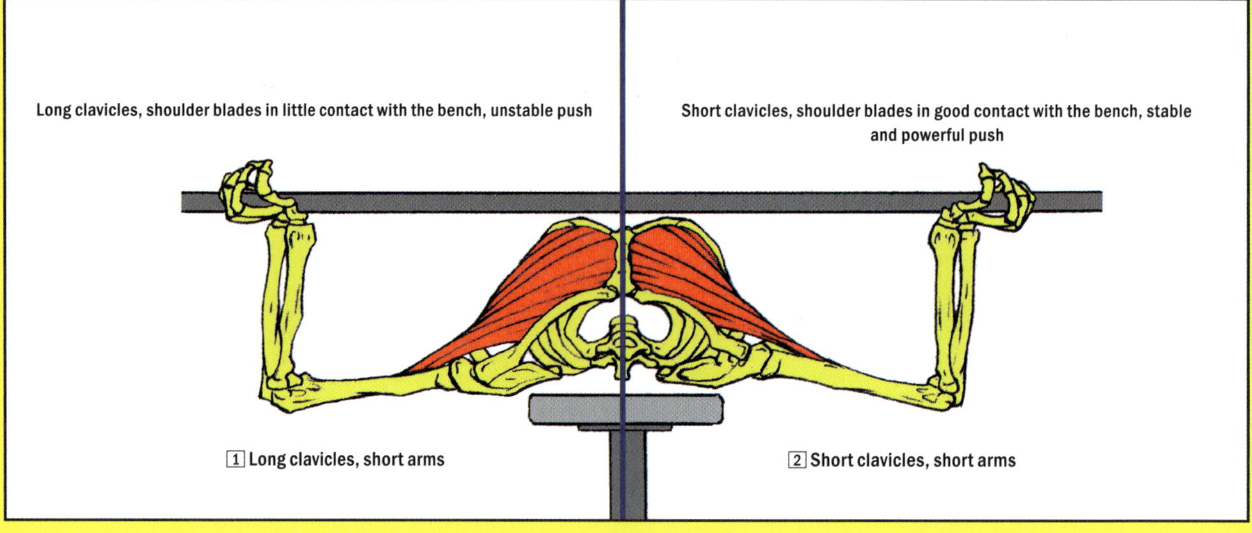

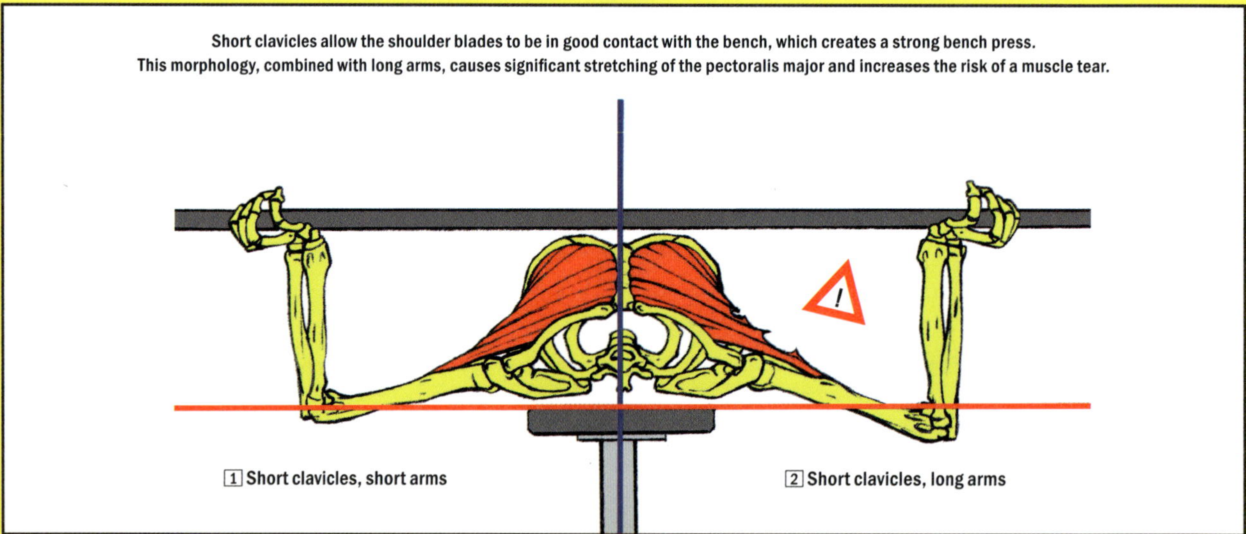

The shoulder width is mainly due to the skeleton and, above all, the length of the clavicles. These bones vary in size and curvature from one individual to another. They are often shorter and curved in women, adapting to the generally more circular and conical shape of their rib cage. Large clavicles enhance the athletic physique and are a certain advantage in many sports; however, in barbell or dumbbell bench presses, they have some disadvantages.

In fact, the narrow width of the bench press backrest is a problem for people with long clavicles. When bench pressing, the shoulder blades will fall outside of the bench and the shoulders will collapse on each side of the backrest. This limits the ability to push vertically with power since the shoulders are not secure on the bench and are in an unstable position. Furthermore, the shoulders collapsing on each side of the bench causes the pectoralis major to overstretch, restricting its power to contract and therefore the possibility of pressing heavy weights.

On the other hand, in people with short clavicles, the shoulder blades will have more contact with the backrest, allowing them to push powerfully and making it easier to press heavy weights.

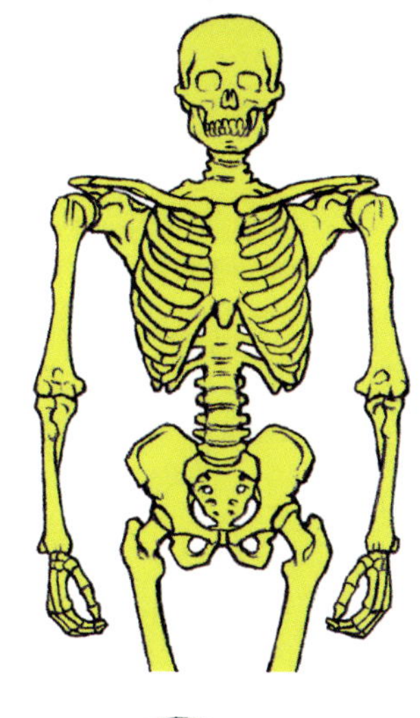

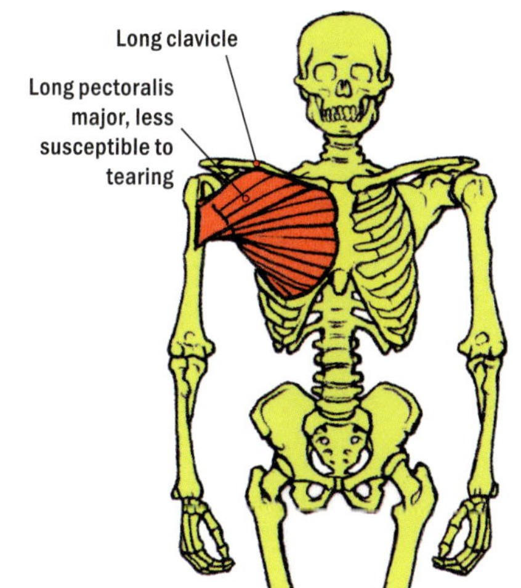

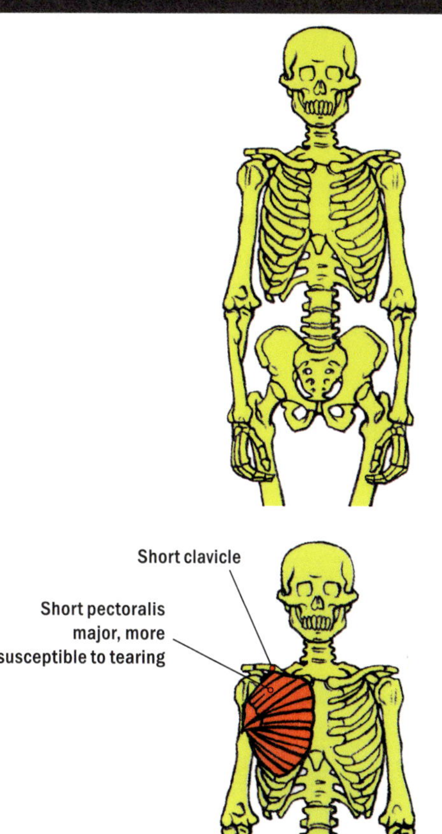

Whether you have short or long clavicles, to have a stable and powerful press, it is important to squeeze the shoulder blades together to increase their contact with the bench. The width of the shoulders primarily depends on the length of the clavicles.

Though people with short clavicles have an advantage in using heavy weights in a bench press, their short pectoralis major muscles are still more prone to excessive stretching and tearing, especially if they also have larger arms.

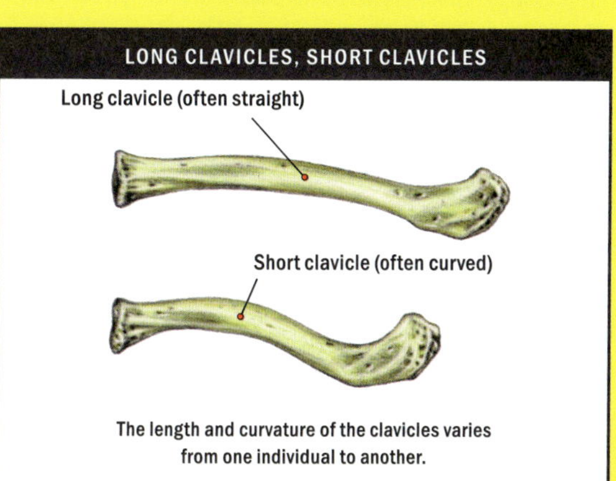

The length and curvature of the clavicles varies from one individual to another.

DECLINE BENCH PRESSES

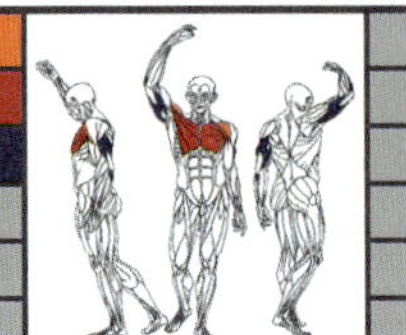

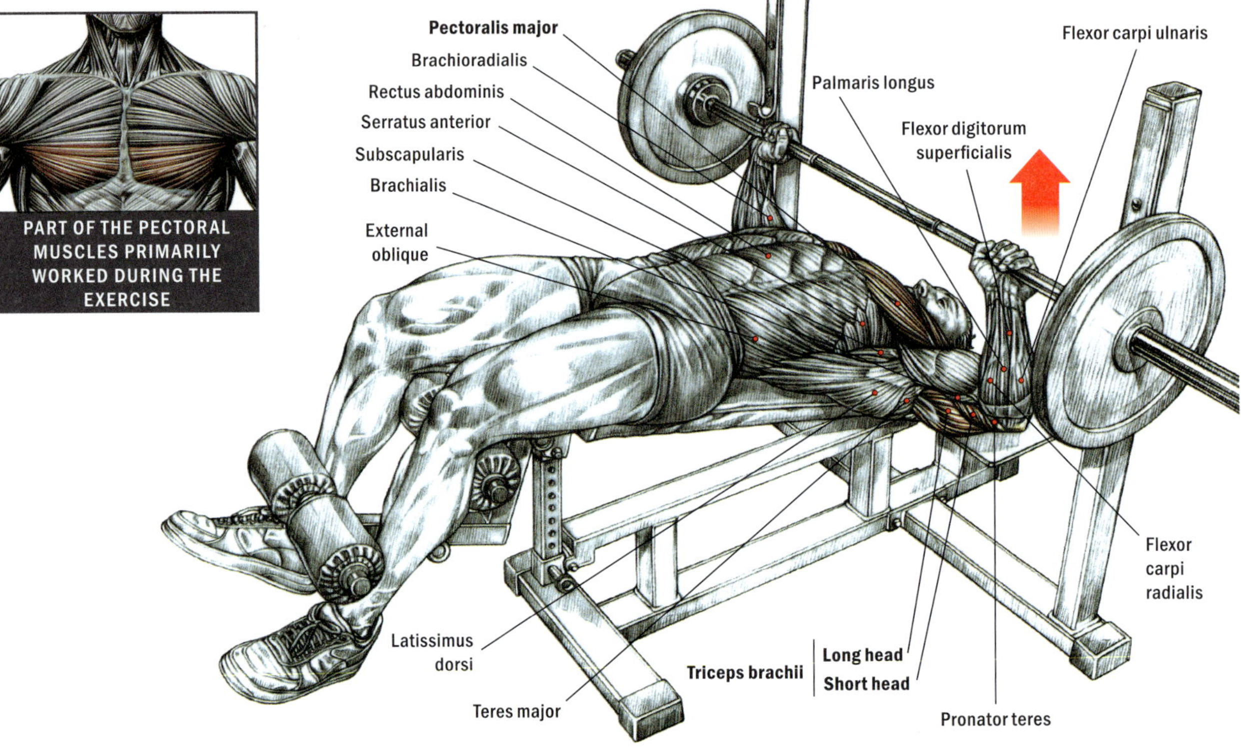

PART OF THE PECTORAL MUSCLES PRIMARILY WORKED DURING THE EXERCISE

Lie on a decline bench (between 20 and 40 degrees), with your head angled down and feet fixed to prevent sliding. Grasp the barbell with an overhand grip that is shoulder width or more:

- Inhale and lower the barbell to your lower chest with control.
- Straighten your arms and exhale at the end of the exercise.

This exercise contracts the pectoralis major (mainly its inferior fibers), triceps brachii, and the anterior deltoid. This exercise is useful for outlining the inferior groove of the pectorals. In addition, using light weights and lowering the bar to the neck makes the pectoralis major more flexible by stretching it correctly. The decline press may be done in a rack.

PERFORMING THE EXERCISE

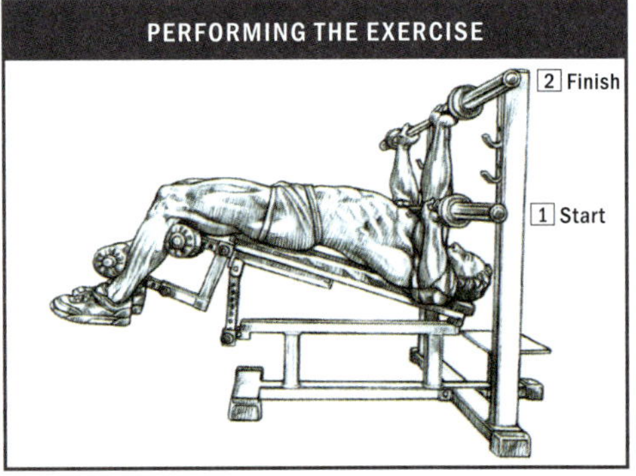

PECTORALIS MAJOR

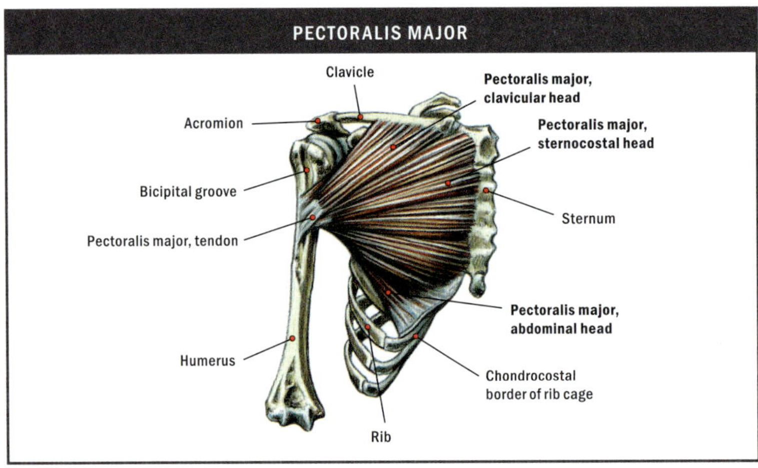

PECTORALIS MAJOR MUSCLE INSERTIONS

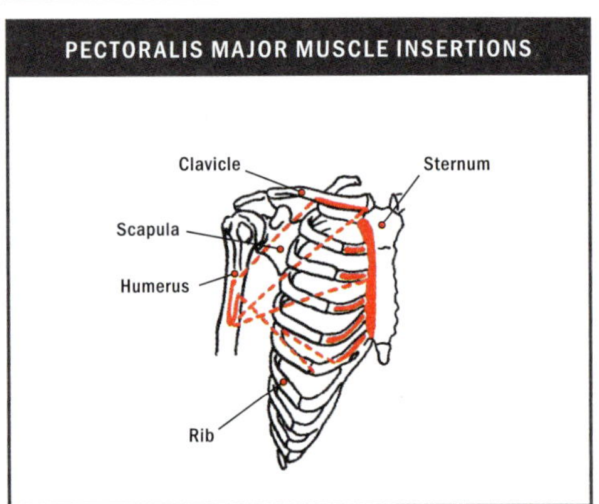

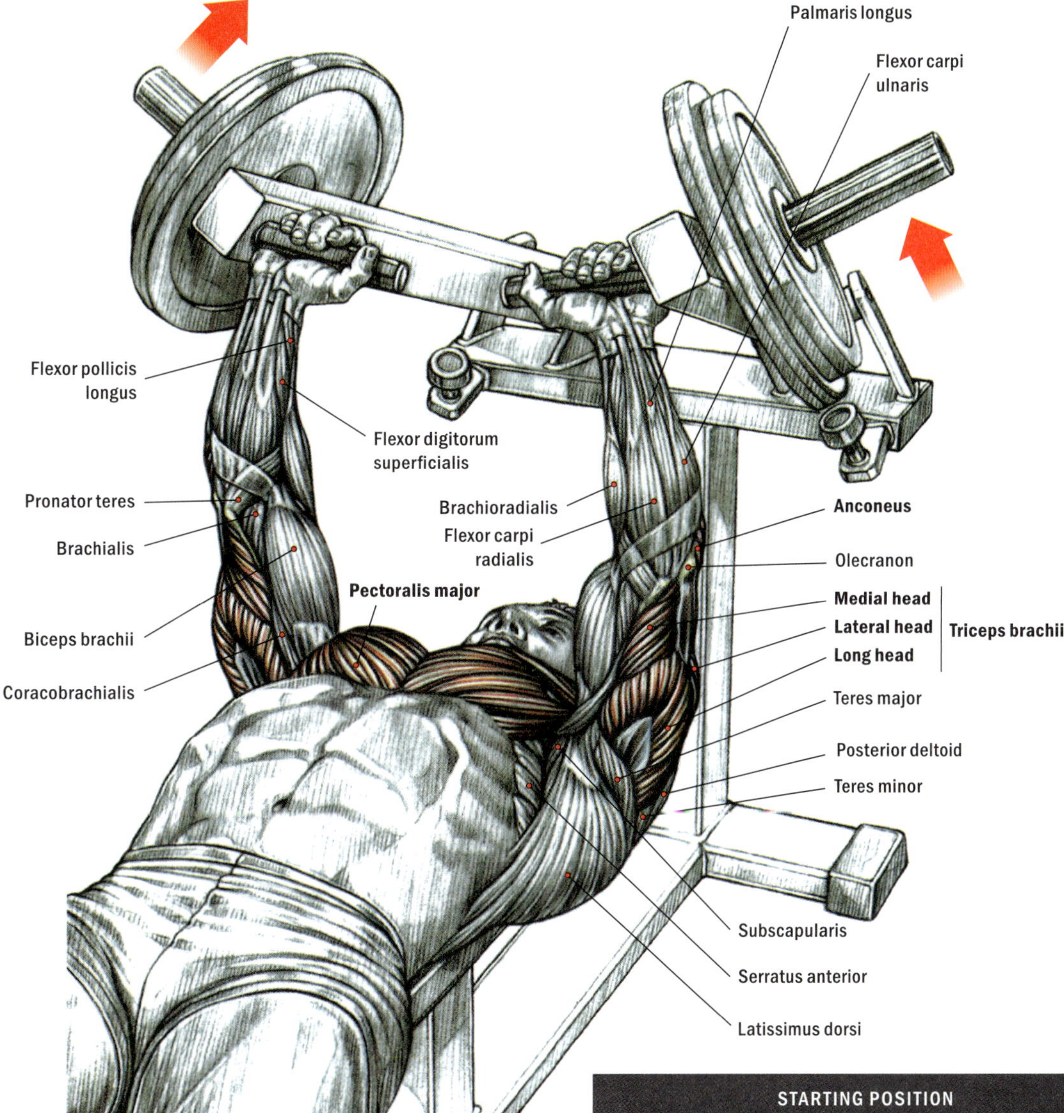

Lie on the machine with your gluteus muscles in contact with the bench and your feet flat on the floor. Grip the handles:

- Inhale and press.
- Exhale at the end of the exercise.

This guided exercise, reminiscent of the dumbbell bench press, focuses the effort on the pectoralis major, mainly on the sternal parts at the end of the exercise.

The triceps and the anterior deltoids are also recruited, although less intensely.

Variation
Arching the back and pushing the chest out places some of the effort onto the lower pectoralis major, but this technique should never be used by people who have back pain.

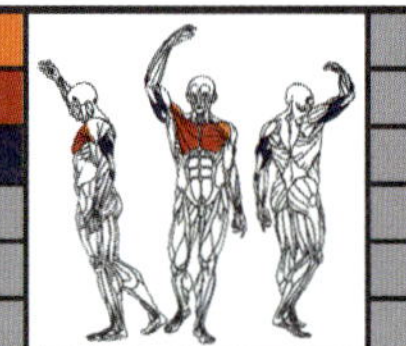

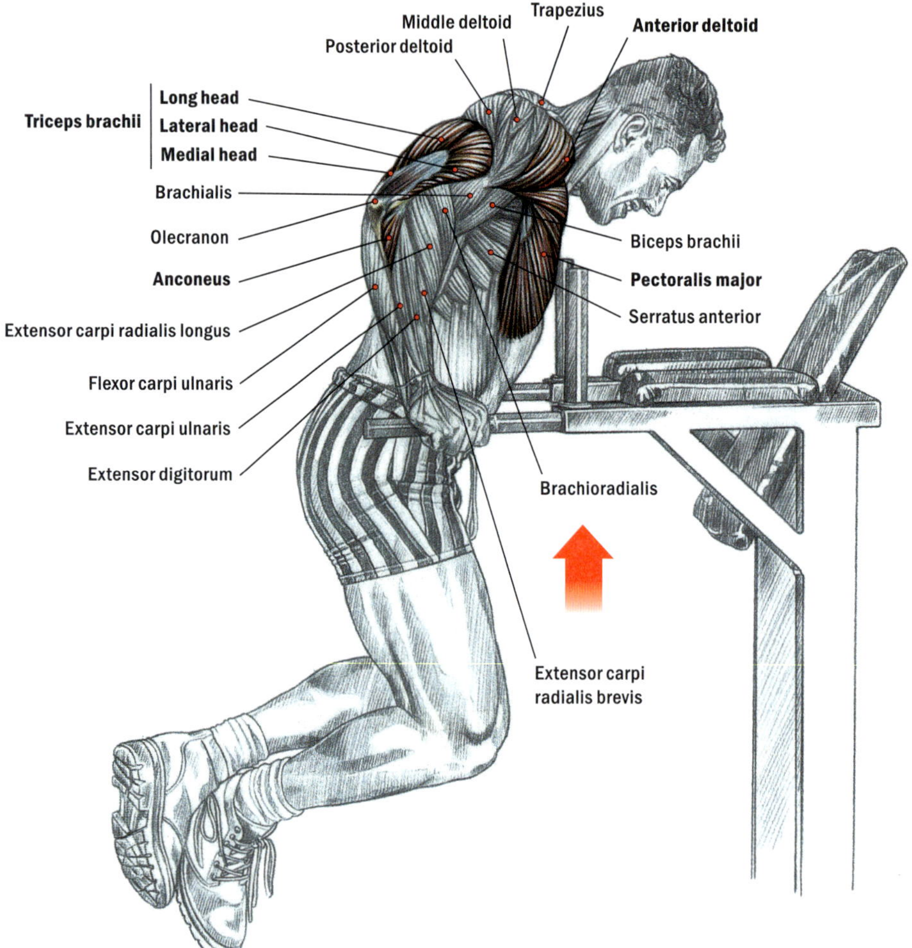

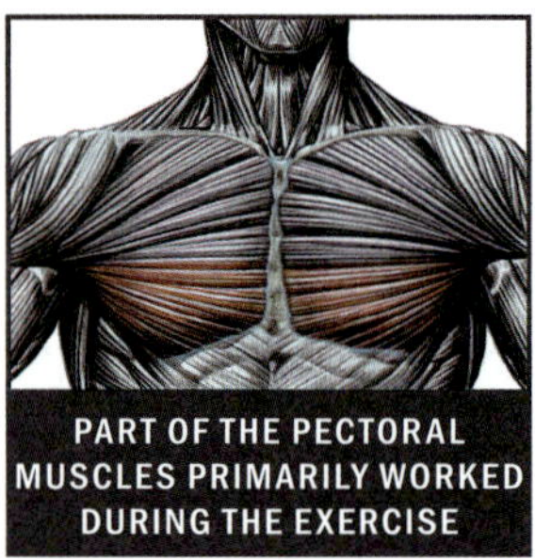

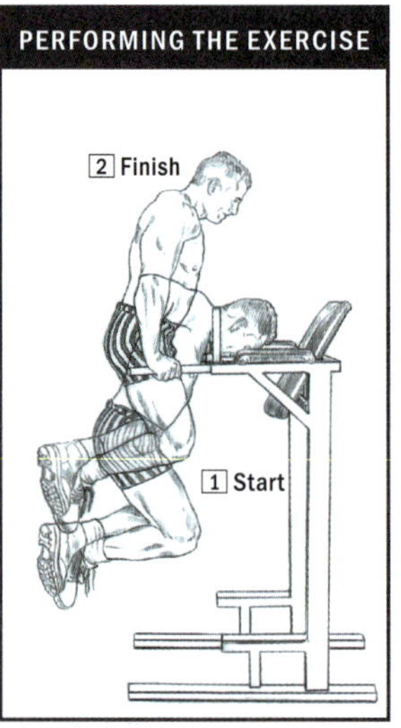

Support yourself on the parallel bars with straight arms and legs hanging:

- Inhale and bend your elbows to bring your chest level with the bars.
- Push up until your arms are straight and exhale at the end of the exercise.

The more the chest is angled forward during the exercise, the more the lower pectorals are worked. Conversely, the more vertical the chest, the more the triceps brachii will be used.

This exercise is excellent for stretching the pectoralis major and for increasing flexibility in the shoulder girdle. However, it is not recommended for beginners because it requires a certain amount of strength. If you are a beginner, use a dips machine to familiarize yourself with the movement.

Sets of 10 to 20 reps provide the best results. For developing more strength and more size, athletes who are used to this exercise can use a weight belt or hang a weight from their legs.

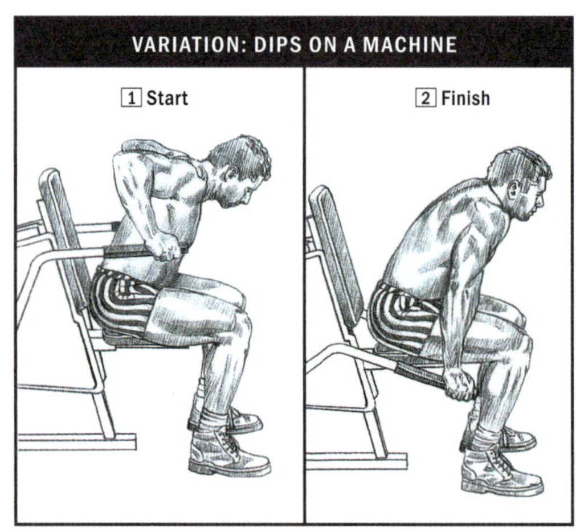

Always do dips carefully to prevent injury to the shoulder joint.

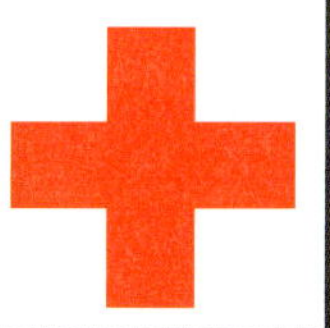

COMPARISON OF A NOT-YET FULLY OSSIFIED STERNUM OF A PREADOLESCENT AND THE STERNUM OF A YOUNG ADULT

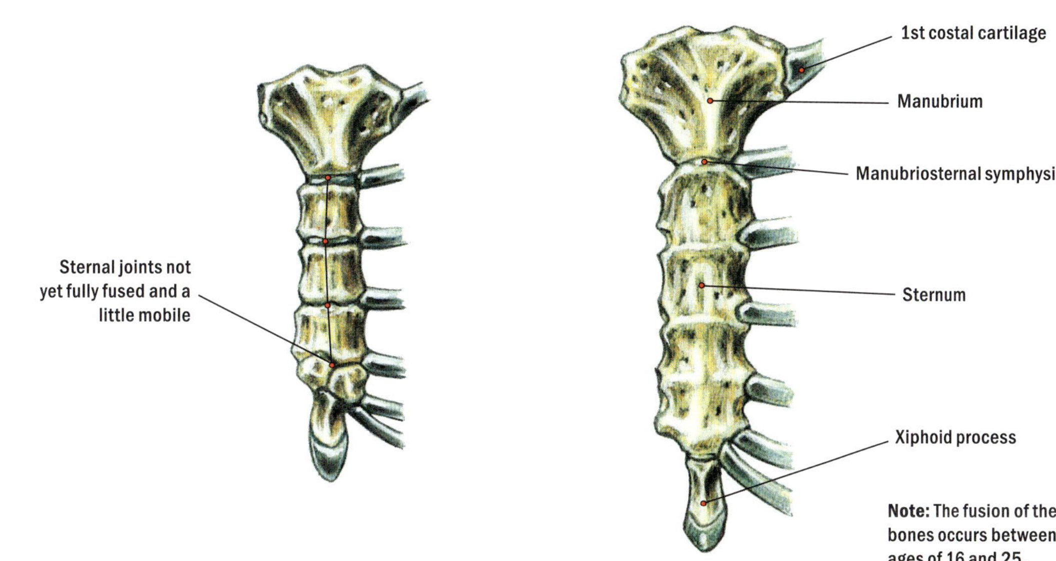

The sternum is not a fixed bone structure. Along with the ribs, it is an actual mobile joint essential for breathing. Like all joints, the sternum can be prone to pain, especially in adolescents and young adults. In fact, in young individuals, the sternum is not yet fully ossified and consists of a set of segments connected to each other by cartilaginous intersections that will disappear with age.

Performing dips tends to pull and open the rib cage. In young people with a not-yet fully ossified sternum, it may cause slight displacements of the segments of the sternum and the attached costal cartilages. Pain can be intense and exacerbated during deep breaths. Cracking, which is often liberating, can be felt when expanding the rib cage and arching the back.

This sternal pathology can also be triggered during bench presses or incline bench presses when the descent of the barbell is not controlled and the barbell hits the rib cage roughly. To prevent pain from persisting, it is best to avoid dips and bench presses with a barbell for some time.

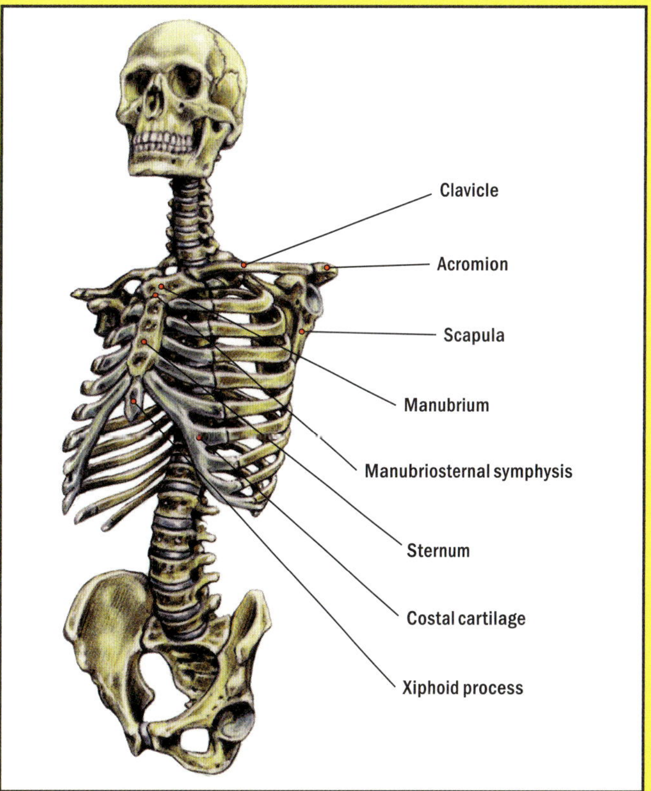

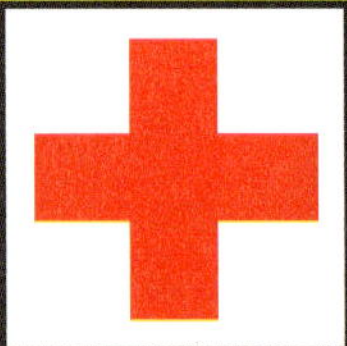

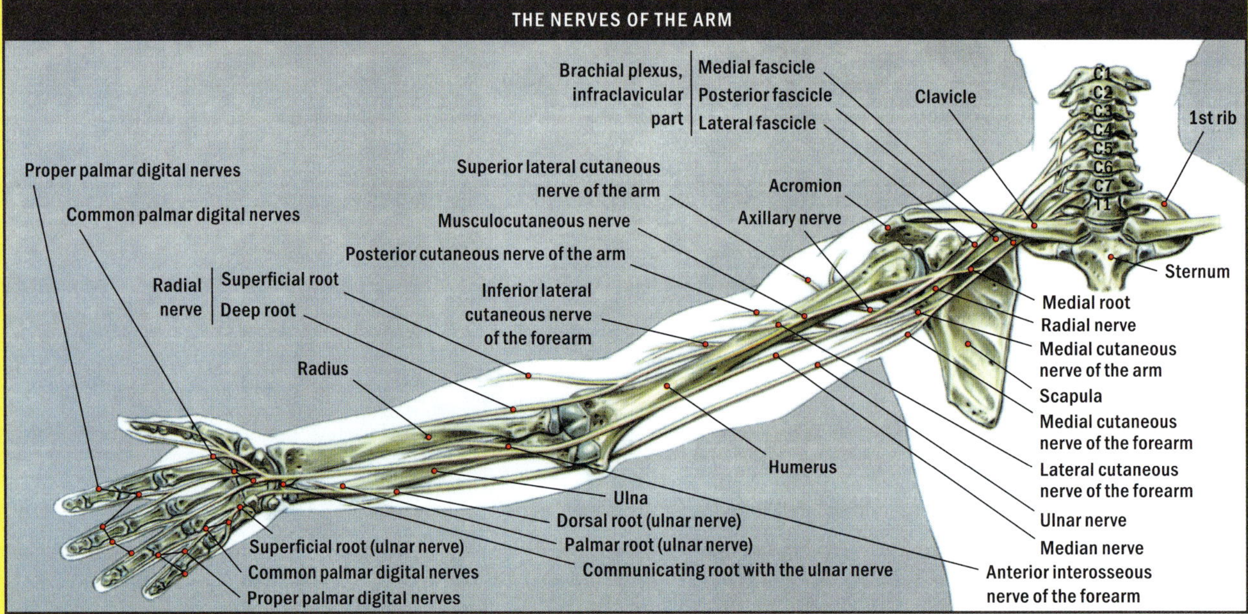

In strength training, a faulty position of the neck during certain exercises may lead to bothersome and incapacitating neuralgia in people predisposed to the condition. These neuralgias manifest as numbness in the arm accompanied by the sensation of pins and needles and sometimes localized numbness.

These symptoms most often appear in the days after doing parallel bar dips (page 100), pec deck rear-delt laterals (page 77), squats (page 168), and deadlifts (page 140), when these movements are done with the neck in extension and the head more or less back. In fact, having the head back can cause spasms and contractions in the deep muscles of the neck, leading to compression of the spinal nerves as they exit from the cervical vertebrae. This compression causes neuralgia that most often affects the brachial plexus at the C4, C5, C6, C7, C8, and T1 vertebrae (C stands for cervical and T for thoracic).

To find out where the affected nerve exits the spine, you need only look at the diagram, then follow the nerve from the area where you feel pins and needles and numbness up to its vertebra.

To avoid neuralgia, do dips or rear-delt exercises on a machine while bringing the head forward and pulling the chin toward the chest. With the squat or deadlift, do the exercise while keeping the neck very straight and looking straight ahead.

If you are experiencing neuralgia, stop doing any exercise that places the head backward with the neck extended.

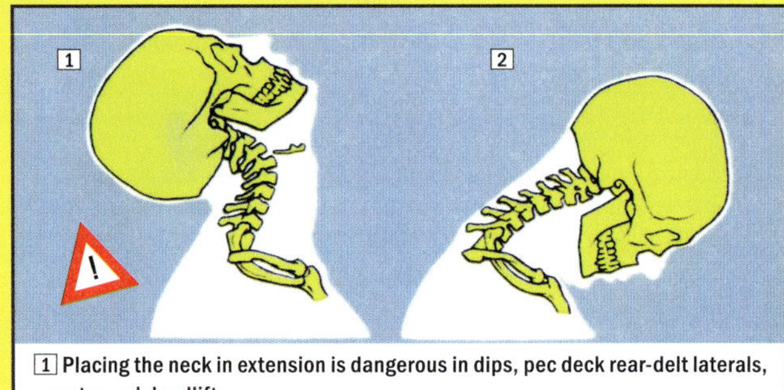

1 Placing the neck in extension is dangerous in dips, pec deck rear-delt laterals, squats, and deadlifts.

2 For people predisposed to cervical neuralgia, positioning the neck forward and the chin against the chest is recommended when doing dips and when doing rear-delt exercises on a machine.

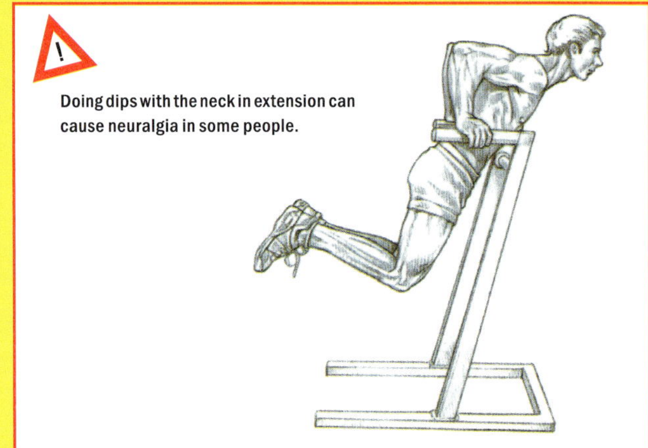

Doing dips with the neck in extension can cause neuralgia in some people.

PUSH-UPS 07

PART OF THE PECTORAL MUSCLES PRIMARILY WORKED DURING THE EXERCISE

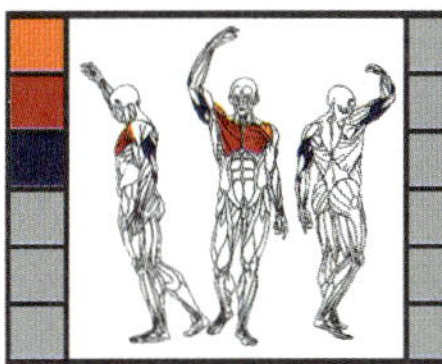

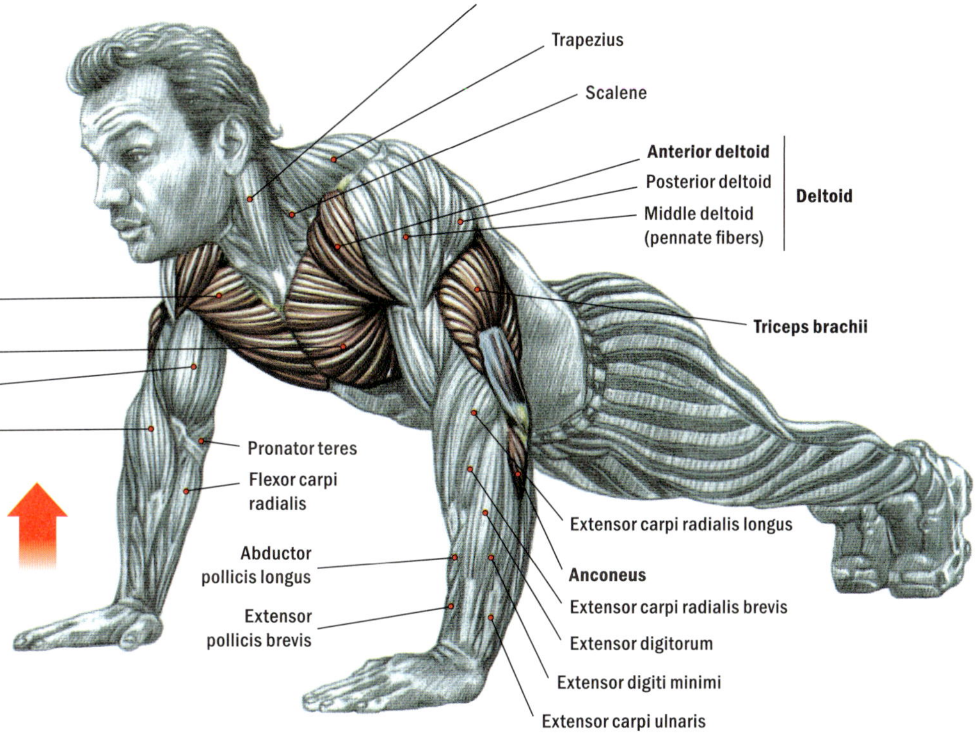

Support yourself on your hands with arms extended, hands shoulder-width (or more) apart, and feet touching or slightly apart:

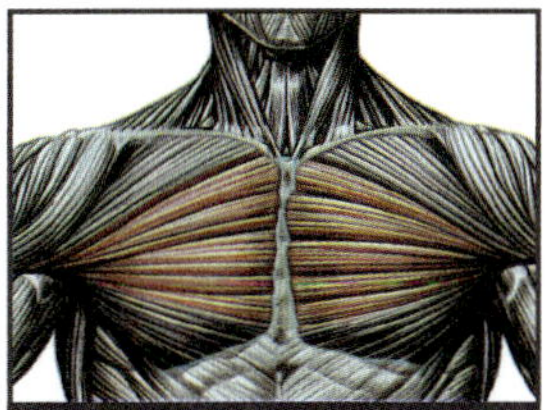

- Inhale and bend your elbows to bring your rib cage close to the ground without arching your lower back excessively.
- Push back up to complete arm extension.
- Exhale at the end of the exercise.

This is an excellent exercise for the pectoralis major and the triceps brachii and can be done anywhere.

STARTING POSITION

Variations

- Varying the angle of the chest focuses the work on different parts of the pectoralis major:
  - Having the feet higher isolates the clavicular head.
  - Having the chest higher isolates the lower part.
- Varying the width of the hands focuses the work on different parts of the pectoralis major:
  - Having the hands spread wide isolates the lateral part.
  - Having the hands closer together isolates the sternal part.

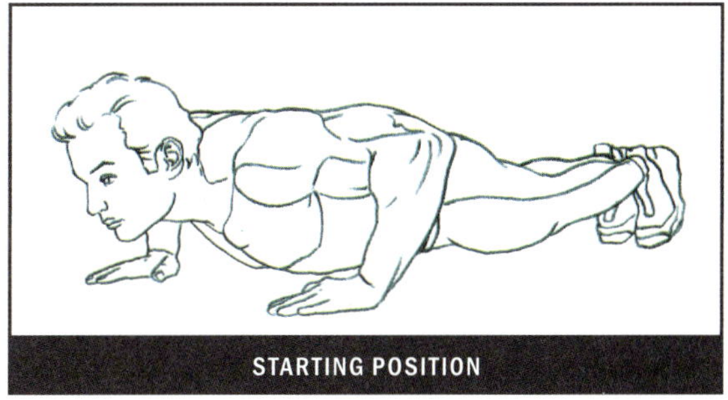

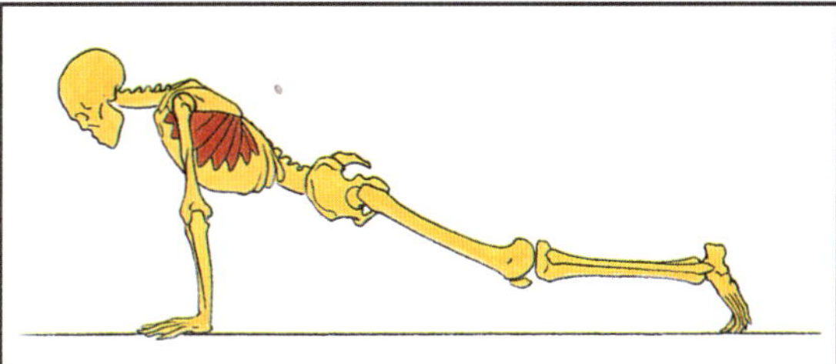

While doing push-ups, the serratus anterior muscles contract and maintain the scapula against the rib cage, locking the arms to the torso.

08 DUMBBELL BENCH PRESSES

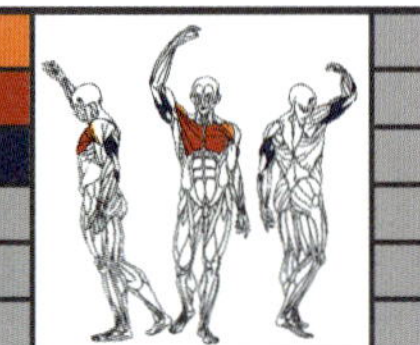

Pectoralis major
Anterior deltoid
Triceps brachii
Humerus

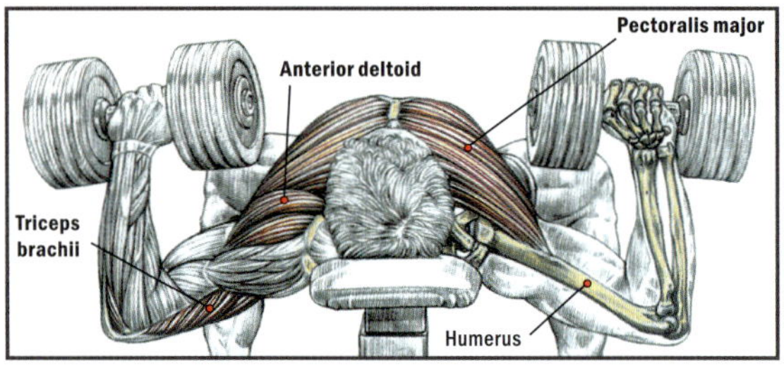

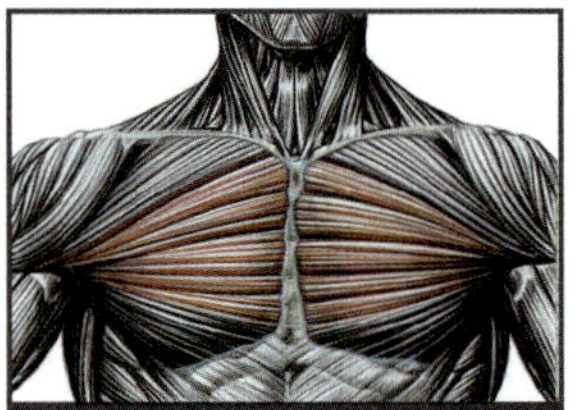

PART OF THE PECTORAL MUSCLES PRIMARILY WORKED DURING THE EXERCISE

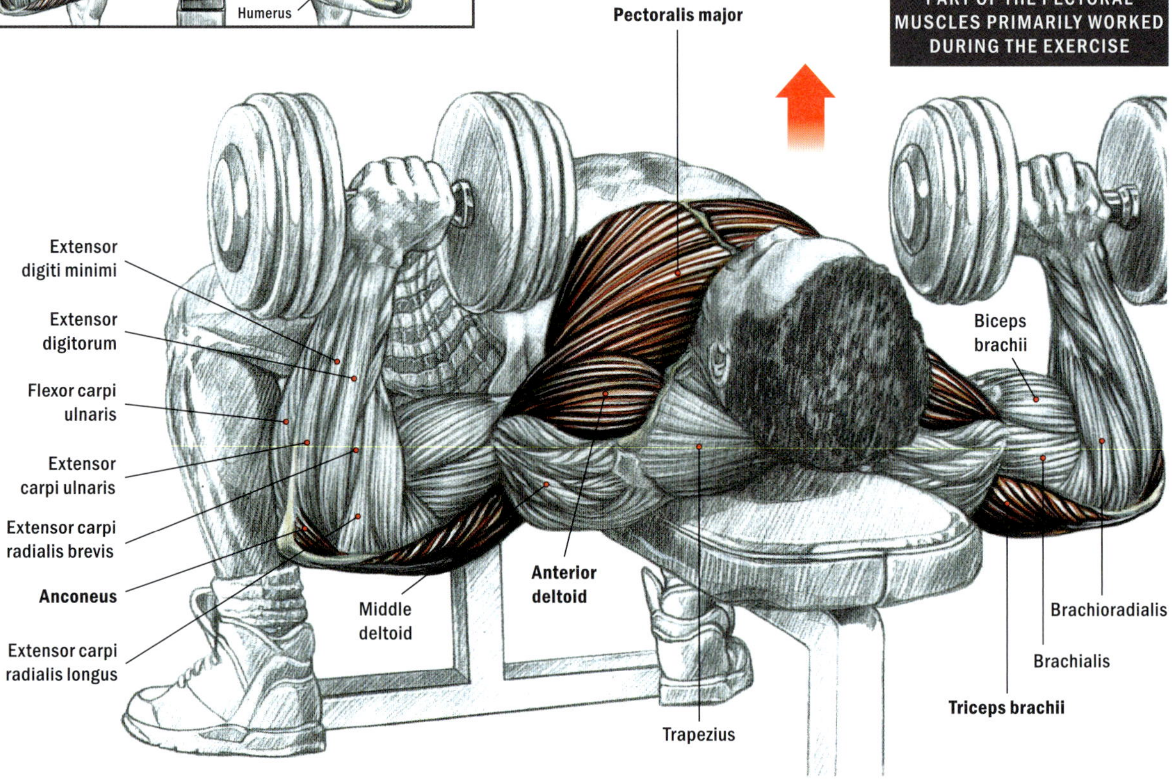

Pectoralis major
Extensor digiti minimi
Extensor digitorum
Flexor carpi ulnaris
Extensor carpi ulnaris
Extensor carpi radialis brevis
Anconeus
Extensor carpi radialis longus
Middle deltoid
Anterior deltoid
Trapezius
Biceps brachii
Brachioradialis
Brachialis
Triceps brachii

Lie faceup on a horizontal bench with your feet flat on the ground for stability and your elbows bent. Hold the dumbbells with an overhand grip at chest level:

- Inhale and extend your arms vertically while rotating your forearms so that your palms face each other.
- Once your hands are facing each other, do an isometric contraction to focus the effort on the sternal head of the pectoralis major.
- Exhale at the end of the exercise.

This exercise is similar to the bench press with a barbell, but with its greater range of motion, it stretches the pectoralis major muscles.

Although not contracted as intensely, the triceps brachii and anterior deltoid are also worked.

VARIATION WITHOUT ROTATING THE FOREARMS

2 Finish
1 Start

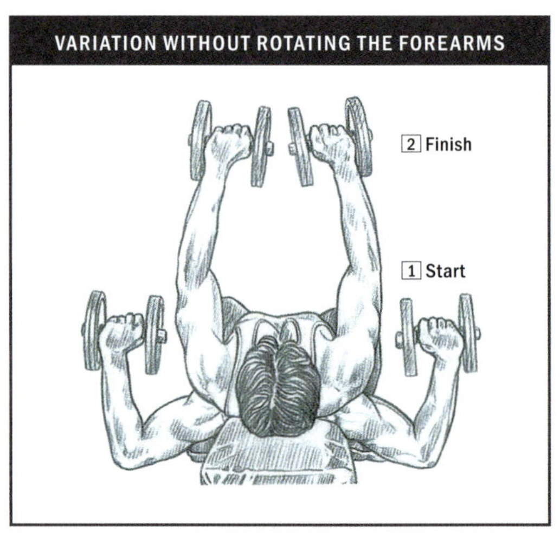

DUMBBELL FLYS 09

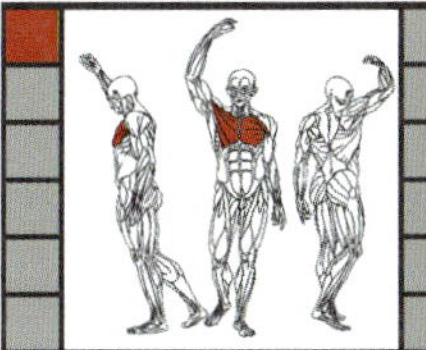

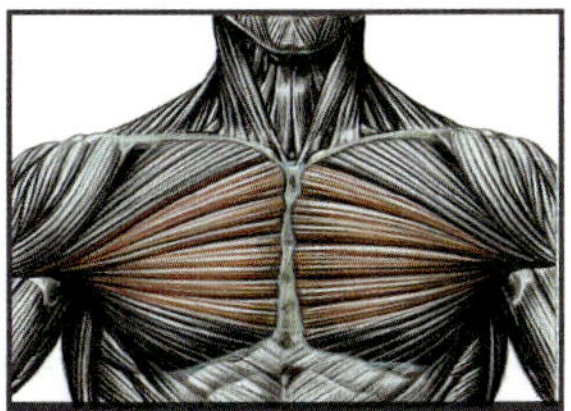

PART OF THE PECTORAL MUSCLES PRIMARILY WORKED DURING THE EXERCISE

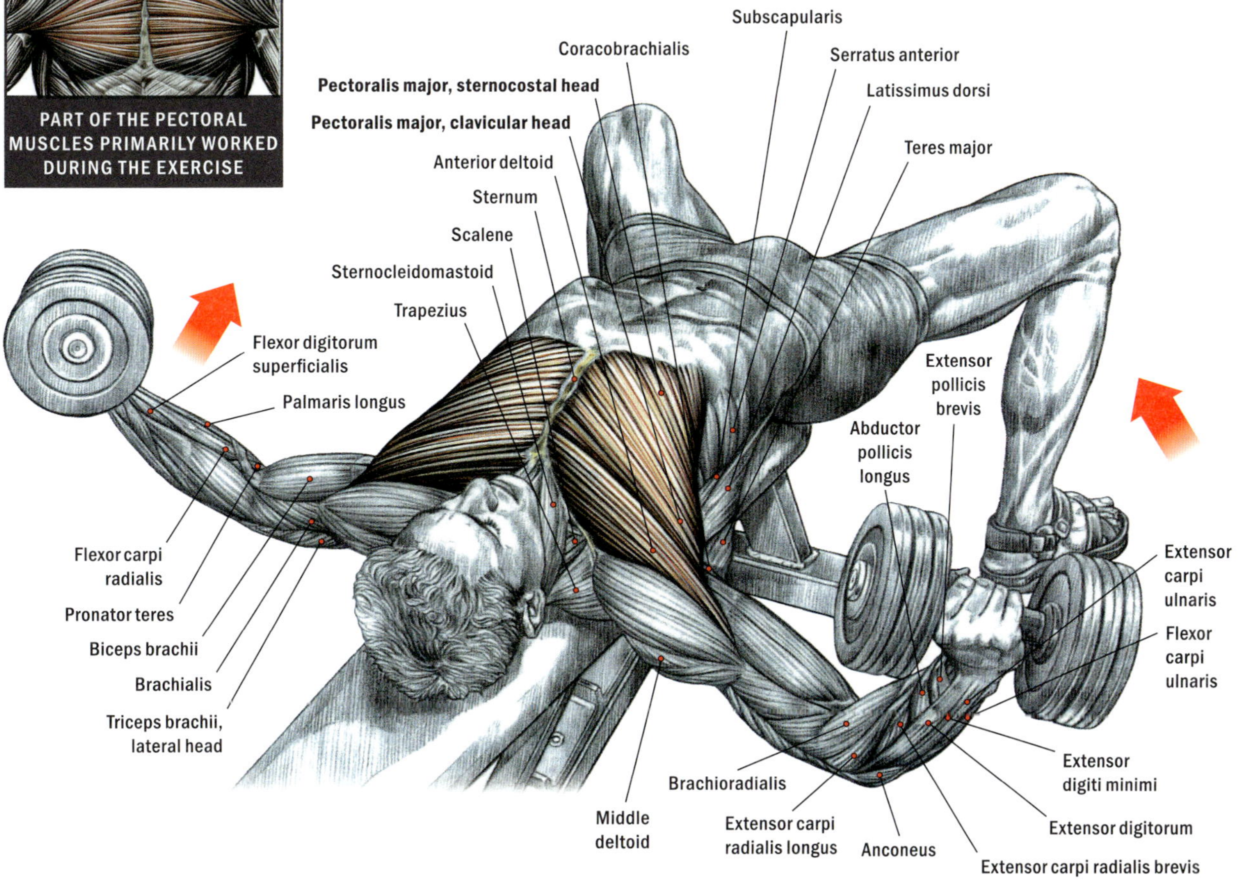

Subscapularis
Coracobrachialis
Serratus anterior
Pectoralis major, sternocostal head
Latissimus dorsi
Pectoralis major, clavicular head
Teres major
Anterior deltoid
Sternum
Scalene
Sternocleidomastoid
Trapezius
Flexor digitorum superficialis
Palmaris longus
Extensor pollicis brevis
Abductor pollicis longus
Extensor carpi ulnaris
Flexor carpi radialis
Pronator teres
Biceps brachii
Brachialis
Triceps brachii, lateral head
Flexor carpi ulnaris
Extensor digiti minimi
Brachioradialis
Middle deltoid
Extensor carpi radialis longus
Anconeus
Extensor digitorum
Extensor carpi radialis brevis

Lie on a narrow bench that will not interfere with shoulder movement and hold a dumbbell in each hand with your arms extended or slightly bent to relieve stress on the joint:

- Inhale and open your arms to a horizontal position.
- Raise your arms to a vertical position while exhaling.
- Do a small isometric contraction at the top of the movement to emphasize the work on the sternal head of the pectoralis major.

This exercise is never performed with heavy weights.

This exercise focuses the work on the pectoralis major. It serves as a basic exercise to increase thoracic expansion, which contributes to increased pulmonary capacity. It also develops muscle flexibility.

To avoid the risk of tearing the pectoral muscles, do this exercise with extreme caution when using heavier weights.

PERFORMING THE EXERCISE

2 Finish
1 Start

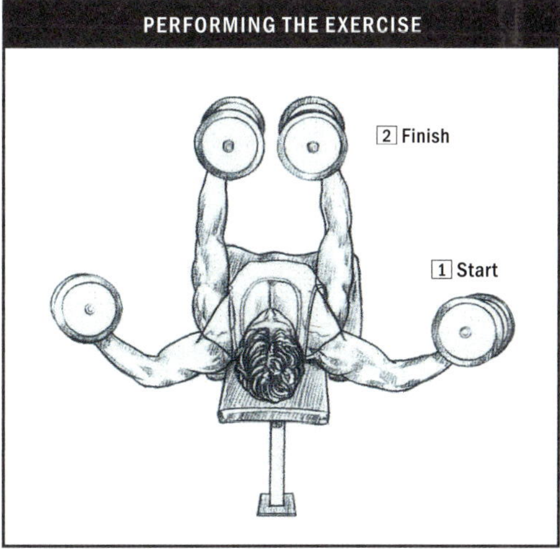

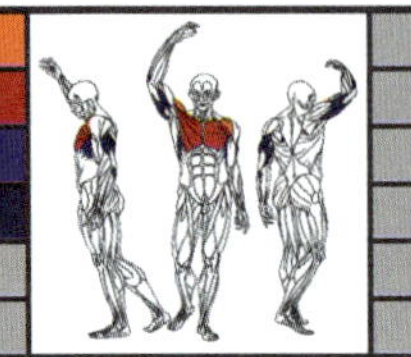

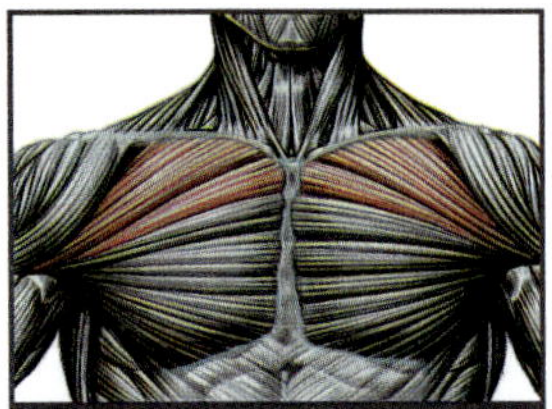

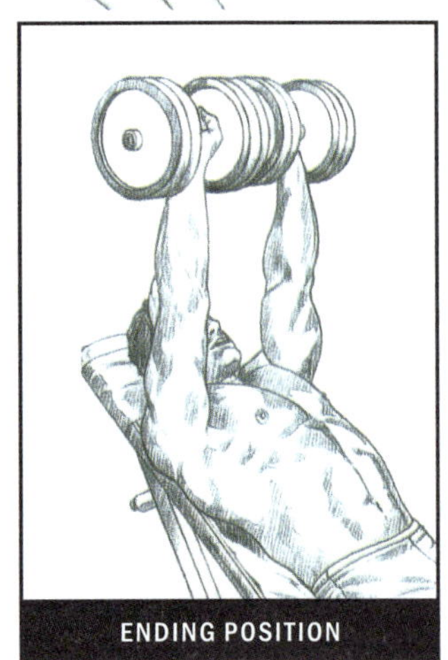

PART OF THE PECTORAL MUSCLES PRIMARILY WORKED DURING THE EXERCISE

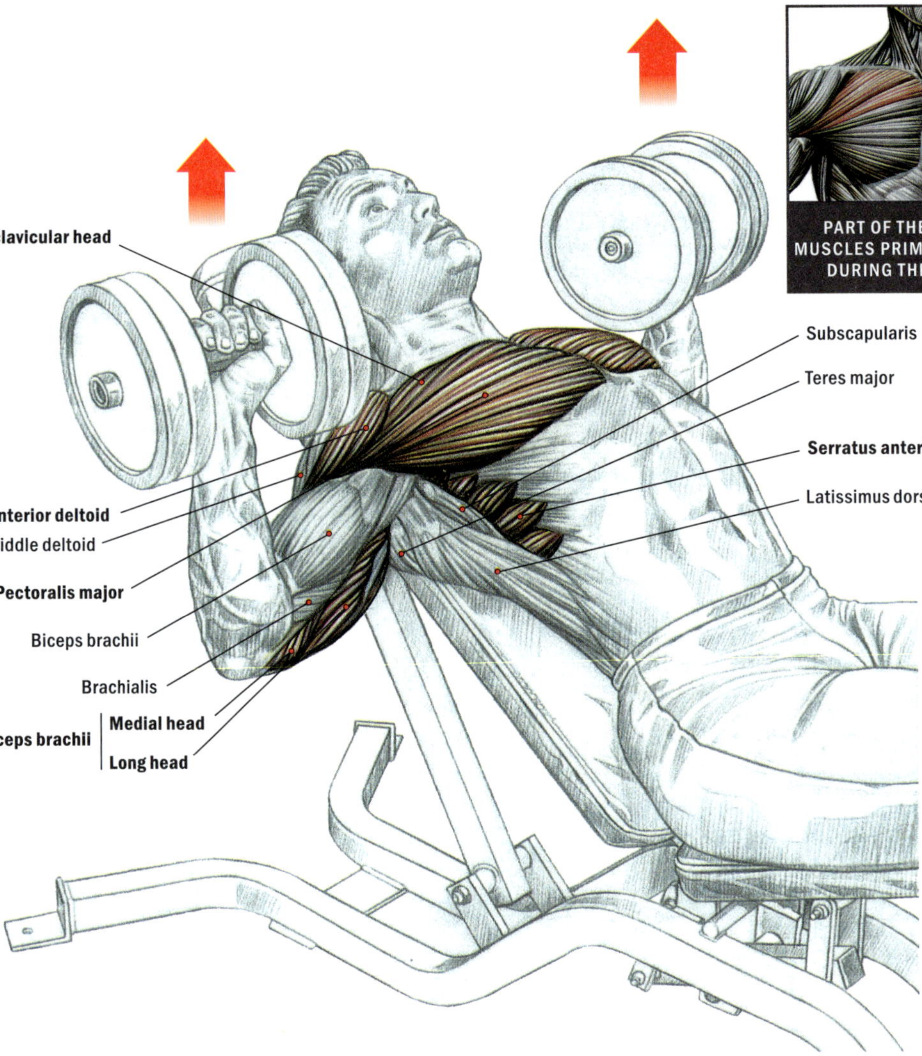

Pectoralis major, clavicular head

Deltoid
- Anterior deltoid
- Middle deltoid

Pectoralis major

Biceps brachii

Brachialis

Triceps brachii
- Medial head
- Long head

Subscapularis

Teres major

Serratus anterior

Latissimus dorsi

Sit on a bench at an angle of no more than 60 degrees (to prevent too much work being done by the deltoids), with your elbows bent.

- Grasp the dumbbells with an overhand grip.
- Inhale and extend your arms vertically, bringing the dumbbells together.
- Exhale at the end of the exercise.

This exercise, which is midway between an incline press and incline dumbbell fly, works the pectorals (mainly the clavicular head) and increases their flexibility. It also works the anterior deltoid, the serratus anterior, and the pectoralis minor (these last two muscles are fixators of the scapula, which stabilize the arm at the torso). It also uses the triceps brachii, but not as intensely as the barbell press does.

Variation

Beginning the press with the hands in an overhand grip and rotating the wrists halfway through the movement so that the dumbbells face each other focuses the effort on the sternal part of the pectoralis major.

ENDING POSITION

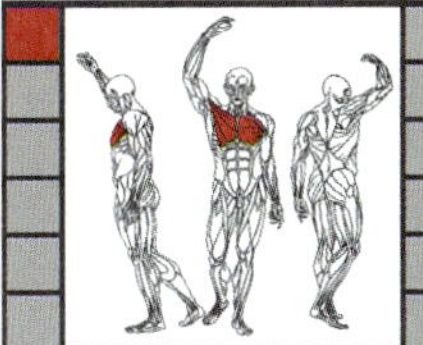

Deltoid

Coracobrachialis

Biceps brachii

Brachialis

Triceps brachii — Medial head

Triceps brachii — Long head

Teres major

Subscapularis

Latissimus dorsi

Serratus anterior

Pectoralis major

Flexor pollicis longus

Extensor carpi radialis longus

Brachioradialis

Flexor digitorum superficialis

Flexor carpi ulnaris

Palmaris longus

Flexor carpi radialis

Biceps brachii, aponeurotic expansion

Medial epicondyle

Pronator teres

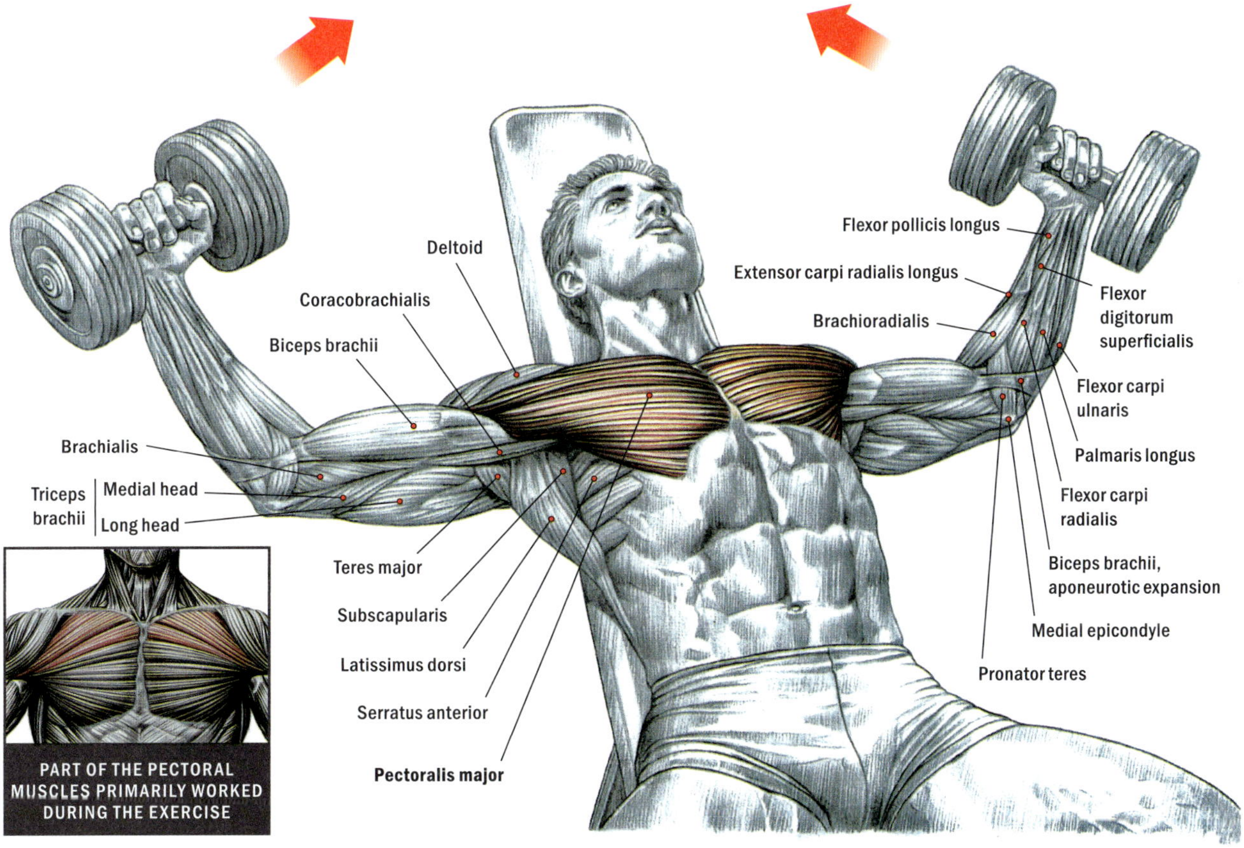

PART OF THE PECTORAL MUSCLES PRIMARILY WORKED DURING THE EXERCISE

Sit on a bench angled between 45 and 60 degrees, with dumbbells in your hands and arms extended or slightly bent to ease stress on your elbows:

- Inhale and bring your arms to a horizontal position.
- Raise your arms to a vertical position while exhaling.

This exercise should not be done with heavy weights. It focuses the effort mainly on the clavicular head of the pectoralis major.

Along with the pullover, it is a fundamental exercise for developing thoracic expansion.

COMPARISON BETWEEN MAN AND A GORILLA

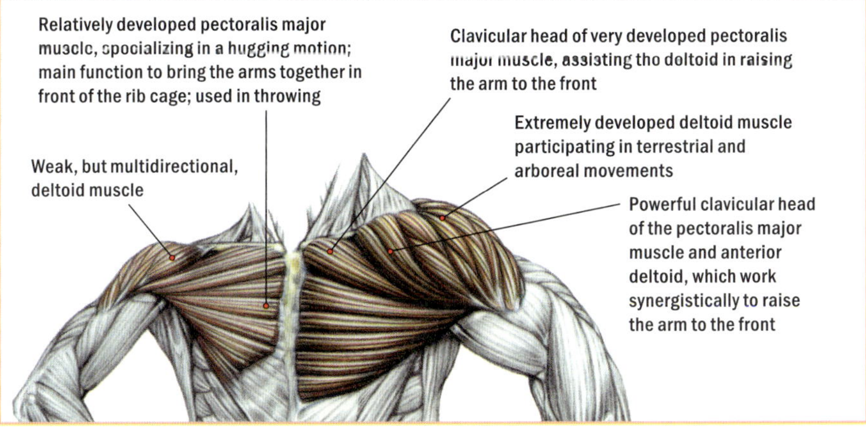

Relatively developed pectoralis major muscle, specializing in a hugging motion; main function to bring the arms together in front of the rib cage; used in throwing

Weak, but multidirectional, deltoid muscle

Clavicular head of very developed pectoralis major muscle, assisting the deltoid in raising the arm to the front

Extremely developed deltoid muscle participating in terrestrial and arboreal movements

Powerful clavicular head of the pectoralis major muscle and anterior deltoid, which work synergistically to raise the arm to the front

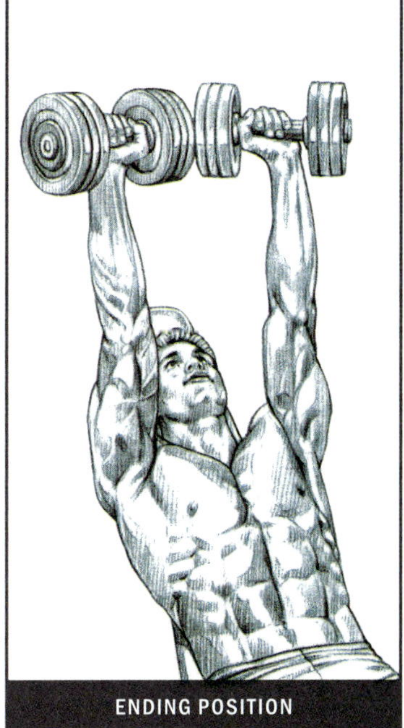

ENDING POSITION

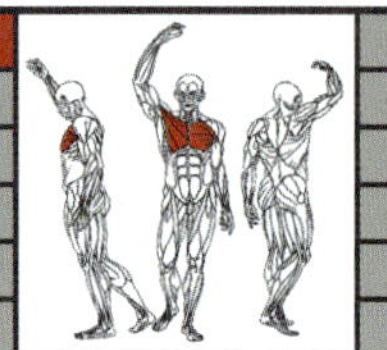

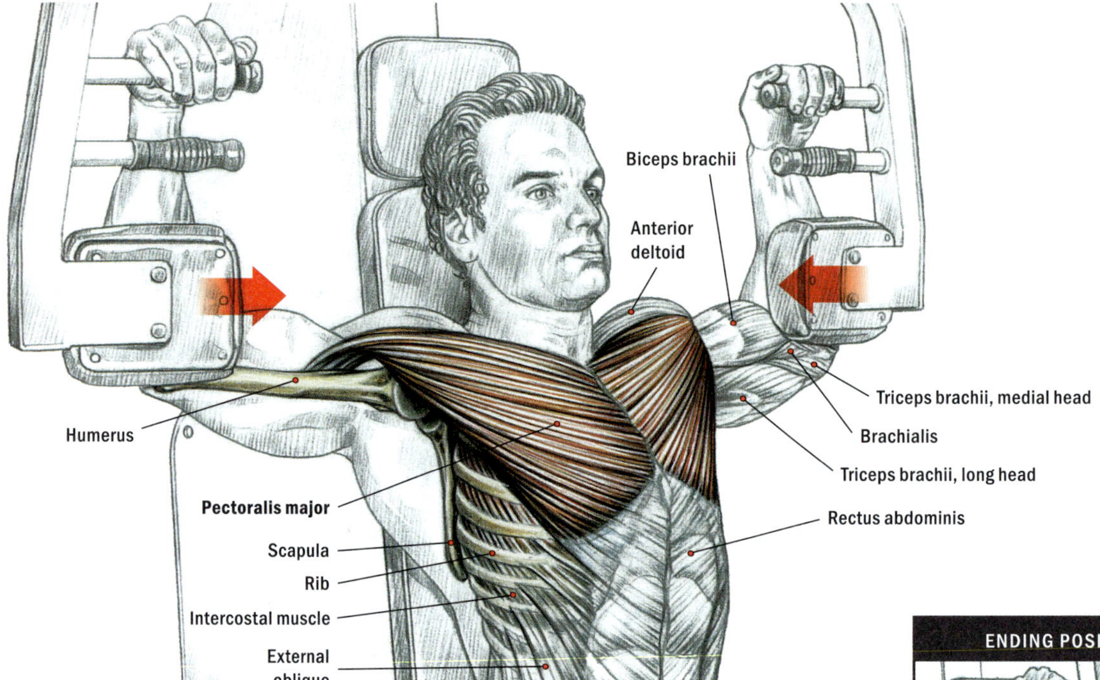

Sit at the machine with your arms open, horizontal, and bent at the elbows. Rest your forearms on the pads, with your forearms and wrists relaxed:

- Inhale and squeeze your arms together.
- Exhale at the end of the exercise.

This exercise works the pectoralis major and stretches it. As the elbows come together, the work is focused on the sternal part of the pectoralis major. This exercise also develops the coracobrachialis and the short head of the biceps brachii. Long sets allow you to pump intensely.

This exercise helps beginners develop enough strength to move onto more complex exercises.

ENDING POSITION

PECTORALIS MAJOR MUSCLE

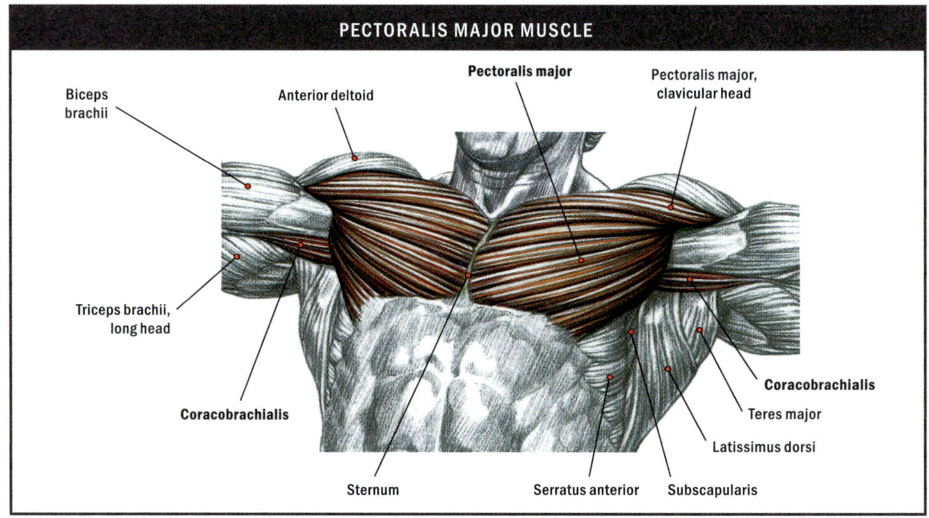

VARIATION ON A MACHINE USING THE HANDS

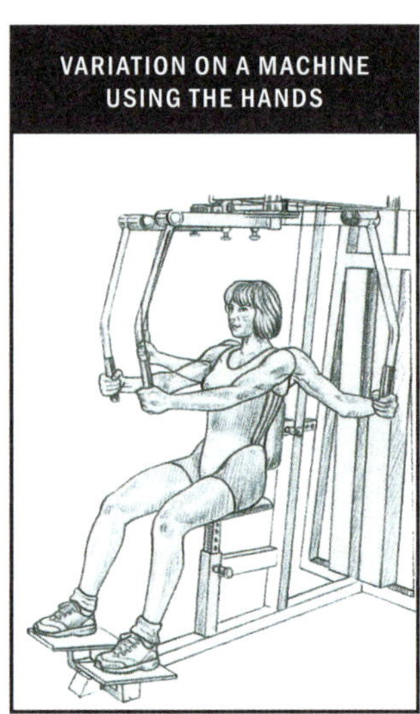

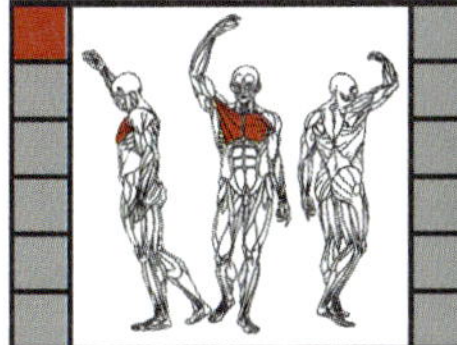

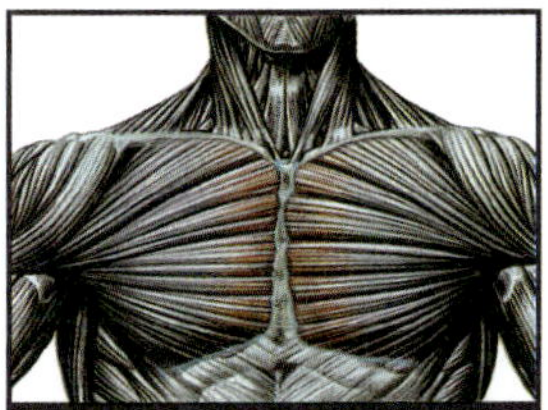

PART OF THE PECTORAL MUSCLES PRIMARILY WORKED DURING THE EXERCISE

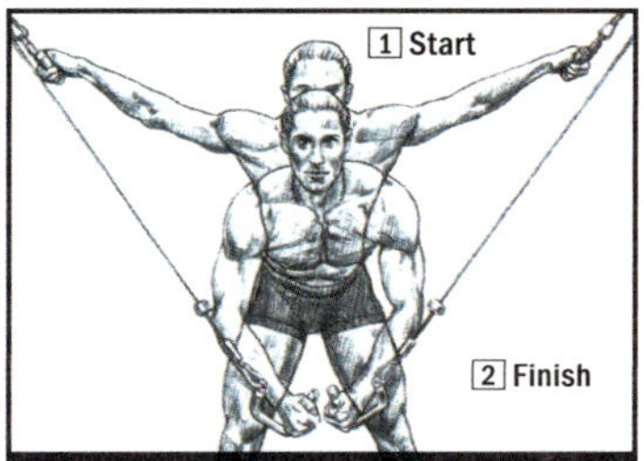

PERFORMING THE EXERCISE

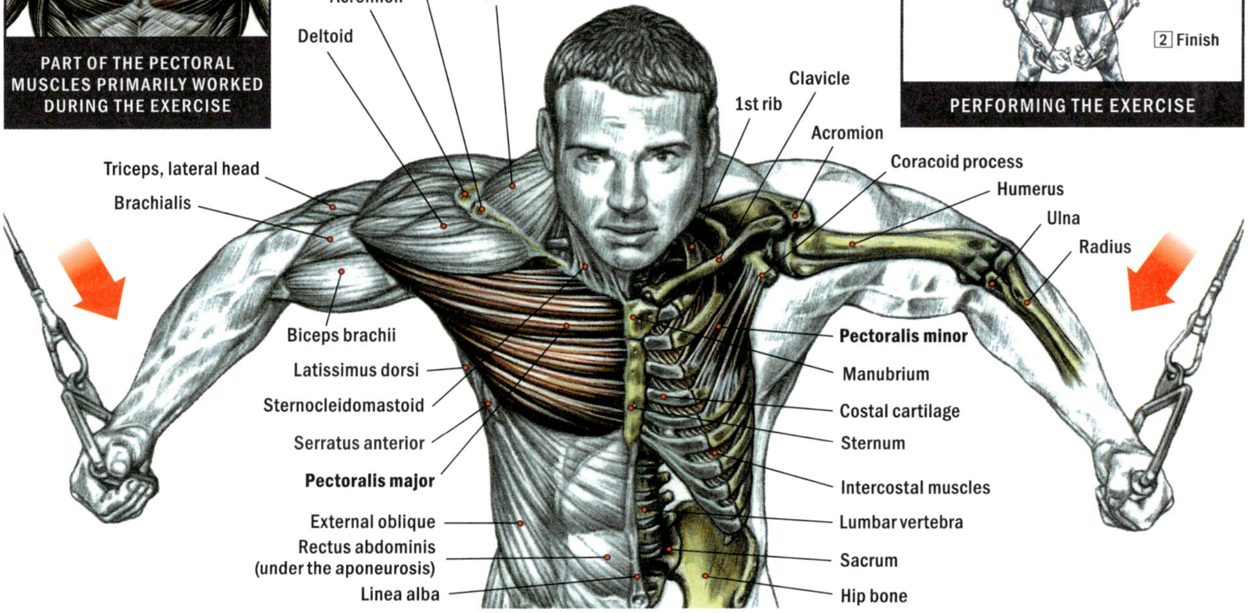

Clavicle
Acromion
Trapezius
Deltoid
Triceps, lateral head
Brachialis
1st rib
Clavicle
Acromion
Coracoid process
Humerus
Ulna
Radius
Biceps brachii
Latissimus dorsi
Sternocleidomastoid
Serratus anterior
Pectoralis major
External oblique
Rectus abdominis
(under the aponeurosis)
Linea alba
Pectoralis minor
Manubrium
Costal cartilage
Sternum
Intercostal muscles
Lumbar vertebra
Sacrum
Hip bone

Stand with your legs slightly apart and lean your torso forward a bit, with your arms spread apart and elbows slightly bent:

- Inhale and squeeze your arms together until the handles touch.
- Exhale at the end of the contraction.
- Return without jerking to the starting position and repeat.

This is an excellent exercise for the pectoralis major muscles. Long sets allow you to develop a good pump. You can work all parts of the pectoralis major by varying the angle of your chest and the working angle of your arms (bringing your arms together at various heights).

STARTING POSITION

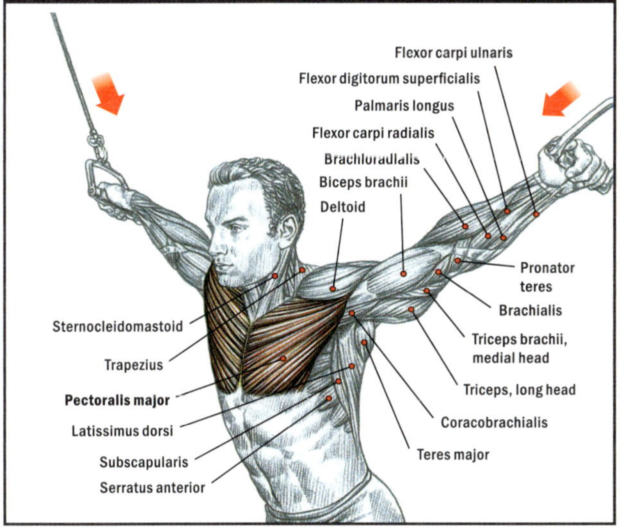

Flexor carpi ulnaris
Flexor digitorum superficialis
Palmaris longus
Flexor carpi radialis
Brachioradialis
Biceps brachii
Deltoid
Sternocleidomastoid
Trapezius
Pectoralis major
Latissimus dorsi
Subscapularis
Serratus anterior
Pronator teres
Brachialis
Triceps brachii, medial head
Triceps, long head
Coracobrachialis
Teres major

Cable crossover flys also contract the pectoralis minor, which is located deeper than the pectoralis major. Besides stabilizing the scapula (shoulder blade), this muscle also pulls the shoulder forward.

ENDING POSITION: VARIATIONS

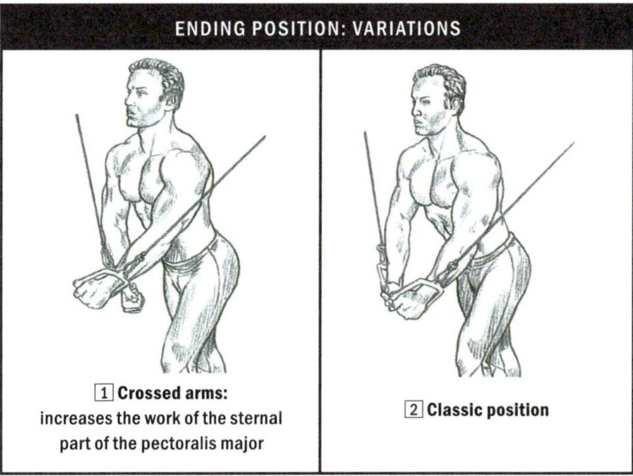

1 **Crossed arms:** increases the work of the sternal part of the pectoralis major

2 **Classic position**

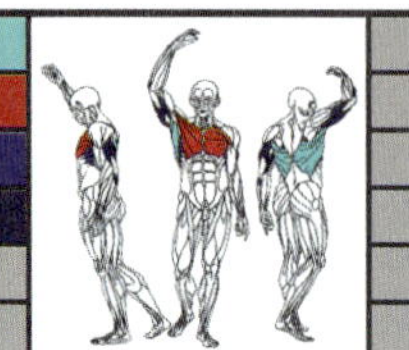

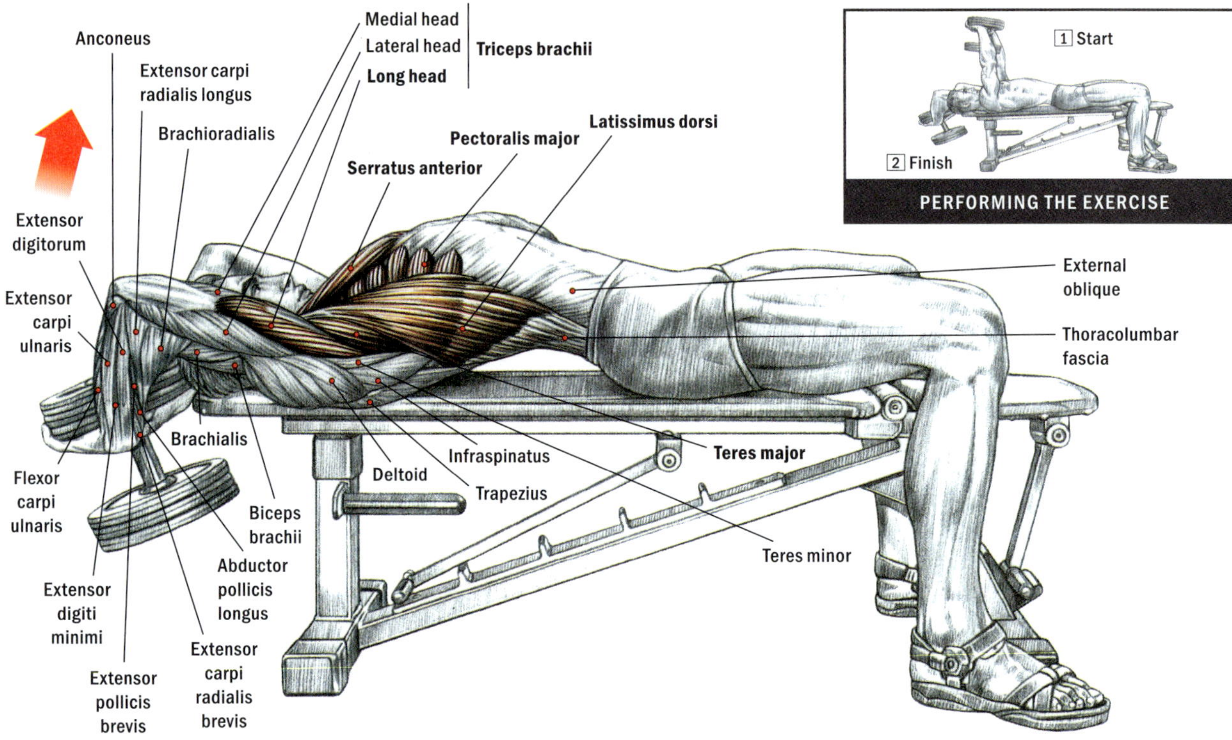

Lie on a bench with your feet flat on the ground and your arms extended. Hold one dumbbell in both hands, with your thumbs and index fingers on the handle and one end of the dumbbell resting on your palms:

- Inhale and lower the dumbbell behind your head, bending slightly at your elbows.
- Exhale and return to the starting position.

This exercise helps develops the bulk of the pectoralis major, the long head of the triceps brachii, the teres major, the latissimus dorsi, the serratus anterior, the rhomboids, and the pectoralis minor. The last three muscles stabilize the scapula so that the humerus can move from a stable base.

If you use this exercise to open the rib cage, you must work with light weights and avoid bending too much at your elbows. If possible, use a convex bench or place yourself across a horizontal bench and position your pelvis lower than the shoulder girdle. Take a deep breath at the beginning of the exercise and breathe out only at the end.

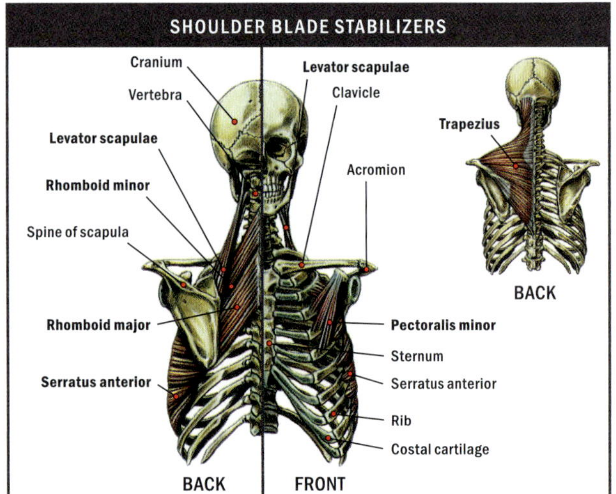

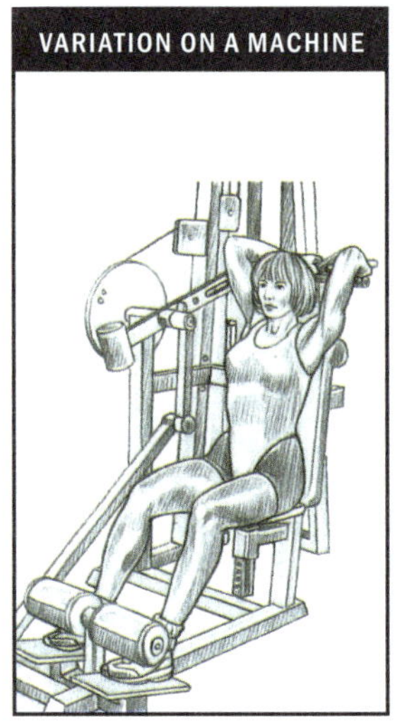

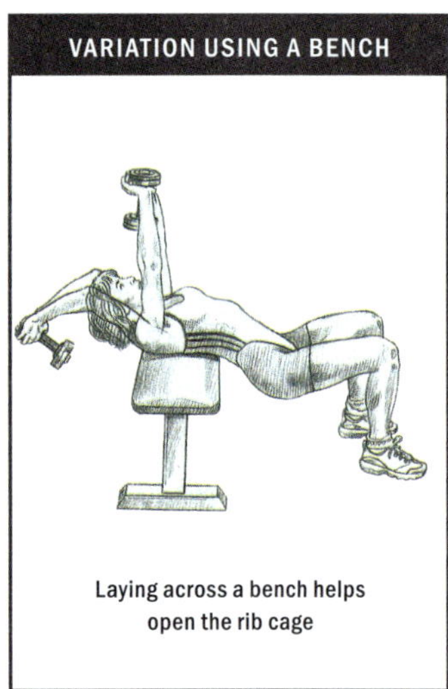

Laying across a bench helps open the rib cage

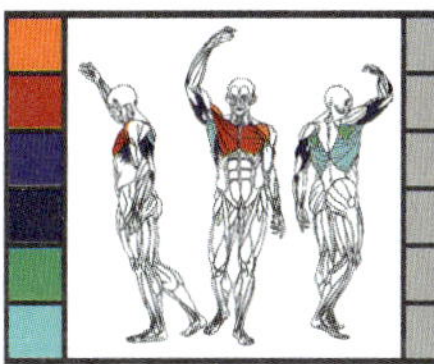

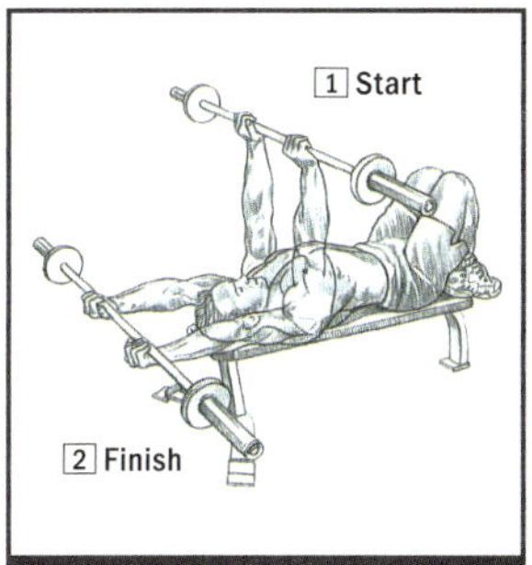

PERFORMING THE EXERCISE

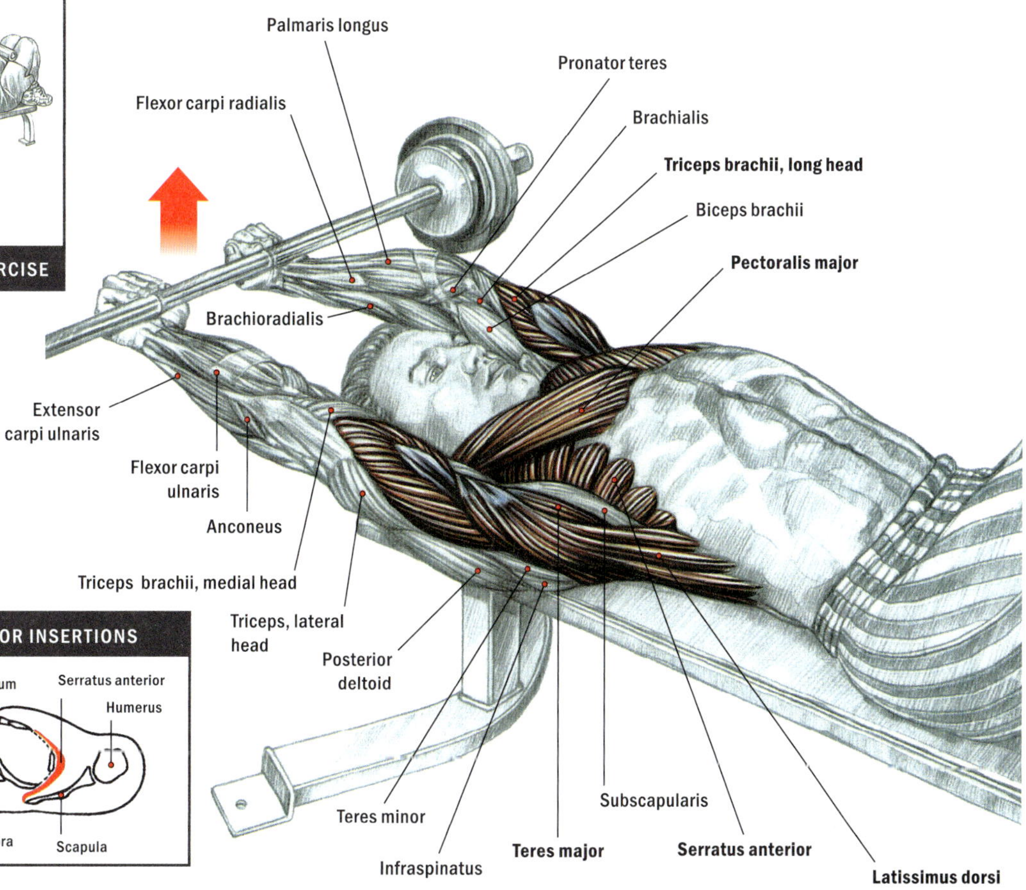

Palmaris longus

Pronator teres

Flexor carpi radialis

Brachialis

Triceps brachii, long head

Biceps brachii

Pectoralis major

Brachioradialis

Extensor carpi ulnaris

Flexor carpi ulnaris

Anconeus

Triceps brachii, medial head

Triceps, lateral head

Posterior deltoid

Teres minor

Infraspinatus

Subscapularis

Teres major

Serratus anterior

Latissimus dorsi

SERRATUS ANTERIOR INSERTIONS

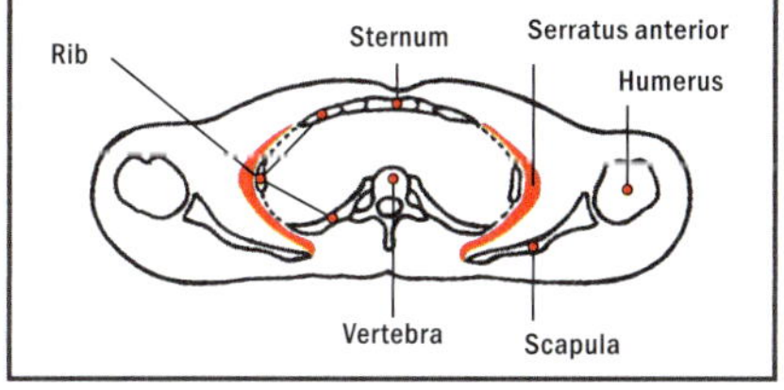

SERRATUS ANTERIOR MUSCLE

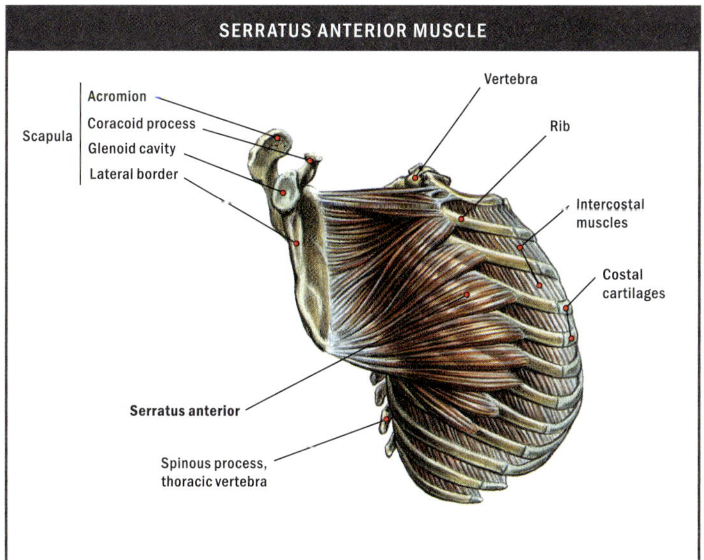

With arms extended, hold the barbell with an overhand grip and hands shoulder-width apart:

- Inhale and expand your chest as much as possible, lowering the barbell behind your head while bending slightly at your elbows.
- Exhale while returning to the starting position.

This exercise develops the pectoralis major, the long head of the triceps brachii, teres major, latissimus dorsi, serratus anterior, and pectoralis minor.

This is an excellent exercise for developing the flexibility to expand the rib cage. It should be performed with light weights using proper form and breathing.

04 # BACK

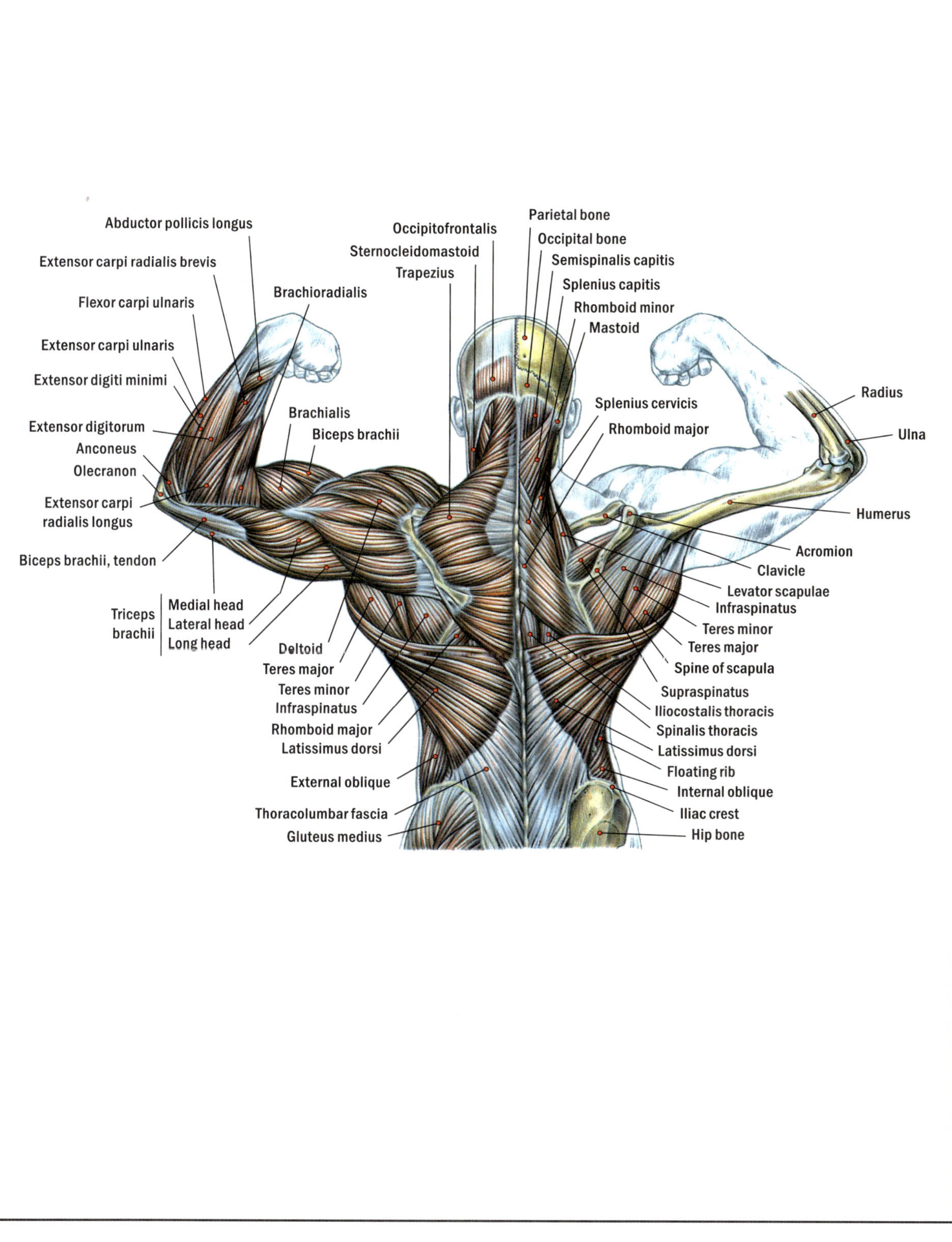

Abductor pollicis longus
Extensor carpi radialis brevis
Flexor carpi ulnaris
Extensor carpi ulnaris
Extensor digiti minimi
Extensor digitorum
Anconeus
Olecranon
Extensor carpi radialis longus
Biceps brachii, tendon
Triceps brachii
Medial head
Lateral head
Long head
Brachioradialis
Brachialis
Biceps brachii
Deltoid
Teres major
Teres minor
Infraspinatus
Rhomboid major
Latissimus dorsi
External oblique
Thoracolumbar fascia
Gluteus medius
Occipitofrontalis
Sternocleidomastoid
Trapezius
Parietal bone
Occipital bone
Semispinalis capitis
Splenius capitis
Rhomboid minor
Mastoid
Splenius cervicis
Rhomboid major
Radius
Ulna
Humerus
Acromion
Clavicle
Levator scapulae
Infraspinatus
Teres minor
Teres major
Spine of scapula
Supraspinatus
Iliocostalis thoracis
Spinalis thoracis
Latissimus dorsi
Floating rib
Internal oblique
Iliac crest
Hip bone

01 CHIN-UPS

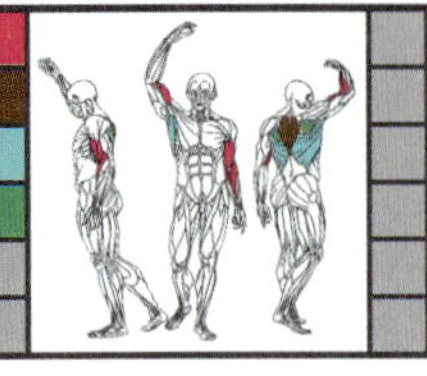

Extensor carpi ulnaris
Extensor digiti minimi
Extensor digitorum
Anconeus
Triceps brachii, lateral head
Pectoralis major
Deltoid
Infraspinatus
Teres minor
Teres major
Subscapularis
Latissimus dorsi
Serratus anterior
Flexor carpi ulnaris
Flexor digitorum
Palmaris longus
Flexor carpi radialis
Brachioradialis
Pronator teres
Triceps brachii, medial head
Brachialis
Triceps brachii, long head
Biceps brachii
Coracobrachialis

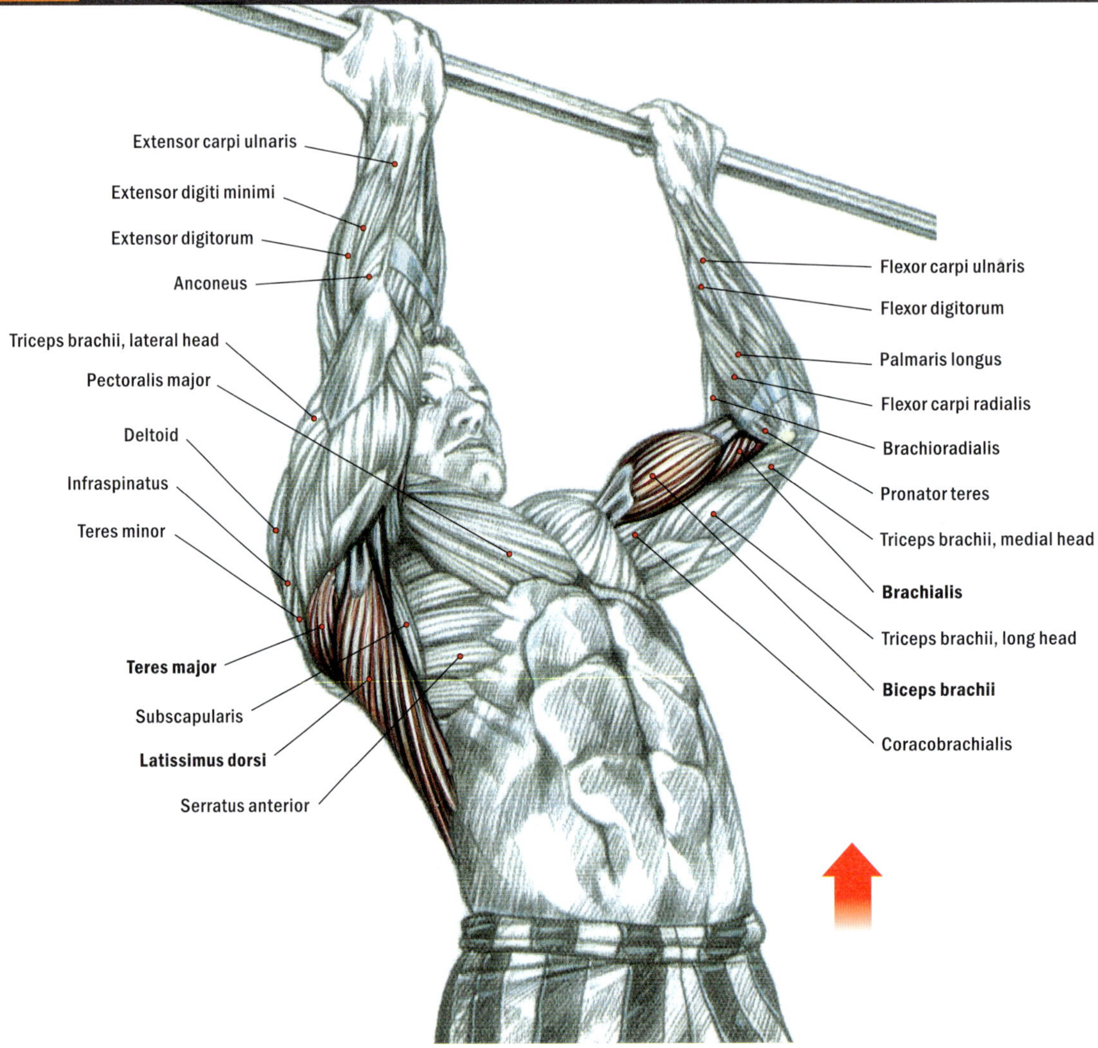

Hang from a bar with an underhand grip and hands shoulder-width apart:

- Inhale and push out your chest as you raise your chin to the bar.
- Exhale at the end of the exercise.

This exercise develops the latissimus dorsi and teres major and is associated with the intense work from the biceps brachii and brachialis. It could, therefore, be included in an arm workout.

This exercise also recruits the middle and lower portions of the trapezius, the rhomboids, and the pectoral muscles. Performing this exercise takes a certain amount of strength; use a high pulley to make it easier.

MUSCLE INSERTIONS ON THE SHOULDER BLADE

Infraspinatus
Trapezius
Teres minor
Levator scapulae
Supraspinatus
Infraspinatus
Serratus anterior
Teres major
Teres minor
Deltoid
Triceps brachii
POSTERIOR VIEW
Biceps brachii
Deltoid
Coracobrachialis
Omohyoid
Supraspinatus
Subscapularis
Serratus anterior
Triceps brachii
Teres major
ANTERIOR VIEW

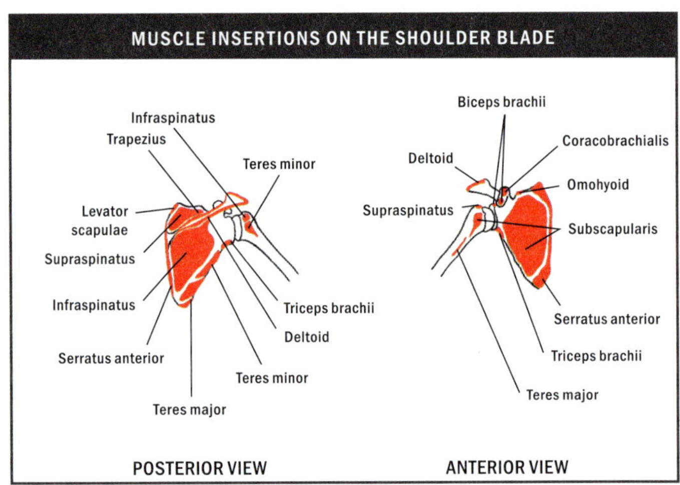

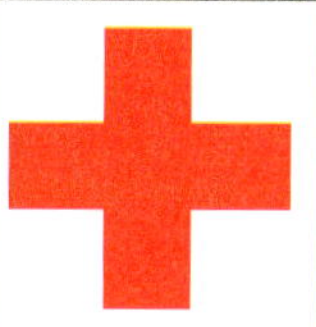

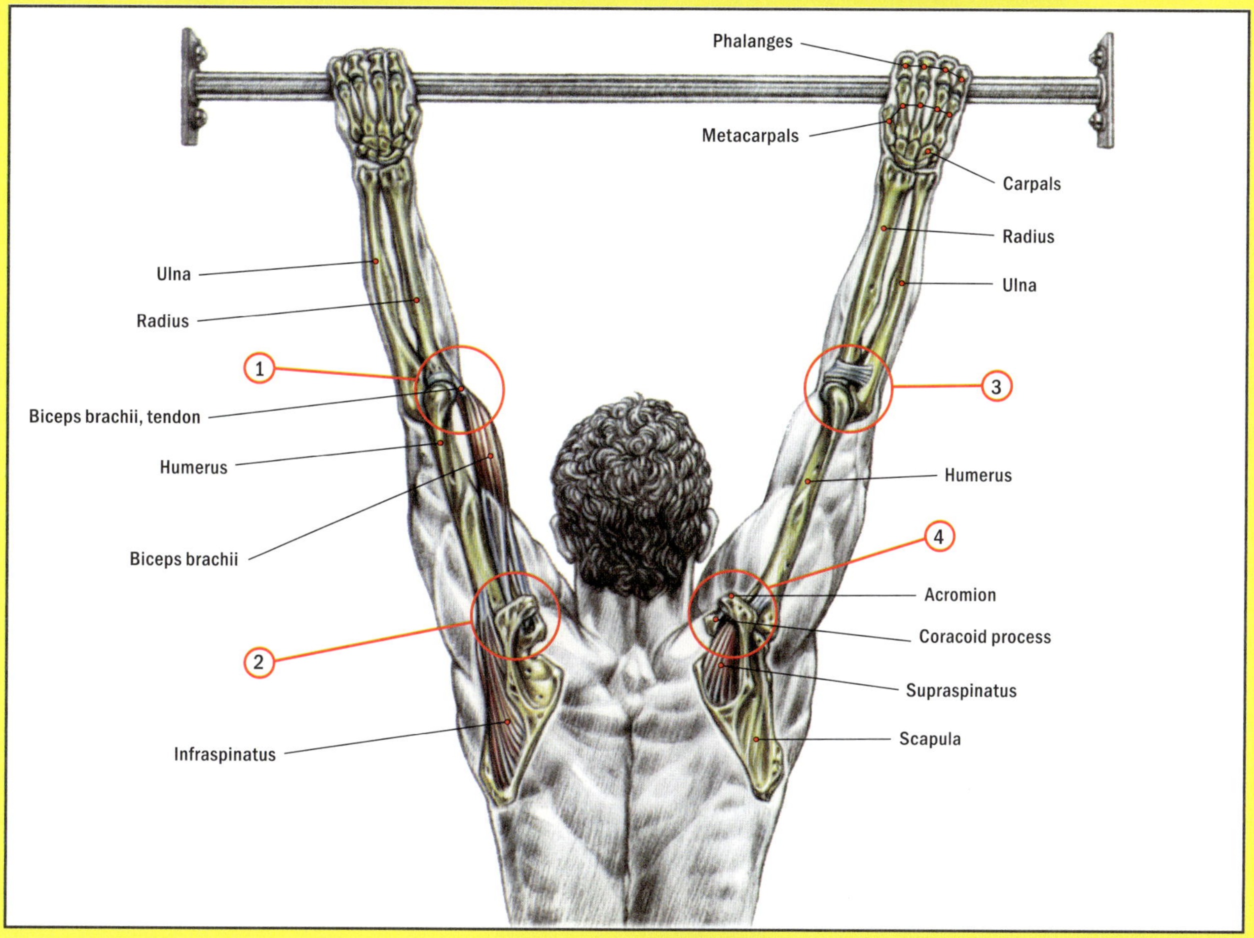

TYPICAL PULL-UP INJURIES

(1) When doing pull-ups, if the movement is poorly controlled in the lower position or during a weighted workout, the distal biceps tendon may be damaged or even ruptured.

(2) During poorly controlled fast descents or weighted workouts on a fixed bar and on machines, the infraspinatus tendon and the shoulder joint capsule can be stretched, resulting in subluxation, which can cause painful instability.

(3) During poorly controlled descents or when the arms are too straight, the elbow ligaments can become overstretched, and the elbow joint can be damaged, creating joint instability.

(4) During repeated pull-ups or in certain individuals with reduced space under the coracoacromial arch, the supraspinatus tendon may be worn down and damaged.

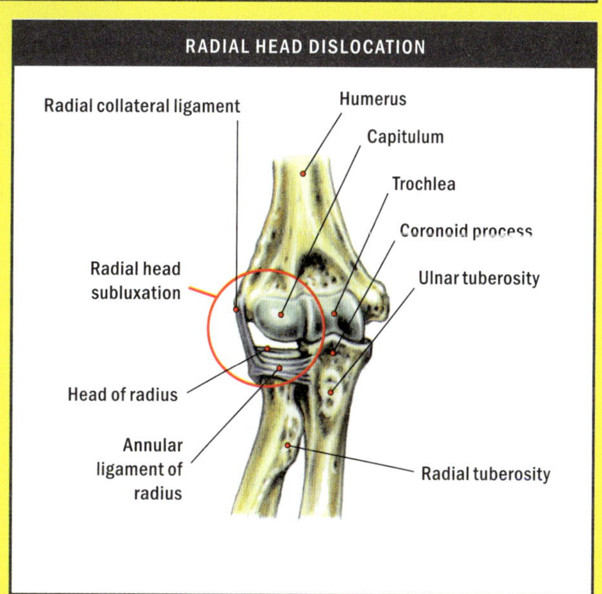

RADIAL HEAD DISLOCATION

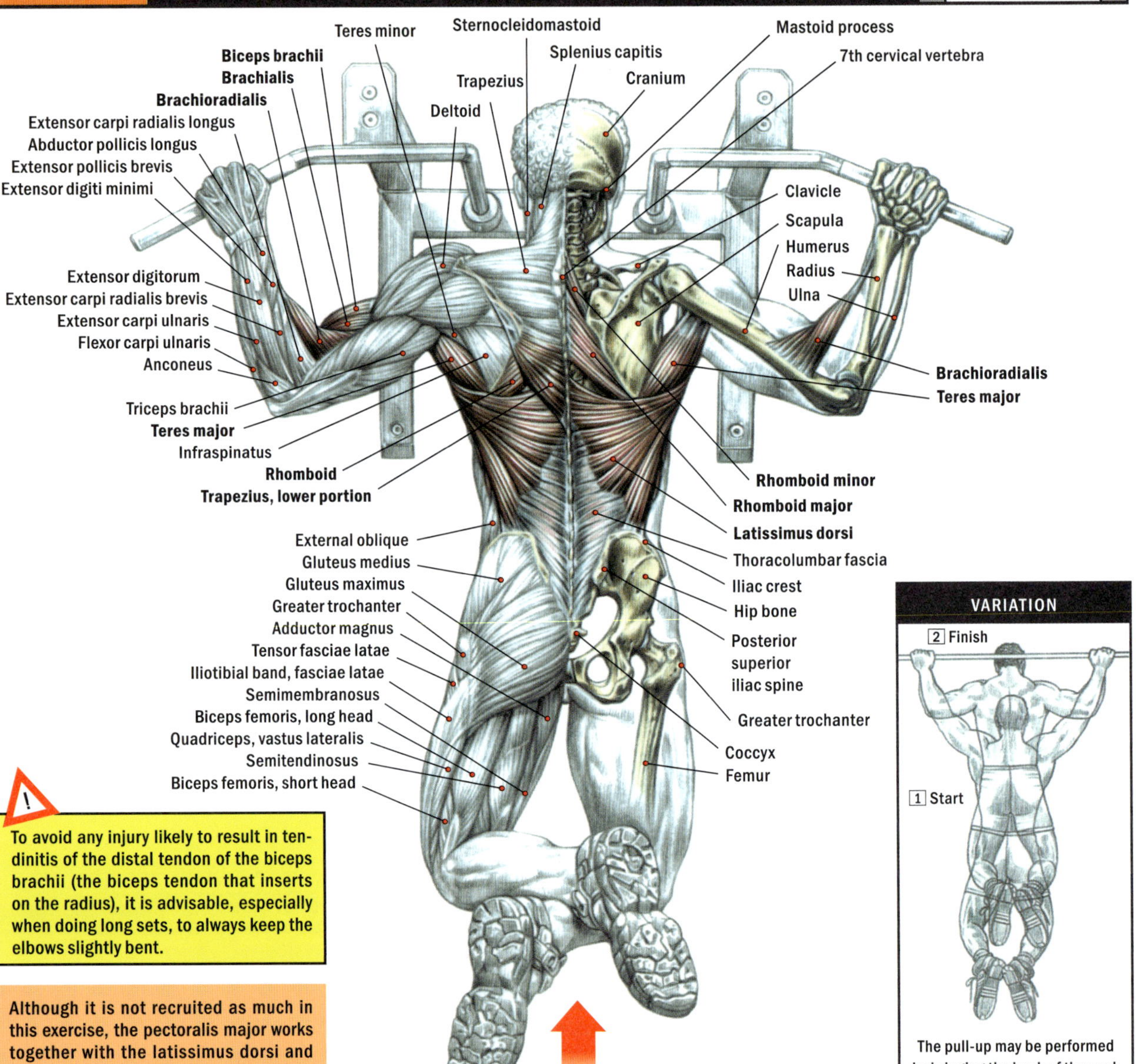

To avoid any injury likely to result in tendinitis of the distal tendon of the biceps brachii (the biceps tendon that inserts on the radius), it is advisable, especially when doing long sets, to always keep the elbows slightly bent.

Although it is not recruited as much in this exercise, the pectoralis major works together with the latissimus dorsi and teres major to close the angle that forms between the arm and the torso.

The pull-up may be performed by bringing the back of the neck underneath the bar.

Hang from a fixed bar with a very wide overhand grip:

- Inhale and pull your chest up almost to the level of the bar.
- Exhale at the end of the exercise.
- Return to the starting position with a controlled descent and then repeat.

This exercise takes a certain amount of strength and is excellent for developing the latissimus dorsi and teres major. When the shoulder blades come together at the top of the chin-up, the exercise also develops the rhomboids and middle and lower portions of the trapezius. It also works the biceps brachii, brachialis, and brachioradialis.

Variations

- To increase the intensity, you can wear a weighted belt.
- Biomechanically, keeping your elbows next to your body during the exercise will primarily work the lateral fibers of the latissimus dorsi to develop the width of your back.
- Bringing your elbows back and sticking your chest out as you raise the chin to the bar will mainly engage the upper and central fibers of your latissimus dorsi and those of the teres major. This variation develops the thickness of the back. When the shoulder blades come together, the rhomboids and the lower portions of the trapezius do equal work.

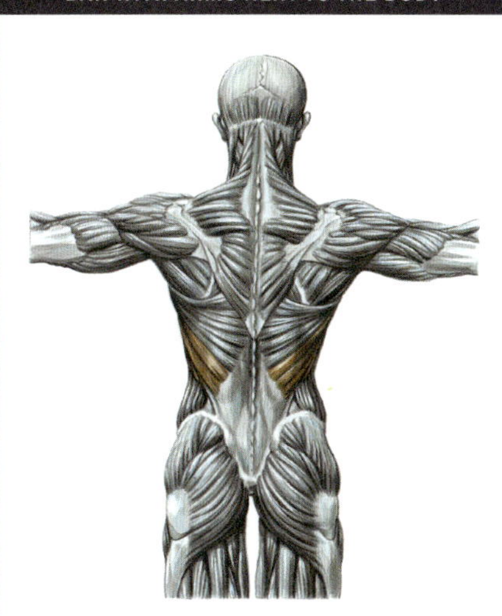

Keeping the elbows alongside the body mainly engages the lateral fibers of the latissimus dorsi and develops the width of the back.

Pulling the elbows back and sticking the chest out to raise the chin to the bar mainly engages the upper and central fibers of the latissimus dorsi. This variation is excellent for developing the thickness of the back.

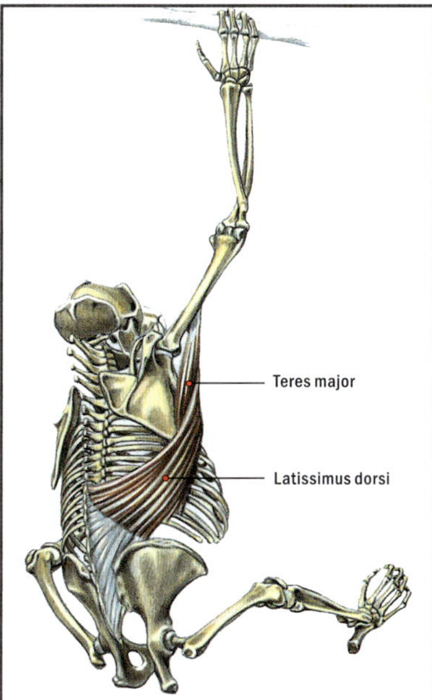

In both monkeys and humans, the latissimus dorsi and teres major are particularly well developed.

COMPARING THE ANATOMY OF A HUMAN AND A GORILLA

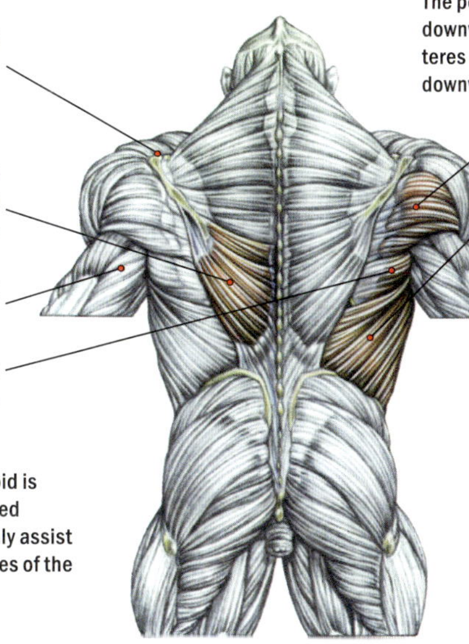

The high positioning of the shoulder joint and small acromion increase circumduction movements of the arm, thereby providing a wider gripping area, which is essential when moving from tree to tree.

The oversized lower trapezius pulls the shoulder blade and arm down and toward the center of the body, making it easier to move from tree to tree.

A long portion of the triceps is overdeveloped to work better in synergy with the back muscles during movement.

The teres major is massive.

The posterior deltoid is massive and positioned downward, working more effectively with the teres major and latissimus dorsi to pull in a downward direction when moving through trees.

The massive latissimus dorsi inserts farther down on the humerus, intensifying the pulling power.

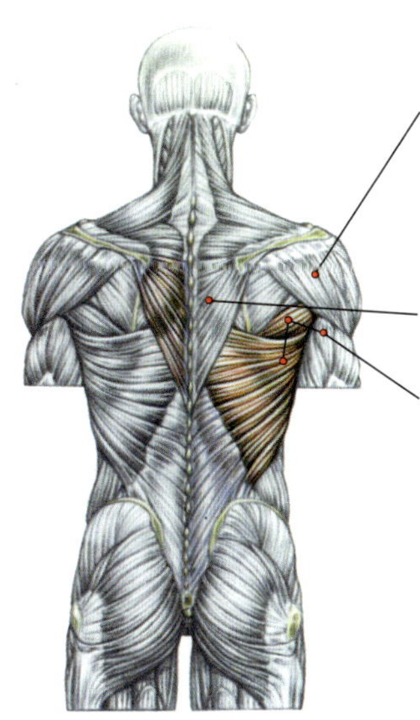

The posterior deltoid is small and positioned upward and can only assist in the last few inches of the pulling action.

The lower trapezius is very understated.

The triceps, teres major, and latissimus dorsi are less developed, but they insert closer to the shoulder joint, which provides speed at the expense of strength (this transforms the arm into an efficient weapon but lessens the strength that is useful for moving through trees).

Originally, the teres major and latissimus dorsi muscles of our far-off ancestors helped them move around on all fours by helping them to push off with the front paws.

As our ancestors became tree climbers, these muscles became powerful, specializing in vertical displacement. Returning to the ground, our more recent ancestors began moving around on two feet; however, they retained the ability to climb. For this reason, we possess powerful back muscles that are capable of pulling our bodies up, which is why we can still climb trees.

The main difference between our locomotor mechanism and that of our close simian relatives is the development of lower extremities that allow us to walk on two legs. Our chest and upper extremities have basically the same structure, and while gorillas have big arms, we have big legs.

PULL-UP RANGE OF MOTION AND LEVEL OF THE SHOULDER BLADES

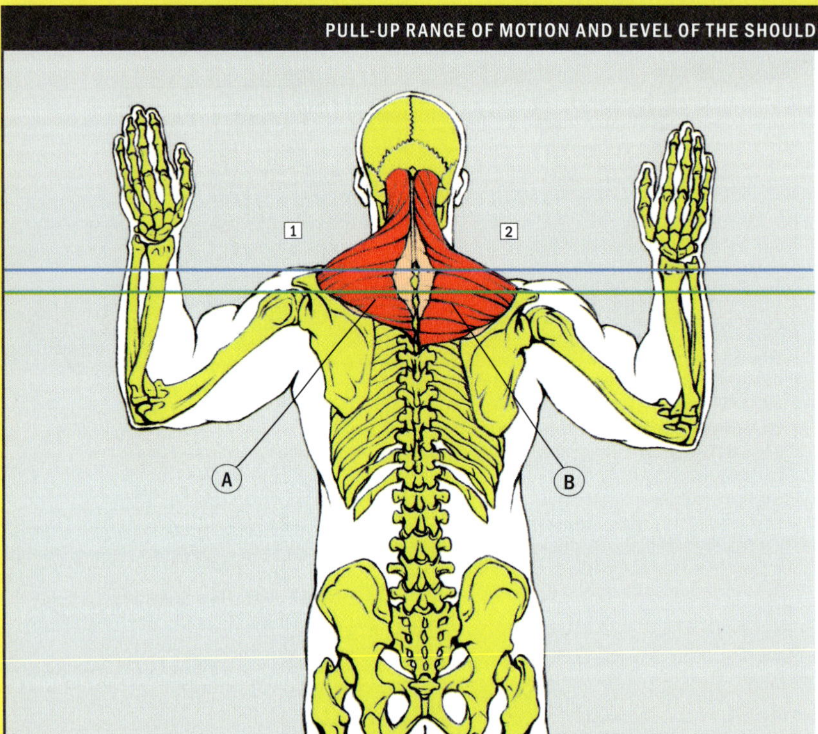

Given the same spine length:

[1] The higher the shoulder blade sits (the neck seems almost nonexistent), the harder it will be to raise the head above the bar.

[2] The lower the shoulder blade sits (the neck seems long), the easier it will be to raise the chin above the bar (so it will be easier to lift the chin over the bar).

(A) Short trapezius, high shoulder blade

(B) Long trapezius, low shoulder blade

TWO MAIN FACTORS LIMIT A FULL RANGE OF MOTION (BRINGING THE CHIN ABOVE THE BAR)

[1] Muscle weakness in the lower trapezius and rhomboids prevents the complete internal tilt of the shoulder blade, thereby limiting the ascent of the chest.

[2] Narrow clavicles associated with overdeveloped muscles in the middle part of the back restrict the ascent of the chest because the muscles in the middle back compress each other.

(A) Lower and middle trapezius

(B) Rhomboid

(C) Scapula

1 MORPHOLOGY THAT MAKES PULL-UPS EASIER

- The shorter the forearms are, the less the distance to bring the chin up to the bar.

- The narrower the clavicles are, the less mobile the shoulder blades will be. This means the lower trapezius and rhomboids do not have to work as hard. This saves energy, which makes longer sets possible.

- The longer, more bent, and less flexible the fingers are, the more they act like hooks that help you hold onto the bar easily.

- The farther from the shoulder the latissimus dorsi inserts on the humerus, the better the leverage, but the slower the downward movement of the arm. This corresponds to the original function of the dorsal muscles (pulling up into trees).

- The lighter the lower limbs are, the easier it is to do sets of pull-ups.

- The stronger the finger flexor muscles are, the easier it is to maintain the hold on the bar.

2 MORPHOLOGY THAT MAKES PULL-UPS HARDER

- The longer the forearms are, the greater the range of motion will be.

- The wider the clavicles are, the more likely the shoulder blades will be mobile, making it difficult to start a pull-up and forcing the trapezius and rhomboids to intervene. This wastes energy and limits the number of repetitions.

- The heavier your body weight—and leg weight, especially—is, the harder it will be to do pull-ups if your bone morphology is not optimal.

- The shorter and more flexible the fingers are, the more difficult it is to maintain the hold on the bar.

- The closer to the shoulder that the latissimus dorsi inserts, the worse the leverage, but the faster the downward movement of the arm.

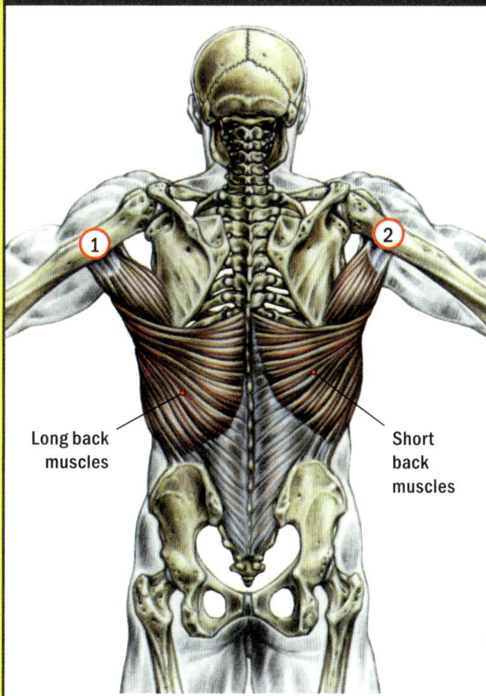

① The farther from the shoulder joint the latissimus dorsi and teres major insert, the longer the back muscles will be and the better you will be at pull-ups.

② The closer to the shoulder joint the latissimus dorsi and teres major insert, the faster you will be on each pull-up; however, you will find it harder to do a large number of them in a row. Because of their original purpose as muscles specialized for movement through trees, the latissimus dorsi are essentially built for strength rather than speed.

1 Long forearm, short humerus   2 Short forearm, long humerus

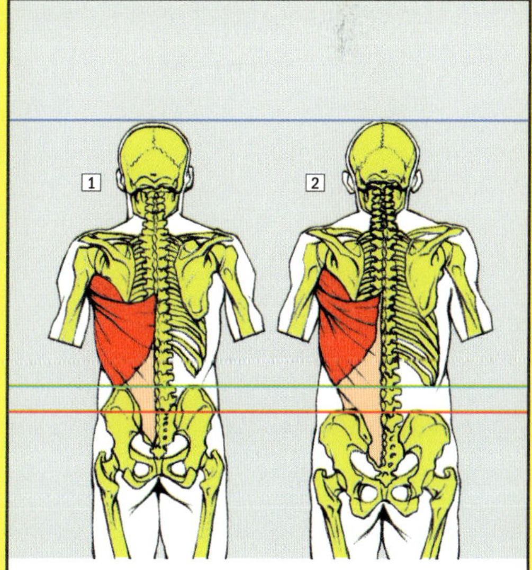

Even when they are the same length, the back muscles can appear longer or shorter depending on the length of the chest.

1 Short chest
2 Long chest

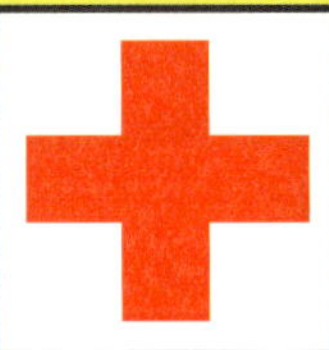

PULL-UPS AND INJURY TO THE LONG THORACIC NERVE

INJURY TO LONG THORACIC NERVE DURING PULL-UPS

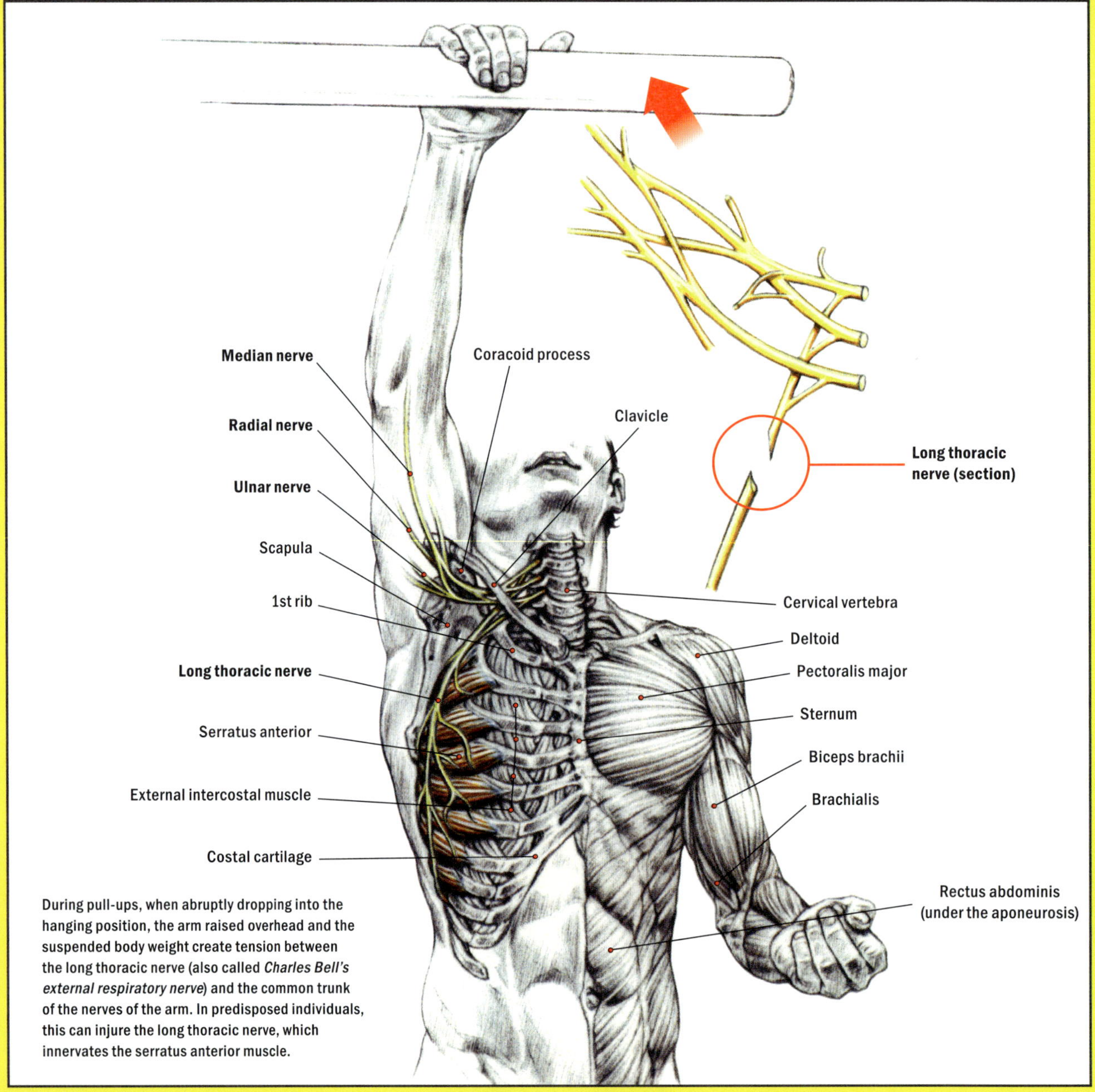

During pull-ups, when abruptly dropping into the hanging position, the arm raised overhead and the suspended body weight create tension between the long thoracic nerve (also called *Charles Bell's external respiratory nerve*) and the common trunk of the nerves of the arm. In predisposed individuals, this can injure the long thoracic nerve, which innervates the serratus anterior muscle.

Pull-ups can, in some predisposed individuals, lead to nerve damage. The main injury observed is a total or partial rupture of the long thoracic nerve (or Charles Bell's external respiratory nerve), the motor nerve innervating the serratus anterior muscle. The long thoracic nerve originates from the cervical nerve roots C5, C6, and, usually, C7. It runs through the serratus anterior muscle and innervates, via its branches, all the digitations of this muscle.

During pull-ups, if the descent is rough and uncontrolled, the tension between the brachial plexus, the common root of the nerves predominantly innervating the arm and above, and the long thoracic nerve, which inserts at the base of the brachial plexus and descends, is so strong that the latter may totally or partially rupture, causing a complete or limited paralysis of the serratus anterior muscle. If the nerve damage is only partial, the serratus anterior muscle can sometimes recover its motor function.

ACTIONS OF THE SERRATUS ANTERIOR MUSCLE

CLINICAL ASPECT, VIEWED FROM THE BACK, WITH ARMS IN FRONT, OF A PARTIAL SHOULDER PARALYSIS CAUSED BY AN INJURY TO THE LONG THORACIC NERVE

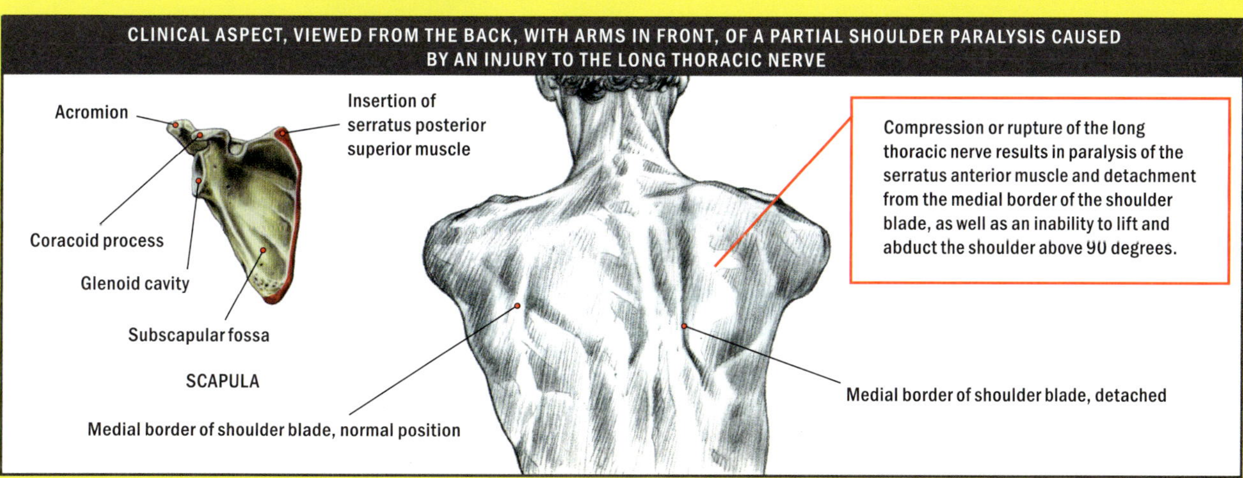

If the nerve rupture is complete, the serratus anterior can no longer perform its function, which is usually to move the shoulder forward while holding the shoulder blade against the rib cage, resulting in a detachment from the medial border of the shoulder blade. This detachment is accompanied by progressive and irreversible atrophy of the serratus anterior and shoulder instability. This can sometimes be offset by specific training of the rhomboids and the middle and lower parts of the trapezius.

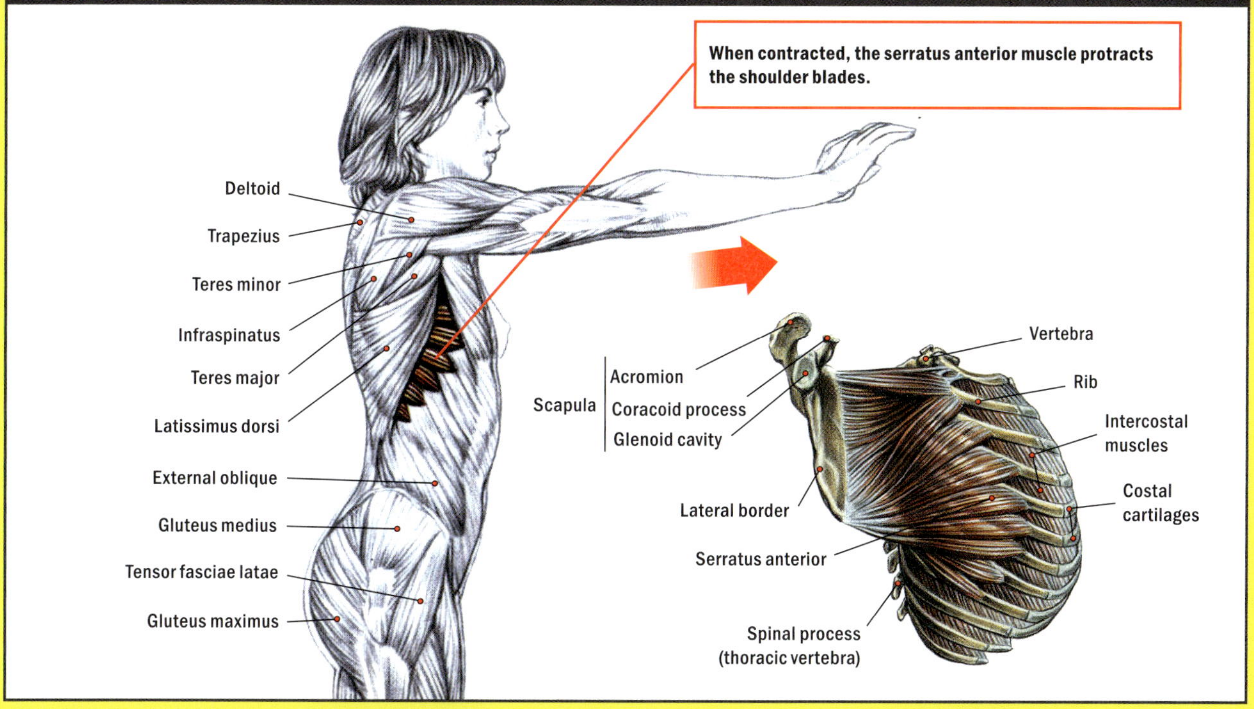

This injury is uncommon, as few people in everyday life find themselves suddenly hanging from something, but it is recurrent in bodybuilding, CrossFit, and street workouts, as well as in military training that includes pull-up exercises.

The rupture of the long thoracic nerve mainly affects individuals with wide clavicles, a morphology that accentuates, during the vertical lifting of the arm, the arm's movement and the tension of the thoracic nerve where it inserts at the root of the brachial plexus.

Finally, the rupture of the long thoracic nerve is often due to abnormal adhesions on its path that prevent it from sliding freely between the fascia and the muscles. These adhesions increase the tension at its root and, consequently, the risk of rupture.

To limit the risk of injury, it is important to not let yourself fall abruptly during pull-ups, to maintain control of your descent, and to regularly hang from a bar in a comfortable manner, in order to proactively break up any adhesions.

While abruptly hanging from the bar can put tension on the long thoracic nerve and sever it, the nerve can be also be damaged during overhead presses from compression between the clavicle and the first rib. The symptoms of this injury are often similar to a rupture, but the prognosis is generally less serious, and total recovery can be achieved.

STRETCHING THE LATISSIMUS DORSI AND TERES MAJOR

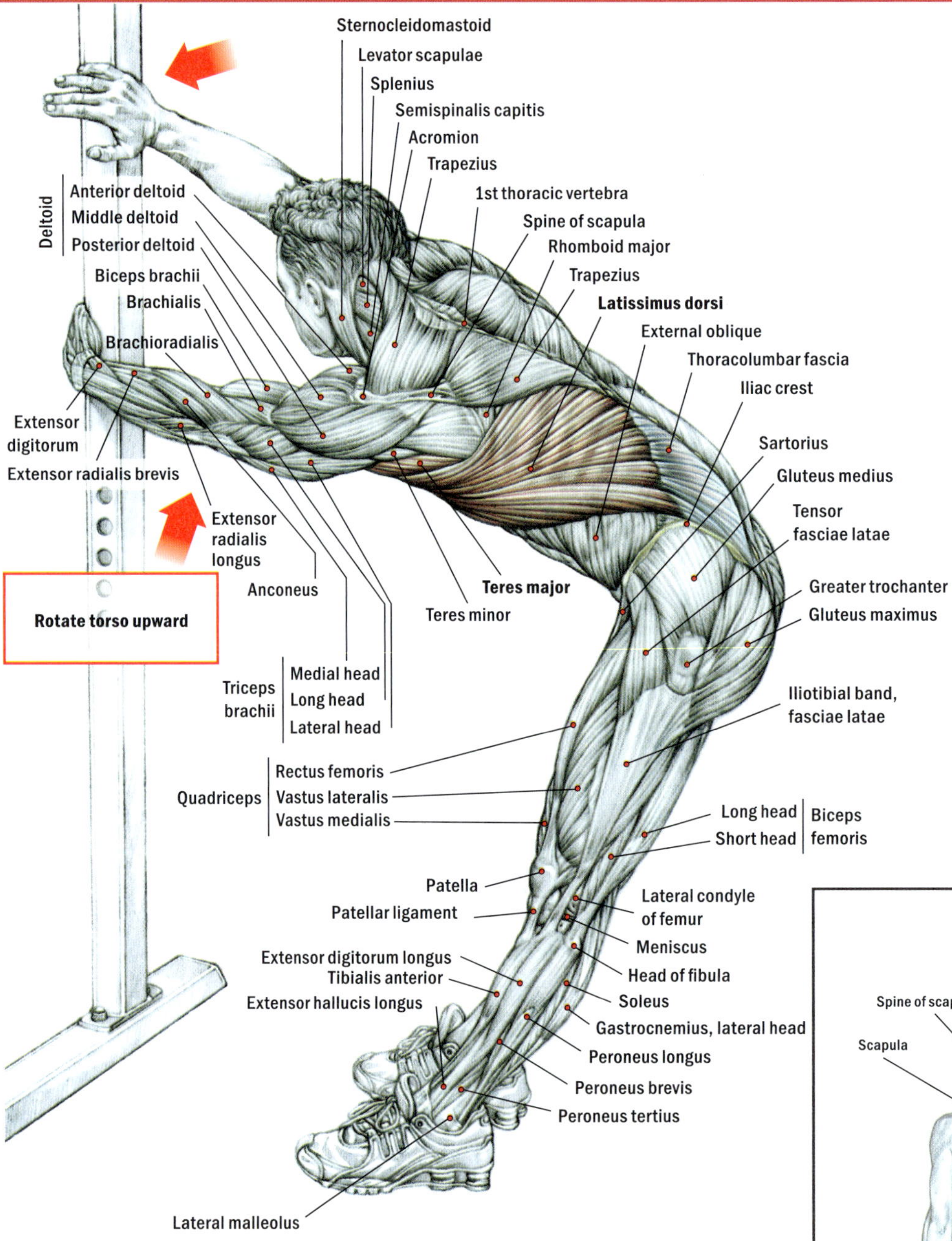

Sternocleidomastoid
Levator scapulae
Splenius
Semispinalis capitis
Acromion
Trapezius
1st thoracic vertebra
Spine of scapula
Rhomboid major
Trapezius
Latissimus dorsi
External oblique
Thoracolumbar fascia
Iliac crest
Sartorius
Gluteus medius
Tensor fasciae latae
Greater trochanter
Gluteus maximus
Iliotibial band, fasciae latae
Deltoid
Anterior deltoid
Middle deltoid
Posterior deltoid
Biceps brachii
Brachialis
Brachioradialis
Extensor digitorum
Extensor radialis brevis
Extensor radialis longus
Anconeus
Rotate torso upward
Teres major
Teres minor
Triceps brachii
Medial head
Long head
Lateral head
Quadriceps
Rectus femoris
Vastus lateralis
Vastus medialis
Long head
Short head
Biceps femoris
Patella
Patellar ligament
Lateral condyle of femur
Meniscus
Head of fibula
Extensor digitorum longus
Tibialis anterior
Extensor hallucis longus
Soleus
Gastrocnemius, lateral head
Peroneus longus
Peroneus brevis
Peroneus tertius
Lateral malleolus

Stand with your legs slightly apart:

- Lean your torso forward. Keep your arms straight and grasp a stable support such as a machine or the frame of a squat cage.
- Place the palm of your other hand higher up on the support. Keep your arm straight and gradually push harder against the machine while simultaneously pulling with the other arm.

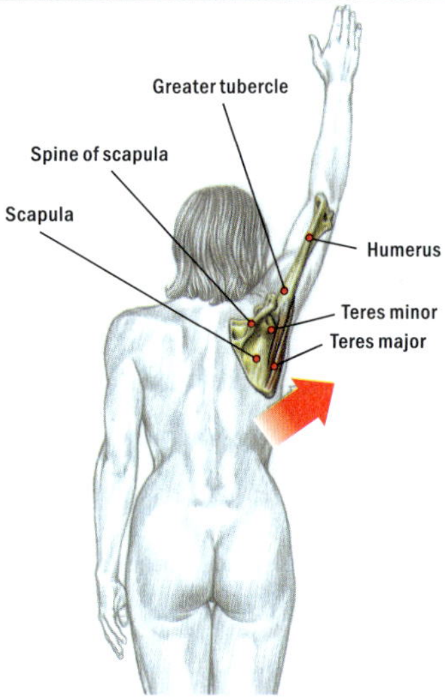

Greater tubercle
Spine of scapula
Scapula
Humerus
Teres minor
Teres major

When the arm is raised, the teres minor and teres major stretch and bring the interior border of the scapula toward the outside of the body.

INSERTIONS OF LATISSIMUS DORSI AND TERES MAJOR ON THE HUMERUS: ANTERIOR VIEW

ANTERIOR VIEW

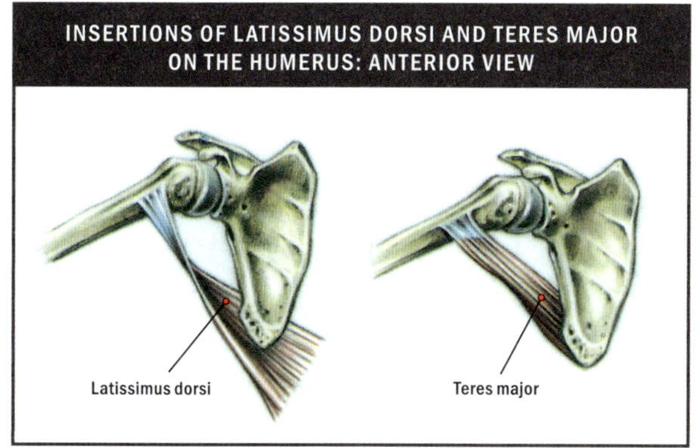

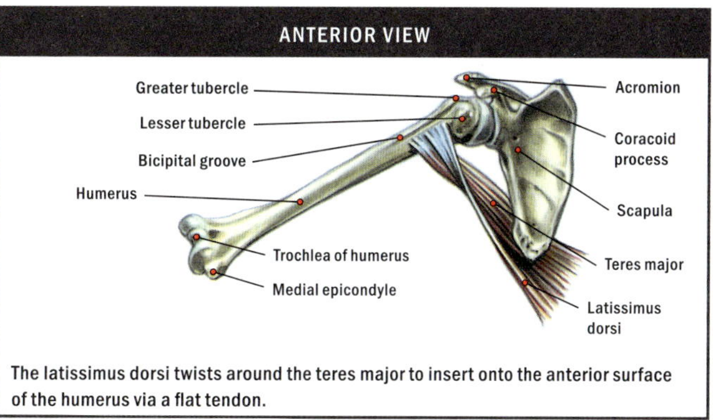

The latissimus dorsi twists around the teres major to insert onto the anterior surface of the humerus via a flat tendon.

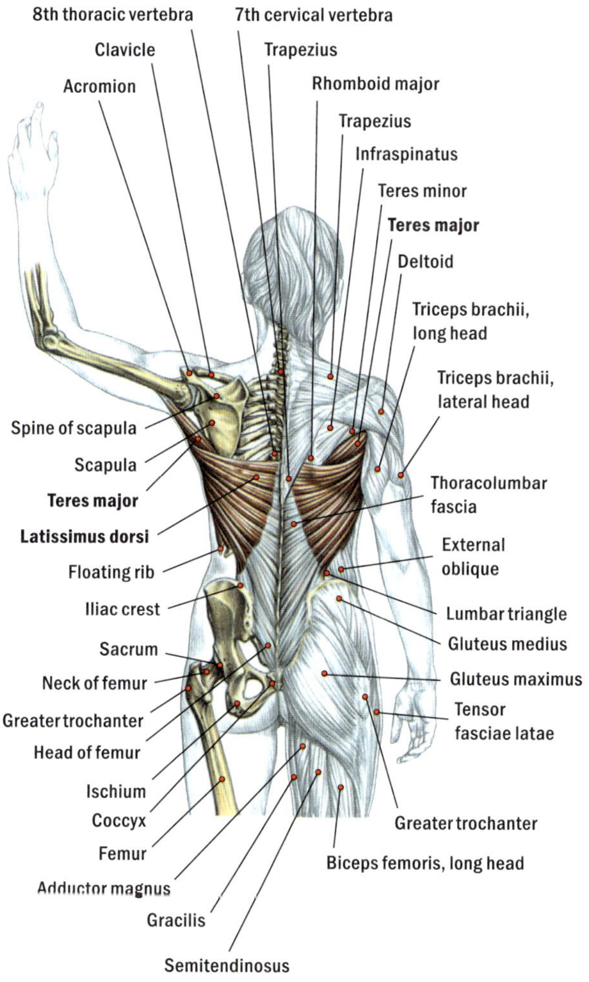

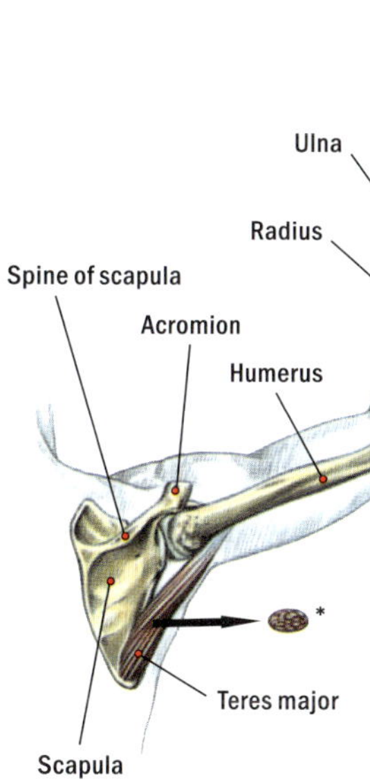

*The teres major gets its name from its round transverse section (from the Latin *teres*, meaning rounded).

To accentuate the stretch of the latissimus dorsi and teres major, rotate your torso while trying to slowly raise your lowest shoulder.

When practiced regularly and incorporated between the first sets of back exercises, this stretch helps prevent tears in the latissimus dorsi and teres major, which can occur during high-pulley exercises with heavy weight or during weighted pull-ups.

03 LAT PULL-DOWNS

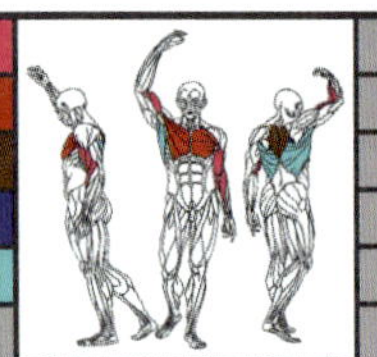

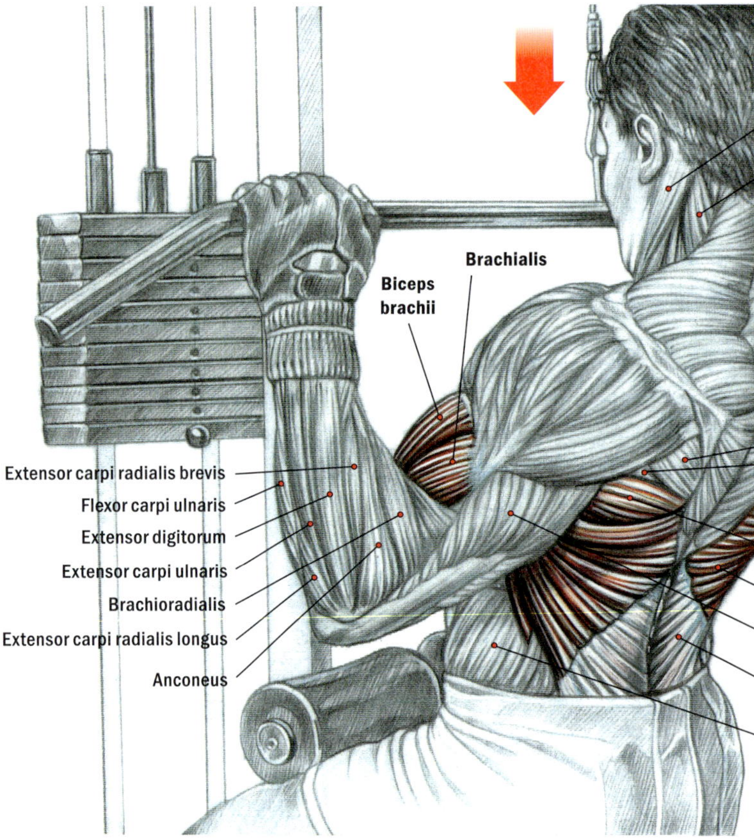

Sternocleidomastoid
Splenius
Brachialis
Biceps brachii
Trapezius
Deltoid
Infraspinatus
Teres minor
Extensor carpi radialis brevis
Flexor carpi ulnaris
Extensor digitorum
Extensor carpi ulnaris
Brachioradialis
Extensor carpi radialis longus
Anconeus
Teres major
Latissimus dorsi
Triceps brachii
Aponeurosis of latissimus dorsi
External oblique

2 Finish
1 Start

VARIATION: WITH A WIDE BAR USING A SEMIPRONATED GRIP

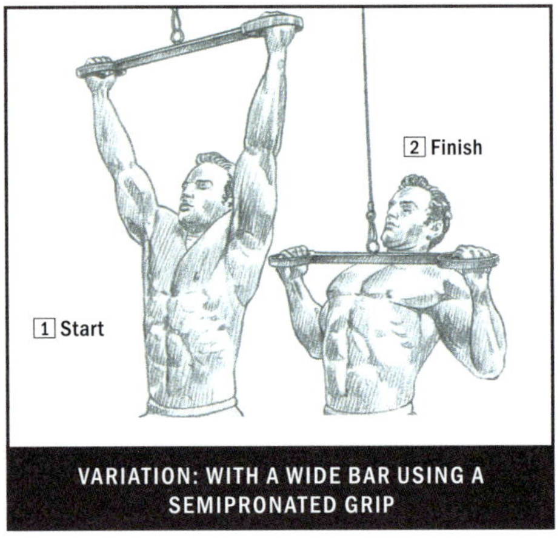

Sit facing the machine with your legs positioned under the pads, gripping the bar with a wide overhand grip:

- Inhale and pull the bar down to your sternal notch while pushing your chest out and pulling your elbows back.
- Exhale at the end of the exercise.

This exercise, which is excellent for developing the width of the back, mainly works the upper and central fibers of the latissimus dorsi. The middle and lower portions of the trapezius, the rhomboids, the biceps brachii, the brachialis, and, to a lesser extent, the pectorals are also working.

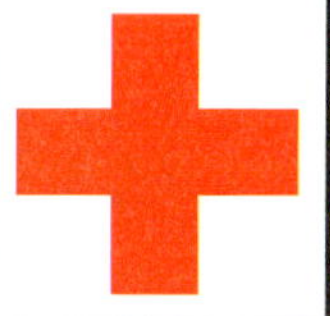

The labrum is a rim of cartilage located around the glenoid cavity; it is designed to increase the depth of this cavity, which houses the head of the humerus and improves its stability.

With time, and during certain strength training exercises, the labrum can deteriorate, causing instability of the arm, which is often felt as a small dislocation in the shoulder joint. The cause of this sensation is most often related to a detachment of the upper part of the labrum, caused by excessive tension on the long head of the biceps, which attaches to it. This pathology is known as a *superior labrum anterior posterior tear* or by its acronym, *SLAP tear*.

This labrum injury is often the result of several types of strength training exercises that create intense stretching stress on the tendon of the long head of the biceps, such as pull-ups and pull-downs (where the arms are extended and the movement is initiated with a violent jerk), upright rows, and heavy deadlifts.

While a very slight labrum detachment can sometimes resolve itself with rest, when the detachment is too substantial, total recovery is often not possible, even with surgery. Thus, it is important, if there is the slightest sensation of dislocation of the arm in the shoulder joint, to temporarily stop doing any exercises that might accentuate a labrum detachment. Focus on strengthening the rotator cuff muscles so as to properly stabilize the humerus in the glenoid cavity and moderate the intensity of any stretching exercises for the biceps and shoulders.

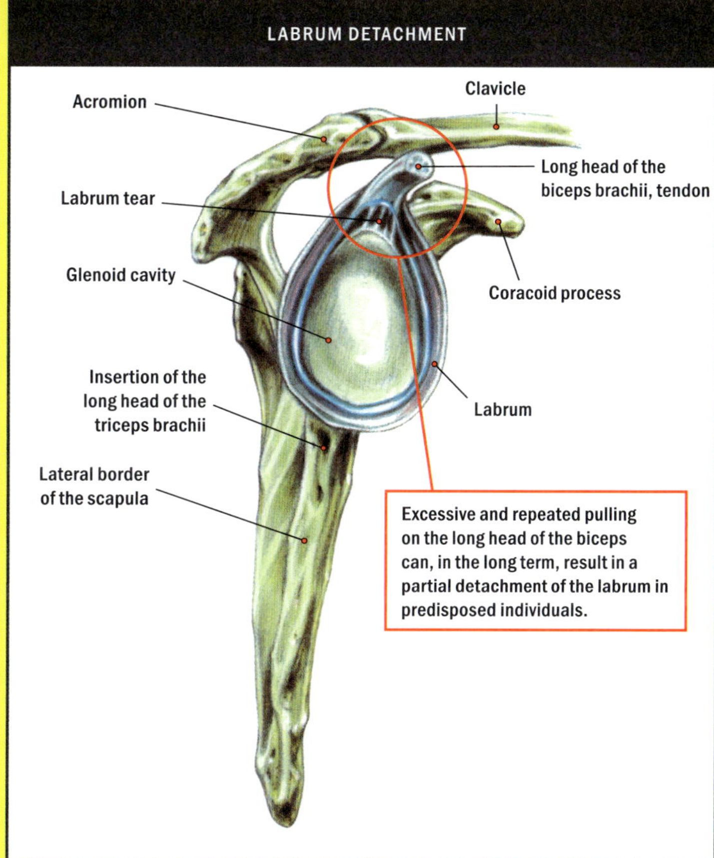

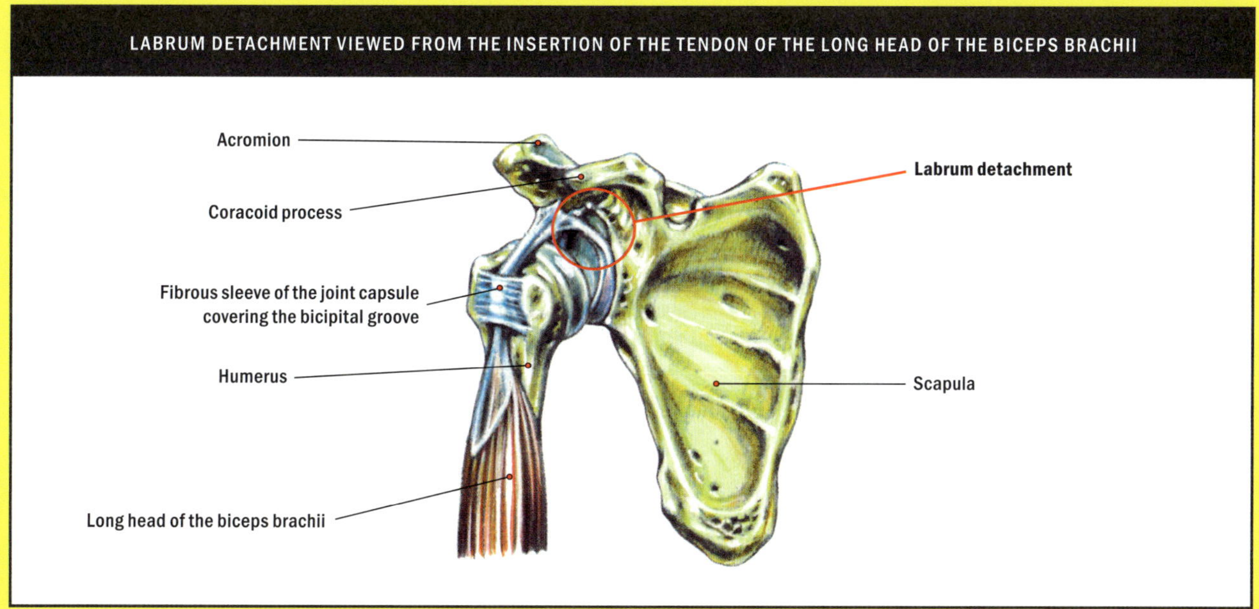

04 PULL-DOWNS BEHIND THE NECK

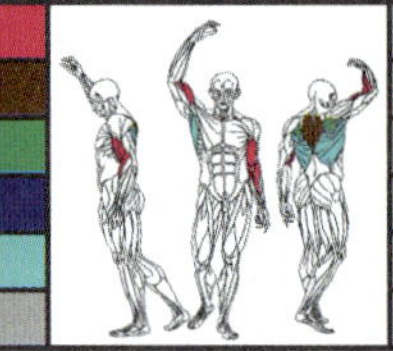

Splenius
Sternocleidomastoid
Spine of scapula
Trapezius
Deltoid
Trapezius, lower portion
Biceps brachii
Brachioradialis
Brachialis
Triceps brachii
Extensor carpi radialis brevis
Extensor carpi ulnaris
Flexor carpi ulnaris
Extensor digitorum
Anconeus
Olecranon
Teres minor
Rhomboid
Extensor carpi radialis longus
Teres major
Infraspinatus
Aponeurosis of latissimus dorsi
Latissimus dorsi
External oblique
Hip bone

1 Start
2 Finish

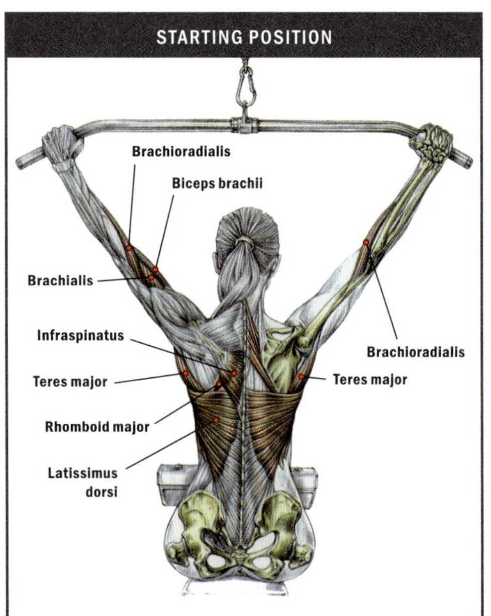

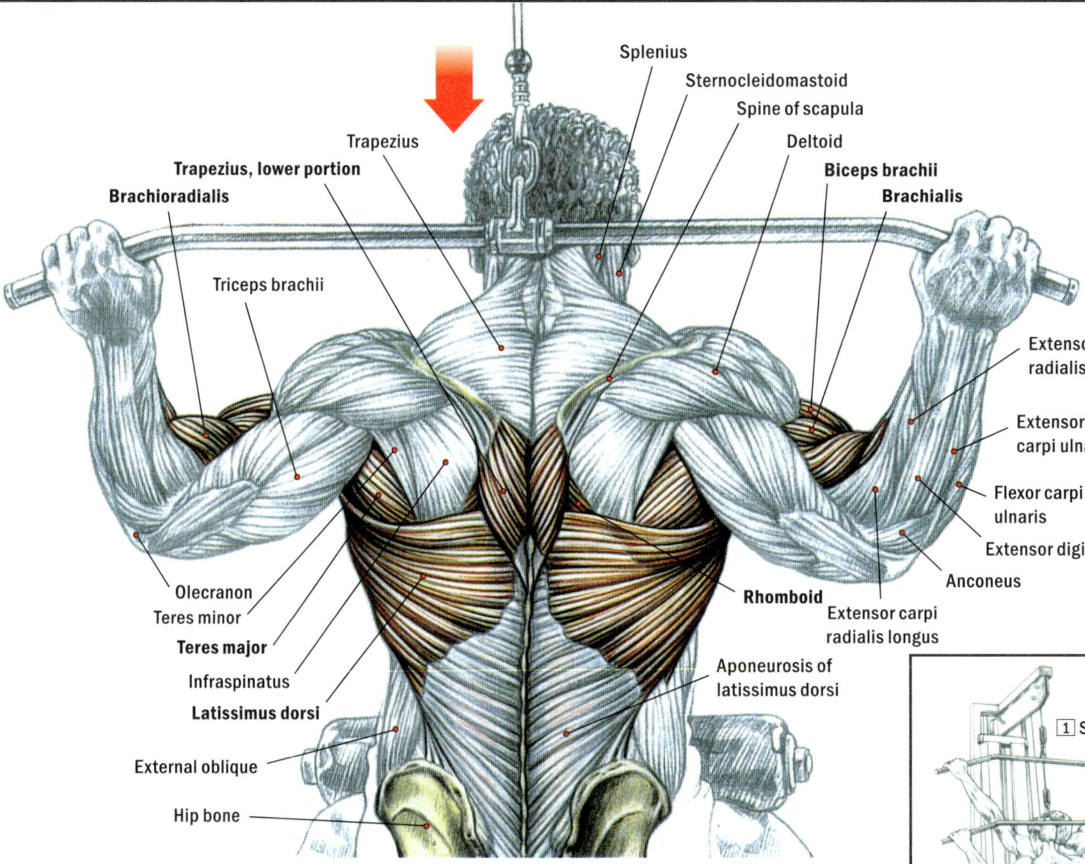

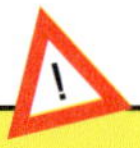

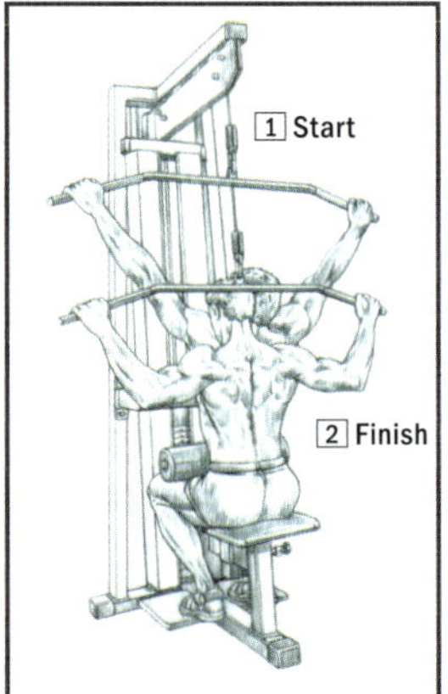

PERFORMING THE EXERCISE

STARTING POSITION

Brachioradialis
Biceps brachii
Brachialis
Infraspinatus
Brachioradialis
Teres major
Teres major
Rhomboid major
Latissimus dorsi

Sit facing the machine with your thighs positioned under the pads. Grasp the bar with a wide overhand grip:

- Inhale and pull the bar down to the back of your neck, bringing your elbows alongside your body.
- Exhale at the end of the exercise.

This is an excellent exercise for developing the width of the back. It works the latissimus dorsi (mainly the lateral and lower fibers) and the teres major muscles. The forearm flexors (biceps brachii, brachialis, and brachioradialis), the rhomboids, and the lower part of the trapezius are also engaged. The latter two muscles come into play when the shoulder blades are pulled together.

Pull-downs behind the neck can help beginners develop enough strength to move on to pull-ups.

1 Start
2 Finish

VARIATION ON A MACHINE WITH A FIXED AXIS

!

In individuals who do not have enough space under the coracoacromial arch, this exercise can cause bursitis. Repeated rubbing of the supraspinatus tendon can eventually lead to abrasion and rupture of the tendon.

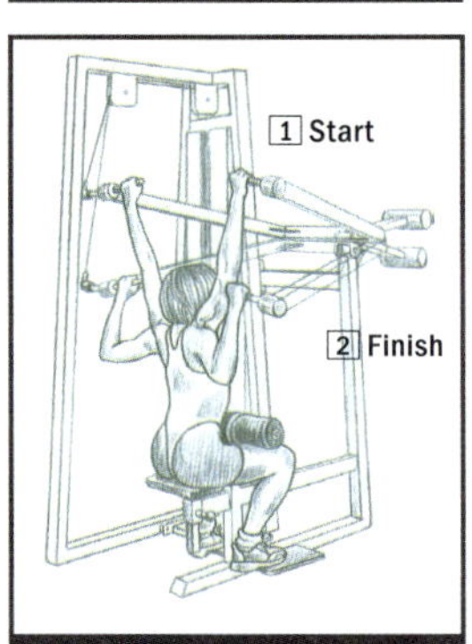

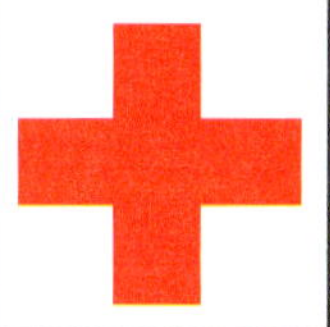

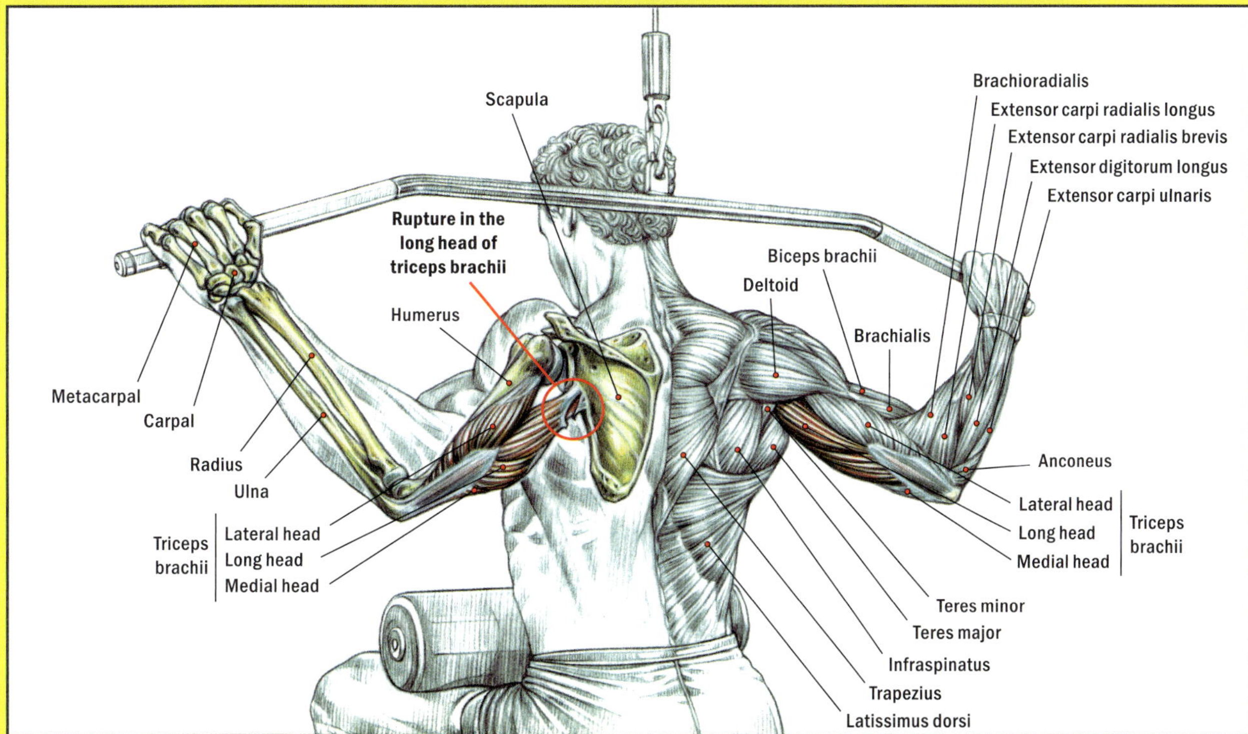

HEAVY STRENGTH TRAINING FOR THE BACK AND INJURY TO THE LONG HEAD OF THE TRICEPS BRACHII

Although it is not the most used muscle when working the back, the long head of the triceps brachii is the most frequently injured muscle during back lat pull-downs with heavy loads or during weighted pull-ups.

Remember that the latissimus dorsi is a powerful, fan-shaped muscle that brings the arm closer to the rib cage; its distal tendon is strongly attached to the humerus. It is the principal climbing muscle.

The long head of the triceps brachii, meanwhile, is a smaller muscle whose main primary function is to extend the forearm. Its secondary function is to bring the arm toward the rib cage to complete the action of the latissimus dorsi.

A tear in the long head of the triceps happens when the muscle is fatigued, often after an improper warm-up. It only takes a sudden relaxation of the latissimus dorsi during weighted pull-ups or weighted pull-downs to immediately shift all the tension to the long head of the triceps. The long head may partially tear, most often close to its insertion on the shoulder blade (fortunately, complete tears are rare).

Unlike shoulder injuries, which are incapacitating and may completely halt upper body training, a tear in the long head of the triceps is less devastating. Despite the injury, it is still possible to do back exercises such as seated rows or T-bar rows. You can also do triceps exercises such as forearm extensions at a high pulley with your elbows next to the body, as long as you begin with lighter weights. However, a brief rest period is recommended before restarting upper body training.

TRICEPS STRETCH

Tearing the long head of the triceps may also occur during bench presses. To prevent this tear, you should warm up with stretching exercises (see pages 46-47) before beginning your training.

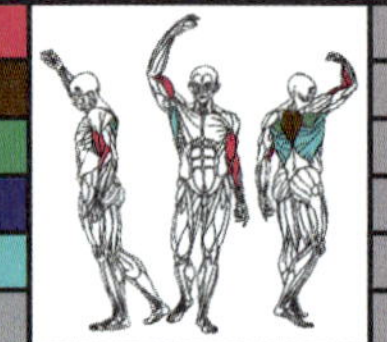

Flexor carpi ulnaris

Extensor carpi ulnaris

Anconeus

Triceps brachii, lateral head

Triceps brachii, long head

Coracobrachialis

Teres minor

Infraspinatus

Teres major

Latissimus dorsi

Subscapularis

Serratus anterior

Pectoralis major

Flexor digitorum

Palmaris longus

Flexor carpi radialis

Brachioradialis

Pronator teres

Brachialis

Triceps brachii, medial head

Biceps brachii

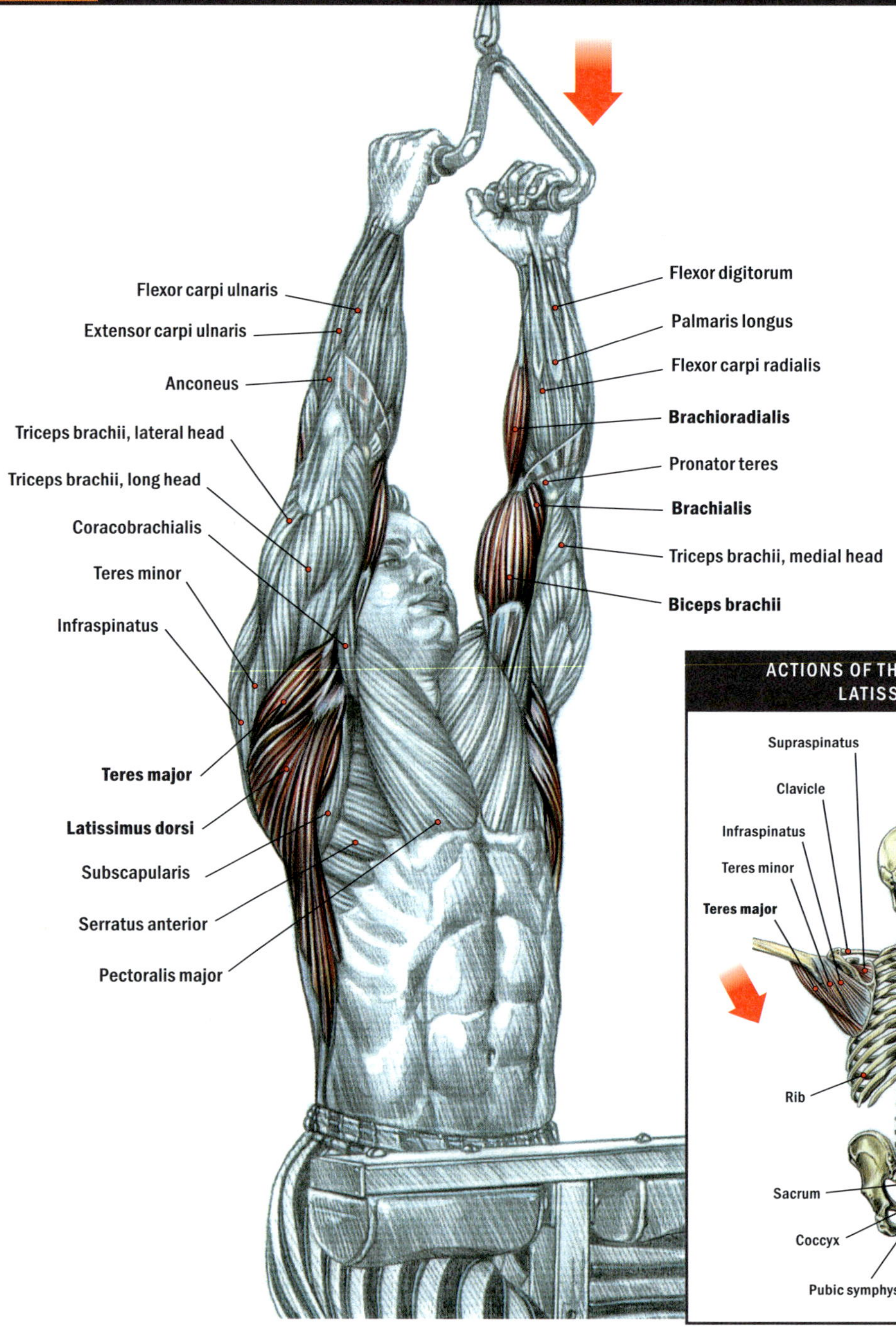

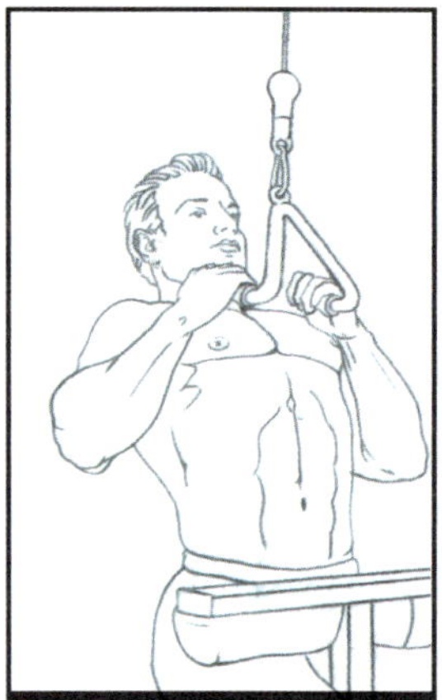

ENDING POSITION

ACTIONS OF THE TERES MAJOR AND LATISSIMUS DORSI

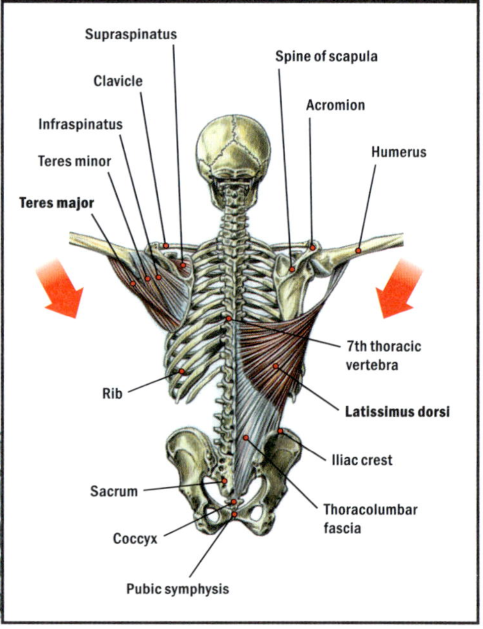

Supraspinatus

Clavicle

Infraspinatus

Teres minor

Teres major

Spine of scapula

Acromion

Humerus

7th thoracic vertebra

Latissimus dorsi

Iliac crest

Thoracolumbar fascia

Rib

Sacrum

Coccyx

Pubic symphysis

Sit and face the machine with your knees positioned under the pads:

- Inhale and bring the handle to your sternum while expanding your chest and leaning your torso slightly backward.
- Exhale at the end of the exercise.

This is an excellent exercise for developing both the latissimus dorsi and the teres major.

When the shoulder blades come together, the rhomboid, the trapezius, and the posterior deltoid contract. As with every pulling exercise, the biceps brachii and the brachialis are engaged, and when the palms face each other, the brachioradialis comes into play.

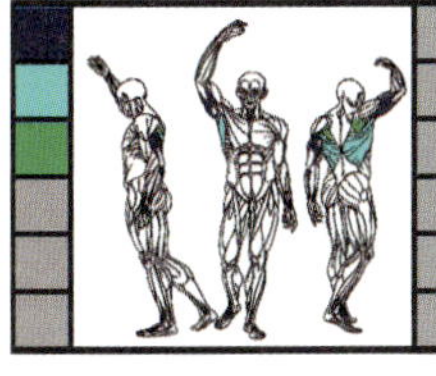

STRAIGHT-ARM PULL-DOWNS 06

Sternocleidomastoid
Splenius capitis
Trapezius
Posterior deltoid
Teres minor
Infraspinatus
Rhomboid
Middle deltoid
Triceps brachii, lateral head
Brachialis
Brachioradialis
Extensor carpi radialis longus
Extensor carpi radialis brevis
Extensor digitorum
Extensor digiti minimi
Teres major
Latissimus dorsi
External oblique
Aponeurosis of latissimus dorsi
Anconeus
Triceps brachii, long head
Triceps brachii, medial head
Flexor carpi ulnaris
Extensor carpi ulnaris

MUSCLES USED

Scapula
Glenoid cavity
Teres major
Latissimus dorsi
Iliac crest
Sacrum
Triceps brachii, lateral head
Triceps brachii, long head
Head of the humerus
10th, 11th, and 12th ribs
Hip bone
Pubis

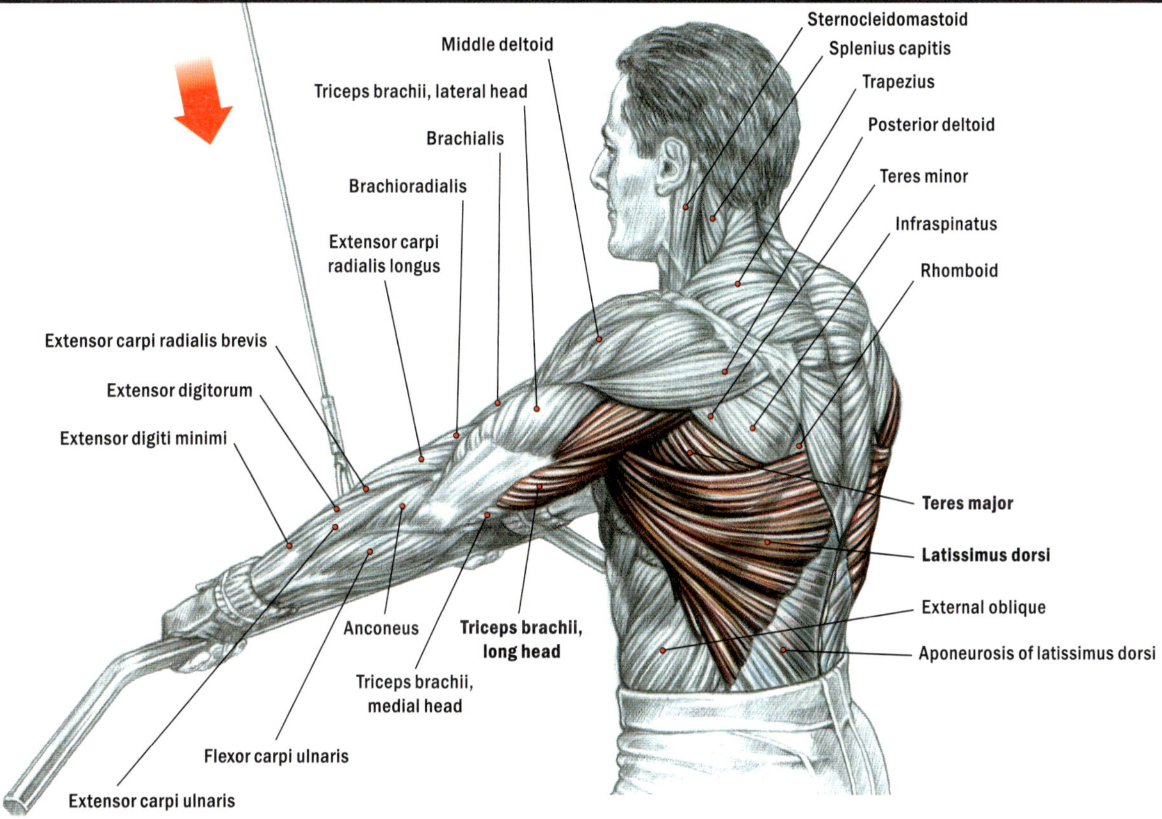

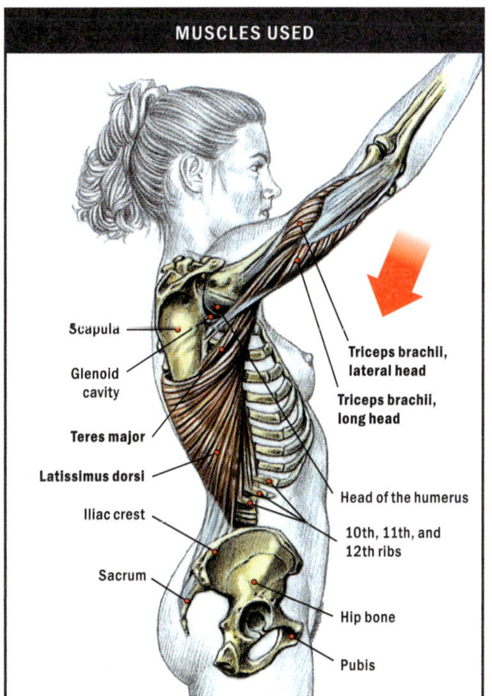

Stand and face the machine with your feet slightly apart. Grip the bar with an overhand grip with your arms extended and shoulder-width apart:

- Stabilize your back and contract the core. Inhale and bring the bar to your thighs, keeping your arms extended (your elbows can be slightly bent).
- Exhale at the end of the exercise.

This exercise, which works the latissimus dorsi, also strengthens the teres major and the long head of the triceps, which are partly responsible for stability in the arm–trunk hinge.

This exercise strengthens the long head of the triceps, which helps to protect the shoulder joint and decrease the risk of dislocation if the shoulder joint has hyperlaxity.

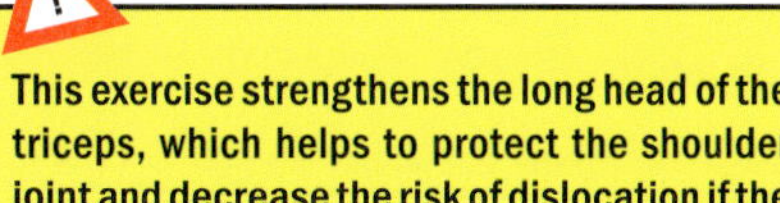

Many swim coaches use this exercise to develop a powerful crawl stroke in their swimmers.

PERFORMING THE EXERCISE

1 Start
2 Finish

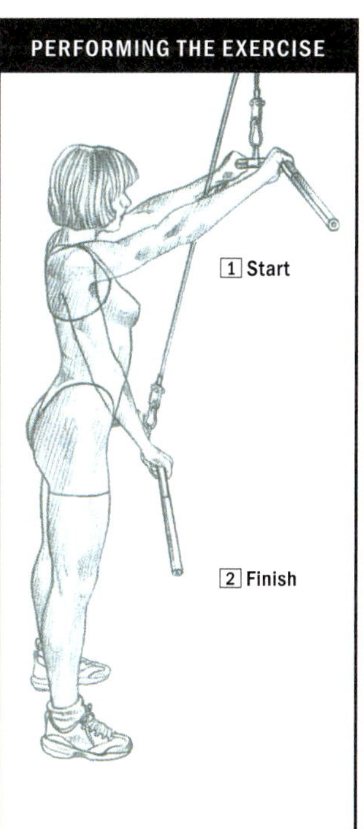

07 CLOSE-GRIP SEATED ROWS WITH A SEMIPRONATED GRIP

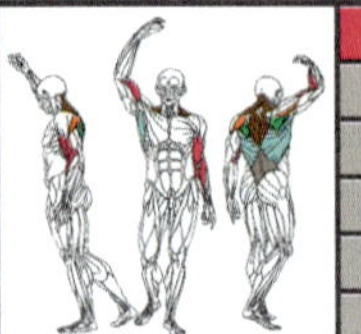

Sternocleidomastoid
Splenius capitis
Levator scapulae
Spine of scapula
Trapezius
Rhomboid major
Infraspinatus
Posterior deltoid
Middle deltoid
Long head
Lateral head
Medial head
Triceps brachii
Brachioradialis
Extensor carpi radialis longus
Extensor carpi radialis brevis
Extensor digitorum
Extensor pollicis brevis
Abductor pollicis longus
Extensor carpi ulnaris
Extensor digiti minimi
Anconeus
Flexor carpi ulnaris
Teres minor
Teres major
Pectoralis major
Latissimus dorsi
Serratus anterior
External oblique
Erector spinae (under the thoracolumbar fascia)

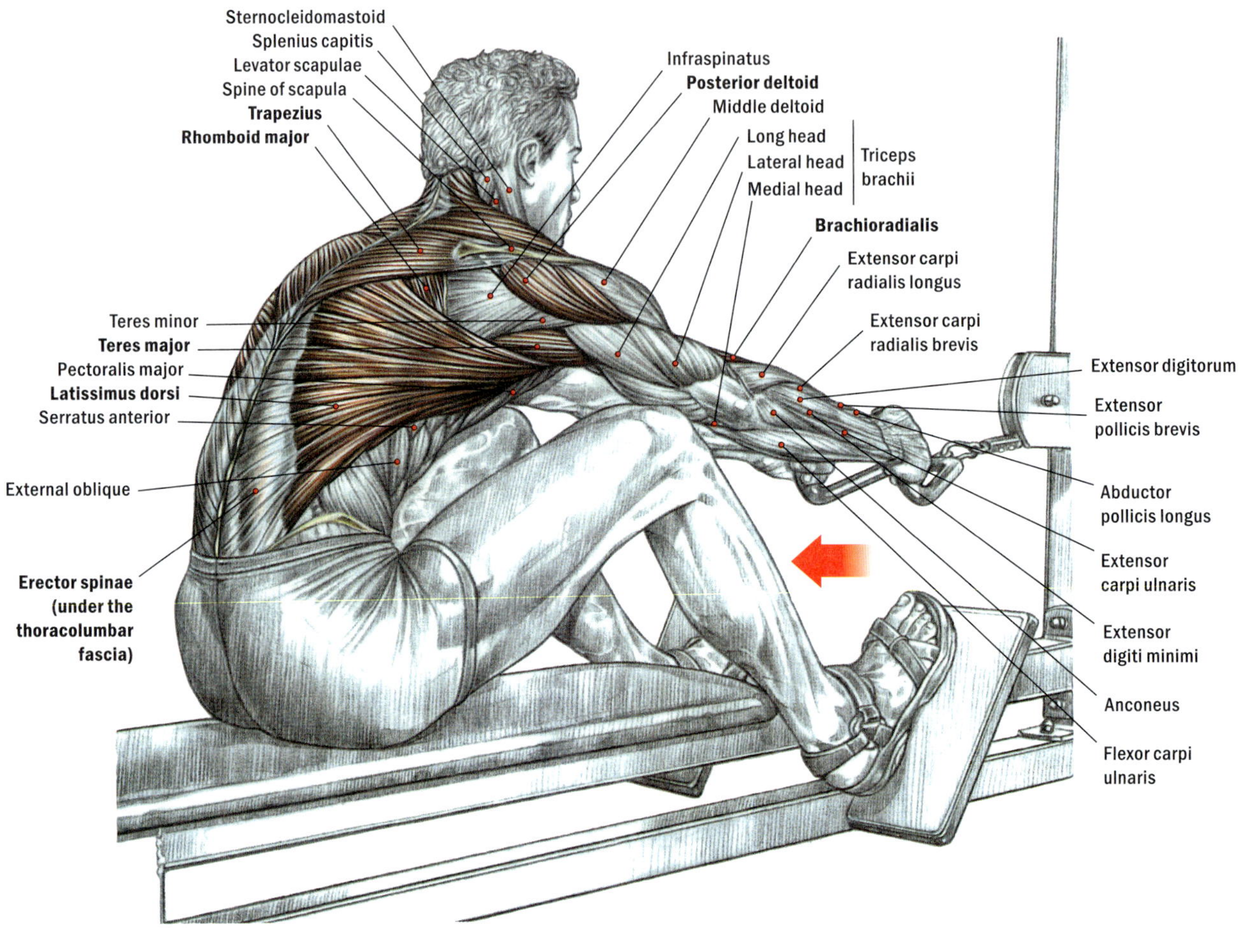

Sit facing the machine, with your feet resting on the footrests and your torso leaning forward:

- Inhale and bring the handle to the base of your sternum by straightening your back and pulling your elbows back as far as possible.
- Exhale at the end of the exercise and return smoothly to the starting position.

This is an excellent exercise for working the thickness of the back. It focuses the effort on the latissimus dorsi, teres major, posterior deltoid, biceps brachii, and brachioradialis. At the end of the movement when the shoulder blades come together, it focuses on the trapezius and rhomboids. As the chest lifts, the spinal muscles (or erector spinae) also contribute to the effort.

During the negative phase of this exercise, allowing the weight to pull you helps develop flexibility throughout the back.

2 Finish
1 Start

PERFORMING THE EXERCISE

To prevent back injury, never round your back when performing seated rows with heavy weights.

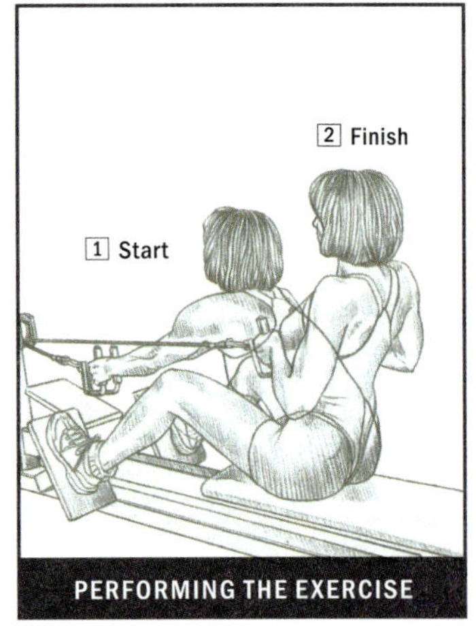

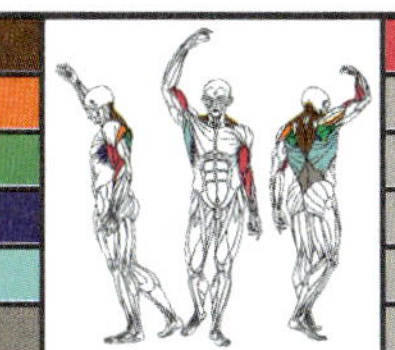

Thyroid cartilage
Sternocleidomastoid
Splenius capitis
Levator scapulae
Scalene
Spine of scapula
Trapezius
Posterior deltoid
Teres minor
Rhomboid
Infraspinatus
Teres major
Latissimus dorsi
Serratus anterior
External oblique

Anterior deltoid
Pectoralis major
Extensor carpi radialis longus
Middle deltoid
Coracobrachialis
Extensor carpi radialis brevis
Extensor digitorum
Extensor digiti minimi
Brachialis
Extensor carpi ulnaris
Biceps brachii
Brachioradialis
Pronator teres
Flexor carpi radialis
Palmaris longus
Flexor digitorum superficialis
Flexor carpi ulnaris
Abductor pollicis brevis
Dorsal interossei
Abductor digiti minimi

Triceps brachii | Long head
Lateral head
Medial head
Anconeus

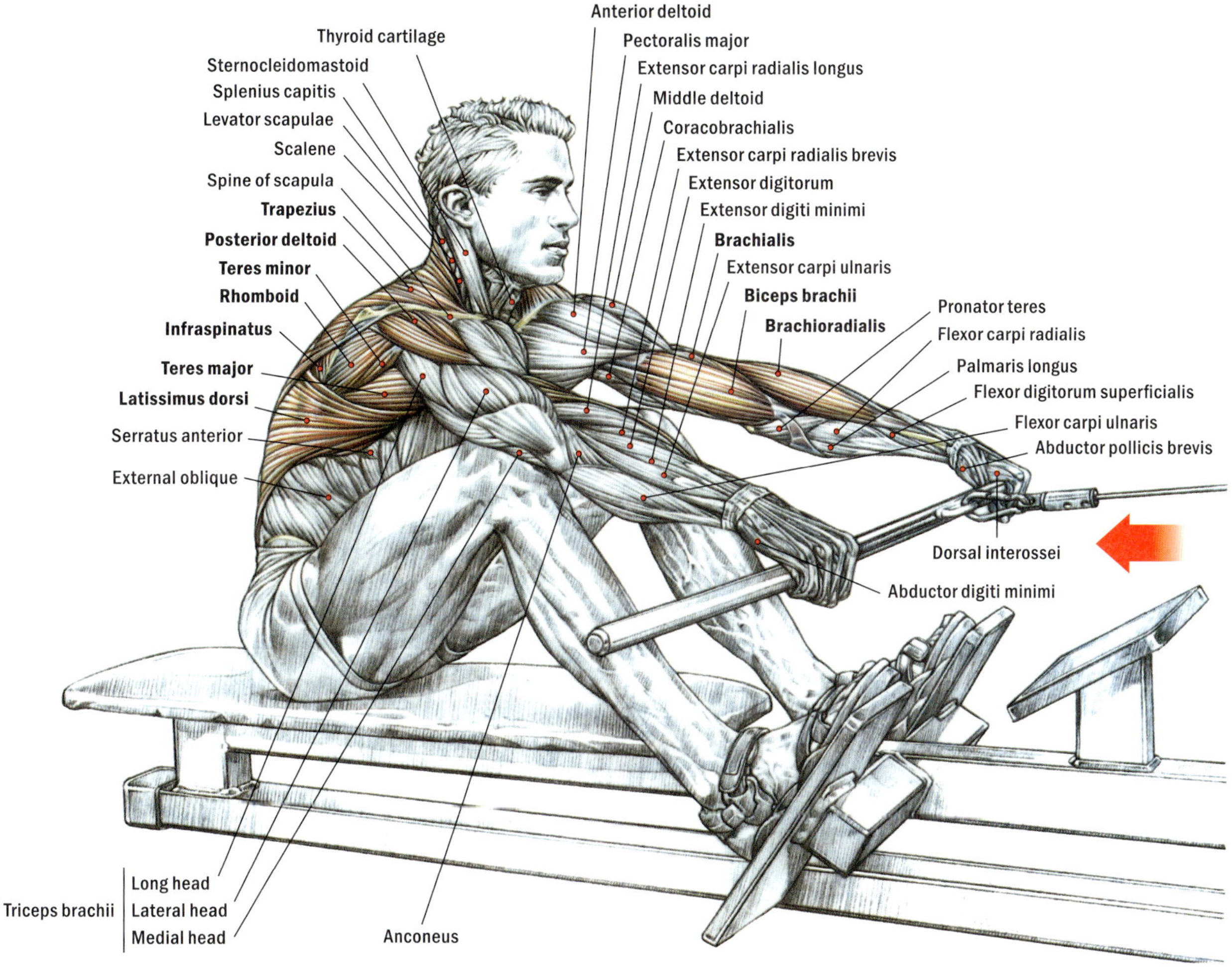

Sit facing the machine with your feet on the footrests and your torso leaning forward. Grasp the bar with an overhand grip (thumbs to the inside) wider than shoulder-width apart:

- Inhale and pull the bar to your chest, straightening your back and keeping your elbows raised.
- Exhale at the end of the exercise and return smoothly to the starting position.

This is an excellent exercise for working the upper back and the back of the shoulders. The main muscles worked are the latissimus dorsi, the teres major, the posterior deltoid, the infraspinatus, the teres minor, and the arm flexors (biceps brachii, brachialis, and brachioradialis). When the shoulder blades come together, the exercise works the rhomboids and the middle part of the trapezius.

As the chest straightens, the spinal muscles (or erector spinae) are also engaged.

To prevent back injury, never round your back when performing seated rows with heavy weights.

Variation

Holding the bar with an underhand grip (thumbs to the outside) will work the lower portion of the trapezius, the rhomboids, and the biceps brachii more intensely.

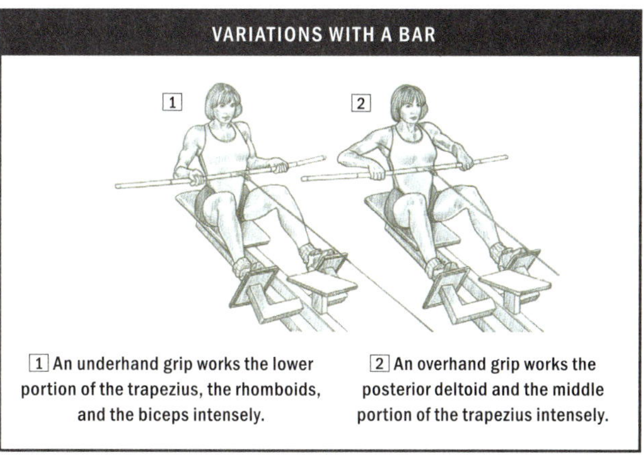

VARIATIONS WITH A BAR

1 An underhand grip works the lower portion of the trapezius, the rhomboids, and the biceps intensely.

2 An overhand grip works the posterior deltoid and the middle portion of the trapezius intensely.

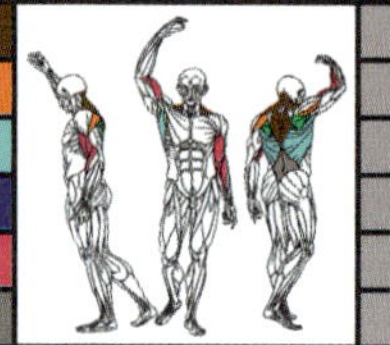

Trapezius — Cervical vertebra — Levator scapulae — Splenius

Rhomboid major
Infraspinatus
Latissimus dorsi
Thoracolumbar fascia
Teres major
Serratus anterior
Pectoralis major
External oblique

Triceps brachii — Long head / Lateral head / Medial head

Anconeus

Extensor carpi ulnaris

Flexor carpi ulnaris

Sternocleidomastoid
Spine of scapula
Teres minor
Anterior deltoid
Posterior deltoid | **Deltoid**
Middle deltoid
Biceps brachii
Brachialis
Brachioradialis
Extensor carpi radialis longus

Extensor carpi radialis brevis

Extensor digiti minimi — Extensor pollicis brevis — Extensor pollicis longus — Abductor pollicis longus

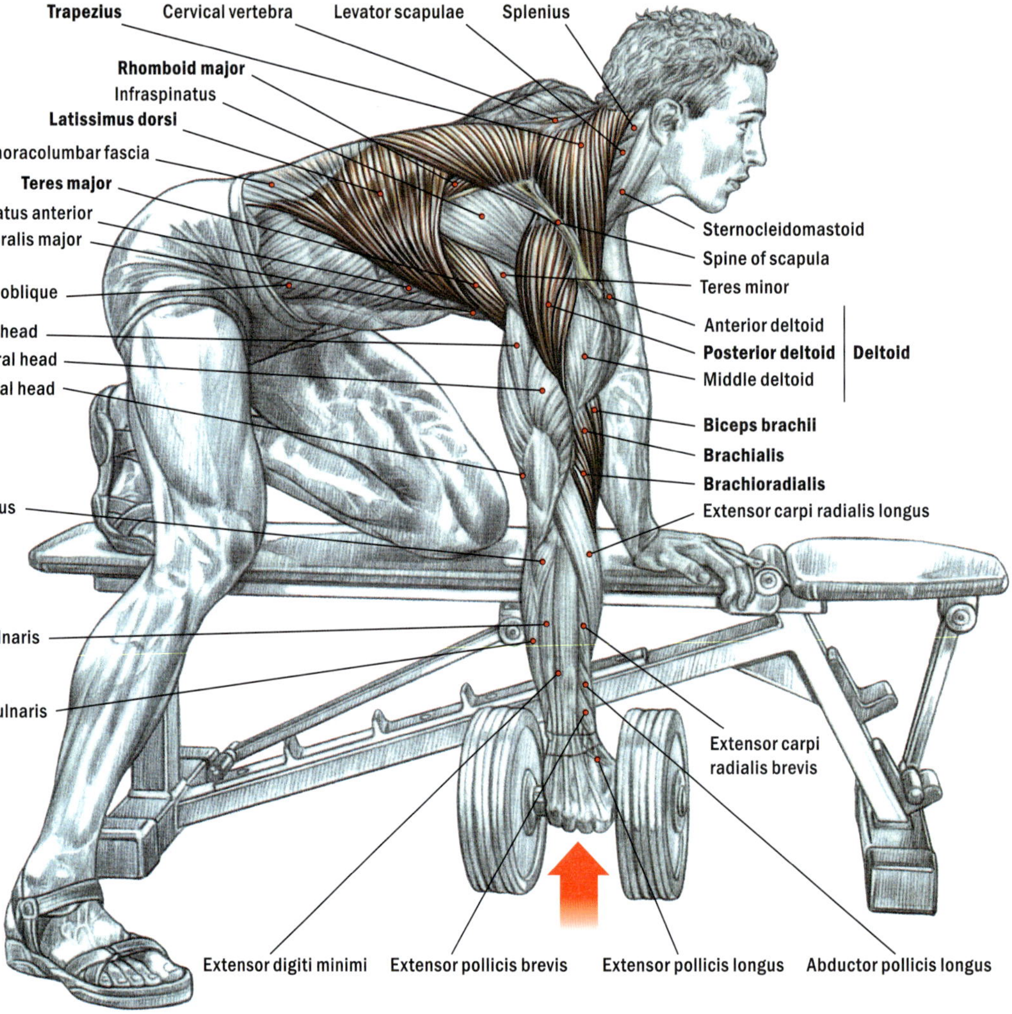

Grasp a dumbbell with your palm facing in; use the opposite hand and knee on the bench to support your back:

- Stabilize your back, inhale, and pull the dumbbell as high as possible, keeping your arm next to your body and bringing your elbow backward.
- Exhale at the end of the exercise.

To maximize the contraction, rotate your torso slightly at the end of the row. This exercise mainly works the latissimus dorsi, teres major, and posterior deltoid. At the end of the contraction, it works the trapezius and rhomboids. The forearm flexors (biceps brachii, brachialis, and brachioradialis) are also engaged.

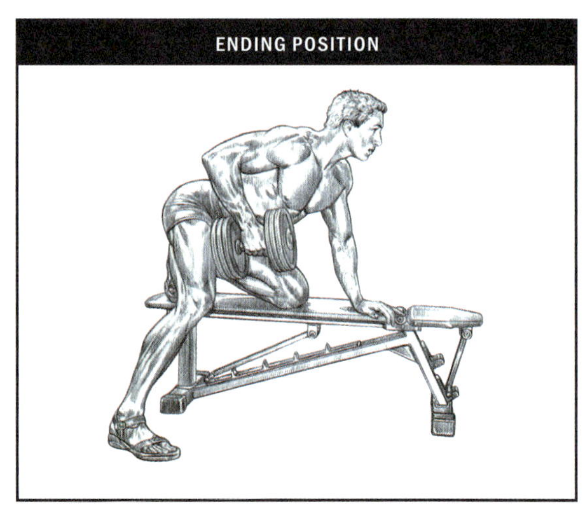

ENDING POSITION

BENT-OVER DUMBBELL ROWS 10

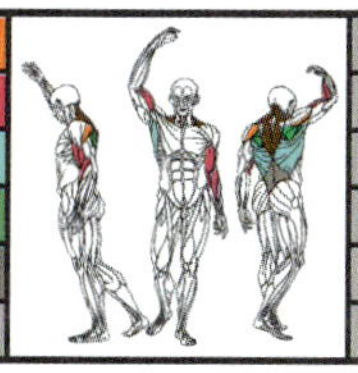

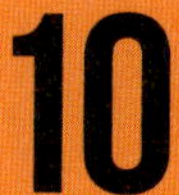

Sternocleidomastoid
Splenius capitis
Levator scapulae
Scalene
Trapezius
Infraspinatus
Rhomboid
Teres minor
Teres major
Latissimus dorsi
Erector spinae (under the aponeurosis)
External oblique
Gluteus medius
Gluteus maximus
Tensor fasciae latae
Rectus femoris
Vastus lateralis
Semitendinosus
Fasciae latae
Long head
Short head
Biceps femoris
Quadriceps, vastus intermedius
Gastrocnemius, medial head
Gastrocnemius, lateral head
Triceps surae
Soleus
Spine of scapula
Serratus anterior
Pectoralis major
Deltoid
Posterior deltoid
Middle deltoid
Triceps brachii
Long head
Lateral head
Medial head
Brachioradialis
Extensor carpi radialis longus
Anconeus
Flexor carpi ulnaris
Extensor carpi radialis brevis
Extensor digitorum
Extensor digiti minimi
Extensor carpi ulnaris
Extensor digitorum longus
Tibialis anterior
Peroneus longus
Peroneus brevis

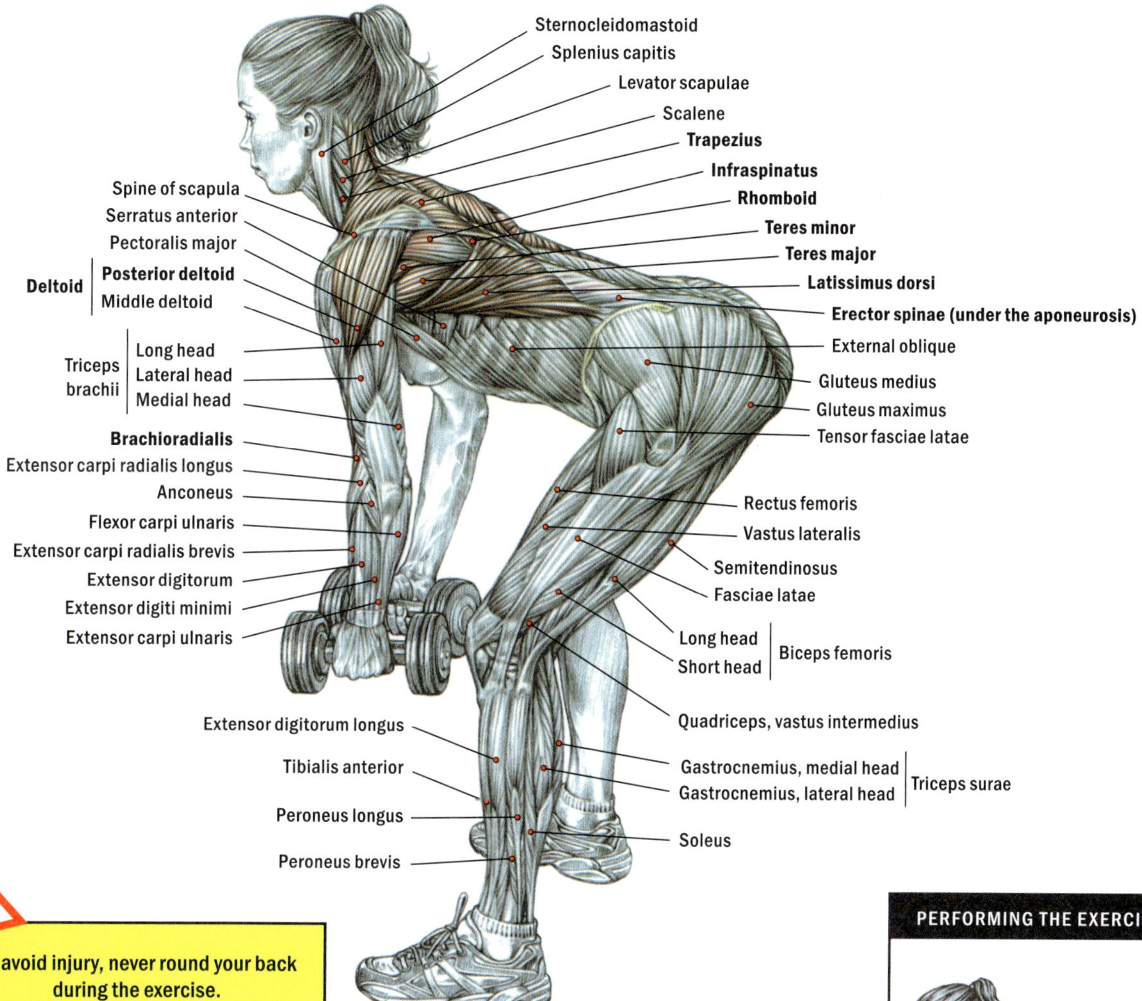

To avoid injury, never round your back during the exercise.

PERFORMING THE EXERCISE

2 Finish
1 Start

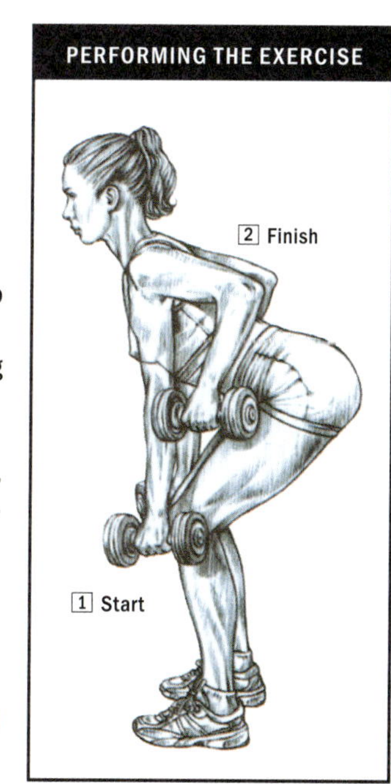

Stand with your legs slightly bent and your chest leaning forward at approximately a 45-degree angle. Keep your back very flat and hang your arms by your sides. Hold a dumbbell in each hand with palms facing in:

- Inhale and isometrically contract your abdominal core. Pull the dumbbells as high as possible, keeping your elbows close to your body. Squeeze your shoulder blades together at the end of the exercise.
- Return to the starting position and exhale.

This exercise recruits the latissimus dorsi, teres major, posterior deltoid, forearm flexors (biceps brachii, brachialis, and brachioradialis), and, when the shoulder blades come together, the rhomboids and trapezius. The tilted position of the chest works the spinal muscles isometrically.

Variations

By varying the angle of the chest, it is possible to focus on working specific parts of the back:

- Keeping the chest up mainly works the upper portion of the trapezius.
- Keeping the torso closer to a horizontal position works the latissimus dorsi, teres major, rhomboids, and middle and lower portions of the trapezius.

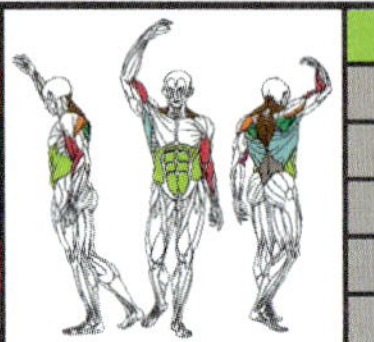

Sternocleidomastoid
Splenius
Levator scapulae
Scalene
Trapezius
Posterior deltoid
Infraspinatus
Rhomboid major
Teres minor
Teres major
Latissimus dorsi

Deltoid — Middle deltoid
Anterior deltoid
Triceps brachii
Brachialis
Biceps brachii
Brachioradialis
Pectoralis major
Extensor carpi radialis longus
Anconeus
Extensor carpi radialis brevis
Extensor digitorum
Extensor carpi ulnaris
Flexor carpi ulnaris
Palmaris longus

Erector spinae (under the thoracolumbar fascia)
Iliac crest
External oblique
Gluteus medius
Tensor fasciae latae
Gluteus maximus
Greater trochanter
Rectus femoris
Vastus lateralis | Quadriceps
Iliotibial band, fasciae latae
Semitendinosus
Long head | Biceps femoris
Short head
Semimembranosus

Gastrocnemius, medial head
Gastrocnemius, lateral head
Soleus
Peroneus longus
Peroneus brevis

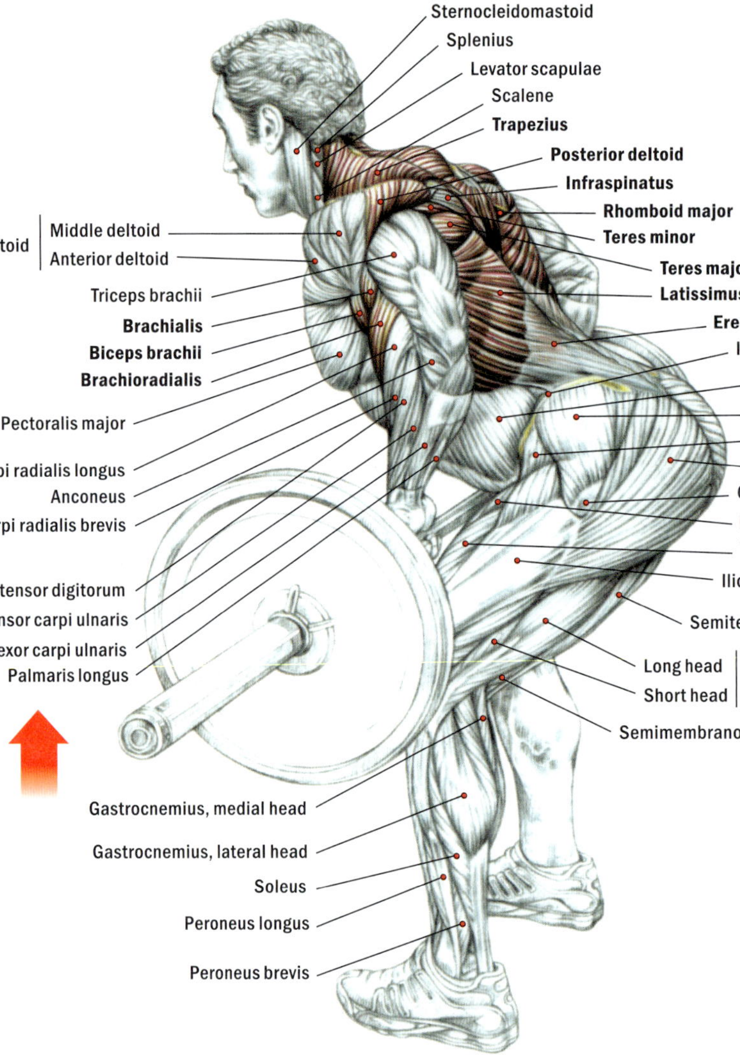

Stand with your legs slightly bent and lean forward 45 degrees at the waist, keeping your back straight. Extend your arms and grasp the bar in an overhand grip with your hands wider than shoulder-width apart.

- Inhale and hold your breath as you brace your core and pull the barbell up to your chest.
- Return to the starting position and exhale.

This exercise contracts the latissimus dorsi, teres major, posterior deltoid, and the forearm flexors (biceps brachii, brachialis, brachioradialis). When the shoulder blades come together, the rhomboids and trapezius contract.

Leaning your torso forward engages your spinal and abdominal muscles in an isometric contraction. It should be noted that varying your hand position in width and grip (overhand or underhand), in addition to changing the angle of your torso, allows you to work your back from a variety of angles.

To avoid injury, never round your back during the exercise.

PERFORMING THE EXERCISE

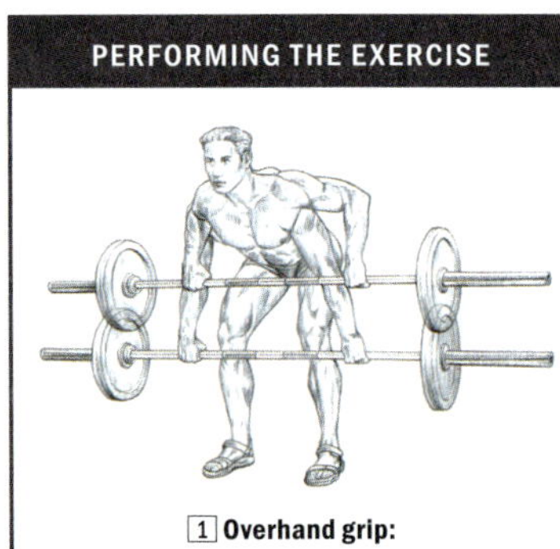

1 Overhand grip:
This method emphasizes the latissimus dorsi, the rhomboids, and the lower and middle portions of the trapezius.

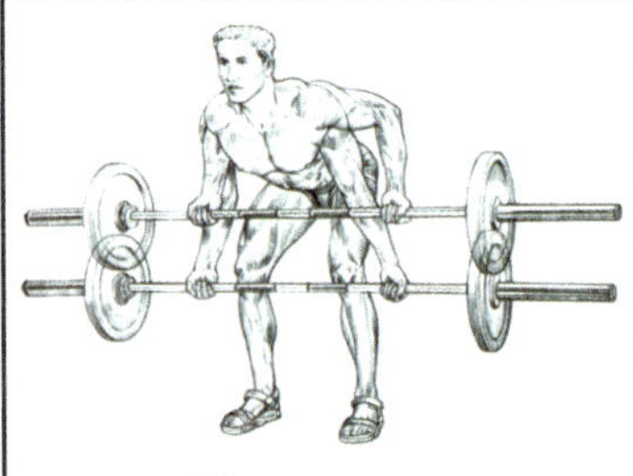

2 Underhand grip:
This variation emphasizes the latissimus dorsi, the upper portion of the trapezius, and the biceps brachii.

CLOSE-GRIP UPRIGHT ROWS 12

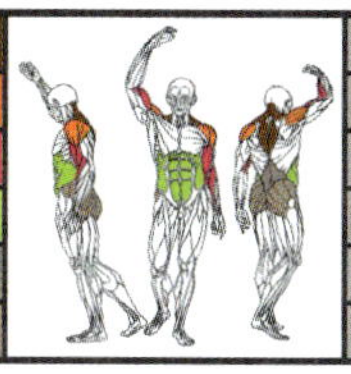

Brachialis
Brachioradialis
Extensor carpi radialis longus
Triceps brachii
Lateral head
Long head
Medial head
Sternocleidomastoid
Semispinalis capitis
Splenius
Levator scapulae
Teres minor
Teres major
Infraspinatus
Rhomboid major
Serratus anterior
Latissimus dorsi
External oblique
Aponeurosis of latissimus dorsi
Middle deltoid
Posterior deltoid
Anterior deltoid
Deltoid
Upper portion
Middle portion
Lower portion
Trapezius

2 Finish
1 Start

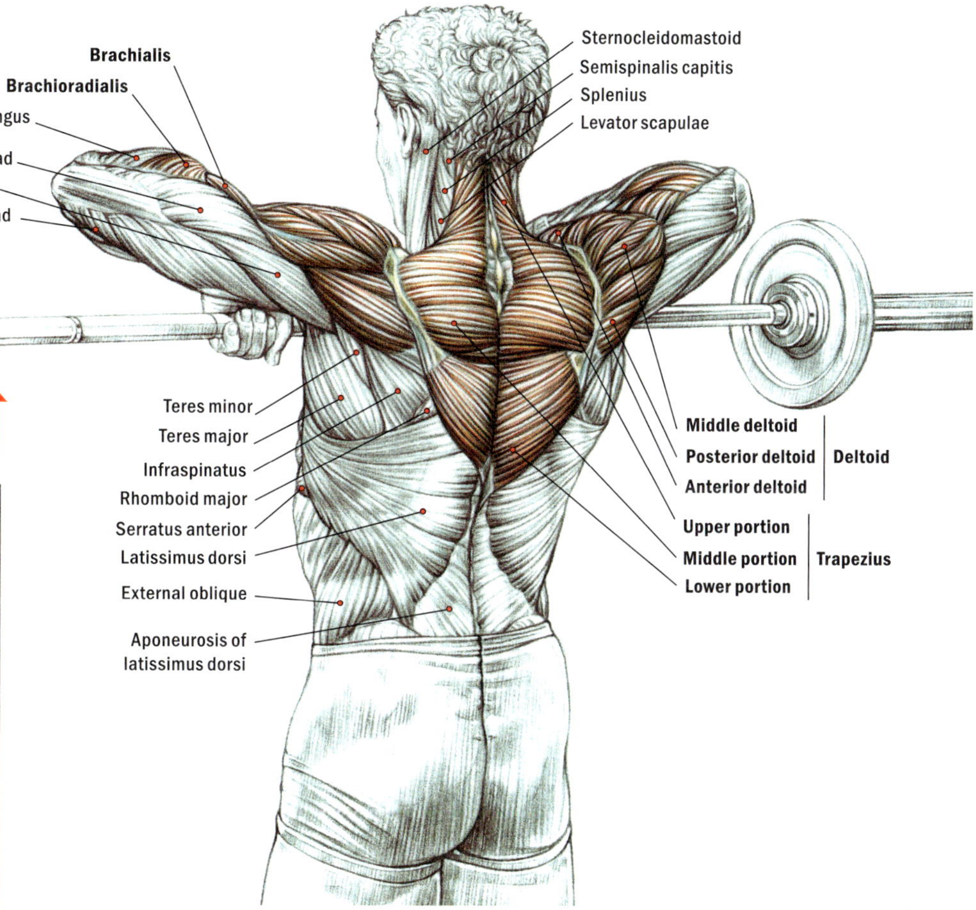

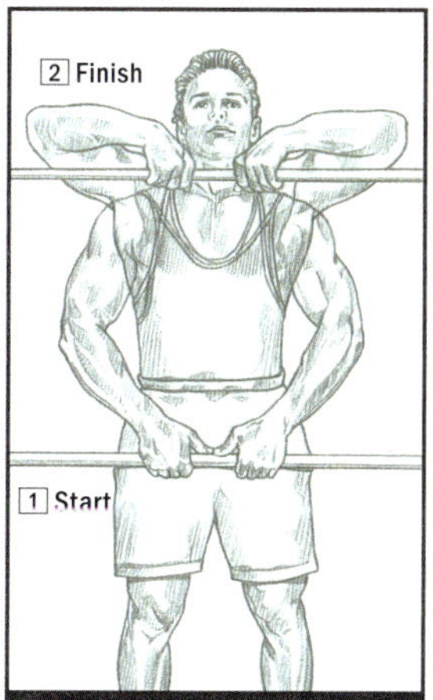

PERFORMING THE EXERCISE

Stand with your legs slightly apart, keeping your back straight and holding the barbell with an overhand grip. The grip should be hand-width apart or slightly wider:

- Inhale and pull the barbell up along the front of your body to your chin, raising your elbows as high as possible.
- Exhale and lower the barbell with a controlled movement.

This exercise works the upper portion of the trapezius as well as the deltoids, levator scapulae, biceps brachii, brachialis, forearm muscles, abdominal muscles, gluteal muscles, and lumbosacral muscles. It is worth noting that, as the grips gets wider, the deltoids work harder than the trapezius muscles.

ACTIONS OF THE TRAPEZIUS MUSCLE

1
2
3

1 Upper portion 2 Middle portion 3 Lower portion

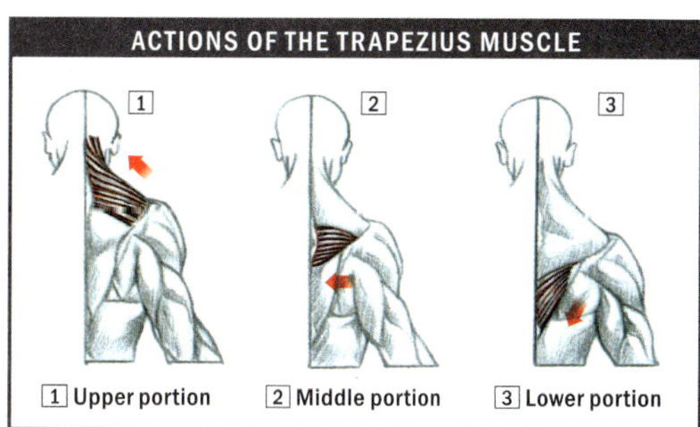

13 T-BAR ROWS

To avoid the risk of injury, never round your back during T-bar rows.

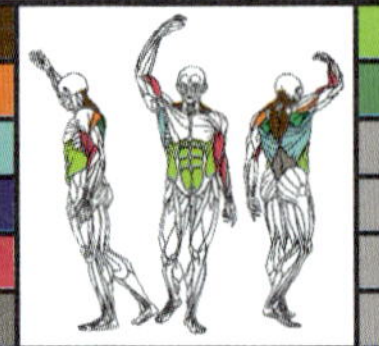

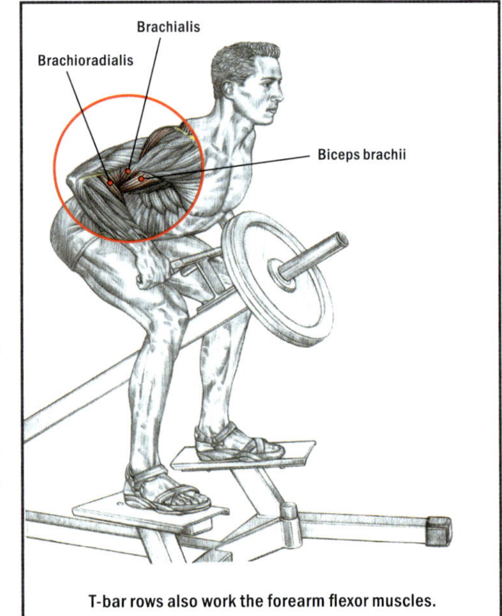

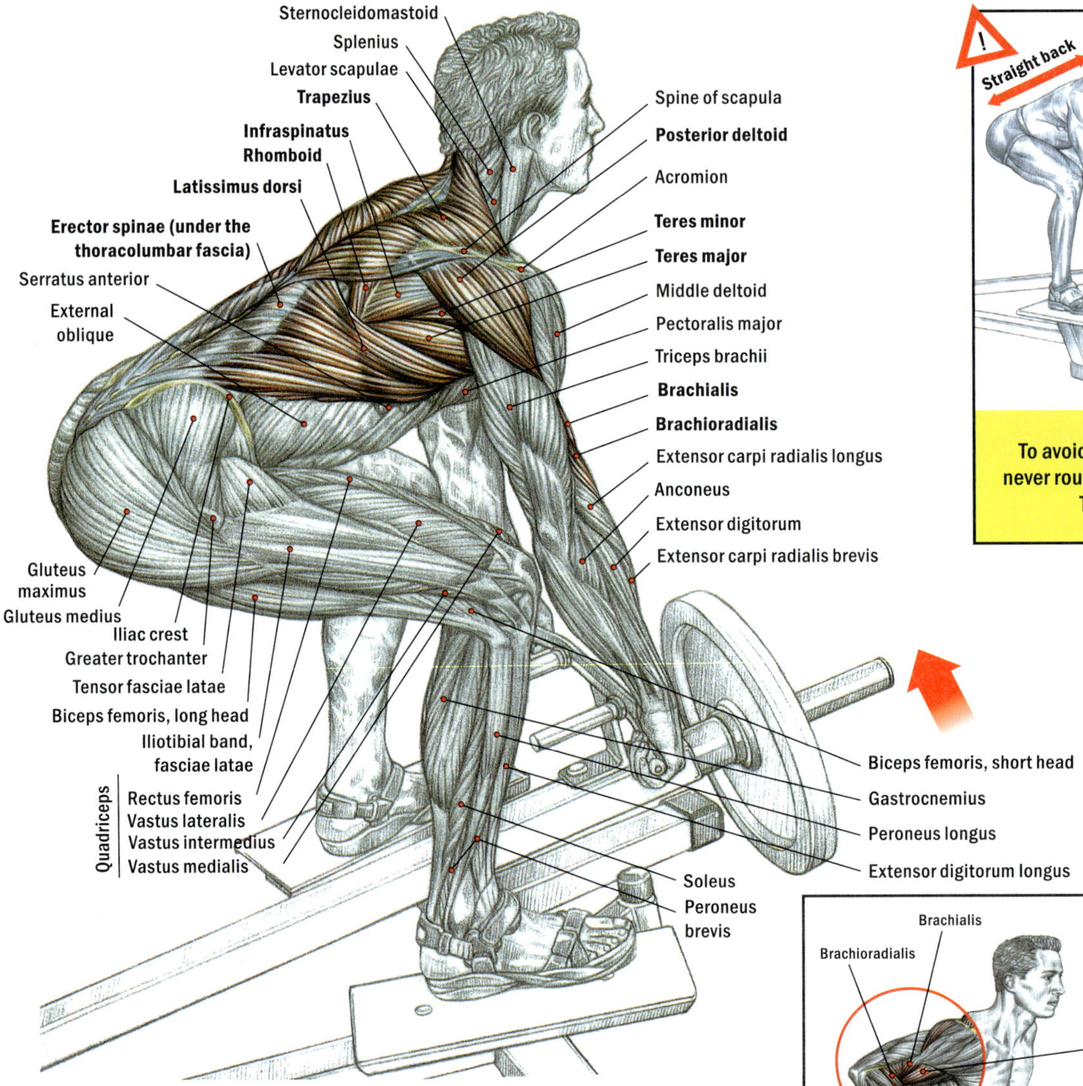

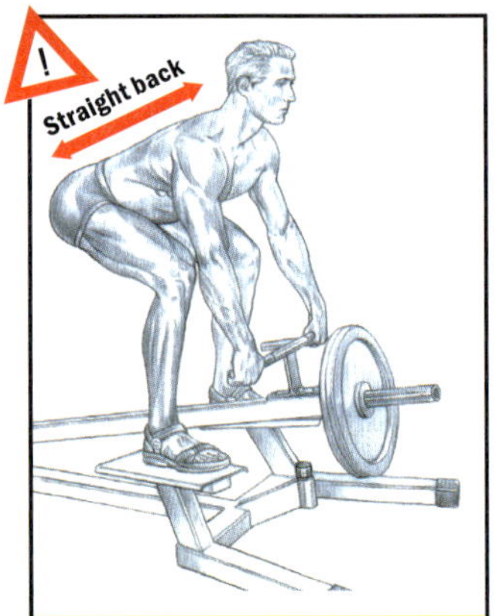

Straddle the bar with your legs slightly bent and lean forward at the waist about 45 degrees with a flat back. Grasp the bar with an overhand grip:

- Inhale and raise the bar to your chest.
- Exhale at the end of the exercise.

This exercise is similar to barbell rows and allows you to concentrate on working your back, since it does not require as much effort to get into the right position. This exercise primarily works the latissimus dorsi, teres major, infraspinatus, rhomboids, trapezius (mainly the middle portion), and the flexors of the forearm.

Leaning the torso forward works the abdominal and spinal muscles isometrically. Using an underhand grip will transfer some of the effort to the biceps brachii and the upper portion of the trapezius at the end of the pull.

Some machines have parallel handles that allow a semipronated grip that is in between and overhand and underhand grip; this will work the forearms—specifically the brachioradialis—more intensely.

T-bar rows also work the forearm flexor muscles.

ABDOMINAL-SUPPORTED T-BAR ROWS

14

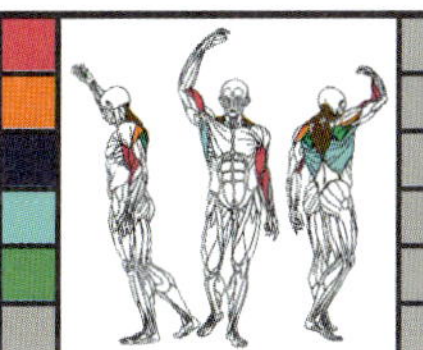

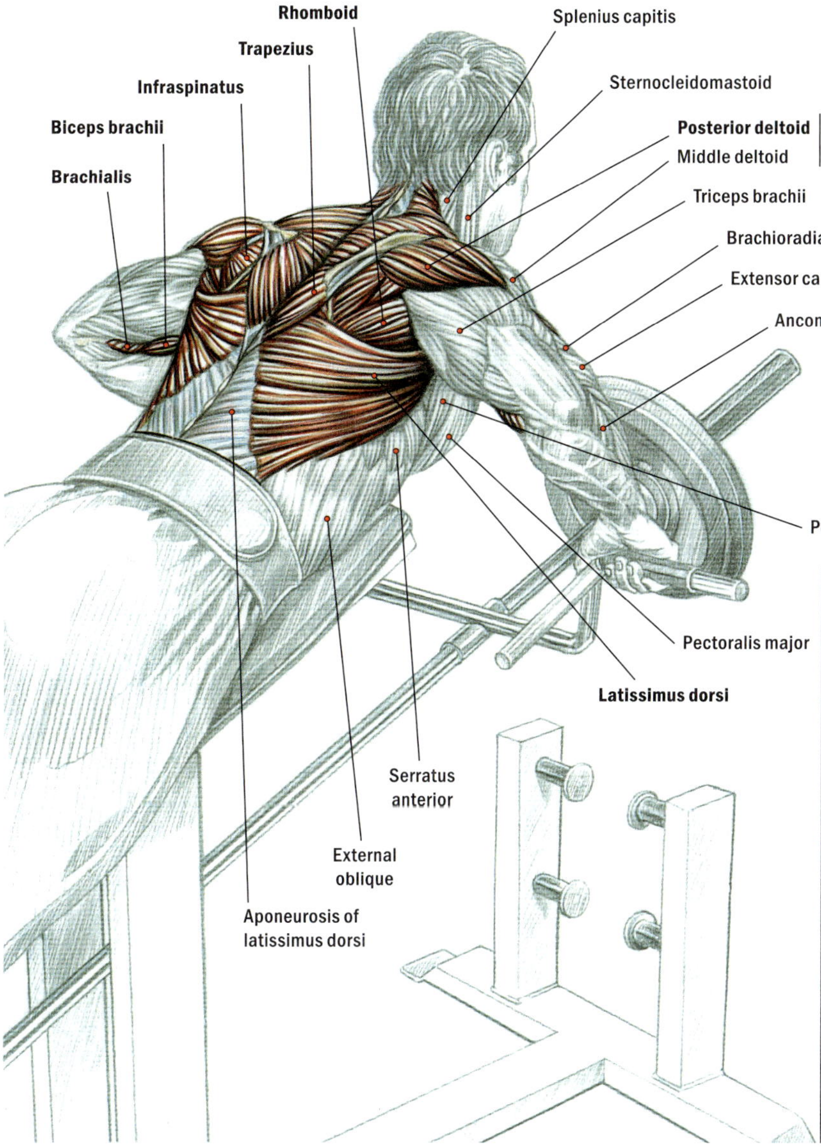

Rhomboid
Trapezius
Infraspinatus
Biceps brachii
Brachialis
Splenius capitis
Sternocleidomastoid
Posterior deltoid
Middle deltoid
Deltoid
Triceps brachii
Brachioradialis
Extensor carpi radialis longus
Anconeus
Pectoralis minor
Pectoralis major
Latissimus dorsi
Serratus anterior
External oblique
Aponeurosis of latissimus dorsi

1 Start
2 Finish

VARIATION USING A SPECIFIC MACHINE THAT REPLICATES THE MOVEMENT DONE WITH A T-BAR

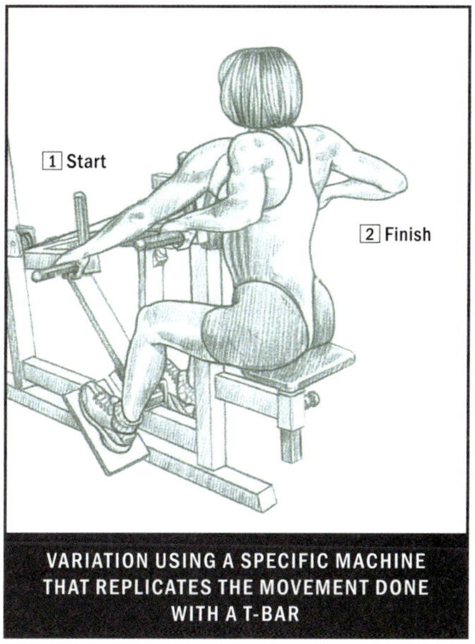

Rest on an incline bench:

- Inhale and bring the bar to your chest with an overhand grip.
- Exhale at the end of the exercise.

This exercise is similar to barbell rows. It allows you to concentrate on working your back, since it does not require as much effort to get into the right position. It mainly works the latissimus dorsi, teres major, posterior deltoid, arm flexors, trapezius, and rhomboids.

Some machines have an abdominal support, which makes positioning easier and eliminates the work of the abdominal and spinal muscles. However, when using heavy weights, the rib cage is compressed against the abdominal-support pad, which interferes with breathing and makes it difficult to do the exercise.

An underhand grip shifts some of the effort to the biceps brachii and the upper portion of the trapezius at the end of the pull.

15 STIFF-LEGGED DEADLIFTS

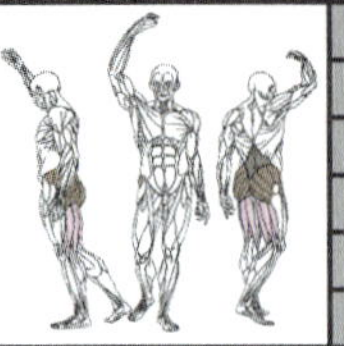

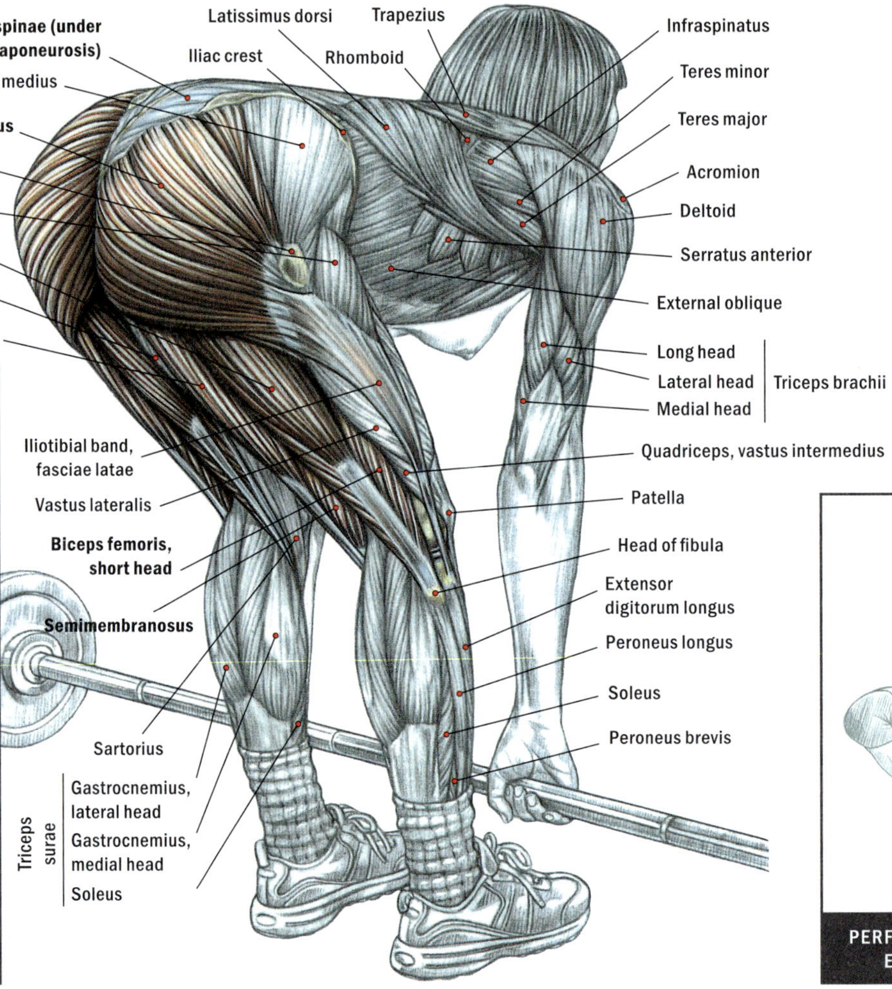

Erector spinae (under the aponeurosis)
Latissimus dorsi
Trapezius
Infraspinatus
Iliac crest
Rhomboid
Teres minor
Gluteus medius
Teres major
Gluteus maximus
Acromion
Greater trochanter
Deltoid
Tensor fasciae latae
Serratus anterior
Biceps femoris, long head
Adductor magnus
External oblique
Semitendinosus
Long head
Lateral head
Medial head
Triceps brachii
Iliotibial band, fasciae latae
Quadriceps, vastus intermedius
Vastus lateralis
Patella
Biceps femoris, short head
Head of fibula
Extensor digitorum longus
Semimembranosus
Peroneus longus
Soleus
Sartorius
Peroneus brevis
Triceps surae
Gastrocnemius, lateral head
Gastrocnemius, medial head
Soleus

ACTION OF THE HAMSTRINGS AND GLUTEUS MAXIMUS WHEN SHIFTING THE PELVIS TO A VERTICAL POSITION

ACTION OF THE HAM-STRINGS
ACTION OF THE GLUTEUS MAXIMUS

2 Finish
1 Start

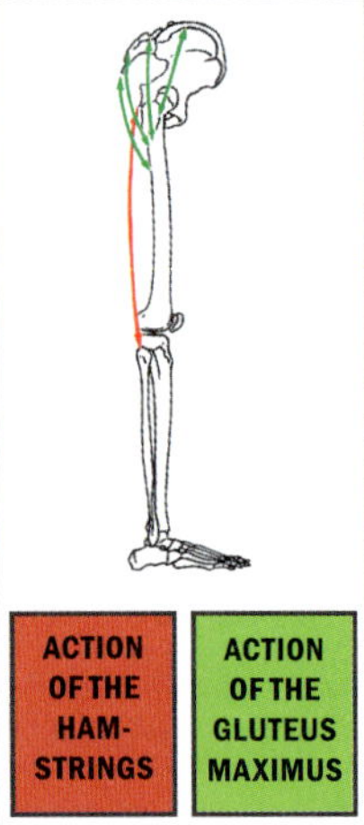

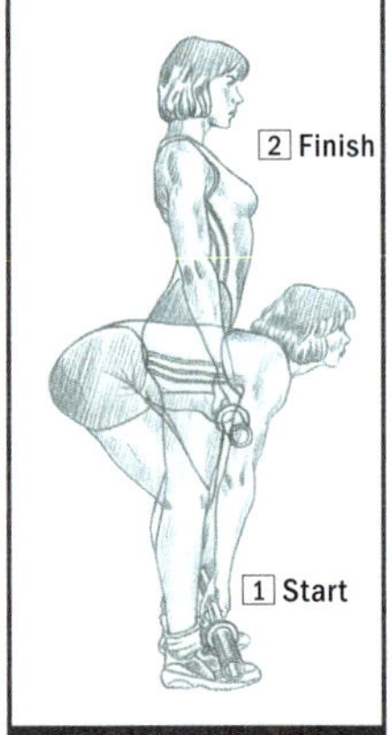

PERFORMING THE EXERCISE

Stand with your feet slightly apart, facing a bar resting on the ground:

- Inhale and bend forward at your waist with your chest forward, back slightly arched, and legs as straight as possible.
- Grasp the bar with an overhand grip. Keeping your arms relaxed and your back stable, lift your torso and stand up straight. The movement should come from your hips. Exhale at the end of the exercise.
- Return to the starting position, but do not set the bar down. Repeat.

To avoid any risk of injury, it is important to keep the back straight during the exercise. This exercise works the deep muscles on either side of the spine that straighten the spine. Raising the torso by tilting the pelvis from front to back works the gluteus maximus and hamstrings (except for the short head of the biceps femoris).

Stiff-legged deadlifts stretch the back of the thighs during the flexing portion of the exercise. To increase the effectiveness of this stretch, you can stand on something so that your feet are higher than the bar.

When done with very light weight, stiff-legged deadlifts can be done to stretch the hamstrings. The heavier the weight, the more the gluteal muscles take over from the hamstrings to straighten the pelvis to a vertical position.

ACTION OF THE HAMSTRINGS

Floating ribs
Lumbar vertebra
Hip bone
Head of femur
Sacrum
Rib
Ischial tuberosity
Neck of femur
Costal cartilage
Greater trochanter
Patella
Biceps femoris, long head
Meniscus
Semitendinosus
Tibial tuberosity
Femur
Head of fibula
Semimembranosus
Tibia
Biceps femoris, short head
Fibula

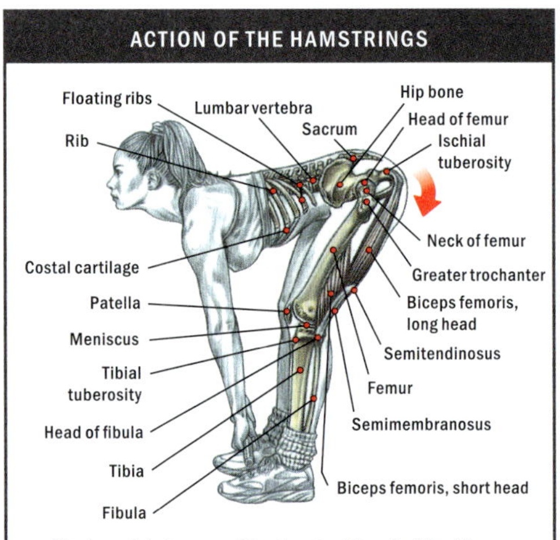

The hamstrings, except for the short head of the biceps femoris, actively participate in tilting the pelvis backward.

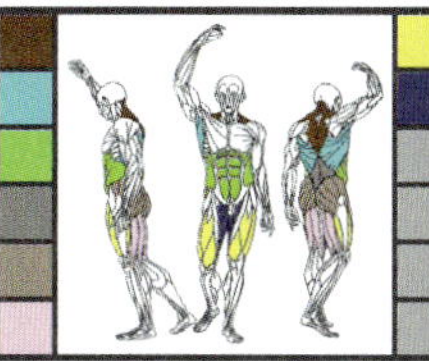

PERFORMING THE EXERCISE

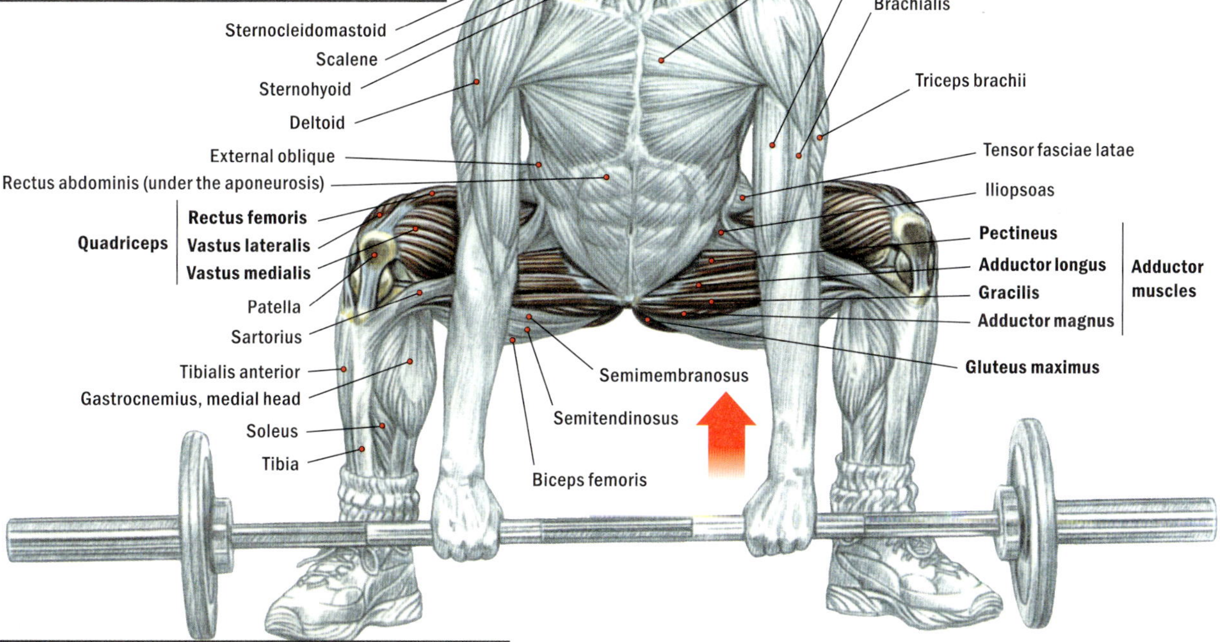

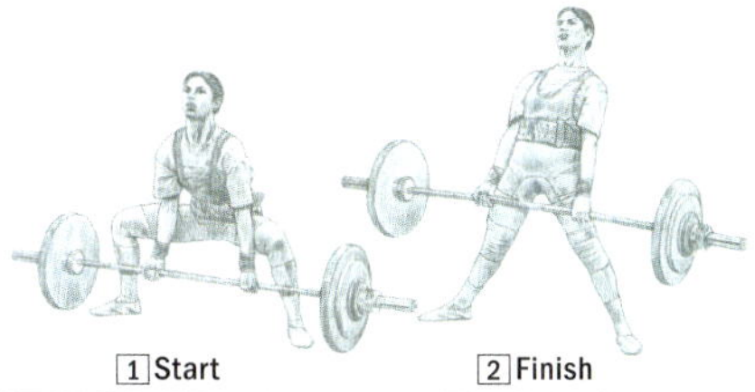

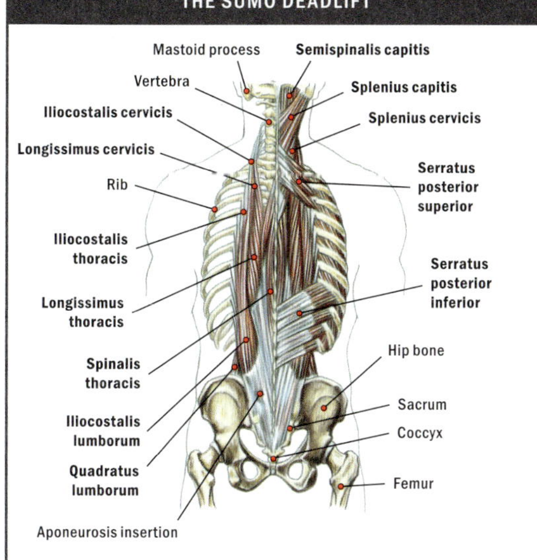

Trapezius
Omohyoid
Pectoralis major
Biceps brachii
Brachialis
Sternocleidomastoid
Scalene
Sternohyoid
Deltoid
External oblique
Rectus abdominis (under the aponeurosis)
Triceps brachii
Tensor fasciae latae
Iliopsoas
Rectus femoris
Quadriceps **Vastus lateralis**
Vastus medialis
Patella
Sartorius
Tibialis anterior
Gastrocnemius, medial head
Soleus
Tibia
Semimembranosus
Semitendinosus
Biceps femoris
Pectineus
Adductor longus **Adductor muscles**
Gracilis
Adductor magnus
Gluteus maximus

DEEP MUSCLES OF THE BACK USED DURING THE SUMO DEADLIFT

Mastoid process
Semispinalis capitis
Vertebra
Splenius capitis
Iliocostalis cervicis
Splenius cervicis
Longissimus cervicis
Rib
Serratus posterior superior
Iliocostalis thoracis
Serratus posterior inferior
Longissimus thoracis
Hip bone
Spinalis thoracis
Sacrum
Iliocostalis lumborum
Coccyx
Quadratus lumborum
Femur
Aponeurosis insertion

Stand facing the bar with your legs apart and toes pointing out but always in line with your knees:

- Bend your legs until the thighs are horizontal to the ground.
- Grasp the bar with an overhand grip about shoulder-width apart (if you are lifting very heavy weights, use a mixed grip—hold the bar with one overhand and one underhand grip—to keep the bar from rolling).
- Inhale, hold your breath, slightly arch your back, contract your core, and straighten your legs to bring your torso up as you pull your shoulders back. Exhale at the end of the exercise.
- Return the bar to the ground while holding your breath. Never round your back.

Contrary to the traditional deadlift, this exercise works the quadriceps and adductor muscles intensely. Because the pelvis is not tilted as much, this exercise works the back less.

When beginning the movement, it is important to slide the bar along the shins. High-repetition counts (10 maximum) with light weights will strengthen the lumbar region and work the thighs and the gluteal muscles.

However, sumo deadlifts should be done with great caution when using heavy weights to avoid injuries to the hip joints, the adductor muscles, and the lumbosacral junction, which works hard during this exercise. The sumo deadlift is one of the three powerlifting movements.

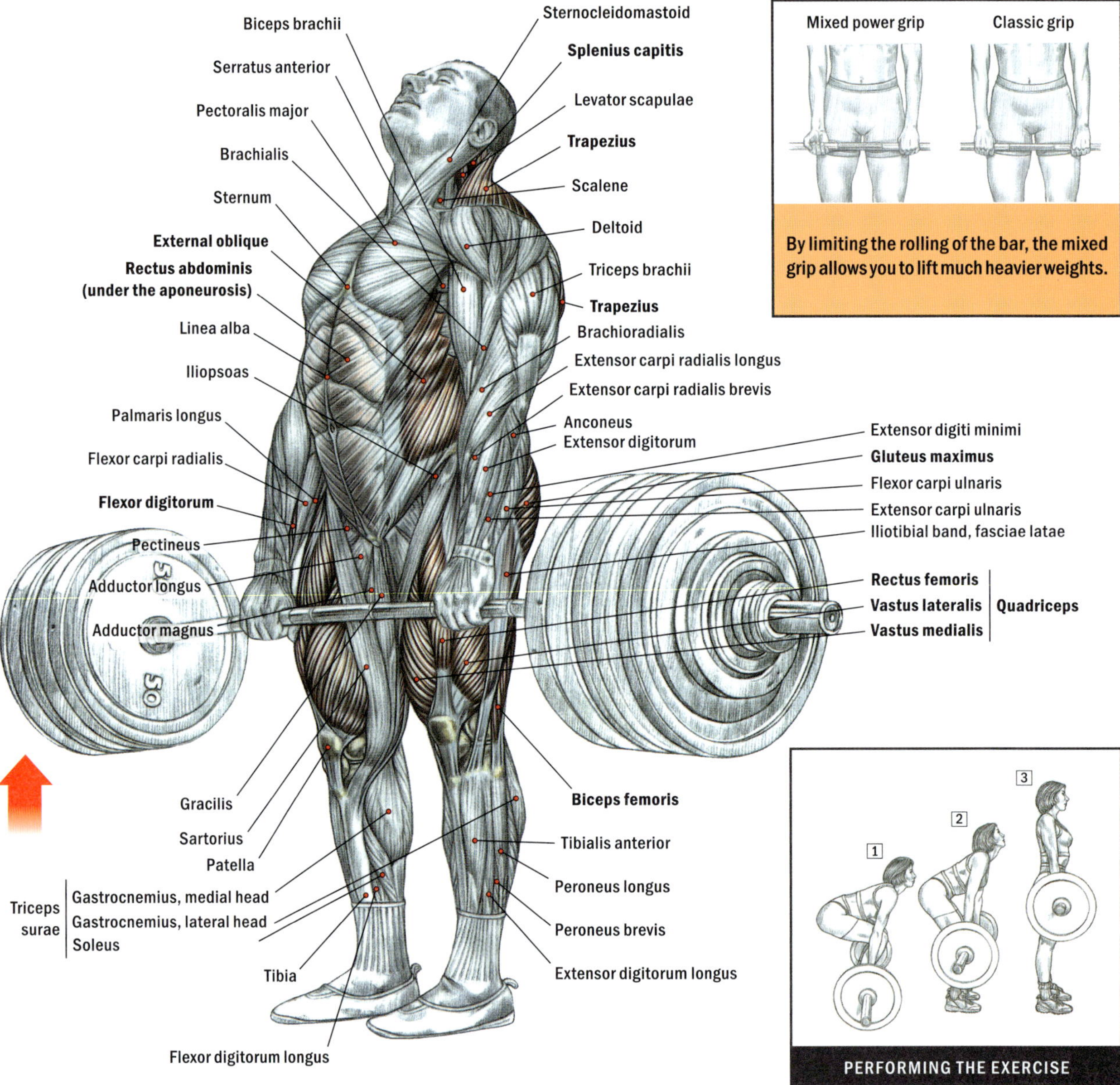

By limiting the rolling of the bar, the mixed grip allows you to lift much heavier weights.

Stand facing the bar with your legs slightly apart and your back stable and slightly arched:

- Bend your knees until your thighs are almost parallel to the floor. This position will vary depending on your morphology and the flexibility of your ankles (for example, the thighs will be horizontal for someone with short thighs and arms, whereas the thighs will be a little above horizontal for someone with long thighs and arms).
- Keeping your arms straight, grab the bar in an overhand grip with your hands slightly more than shoulder-width apart. You can also use a mixed grip (one hand in a pronated grip and the other in a supinated grip) to prevent the bar from rolling, which will allow you to lift a much heavier weight.
- Inhale, hold your breath, contract your core and lower back muscles, and lift the bar by straightening your legs and allowing the bar to slide up the shins.
- When the bar reaches your knees, lift your torso upright while straightening your legs and exhale as you complete the exercise.
- Hold this straightened position for 2 seconds, then place the bar on the floor while keeping your core and lower back muscles contracted.

Throughout the exercise, you must never round your back.

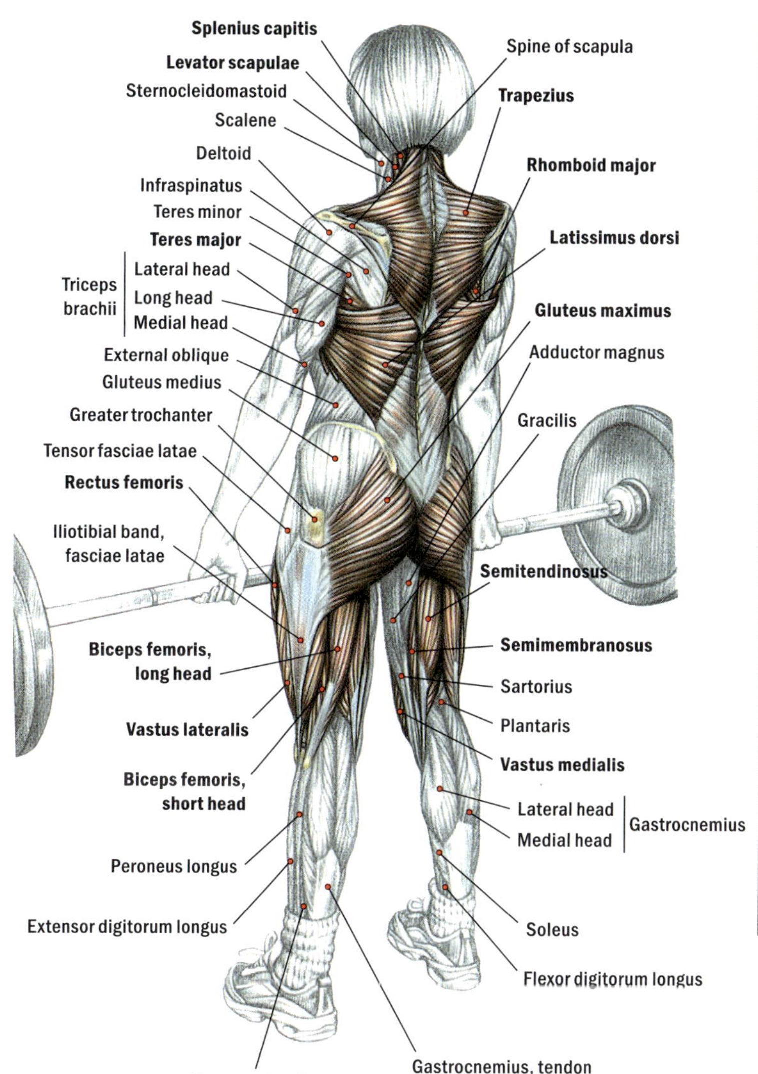

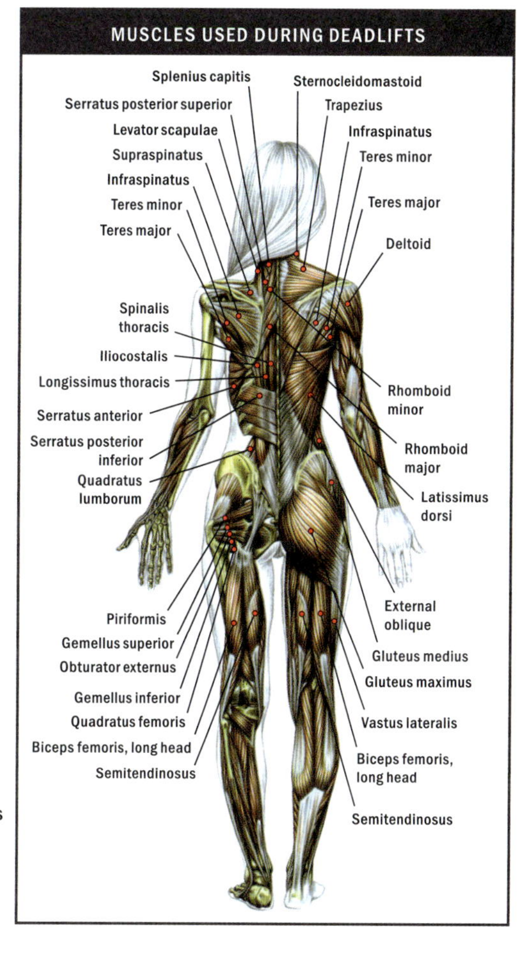

This exercise works nearly every muscle in the body and is very effective for developing the lumbosacral and trapezius muscles. It also works the gluteal muscles and quadriceps intensely. The deadlift, the bench press, and the squat are the exercises done in powerlifting competitions.

> ⚠ No matter what the exercise, as soon as heavy weights are involved, it is essential to brace:
>
> 1. Expand your chest by inhaling deeply and holding your breath to fill the lungs like a balloon. This supports your rib cage and prevents your chest from leaning forward.
> 2. Contract all of your abdominal muscles to support your core and increase intra-abdominal pressure. This prevents your torso from slumping forward.
> 3. Finally, arch your lower back by contracting your lumbar muscles to extend your lower spine.
>
> These three actions together are referred to as *bracing*, which keeps you from rounding your back (vertebral flexion). A rounded back, when lifting heavy weights, can result in a herniated disc (see pages 176-177).

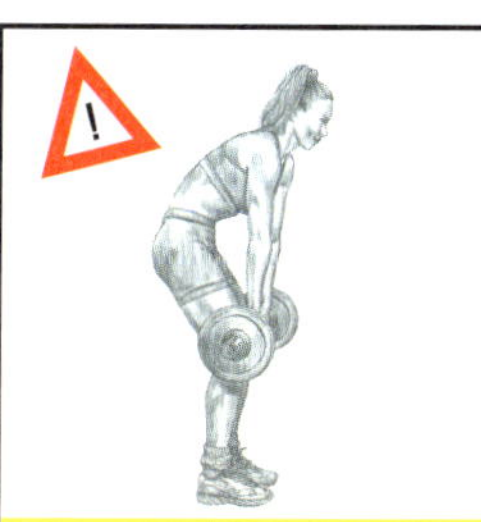

> ⚠ To avoid injury, never round your back during the exercise.

BICEPS BRACHII DISTAL TENDON TEAR

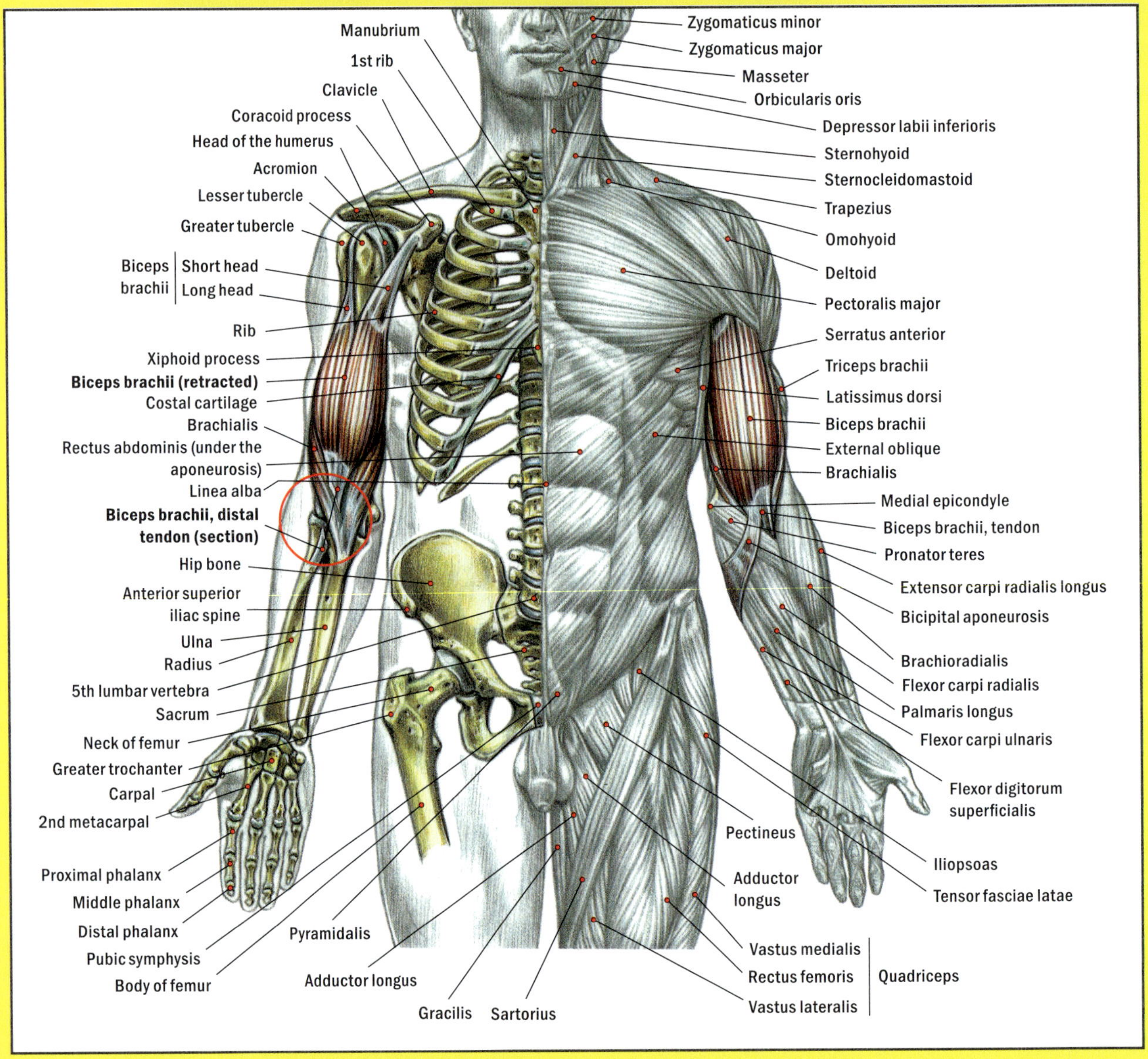

Tearing or rupture of the long head of the biceps brachii is by far the most common serious sport-related biceps injury. Generally, it occurs in a muscle already weakened by tendinitis, after a sudden backward movement of the arm (for example, during a throw). Thus, this injury is relatively common in baseball, tennis, and in all throwing sports. It also occurs in weightlifting during the snatch. During this motion, tension is suddenly placed on the long head of the biceps brachii, which most often tears where its tendon passes through the bicipital groove of the humerus.

Strength training, specifically deadlifts with heavy weights, can cause another characteristic biceps brachii injury.

A common practice when using heavy weights in the deadlift is to use a mixed grip (one overhand grip and one underhand grip) to prevent the bar from rolling in the hands. This technique, although usually safe, can in extremely rare instances cause the tearing or pulling away of the inferior tendon of the biceps brachii where the muscle inserts onto the humerus.

During the positive phase of the deadlift, the effort is mainly exerted by the leg, gluteal, back, and abdominal muscles. The arms hang down relaxed but completely extended, like the cables of a crane.

Unfortunately, the slight shortening of either biceps tendon caused by contracting it to supinate the hand (since the biceps is the strongest supinator) can cause excessive tension, which, along with heavy weights, may cause a tear or a complete rupture of the tendon at the radius.

This injury occurs at the distal attachment, because, as the arms hang next to the body, the tension in the upper muscle is divided between the short and long heads of the biceps brachii, whereas at the bottom of the muscle, only one tendinous insertion supports all of the tension.

In other tendon tears such as in the pectoralis major or the adductors of the thigh, the pain is unbearable and stops the athlete from continuing. By comparison, the pain of a biceps tendon tear is relatively mild despite the seriousness of the injury.

In powerlifting competitions, athletes have actually continued their deadlift despite having just torn a biceps tendon. After the accident, the diagnosis is obvious: Swelling caused by hemorrhaging appears in the front of the arm. But what is most striking is the appearance of the biceps brachii, which retracts into a ball in the upper arm, close to the pectoralis major and the deltoid, revealing the brachialis muscle farther down.

Despite the muscle tear, the brachialis, brachioradialis, extensor carpi radialis longus and brevis, and pronator teres muscles can still flex the arm, just not as powerfully. However, supination of the forearm becomes much more difficult since the end of that kind of movement can only now be done by a single supinator muscle.

If this injury is not immediately treated with surgery to reattach the biceps tendon onto the radius, irreversible retraction of the muscle will occur with fibrous changes. Although it will still be possible to move the arm, there will be permanent loss of strength in flexion and supination.

It is possible to prevent this injury, which is typical when performing deadlifts, by regularly working the biceps. This is not to develop the muscle, but to strengthen its tendon. To that end, when doing curls with a bar, it is advisable to add a few cheat sets by leaning the chest back to give the bar a boost. If practiced regularly, this technique places tension on the distal tendon of the biceps, which ends up strengthening it. Nevertheless, it must still be done carefully and without rounding the back to avoid injury.

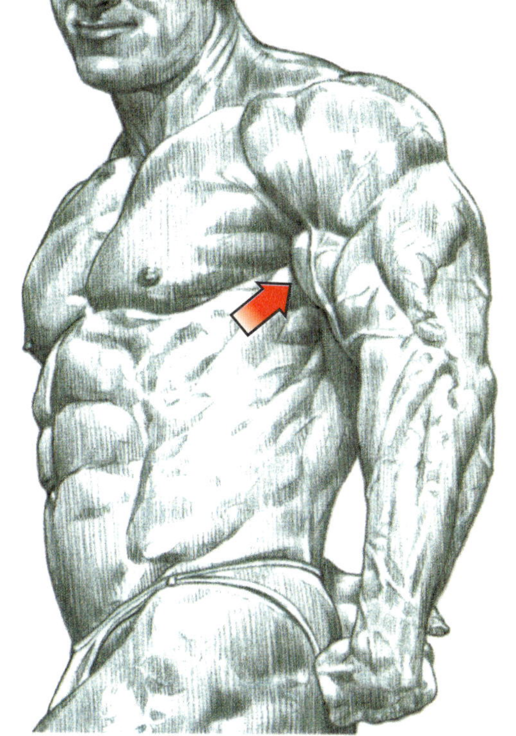

After the distal tendon of the biceps brachii has torn, if surgery to reattach it to the radius is not performed quickly, permanent retraction and atrophy of the muscle will occur.

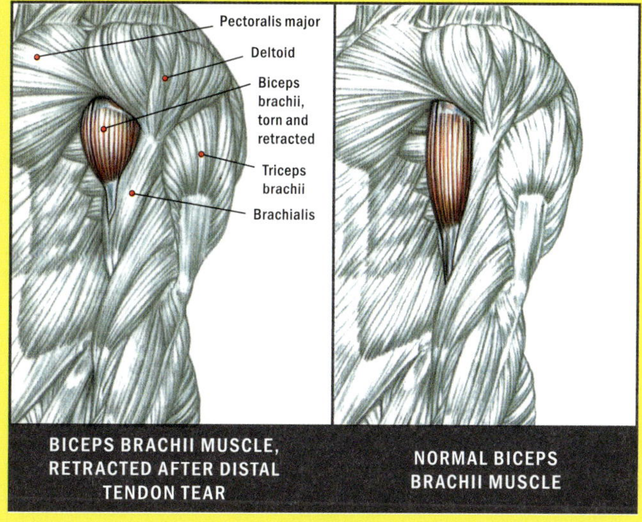

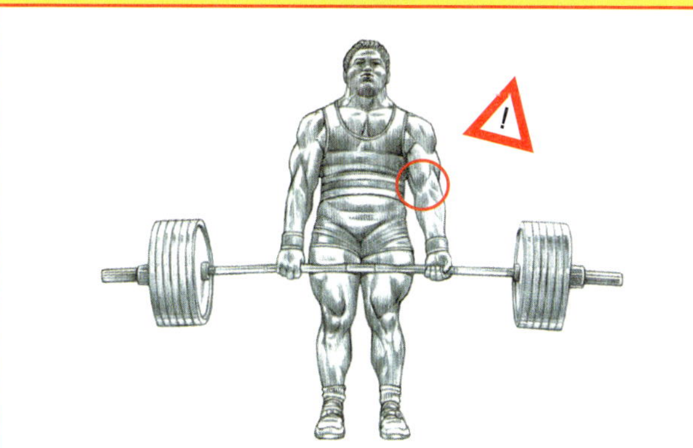

The biceps tendon on the arm of the supinated hand can sometimes tear during an extremely heavy deadlift.

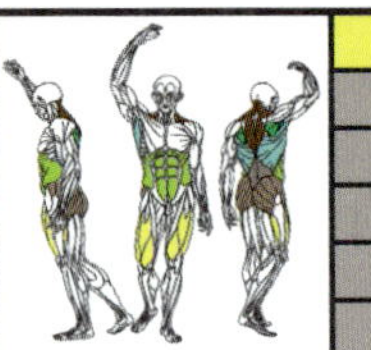

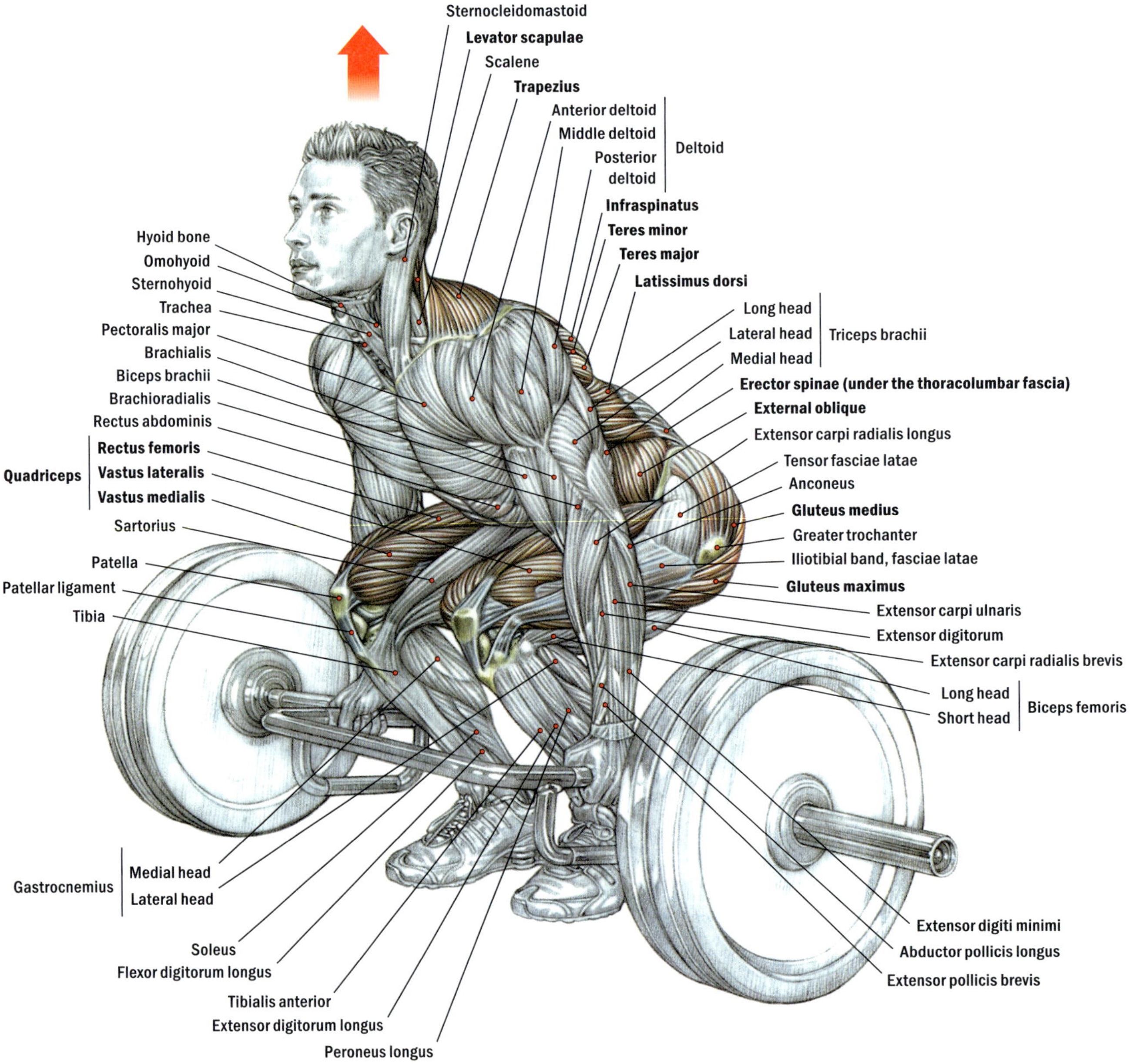

Stand well centered within the bar (be careful because poor centering causes lateral instability). Your legs should be slightly apart and your back stabilized and slightly arched:

- Bend your legs to bring your thighs close to a horizontal position; this position can vary depending on the flexibility of your ankles and individual morphology (for example, for individuals with short thighs and arms, the thighs will be horizontal; for individuals with long thighs and arms, the thighs will be a little above horizontal).

- With your arms extended, grasp the handles of the bar, carefully centering the grip. Remember that, with heavy weights on a trap bar, a badly adjusted grip will push the bar forward or back.
- Inhale, hold your breath, contract your core and lumbar region, and lift the bar by straightening your legs without ever rounding your lower back. Exhale at the end of the exercise.
- Maintain the extension of the body for 2 seconds, then set the bar down while keeping your core and lumbar region contracted.

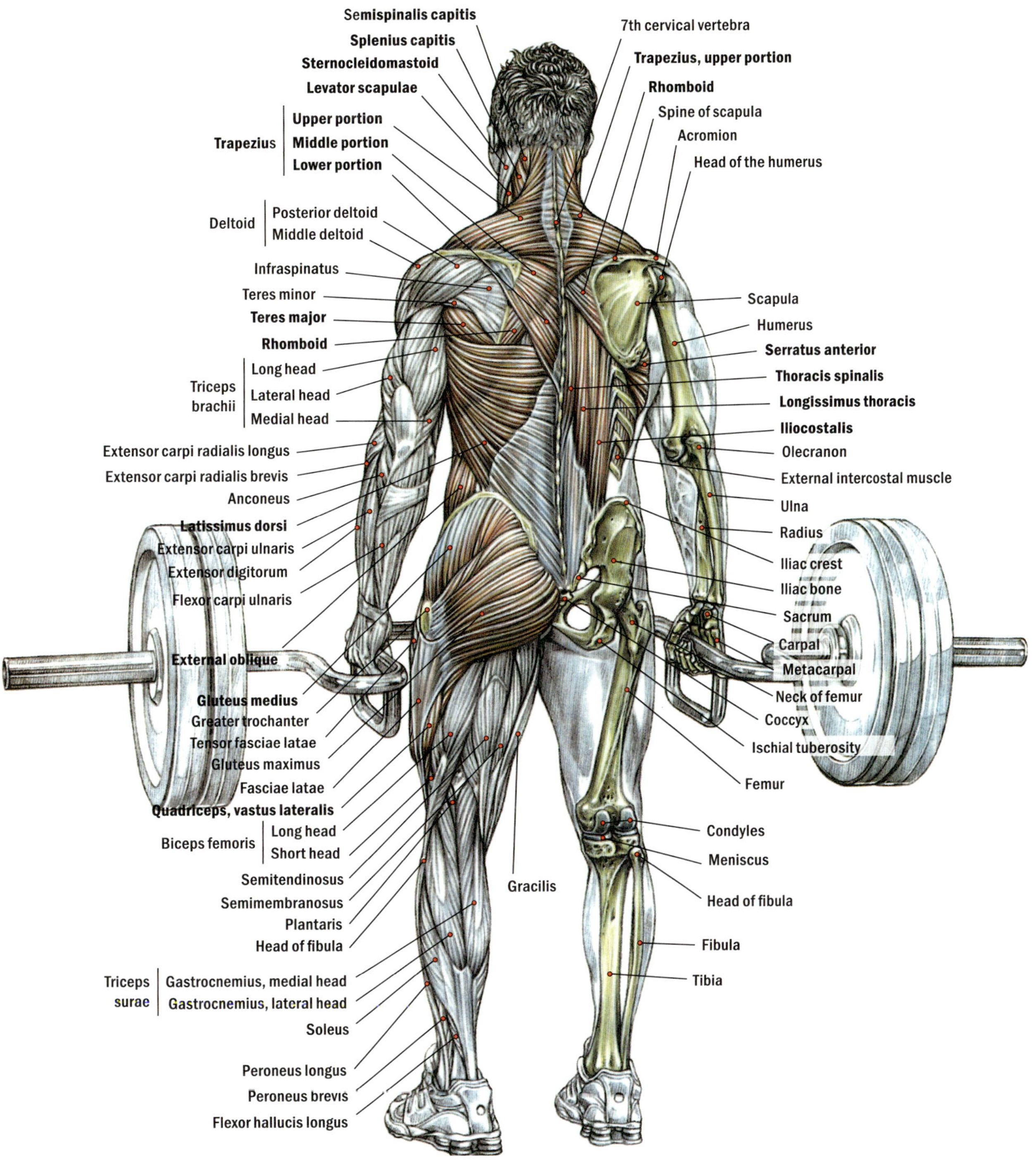

Like the classic deadlift (page 140), the deadlift with a trap bar works all the muscles of the body, but the centered position of the bar enables you to decrease the lean of your torso. This limits the intensity of the work on the lumbar region and the gluteal muscles by transferring some of the effort to the quadriceps. This exercise may, therefore, be included in a specific thigh work program, and in some cases it could replace the squat.

With heavy weights, the upper portion of the trapezius is strongly recruited.

For individuals with lower back pain, this exercise is safer than the traditional deadlift.

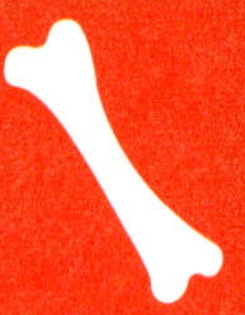

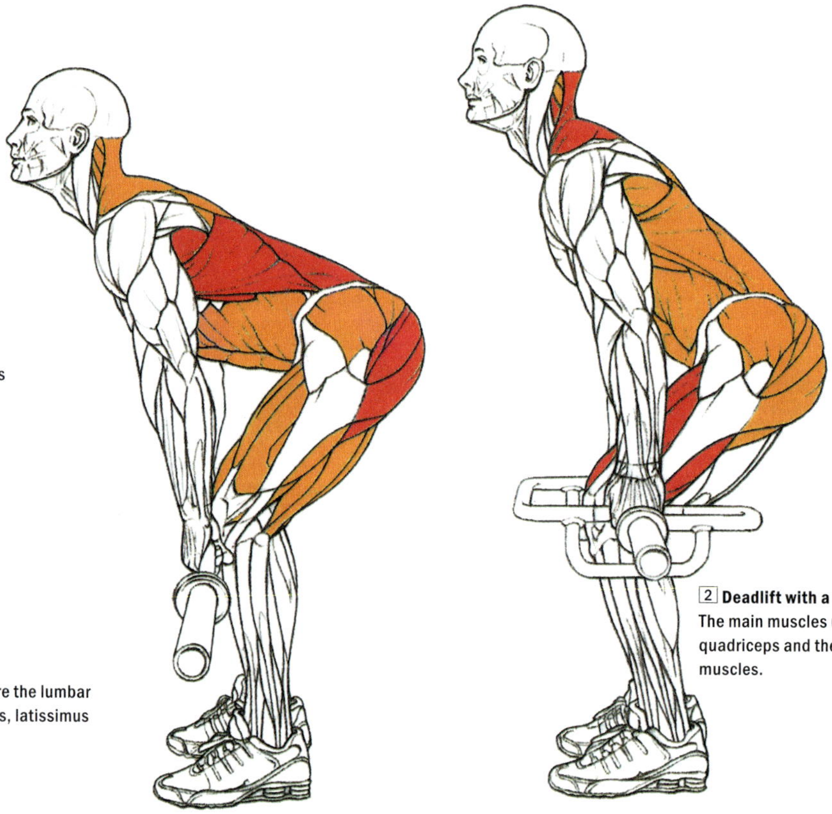

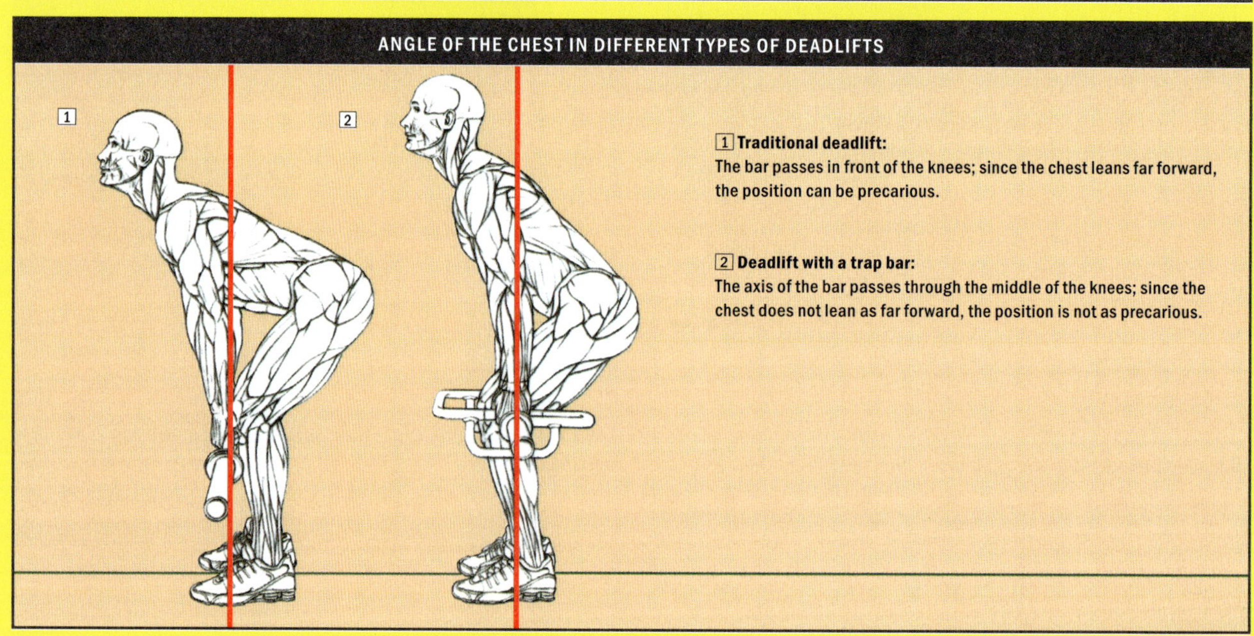
Most recruited muscles
Recruited muscles
1 Traditional deadlift:
The main muscles used are the lumbar muscles, gluteus maximus, latissimus dorsi, and teres major.
2 Deadlift with a trap bar:
The main muscles used are the quadriceps and the upper trapezius muscles.
ANGLE OF THE CHEST IN DIFFERENT TYPES OF DEADLIFTS
1
2
1 Traditional deadlift:
The bar passes in front of the knees; since the chest leans far forward, the position can be precarious.
2 Deadlift with a trap bar:
The axis of the bar passes through the middle of the knees; since the chest does not lean as far forward, the position is not as precarious.

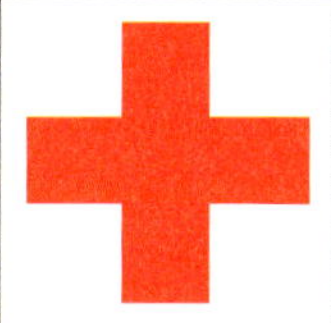

Back pain is the most common problem encountered in the lumbar region. Generally, it is not serious and is most often caused by cramping of the small, deep vertebral muscles that attach to the transverse processes linking the spine.

If, during a poorly executed rotation or extension of the spine, one of these muscles is overstretched or is slightly torn, it will automatically shorten along with its small neighboring muscles and the superficial erector spinae muscles. The back muscles cramp in pain; however, this cramping also limits movements that otherwise might tear or increase a tear in the small deep muscle.

This general shortening of a portion of the back muscles often disappears when the small deep muscle heals. But sometimes the back pain persists, and even after the muscles heal, the local shortening can last several weeks or even years in some individuals.

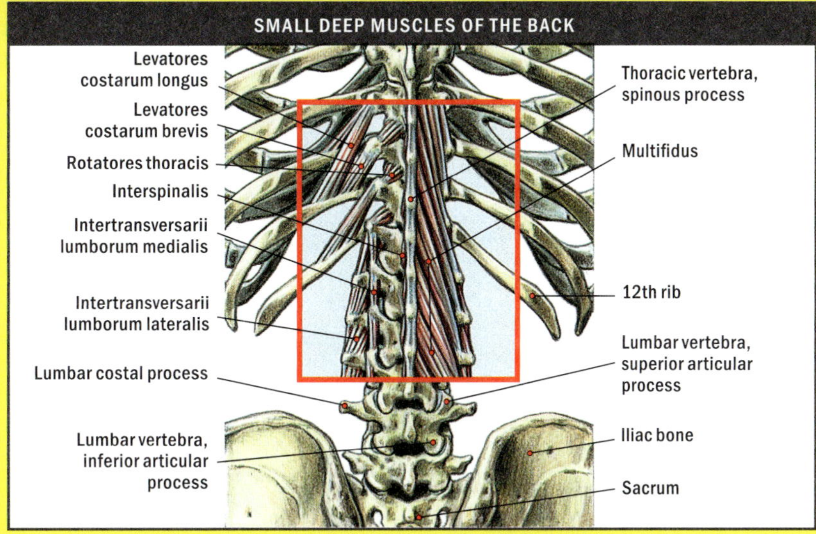

Although not serious in and of itself, lumbago, which is a painful contracture of the back muscles, can be a symptom of serious vertebral injuries such as herniated discs, tears in the paravertebral muscles and ligaments, and fractures.

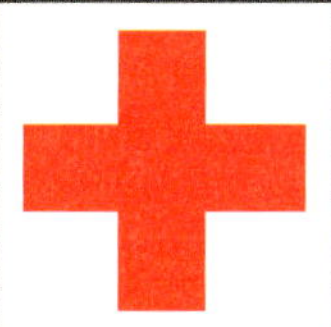

For individuals without back problems, arching the back during an exercise is not risky. In fact, with exercises like squats (page 168) or deadlifts (page 140), where the back tends to round, arching the back can prevent injury. However, for some people, arching the back during an exercise can be very dangerous.

- For individuals suffering from congenital spondylolysis (incomplete fusing of the vertebral arch), putting the lumbar spine in extension can cause the vertebra to slide (spondylolisthesis), which may cause serious nerve compression and lead to sciatica.
- For individuals who are not fully grown or are experiencing osteoporosis, extending the lumbar spine may lead to spondylolysis because of fractures in the vertebral arch. This fracture in the posterior anchoring system of the vertebra may allow the vertebra to slide forward and seriously compress the neural elements (which leads to sciatica).

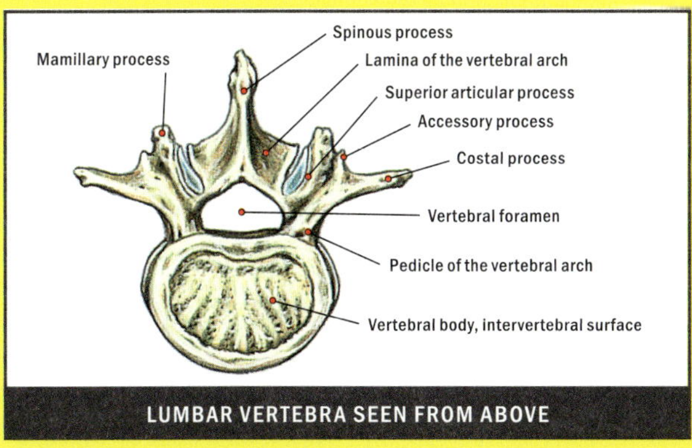

LUMBAR VERTEBRA SEEN FROM ABOVE

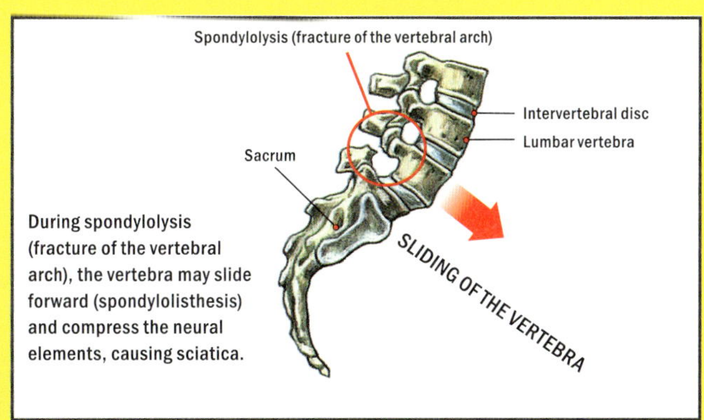

During spondylolysis (fracture of the vertebral arch), the vertebra may slide forward (spondylolisthesis) and compress the neural elements, causing sciatica.

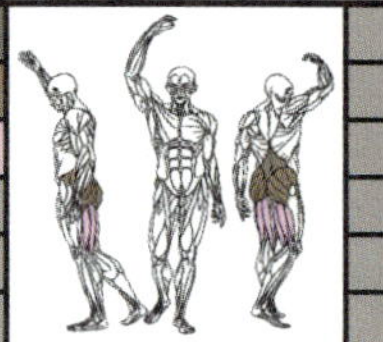

Biceps femoris, short head
Semitendinosus
Gluteus maximus
Iliotibial band, fasciae latae
Gluteus medius
Quadratus lumborum
Iliocostalis lumborum
Latissimus dorsi
Rhomboid major
Teres major
Infraspinatus
Trapezius

Gastrocnemius
Semimembranosus

Quadriceps, vastus lateralis
Biceps femoris, long head
Iliac crest
Thoracis spinalis
Longissimus thoracis
External intercostals
Iliocostalis thoracis
Scapula
Humerus

Soleus
Peroneus longus
Extensor digitorum longus
Tibialis anterior

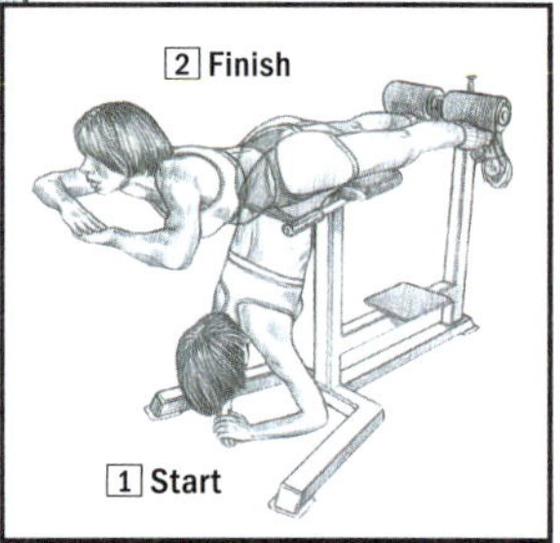

Lie facedown on a Roman chair and secure your ankles under the roller pads. Because the axis of flexion passes through the hip joints, your pubic bone should not rest on the support pad:

- With your torso bent forward, extend your back to a horizontal position while raising your head.
- Continue into hyperextension by arching your lumbar spine. This must be done carefully to protect your lower back.

This exercise mainly develops the group of erector spinae muscles (iliocostalis, longissimus thoracis, spinalis thoracis, splenius, and semispinalis capitis), the quadratus lumborum, and, to a lesser degree, the gluteus maximus and the hamstrings, except for the short head of the biceps femoris. Complete flexion of the torso develops flexibility in the lumbosacral region. Supporting the pelvis on the bench so that the axis is displaced toward the front of the body focuses the movement completely on the lumbosacral area but less intensely given the limited range of motion and the greater power of the lever arm.

To enhance the focus, hold the horizontal position of your torso at the end of the extension for a few seconds. Using an incline bench makes this exercise easier for beginners.

Variations

- Doing back extensions with a bar on the shoulders will stabilize the upper back and focus the effort on the lower part of the erector spinae muscles.
- A back extension machine allows you to focus on the lumbosacral portion of your spinal muscles (see machine back extensions on the following page).
- To increase the intensity, do this exercise while holding a weight plate against your chest or behind your neck.

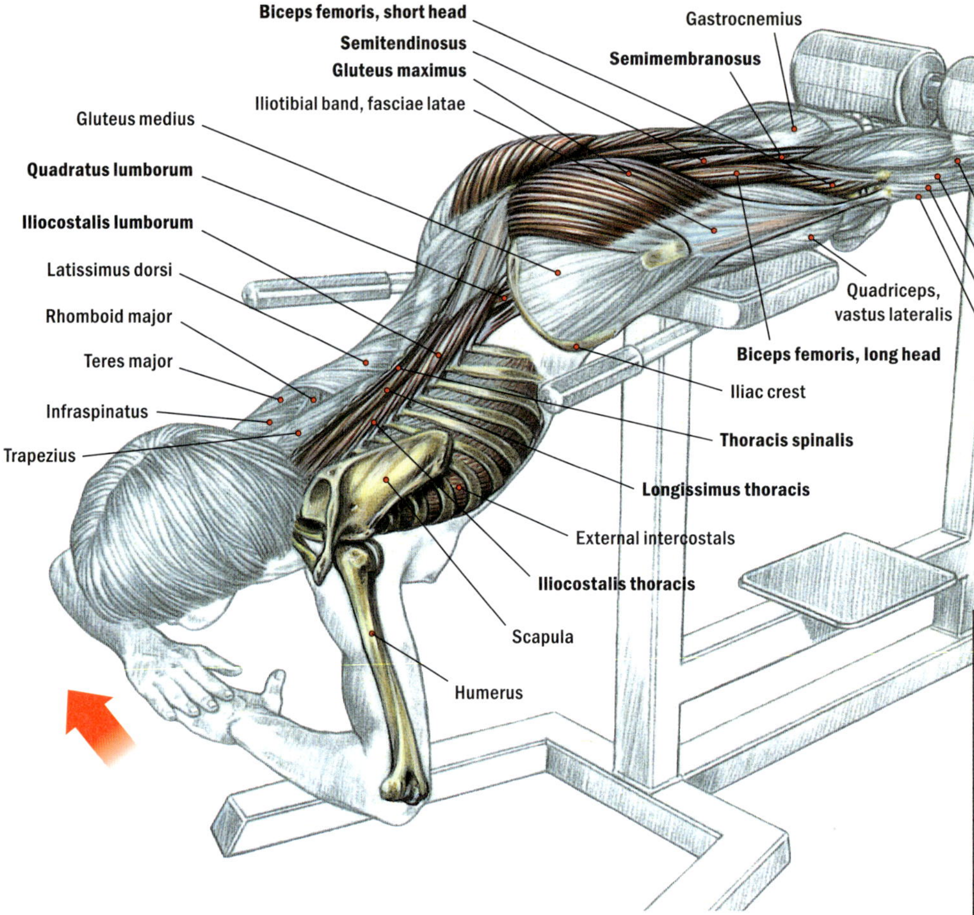

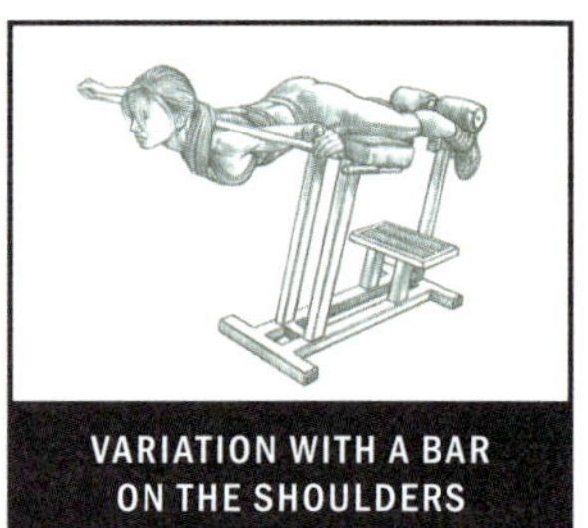

PERFORMING THE EXERCISE

VARIATION WITH A BAR ON THE SHOULDERS

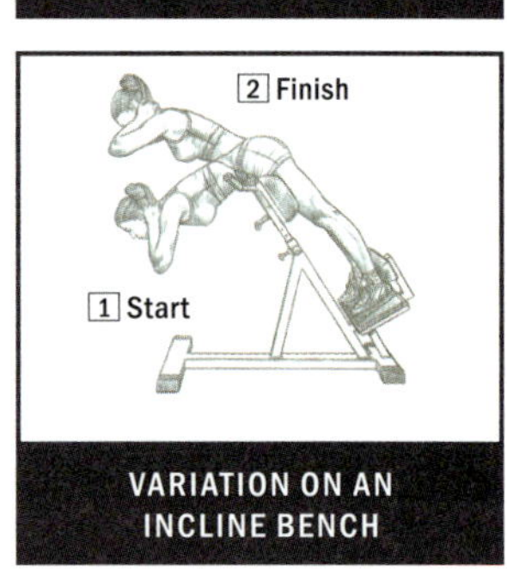

VARIATION ON AN INCLINE BENCH

MACHINE BACK EXTENSIONS 20

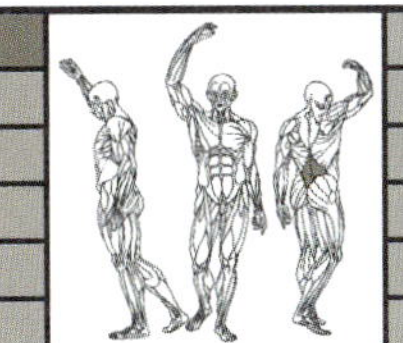

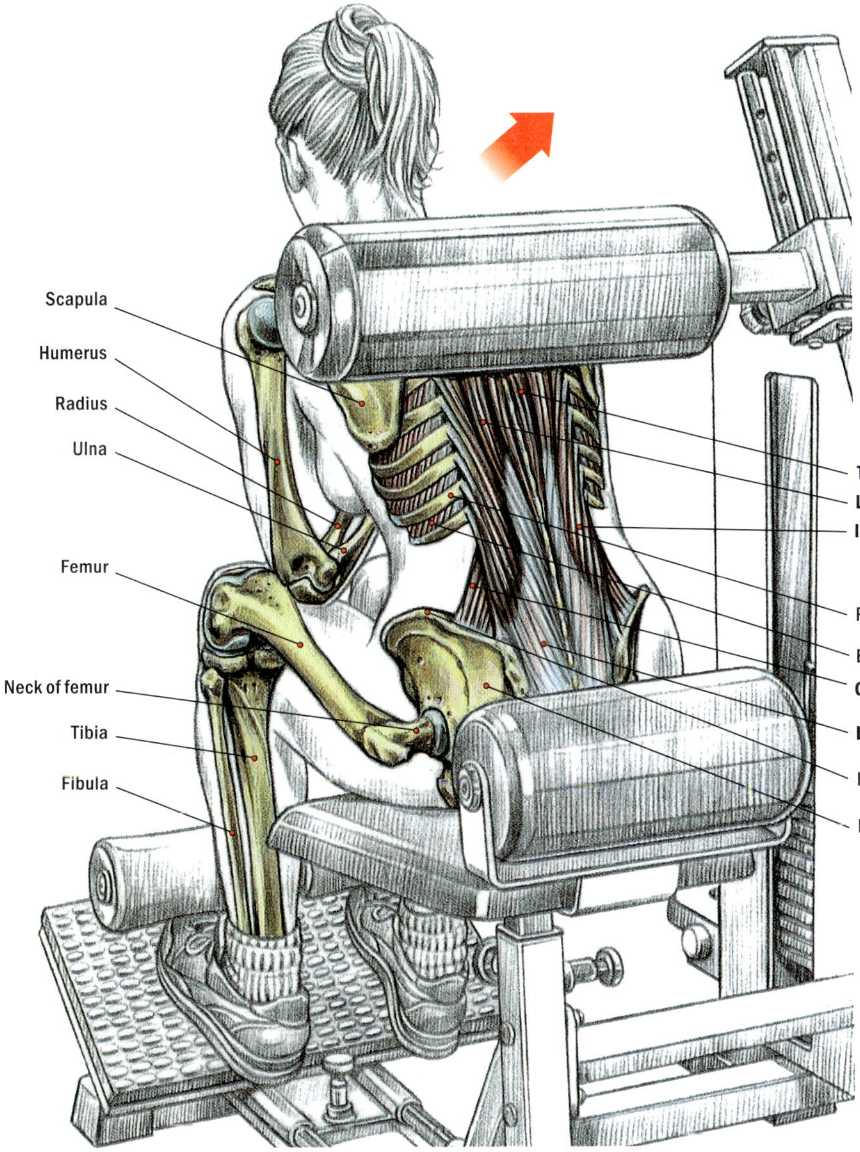

Scapula
Humerus
Radius
Ulna
Femur
Neck of femur
Tibia
Fibula
Thoracis spinalis
Longissimus thoracis
Iliocostalis lumborum
Erector spinae
Rib
External intercostals
Quadratus lumborum
Lumbosacral region (under the aponeurosis)
Iliac crest
Hip bone

1 Start
2 Finish

PERFORMING THE EXERCISE

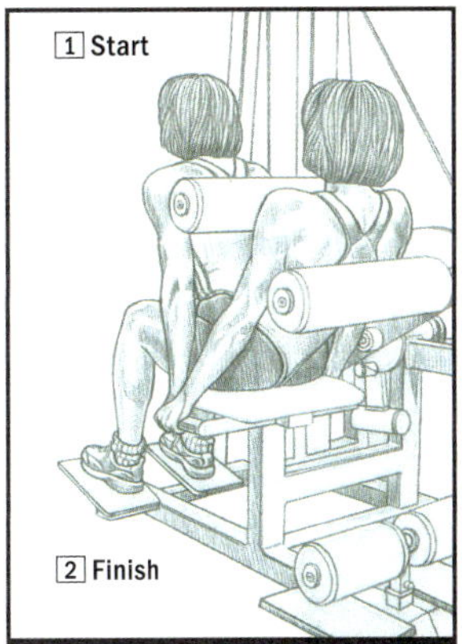

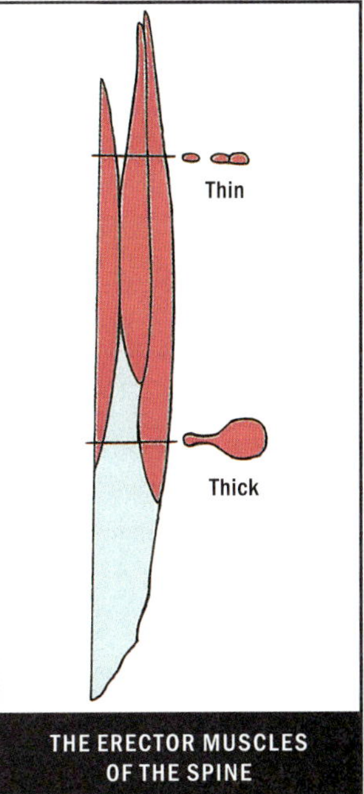

Sit on the machine's seat, with your torso leaning forward and the pad of the machine at shoulder-blade level:

- Inhale and straighten your torso as much as possible.
- Exhale as you slowly return to the starting position and repeat.

This exercise works the erector muscles of the spine, focusing the effort on the lower back, specifically the lumbosacral mass of the spinal muscles. This exercise is excellent for beginners. Done in sets of 10 to 20 reps, it develops the necessary strength to progress to more technically demanding back exercises.

To perform this exercise with heavier weights, reduce the number of repetitions in the set.

You can use the machine to adjust the range of motion and the weight so that you can vary both during the same workout. For example: 2 sets of 15 reps with moderate weights and a full range of motion followed by 2 sets of 7 reps with heavier weights and a smaller range of motion.

Thin
Thick

THE ERECTOR MUSCLES OF THE SPINE

STRETCHING THE BACK AT A PULL-UP BAR

DIAGRAM OF VERTEBRAE

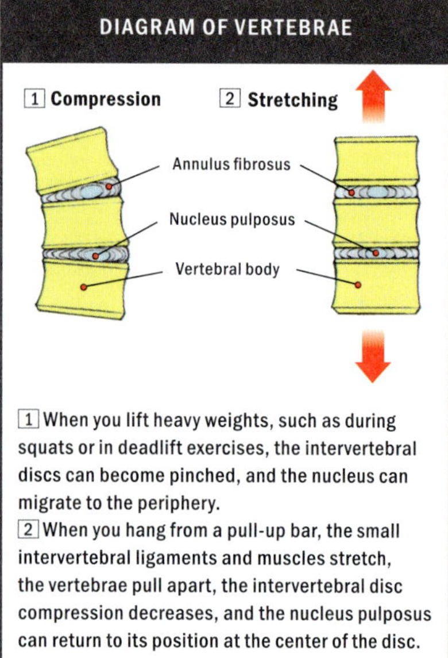

1 When you lift heavy weights, such as during squats or in deadlift exercises, the intervertebral discs can become pinched, and the nucleus can migrate to the periphery.

2 When you hang from a pull-up bar, the small intervertebral ligaments and muscles stretch, the vertebrae pull apart, the intervertebral disc compression decreases, and the nucleus pulposus can return to its position at the center of the disc.

Hang from a pull-up bar with a wide overhand grip (with thumbs facing each other):

- Inhale and exhale slowly, concentrating on relaxing your body. This allows your back muscles to loosen up and the pressure inside the discs to balance. It also relaxes the small paravertebral muscles that interconnect the vertebrae (these are often painfully contracted).
- When you are adequately relaxed, lean your head forward, trying to touch your chin to your chest. This will stretch the upper and middle back.

To enhance the stretch, swing gently or ask a partner to grasp your hips on each side and slowly pull down. This stretch is fundamental. When practiced regularly at the end of squat and heavy deadlift workouts (or any other heavy exercises that compress the spine), it helps, over time, to limit the deterioration of the intervertebral discs and reduces the risk of disc herniation (see pages 176-177).

Variation

If you grip as strongly as you can, the latissimus dorsi and teres major muscles will be stretched more intensely.

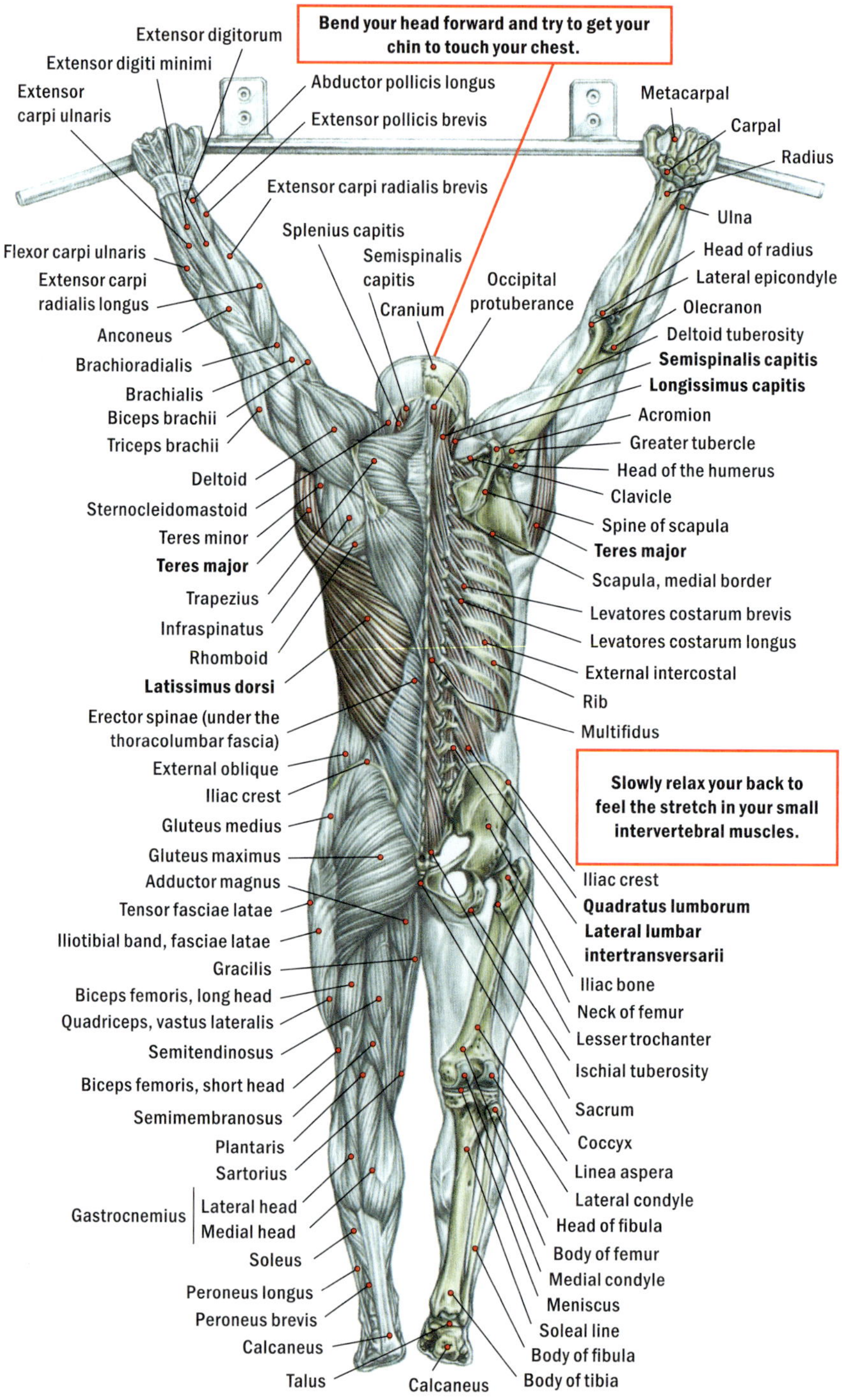

During this exercise, you will often hear cracking of the spine followed by a pleasant feeling of release and relaxation of the spine. These harmless sounds are caused by the release of the paravertebral muscles. Once relaxed, the muscles decompress the small intervertebral and costovertebral joints.

BARBELL SHRUGS 21

ENDING POSITION
TRAPEZIUS CONTRACTED

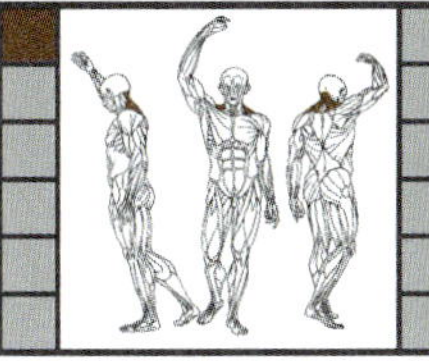

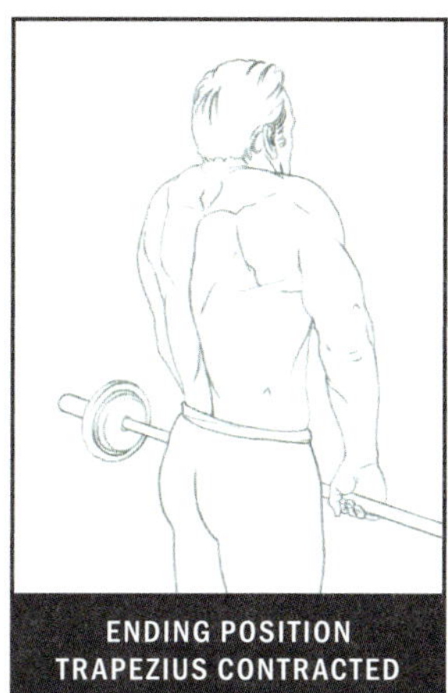

Stand with your legs slightly apart and face the bar, which should either be on the ground or on a rack:

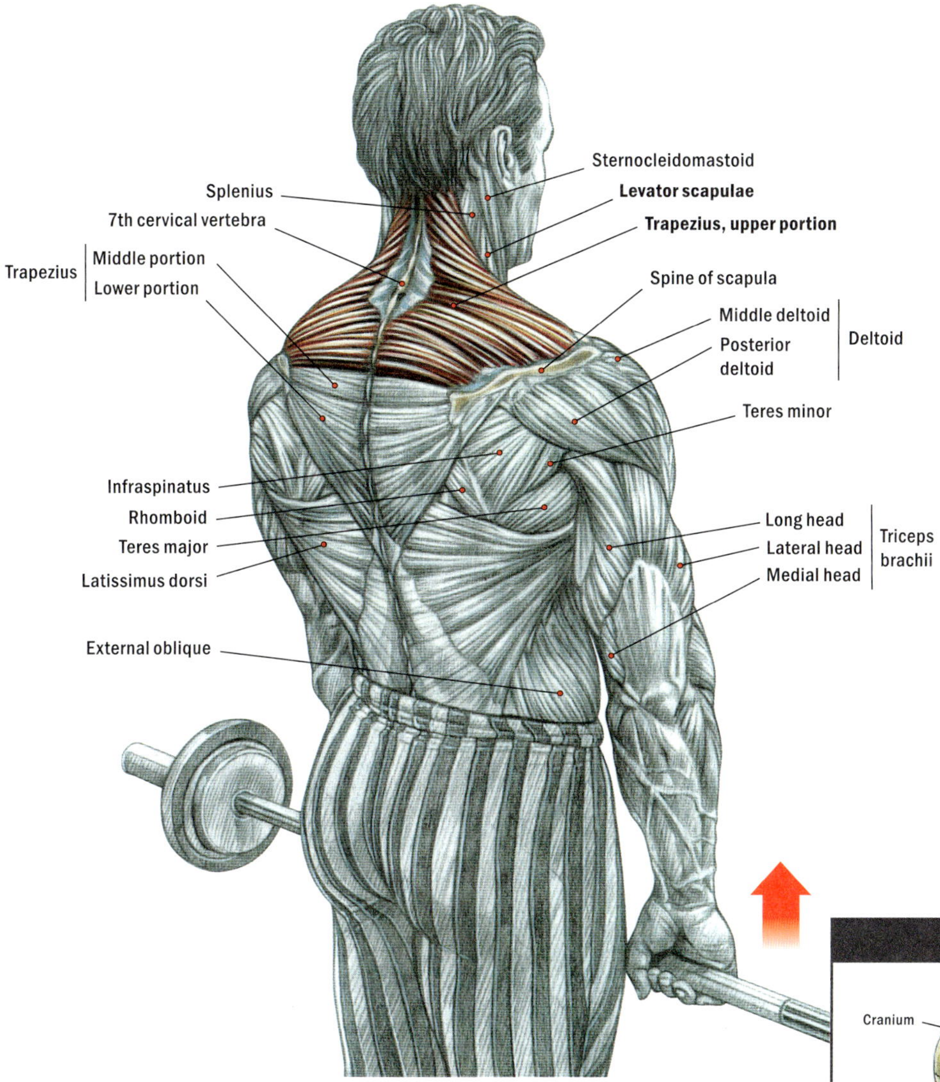

- Grasp the bar with an overhand grip with the hands slightly wider than shoulder-width apart. Use a mixed grip if the weight is heavy.
- Shrug your shoulders while keeping your arms relaxed, back very straight, and abdominal muscles contracted.

This exercise develops the upper portion of the trapezius, specifically its occipital-clavicular fibers, and the levator scapulae.

When working with heavy weights and a mixed grip, it is best to change your grip with each set, so as to balance the work on the trapezius. For example, perform one set with the right hand overhand and the left hand underhand, then switch on the following set.

TRAPEZIUS MUSCLE

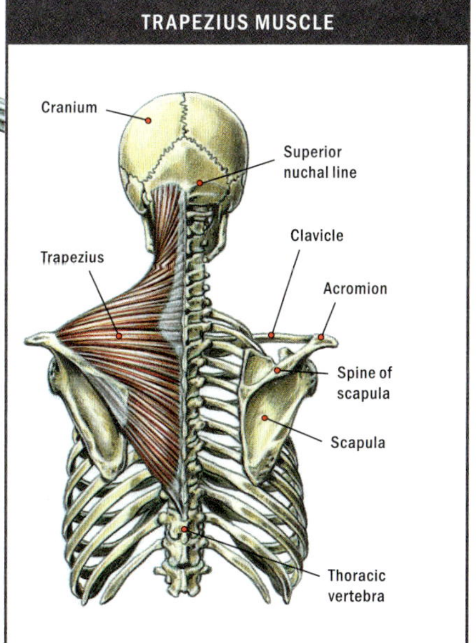

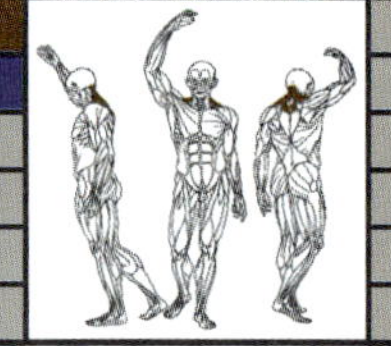

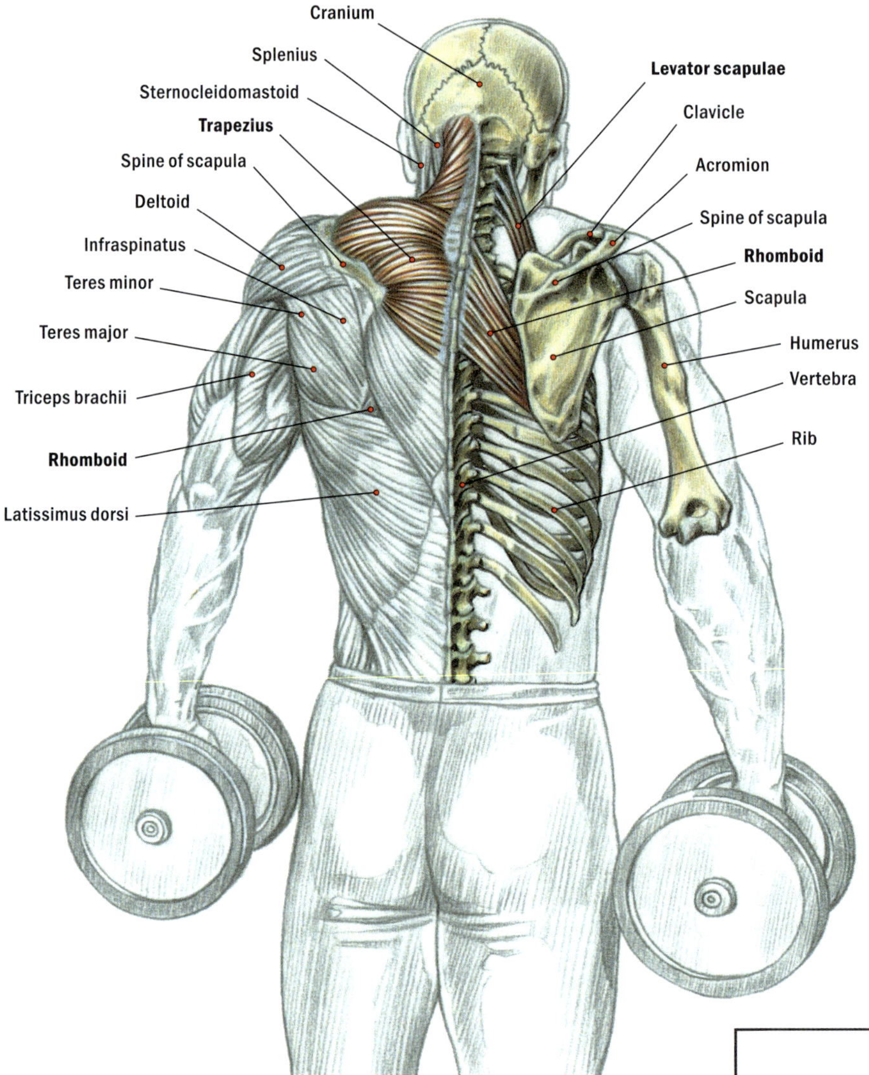

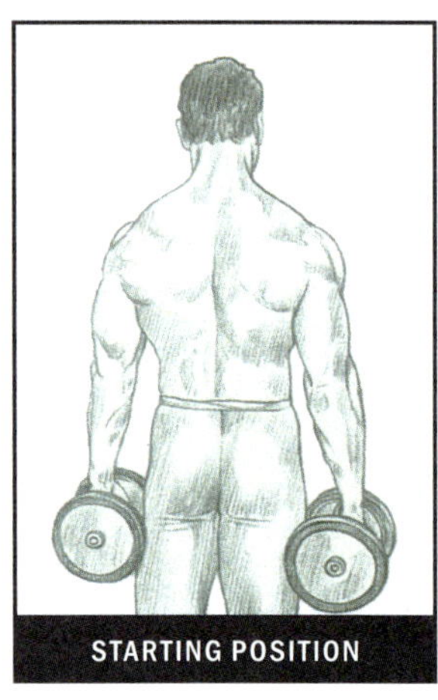

STARTING POSITION

Stand with your legs slightly apart, head upright or bent slightly forward, and arms relaxed at your sides with a dumbbell in each hand:

- Shrug the shoulders with a front-to-back rotation, then return to the starting position.

This exercise contracts the upper, or clavicular, part of the trapezius, the levator scapulae, the middle part of the trapezius, and the rhomboids when squeezing the shoulder blades together and rotating the shoulders to the back.

It is impossible to rotate the shoulders when using heavy weights.

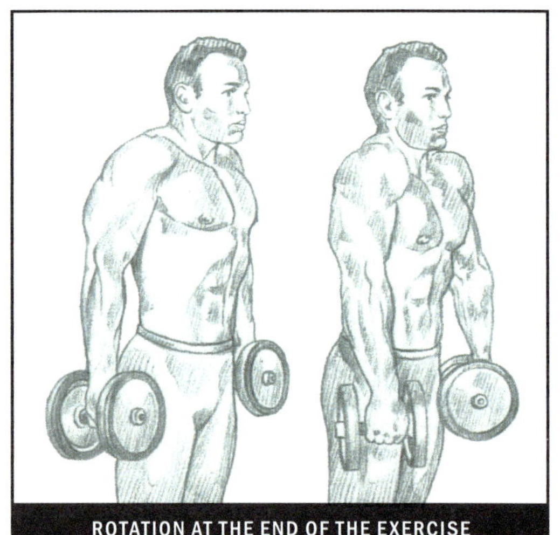

ROTATION AT THE END OF THE EXERCISE

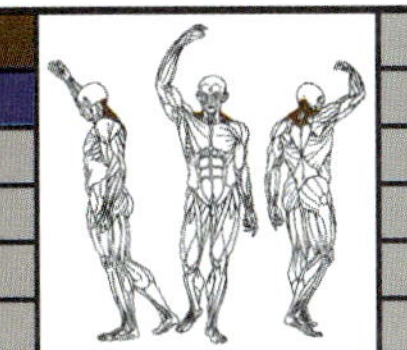

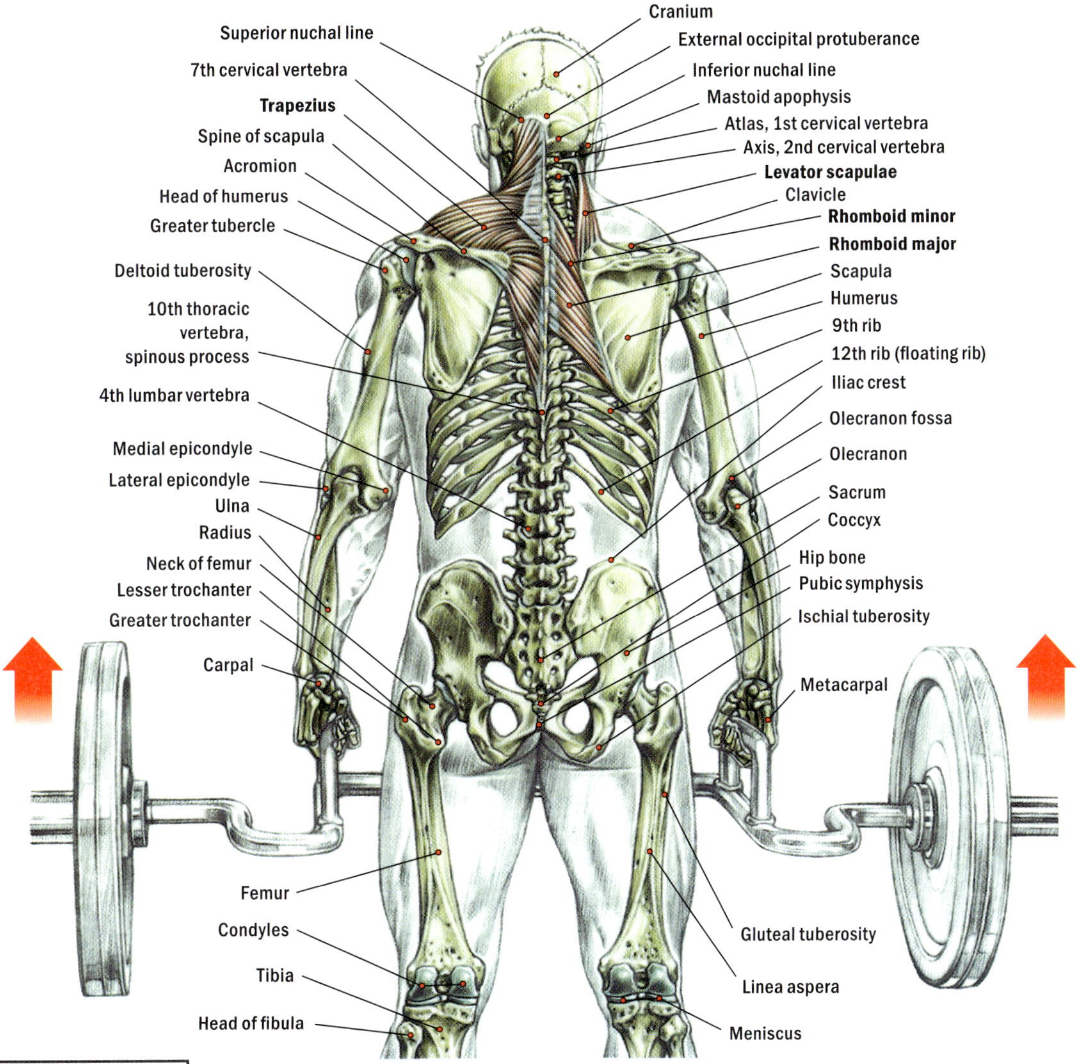

Cranium
Superior nuchal line
External occipital protuberance
7th cervical vertebra
Inferior nuchal line
Trapezius
Mastoid apophysis
Spine of scapula
Atlas, 1st cervical vertebra
Acromion
Axis, 2nd cervical vertebra
Head of humerus
Levator scapulae
Greater tubercle
Clavicle
Rhomboid minor
Deltoid tuberosity
Rhomboid major
10th thoracic vertebra, spinous process
Scapula
Humerus
9th rib
4th lumbar vertebra
12th rib (floating rib)
Iliac crest
Medial epicondyle
Olecranon fossa
Lateral epicondyle
Olecranon
Ulna
Sacrum
Radius
Coccyx
Neck of femur
Hip bone
Lesser trochanter
Pubic symphysis
Greater trochanter
Ischial tuberosity
Carpal
Metacarpal
Femur
Condyles
Gluteal tuberosity
Tibia
Linea aspera
Head of fibula
Meniscus

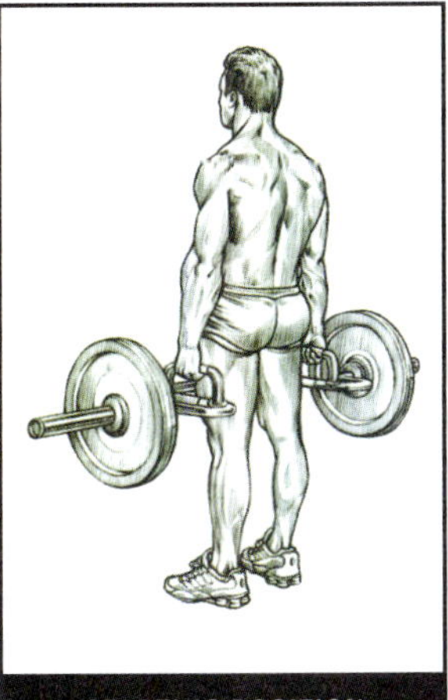

Stand with your legs slightly apart. Face the bar, which should either be on the floor or on a rack:

- Grasp the bar, making sure that your hands are centered (remember that when you have heavy weights on a trap bar, gripping the bar without adjusting your hands properly will cause the bar to swing forward or backward).
- With your head straight or slightly forward, arms relaxed, back very straight, and abdominals contracted, perform shoulder shrugs.

This exercise mainly works the upper portion of the trapezius, which inserts onto the clavicle and the acromion and spine of the scapula and ascends to the superior nuchal line of the cranium. On a deeper level, the minor and major rhomboids and levator scapulae are also engaged.

As the name indicates, the trap bar was initially created to work the trapezius muscles; it allows you to lift much heavier weights than possible with a straight bar or dumbbells without scraping your thighs.

> Individuals with long clavicles will always find it harder to do shoulder shrugs with heavy weights than those individuals with shorter clavicles.

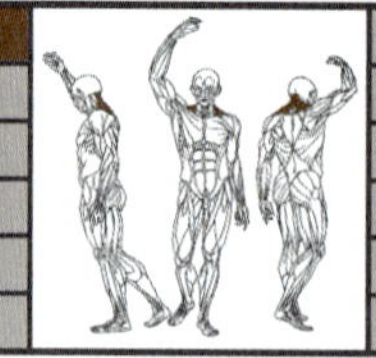

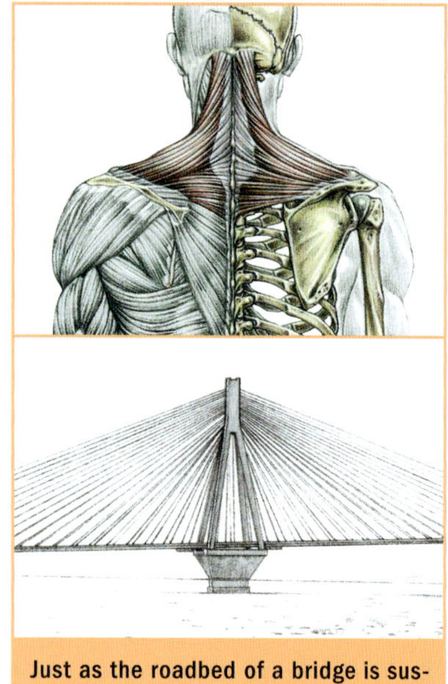

Just as the roadbed of a bridge is suspended by metal cables, the clavicles and shoulder blades are suspended by the trapezius.

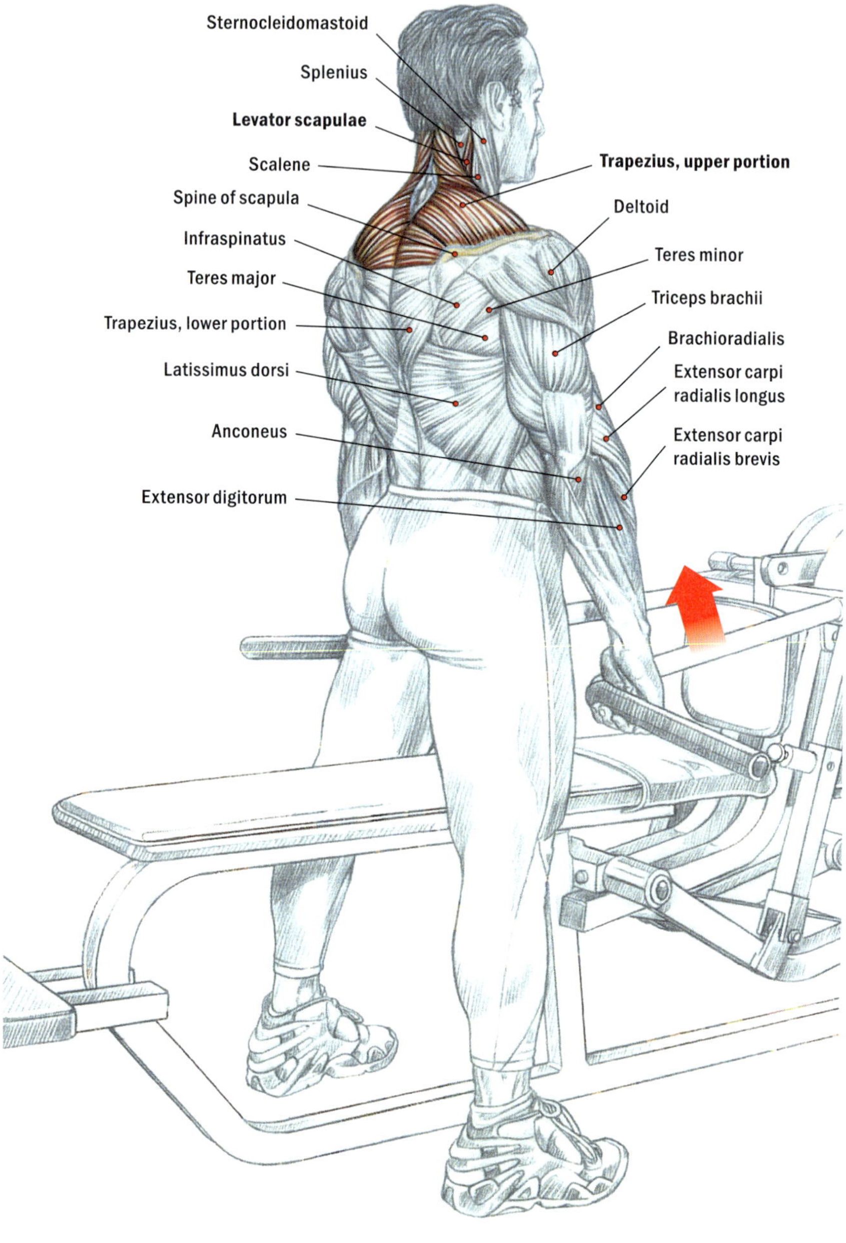

Sternocleidomastoid

Splenius

Levator scapulae

Scalene

Spine of scapula

Infraspinatus

Teres major

Trapezius, lower portion

Latissimus dorsi

Anconeus

Extensor digitorum

Trapezius, upper portion

Deltoid

Teres minor

Triceps brachii

Brachioradialis

Extensor carpi radialis longus

Extensor carpi radialis brevis

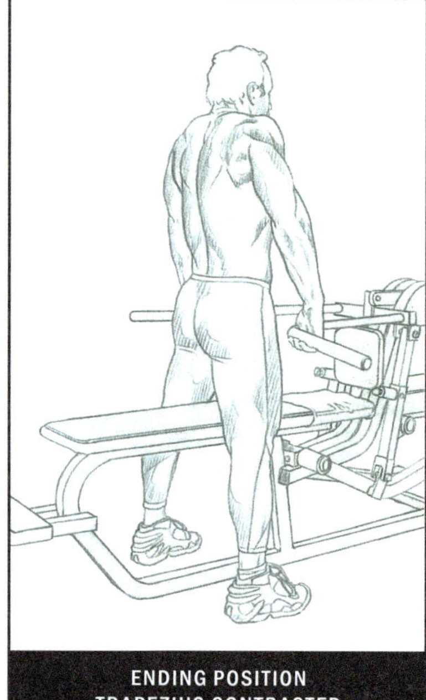

ENDING POSITION
TRAPEZIUS CONTRACTED

Stand facing the machine and hold the handles with an overhand grip slightly wider than shoulder width, or if the machine allows for it, with the palms facing each other:

- Shrug the shoulders, keeping your head and back straight.

This exercise can be done in long sets. It is excellent for developing the upper portion of the trapezius and the levator scapulae.

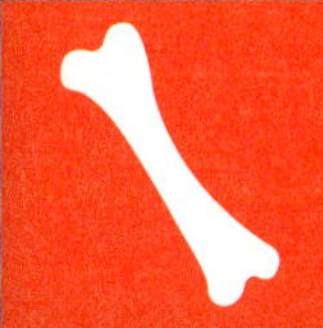

LONG CLAVICLES, LONG UPPER TRAPEZIUS

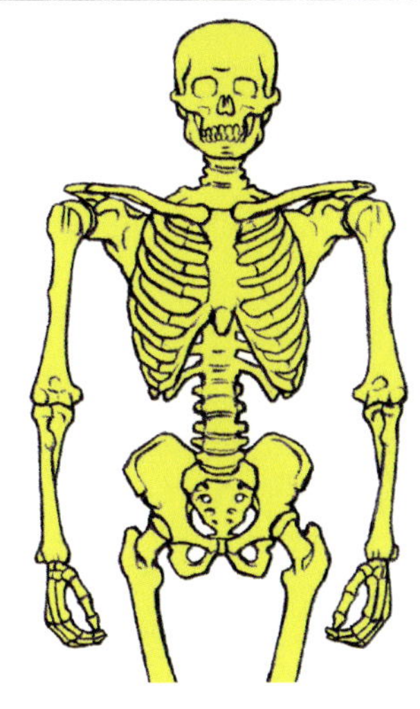

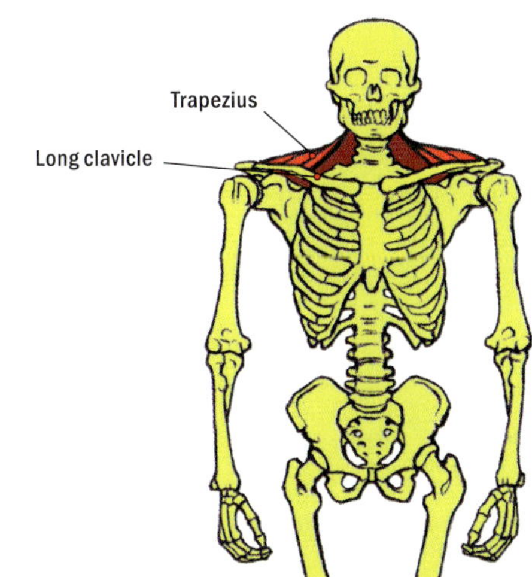

SHORT CLAVICLES, SHORT AND ROUNDED UPPER TRAPEZIUS

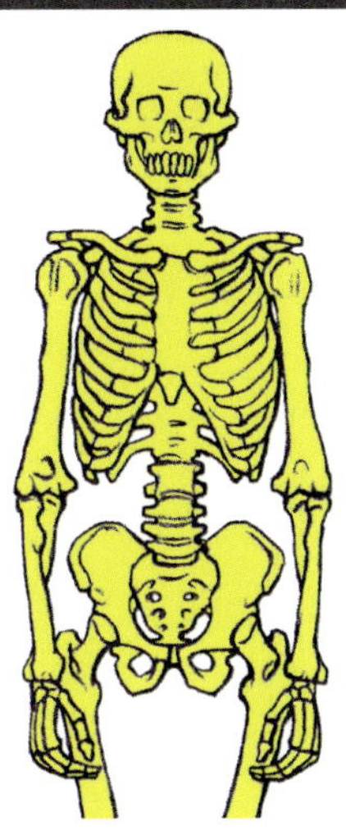

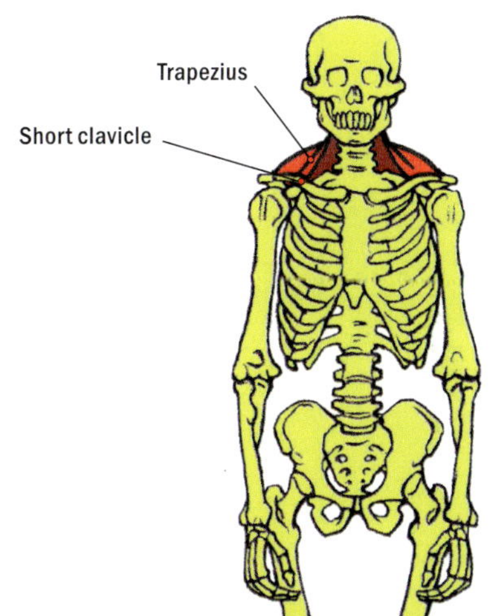

Bone morphology plays an important role in individual shrug strength. The longer the clavicles, the greater the cantilever, and the more difficult it will be to perform a weighted shrug. Thus, an individual with short clavicles can do shrugs with heavy weights better than an individual with long clavicles, but their shrugs will have a smaller range of motion.

Additionally, individuals with short clavicles can develop their trapezius more quickly, but this can give the impression that they have drooping shoulders, with the upper body resembling the shape of a bottle.

LONG CLAVICLES, SHORT CLAVICLES

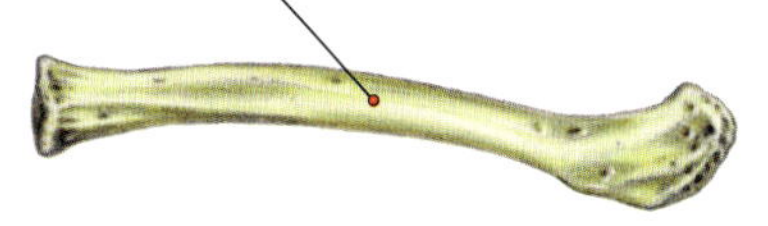

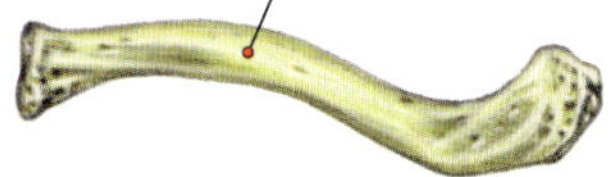

The length and curvature of the clavicles varies from one person to another.

25 DELAVIER'S SHRUGS OR SHRUGS WITH A SMITH MACHINE

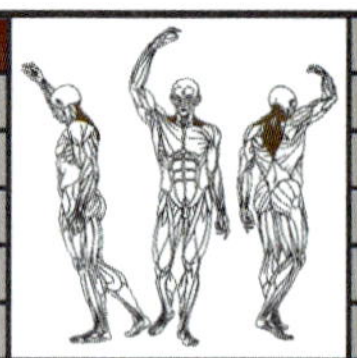

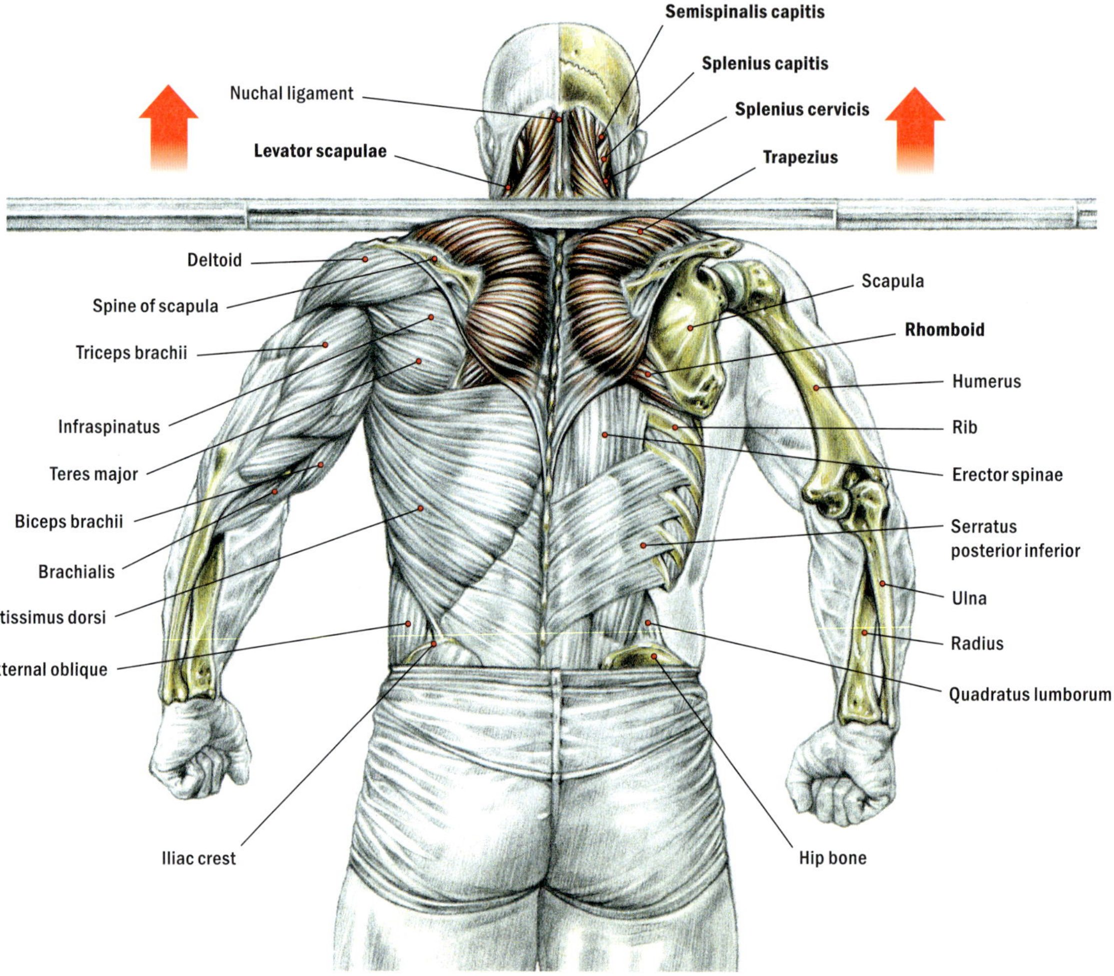

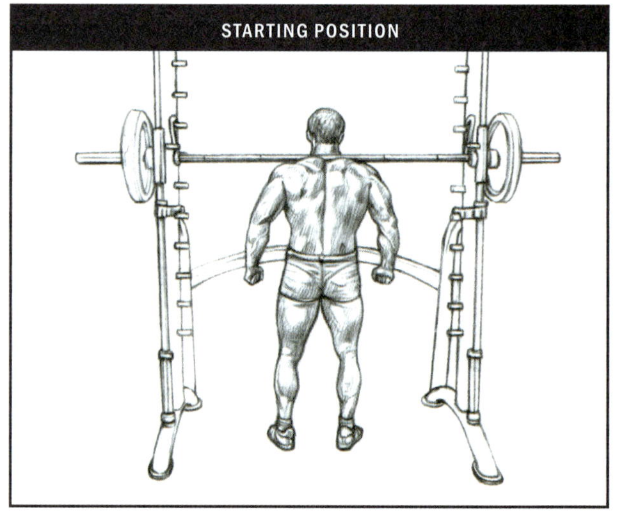

Place the bar of the Smith machine on the rack in line with the middle of your trapezius muscles. Position yourself underneath, with the bar resting on the upper part of your trapezius. Keep your arms at your sides:

- Arch your back slightly, contract your core, inhale, and shrug your shoulders.

This exercise mainly works the upper part of the trapezius but also the middle portion, which is harder to isolate, hence the usefulness of this exercise. On a deeper level, the minor and major rhomboids, levator scapulae, splenius cervicis, splenius capitis, and semispinalis capitis are also engaged.

This is one of the few exercises that work the trapezius without having to hold a weight in the hands, so it can be practiced by individuals with grip problems or disabilities that prevent them from handling heavy weights.

STARTING POSITION

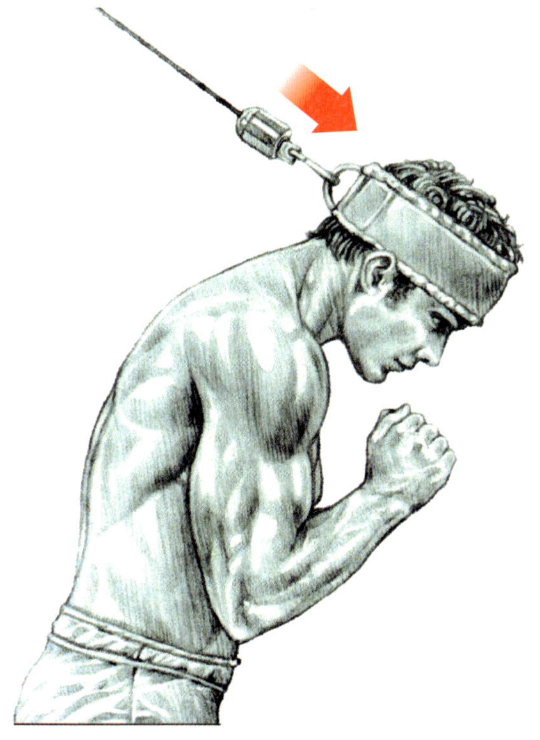

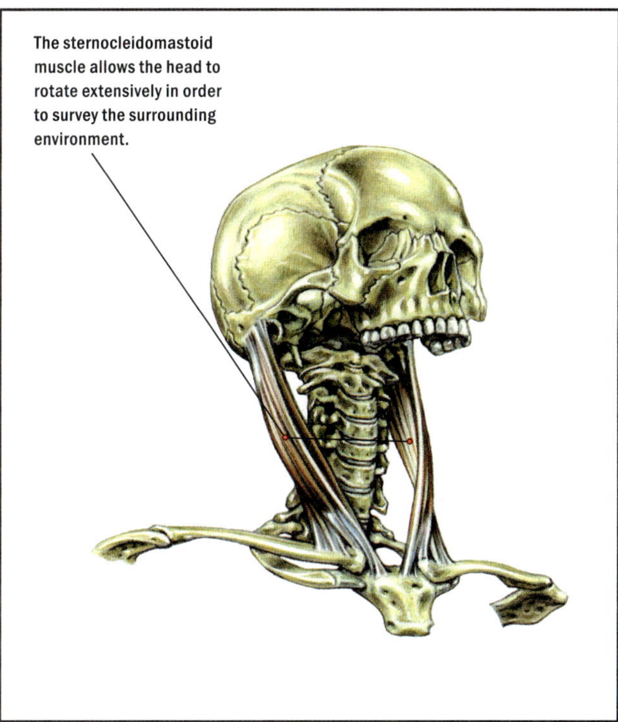

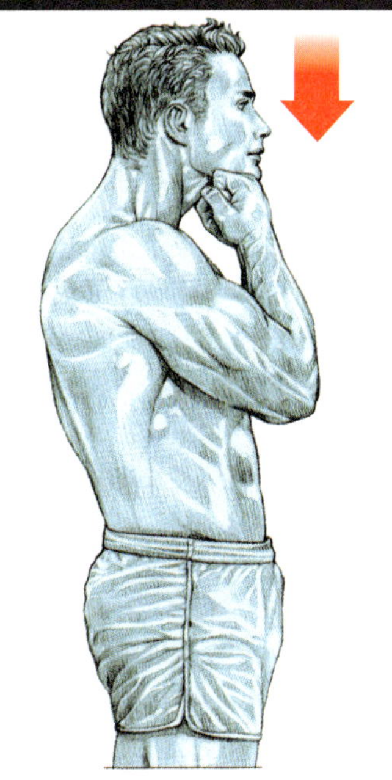

The anterior neck muscles can be worked in an isometric contraction without the need for equipment.

Stand with your back to the machine and a padded strap placed around your forehead. Bend your torso slightly forward:

- Thrust your neck forward with a slight downward chin movement.
- Slowly return to the starting position without moving your head backward.

This exercise mainly works the sternocleidomastoid muscles.

Sets of 20 to 30 reps provide the best results. For safety reasons, this exercise should not be done with heavy weights.

Variation

Stand upright with your head straight and lower your chin very slightly. Position your clenched fists under your chin:

- Using the strength of your neck, push down on your fists as hard as possible, making sure that they provide equal resistance.
- Hold this isometric contraction for 5 seconds and repeat.

This variation mainly works the sternocleidomastoid muscles and the small muscles involved in swallowing.

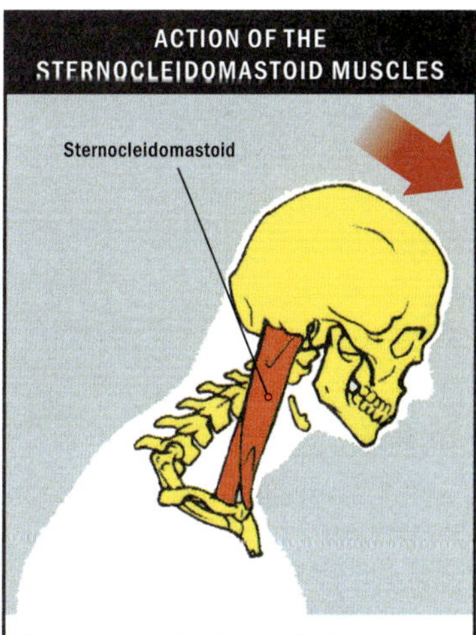

By contracting simultaneously, the sternocleidomastoid muscles project the head forward, as in a headbutt.

With the straightening due to bipedal locomotion, the head, on top of a mobile neck, is like the periscope of a submarine. Through its mobility, it can rotate to scan the horizon and analyze the surrounding environment.

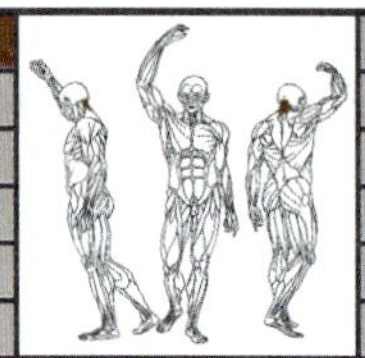

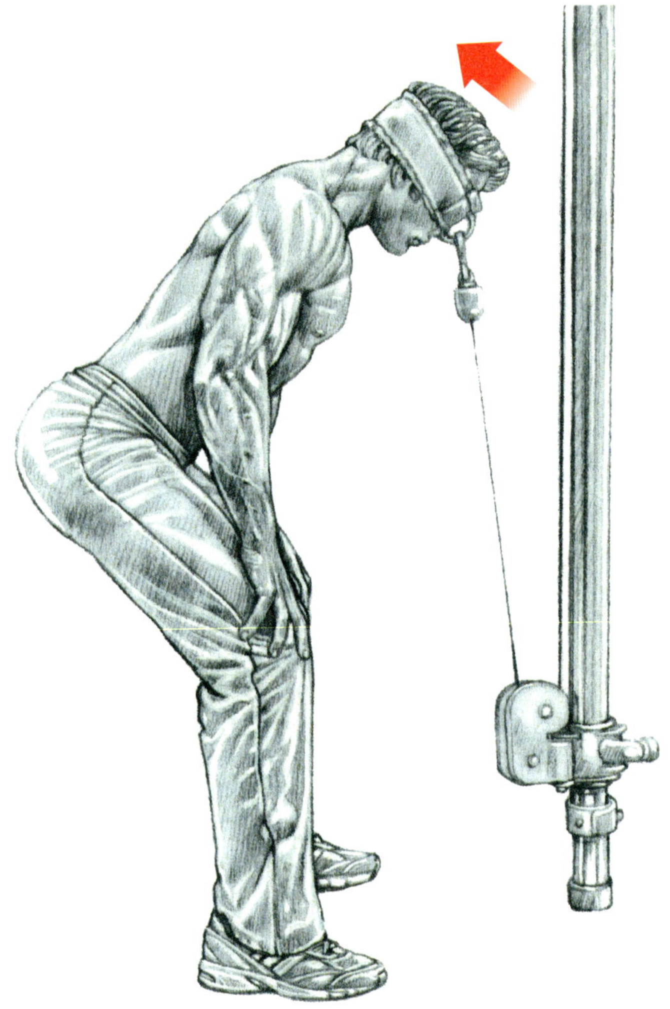

Face the machine with your knees slightly bent and your chest learning forward. Place your hands on your thighs, with your neck bent forward, your chin tucked in, and a padded strap placed around the back of your head:

- Without moving your torso, raise your head gently while ensuring that it does not move too far backward.
- Slowly return to the starting position and repeat.

This exercise mainly works the deep muscles of the neck, which form the lateral border of the nuchal ligament and insert on the vertebral processes. While it should be performed with extreme caution, when done properly, it strengthens the neck and protects the cervical spine from impact. It is preferable not to use heavy weight. Sets of 10 to 20 reps offer the best results.

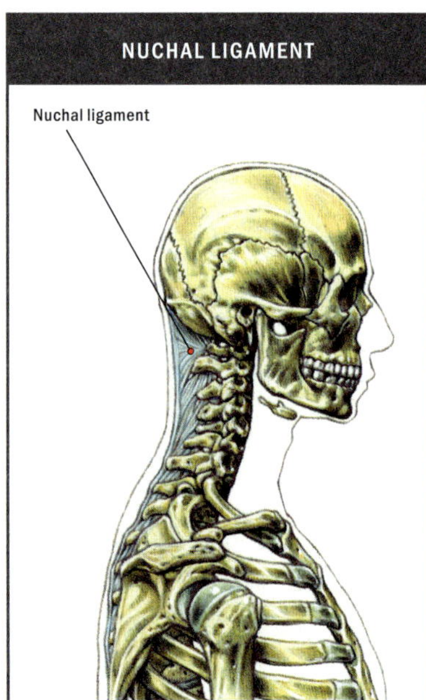

The nuchal ligament extends like a fibrous veil from the base of the skull to the bottom of the neck. Stiffening and protecting the neck, it prevents the range of motion from becoming too large and damaging the spinal cord.

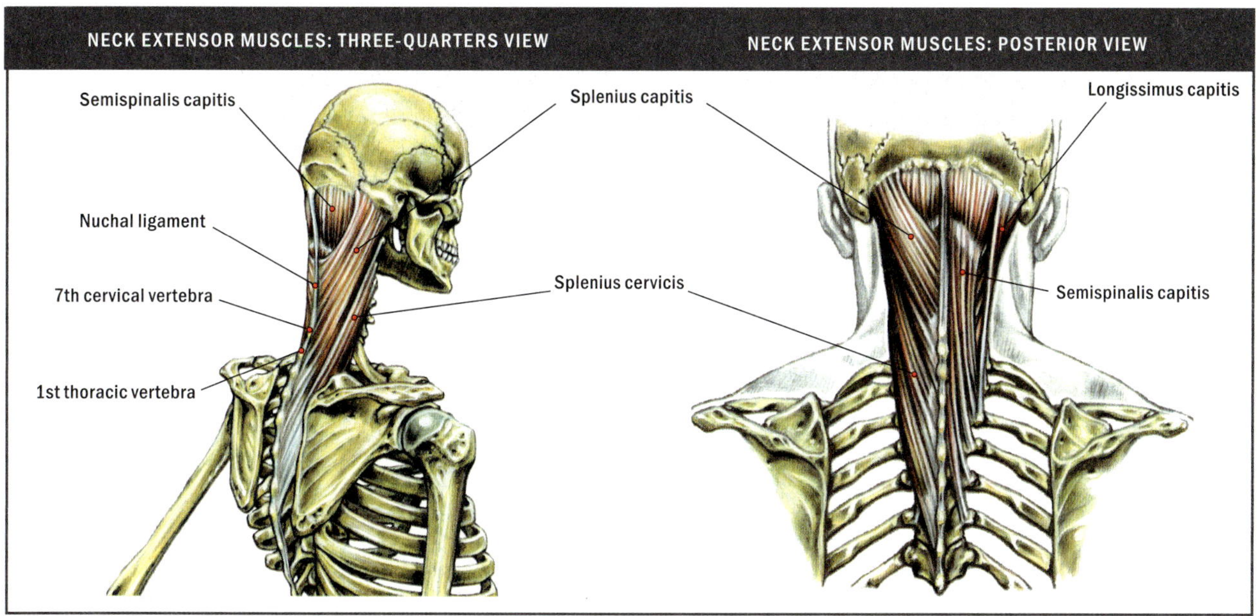

Due to the extensive mobility of the neck and fragility of the cervical spine, it is important to use extreme caution during any neck muscle strengthening exercise. These exercises should be performed slowly and with control. During neck extensions, be careful not to move your head too far backward to avoid nerve compression and compression of the small arteries that pass through the transverse foramen of the cervical vertebrae. This compression may cause dizziness and sometimes loss of consciousness.

ABOUT THE NECK

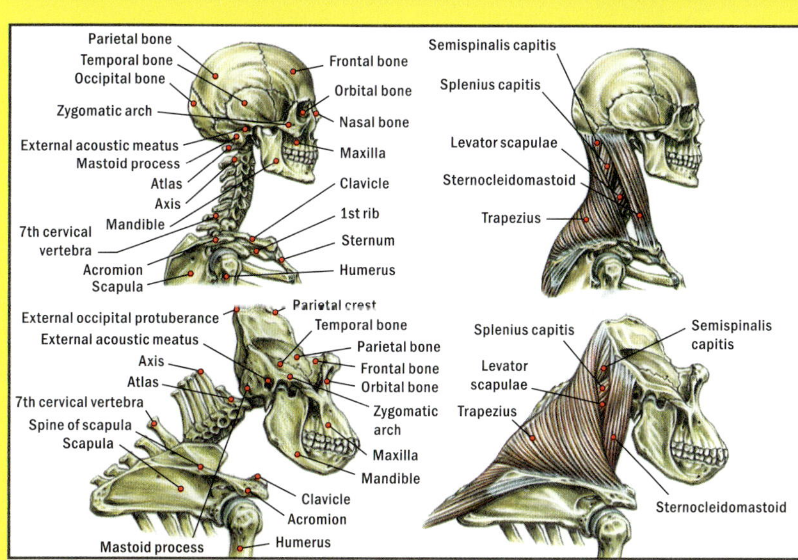

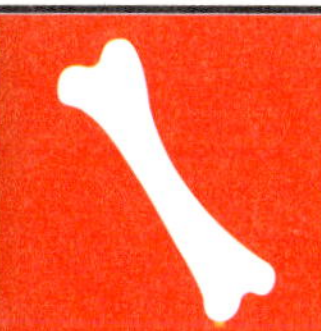

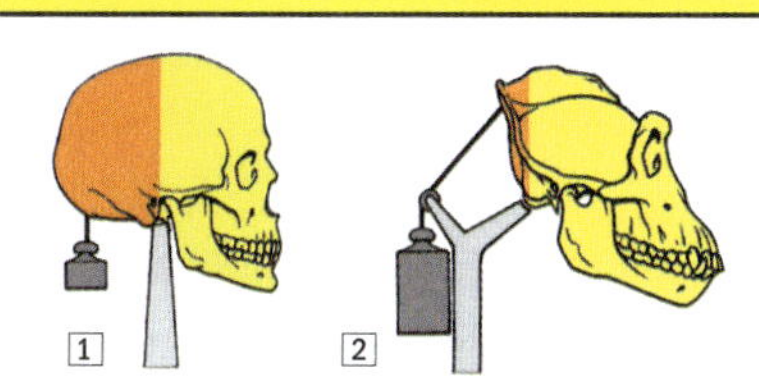

[1] In humans, with the shift to bipedal locomotion, the smaller face and the development of the brain caused the foramen magnum to move toward the center of the skull. The position of the head at the top of the spine requires the muscles of the neck to play only an understated stabilizing role.

[2] In a gorilla, a partial quadruped with a bigger face and a foramen magnum located at the back of the skull, the muscles of the neck are particularly well developed and powerful to prevent the head from falling forward.

In quadrupeds as well as in the great apes, such as the gorilla, the muscles of the neck are particularly strong and developed to maintain the head's position and prevent it from dropping forward.

But in humans, moving to total bipedal locomotion means the body is now upright with the head perched at the top of the spine. The muscles of the neck no longer serve to firmly hold the head up but, rather, to delicately balance the head on the spine.

STRETCHING THE DELTOIDS, TRAPEZIUS, AND NECK

Leaning the head to the opposite side of the shoulder being stretched will accentuate the stretch of the trapezius and the muscles of the neck.

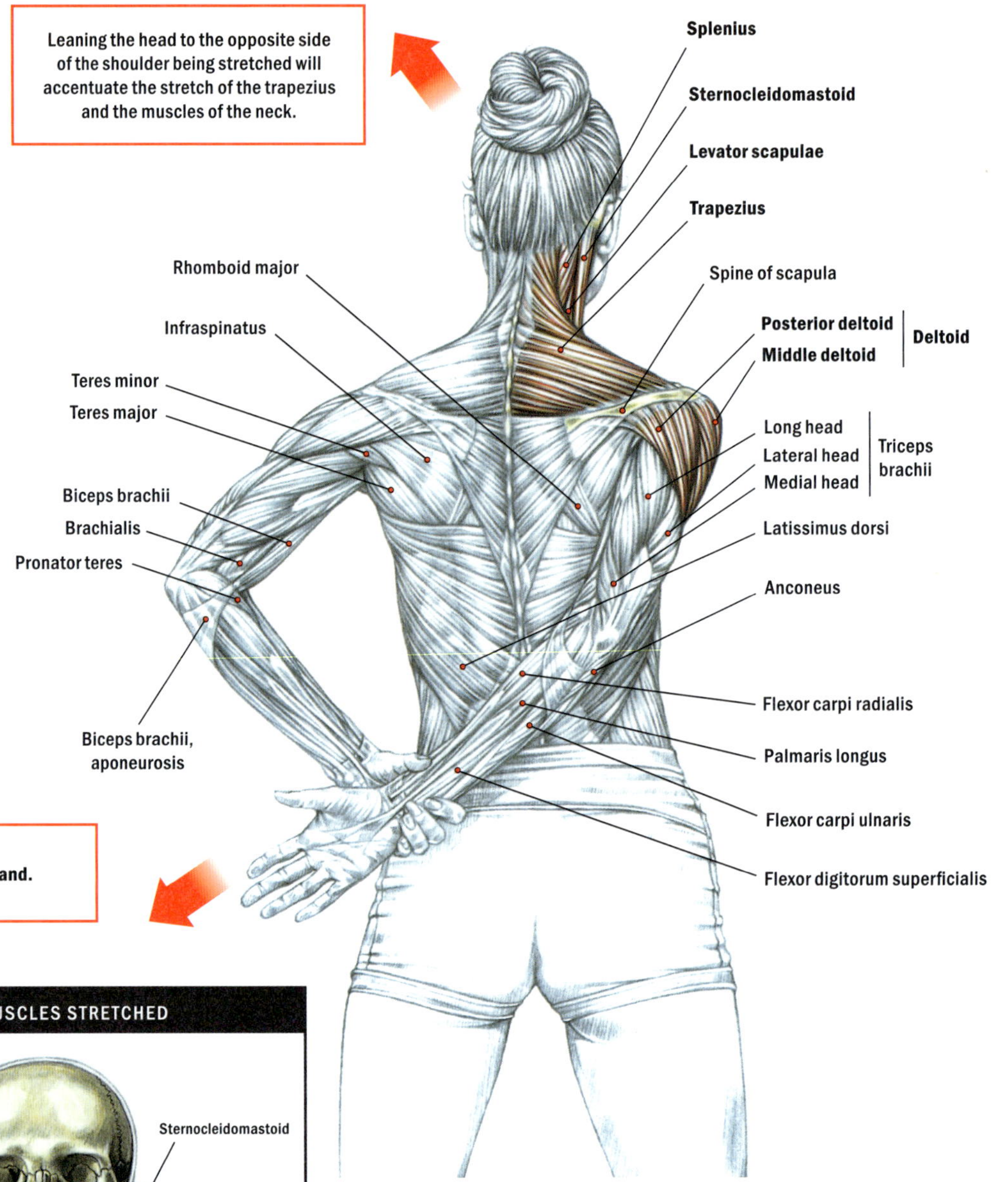

Pull slowly on the hand.

NECK MUSCLES STRETCHED

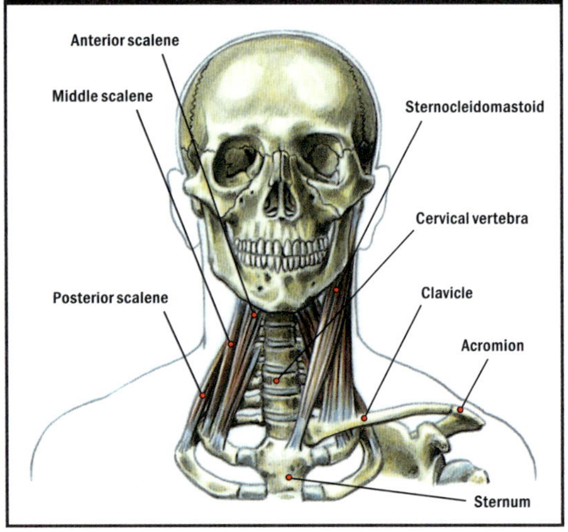

Stand with your legs slightly apart and your back very straight. Place one arm behind your back and clasp that wrist with your other hand. Pull the arm slowly down and toward the outside of your body to feel the deltoid being stretched (mainly the posterior and middle portions), as well as the trapezius.

Variation

To feel the stretch more in your neck, do this stretch while slowly bending your head to the opposite side. This variation allows you to stretch the deep complex muscles along your cervical spine as well as your scalene and sternocleidomastoid.

STRETCHING THE TRAPEZIUS AND NECK

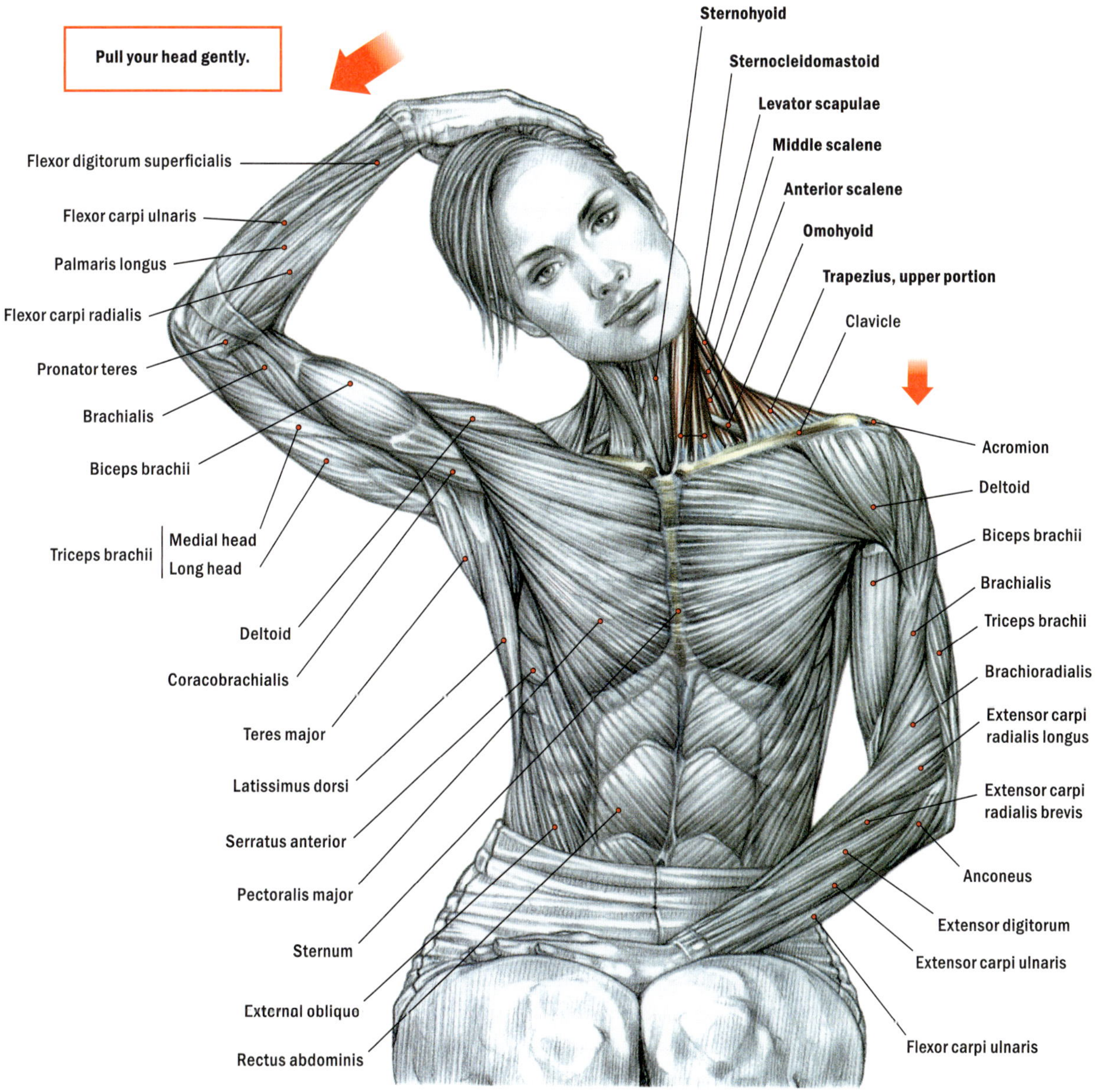

Pull your head gently.
Sternohyoid
Sternocleidomastoid
Levator scapulae
Middle scalene
Anterior scalene
Omohyoid
Trapezius, upper portion
Clavicle
Acromion
Deltoid
Biceps brachii
Brachialis
Triceps brachii
Brachioradialis
Extensor carpi radialis longus
Extensor carpi radialis brevis
Anconeus
Extensor digitorum
Extensor carpi ulnaris
Flexor carpi ulnaris
Flexor digitorum superficialis
Flexor carpi ulnaris
Palmaris longus
Flexor carpi radialis
Pronator teres
Brachialis
Biceps brachii
Triceps brachii
Medial head
Long head
Deltoid
Coracobrachialis
Teres major
Latissimus dorsi
Serratus anterior
Pectoralis major
Sternum
External oblique
Rectus abdominis

Place one hand over your head and pull your head gently, bending your head to the side. This stretches the sternocleidomastoid, scalene group, upper portion of the trapezius, splenius capitis, and splenius cervicis. More deeply, it stretches the semispinalis capitis as well as the small muscles of the spine such as the longissimus cervicis, rectus capitis anterior, rectus capitis lateralis, and longus capitis.

Always do this stretch gradually, pulling carefully on your head.

To feel the stretch better in the upper portion of the trapezius, try to lower the shoulder of the inactive arm at the same time.

05 LEGS

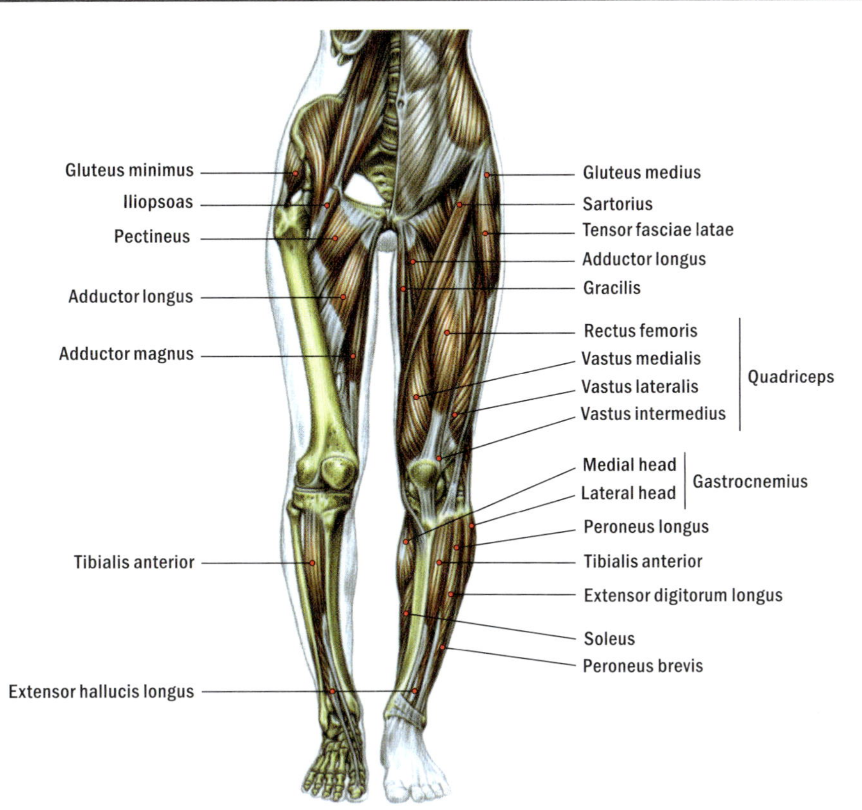

Gluteus minimus
Iliopsoas
Pectineus
Adductor longus
Adductor magnus
Tibialis anterior
Extensor hallucis longus
Gluteus medius
Sartorius
Tensor fasciae latae
Adductor longus
Gracilis
Rectus femoris
Vastus medialis
Vastus lateralis
Vastus intermedius
Quadriceps
Medial head
Lateral head
Gastrocnemius
Peroneus longus
Tibialis anterior
Extensor digitorum longus
Soleus
Peroneus brevis

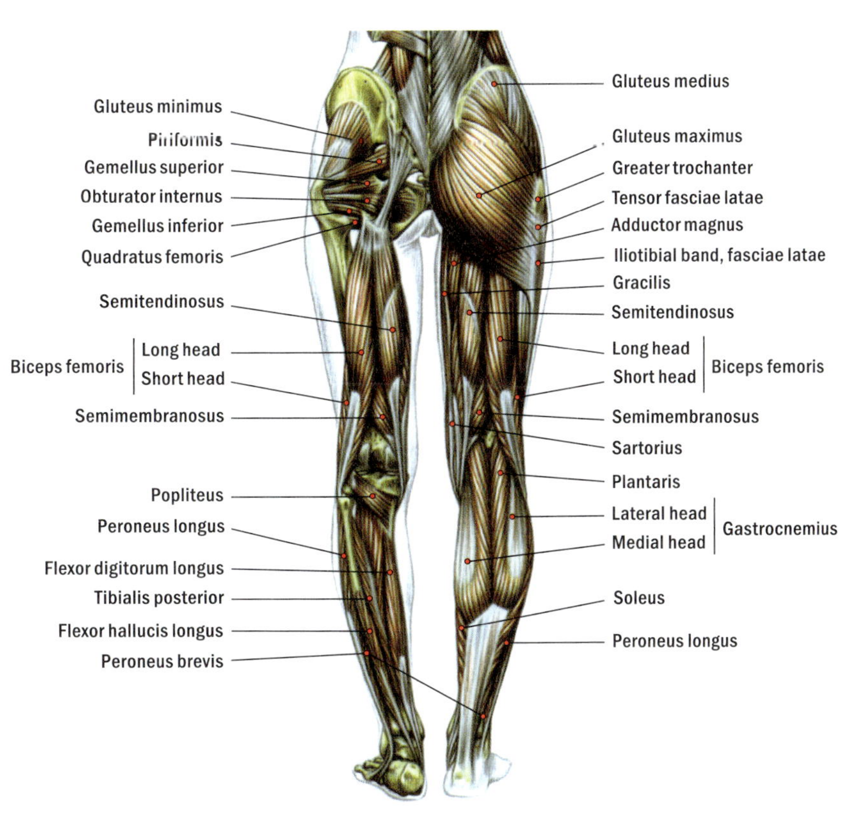

Gluteus minimus
Piriformis
Gemellus superior
Obturator internus
Gemellus inferior
Quadratus femoris
Semitendinosus
Biceps femoris
Long head
Short head
Semimembranosus
Popliteus
Peroneus longus
Flexor digitorum longus
Tibialis posterior
Flexor hallucis longus
Peroneus brevis
Gluteus medius
Gluteus maximus
Greater trochanter
Tensor fasciae latae
Adductor magnus
Iliotibial band, fasciae latae
Gracilis
Semitendinosus
Long head
Short head
Biceps femoris
Semimembranosus
Sartorius
Plantaris
Lateral head
Medial head
Gastrocnemius
Soleus
Peroneus longus

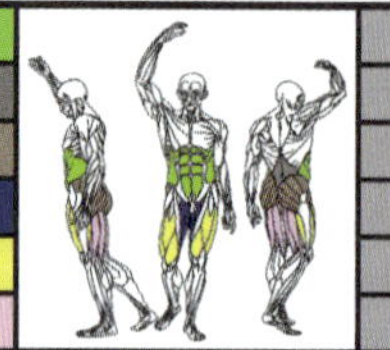

STARTING POSITION

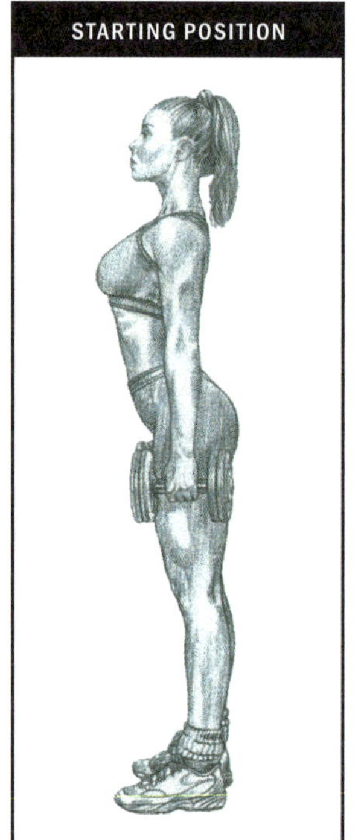

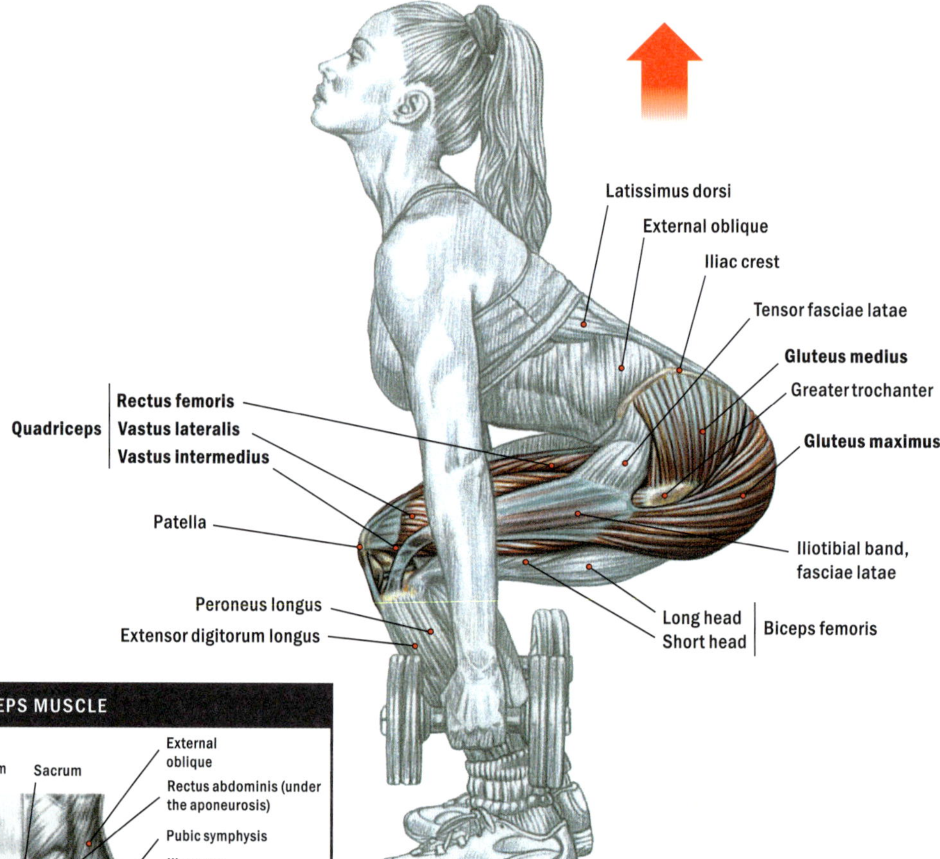

QUADRICEPS MUSCLE

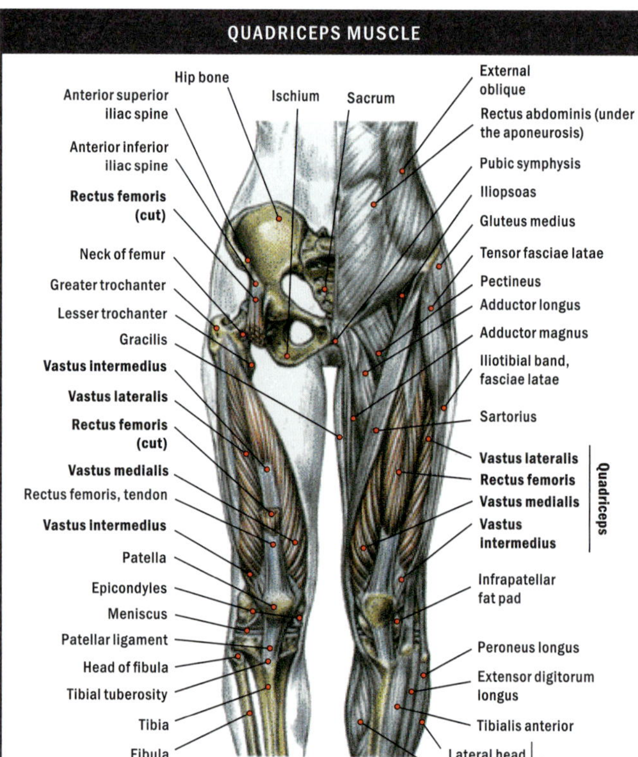

Stand with your feet slightly apart, a dumbbell in each hand, and your arms relaxed:

- Look straight ahead, inhale, arch your back slightly, and bend your knees.
- When your thighs are horizontal, straighten your legs to return to the starting position.
- Exhale at the end of the exercise.

This exercise mainly works the quadriceps and the gluteus muscles.

There is no real point in working with heavy weights here. Working with moderate weights in sets of 10 to 15 reps provides the best results.

SUMO DUMBBELL SQUATS 02

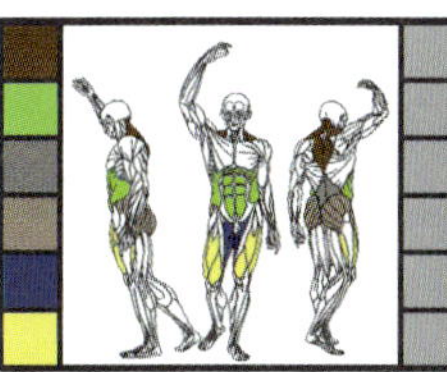

STARTING POSITION

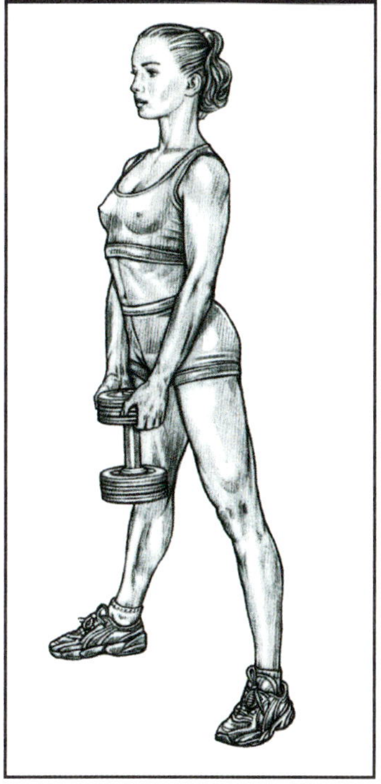

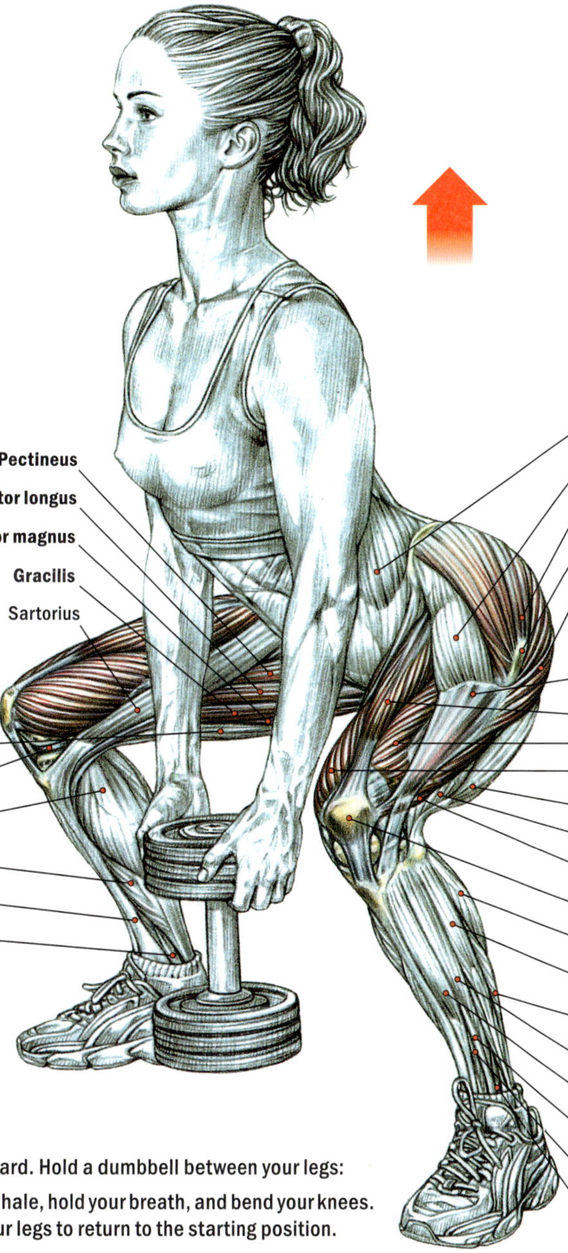

Stand with your legs apart and feet pointing outward. Hold a dumbbell between your legs:

- Look straight ahead, arch your back slightly, inhale, hold your breath, and bend your knees.
- When the thighs are horizontal, straighten your legs to return to the starting position.
- Exhale at the end of the exercise.

This exercise works the quadriceps as well as the gluteus muscles.

This sumo position works the adductors.

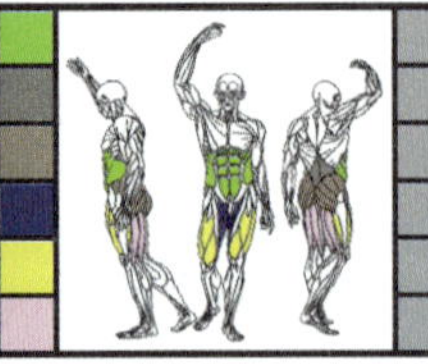

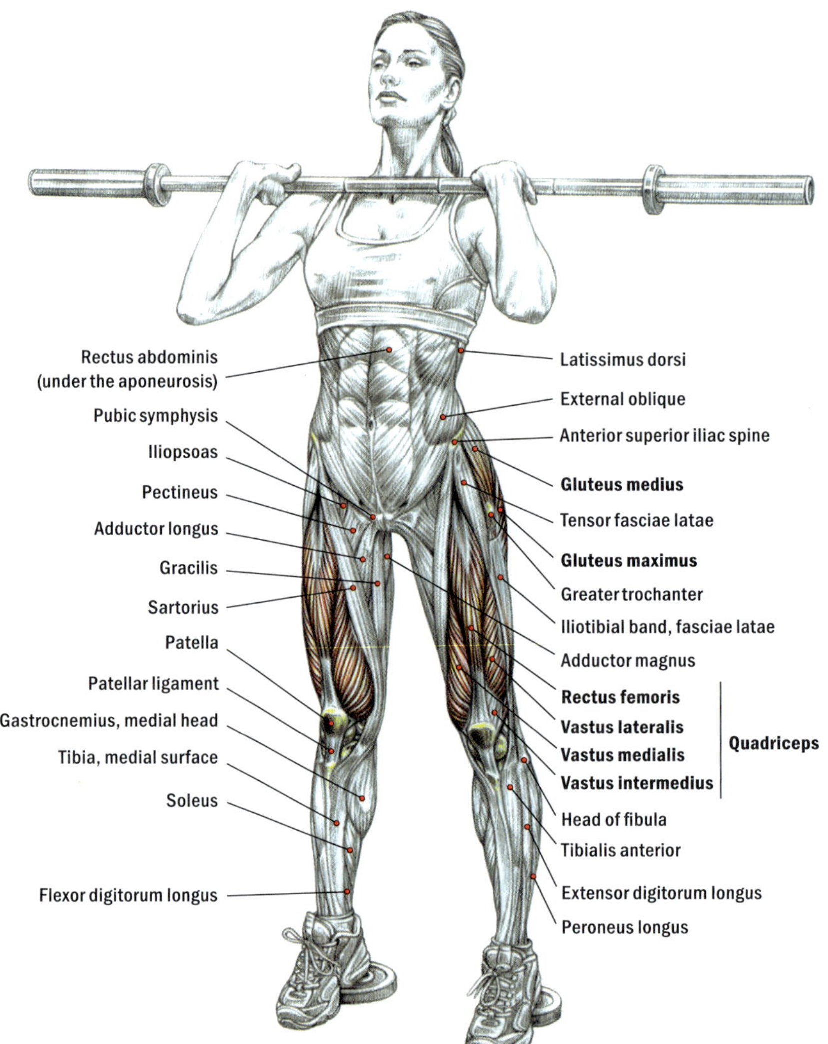

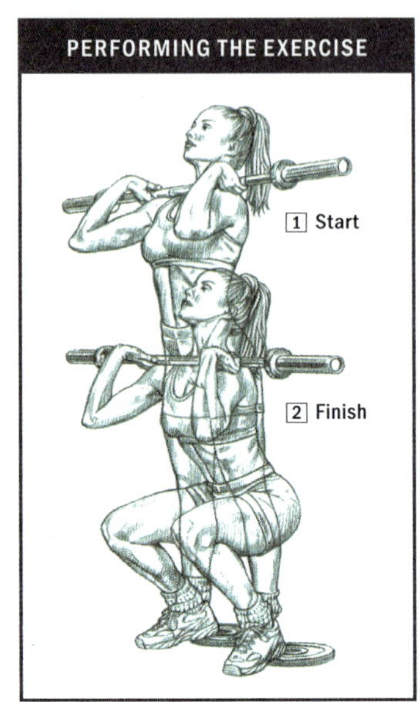

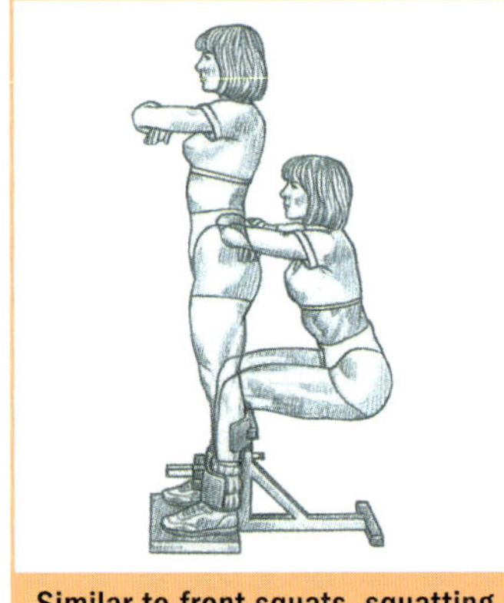

Similar to front squats, squatting with the legs held by equipment focuses a major part of the work on the quadriceps muscles.

Stand with your legs about shoulder-width apart and hold the bar with an overhand grip as it rests on your upper pectoral muscles and your anterior deltoids:

- Take a deep breath to maintain intrathoracic pressure, which prevents your torso from slumping forward, slightly arch your lower back, engage the core, and bend your knees to lower your thighs until they are parallel to the floor.
- Return to the starting position and exhale at the end of the exercise.

To prevent the barbell from sliding forward, stick out your chest and raise your elbows as high as possible.

The barbell's position at the front prevents your torso from bending forward, so your back will always be straight. To make the exercise easier, you can put something under your heels.

This type of squat puts most of the work on the quadriceps and is always done with lighter weights than the traditional squat. This comprehensive exercise also works the gluteus muscles, hamstrings, abdominal muscles, and the erector spinae. It is frequently used in weight training because it corresponds perfectly with the work the thighs do during clean and jerks and at the end of a snatch.

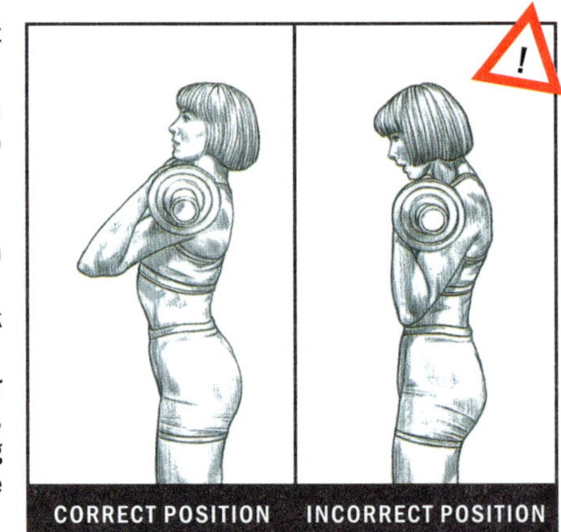

HERNIAS

DIFFERENT TYPES OF HERNIAS

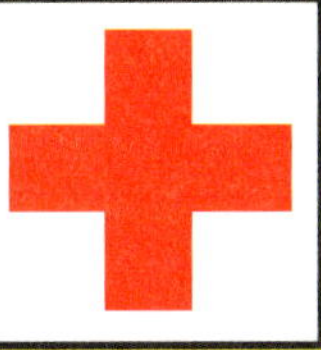

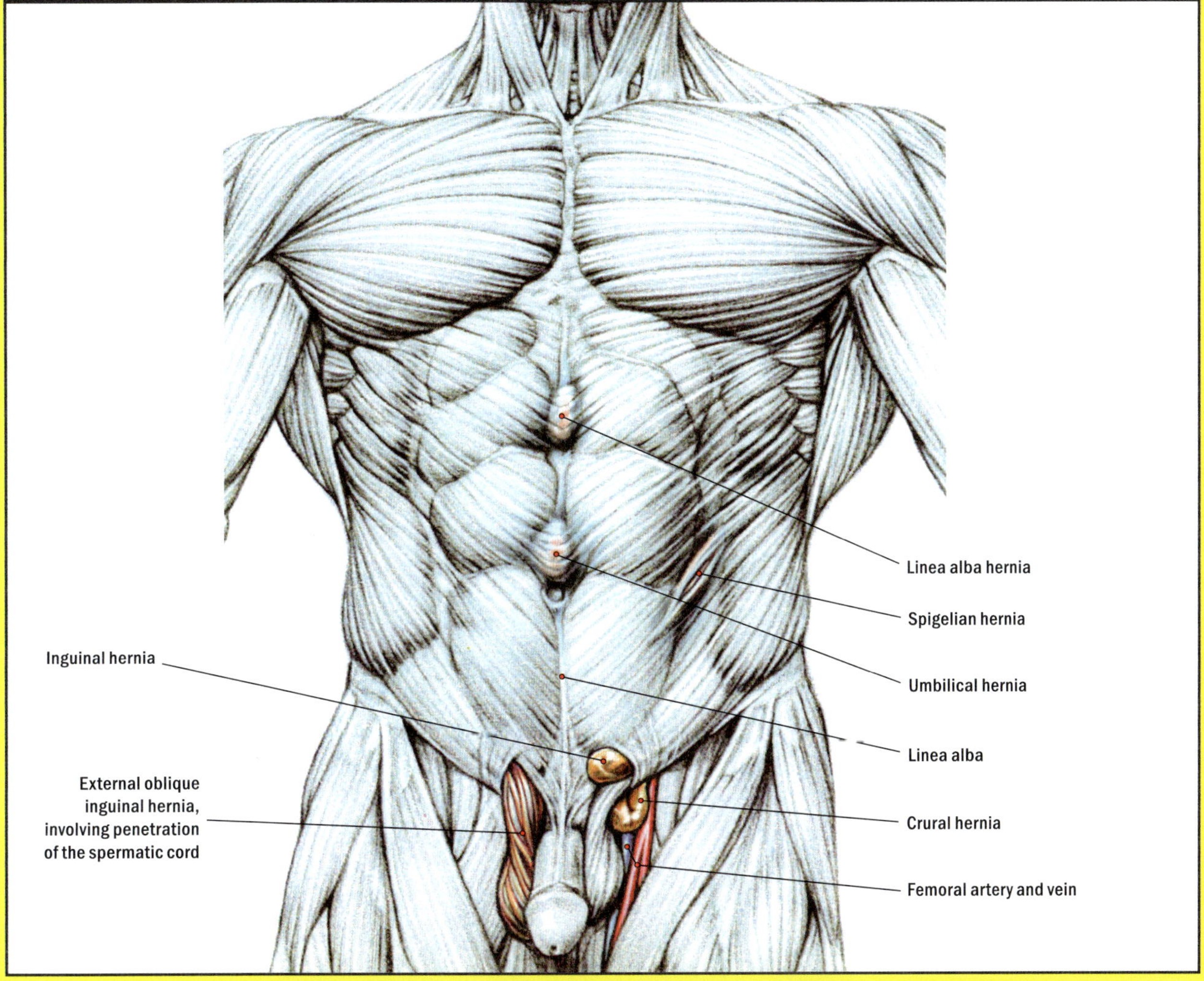

Although hernias affecting the abdominal wall and the crural and inguinal regions are often due to an individual fragility resulting from a structural defect in the supporting connective tissue, working with heavy weights in squat, press, and deadlift exercises significantly increases the risk of hernias because of the internal pressure it generates.

Like torn tissue, a hernia never repairs itself, and it can only get worse. It is important, therefore, to consult a surgeon after your diagnosis to determine if an operation is necessary. Umbilical and abdominal hernias, which often involve the linea alba, are less likely to cause complications, but inguinal and crural hernias can have dramatic consequences without an operation to repair them.

In fact, a loop of intestine can pass through the hole in the fascia and become twisted, blocking the blood supply and intestinal digestion. This is known as a *strangulated hernia*. This is a medical emergency, the seriousness of which depends on the intestinal obstruction and ischemia of the strangulated intestines. Surgery should be done as soon as possible.

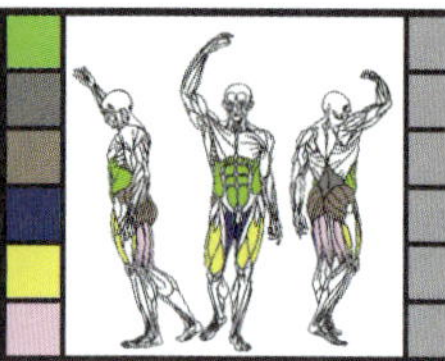

Quadriceps
- Vastus lateralis
- Rectus femoris
- Vastus intermedius
- Vastus medialis

- Sartorius
- Patella
- Patellar tendon

- Gastrocnemius, medial head
- Tibia
- Soleus

- External oblique
- Iliac crest
- **Gluteus medius**
- Tensor fasciae latae
- Greater trochanter
- **Gluteus maximus**
- Fasciae latae
- Short head / Long head — Biceps femoris
- Gastrocnemius, lateral head
- Soleus
- Peroneus longus
- Peroneus brevis
- Extensor digitorum longus
- Tibialis anterior

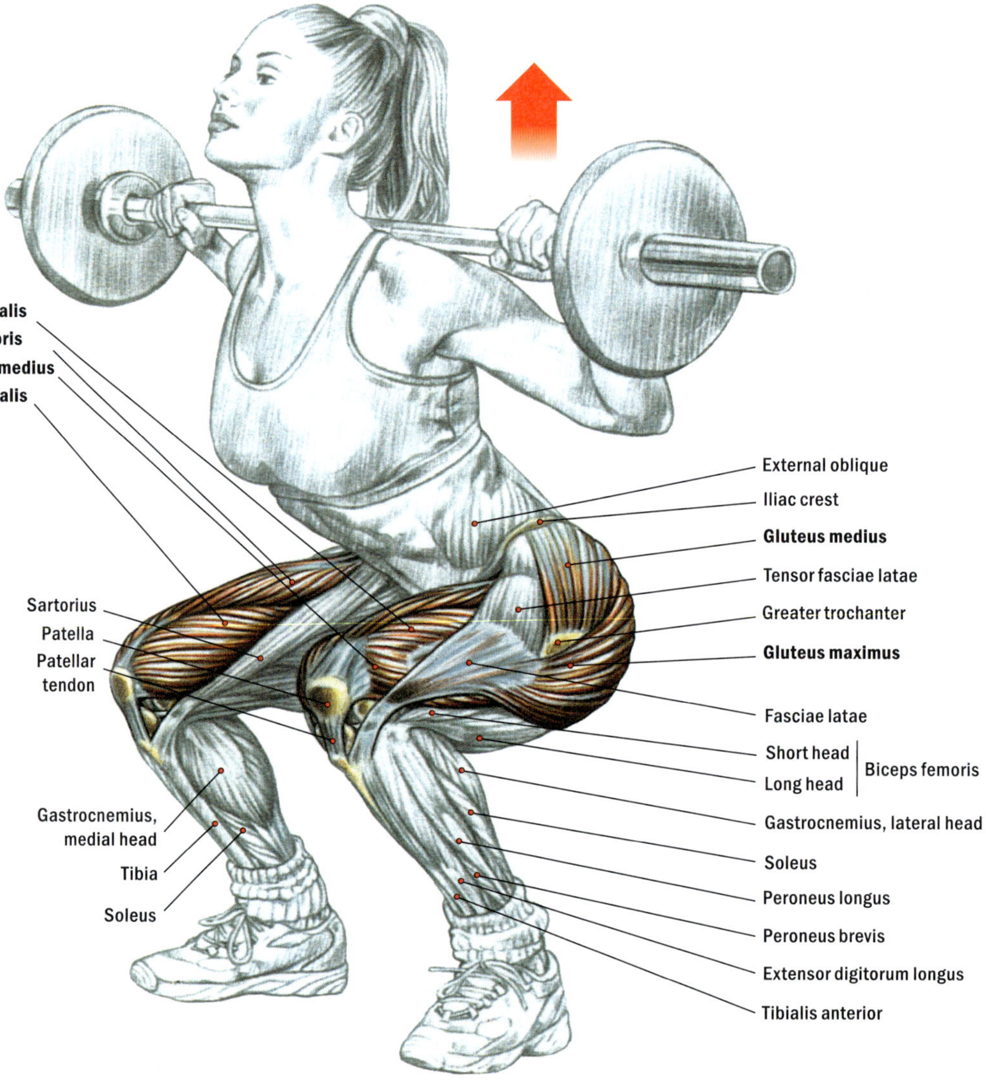

TWO WAYS TO HOLD THE BARBELL

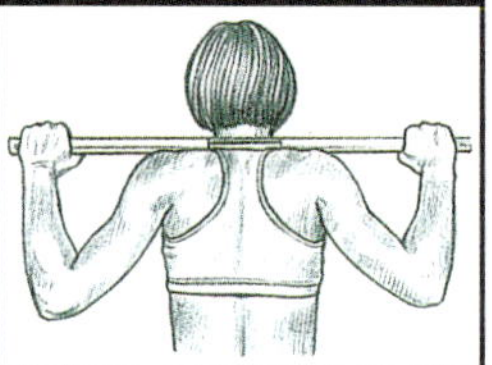

Resting on the trapezius muscles

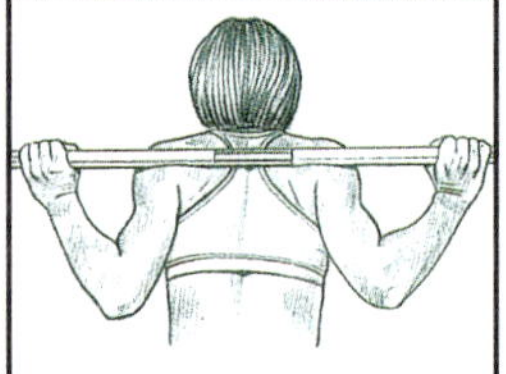

Resting on the deltoid and trapezius, like a powerlifter

The squat is the number one strength training exercise: It works almost the entire muscular system, as well as the cardiovascular system. It helps develop thoracic expansion, and therefore, respiratory capacity:

- With the barbell resting on a stand, slide under the bar and place it on your trapezius, slightly higher than the posterior deltoid. Grasp the bar firmly with your hands at a comfortable width and keep your elbows back.
- Take a deep breath (to maintain intrathoracic pressure and prevent your torso from slumping forward), arch your back slightly by rotating your pelvis forward, engage your core, look straight ahead, and remove the barbell from the stand.
- Take a couple of steps back and stop with your feet parallel to each other (or toes pointing slightly outward) and about shoulder-width apart. Bend forward (the axis of flexion should pass through the hip joints), controlling your descent and keeping your back straight at all times to prevent injury.
- When your thighs are parallel to the floor, straighten your legs and lift your torso to return to the starting position. Exhale at the end of the exercise.

The squat mainly works the quadriceps, glutes, adductors, erector spinae, abdominal muscles, and hamstrings.

The squat is one of the best exercises for developing the shape of the buttocks. To feel the gluteus muscles working, it is important to lower the thighs until they are parallel to the floor.

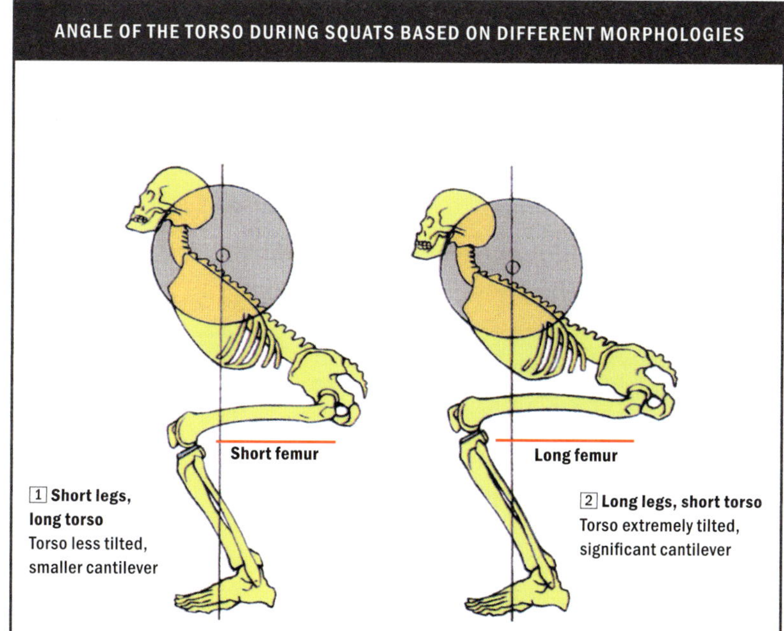

Variations

- People with rigid ankles or long femurs can place a block under their heels to stop the torso from tilting too much. This variation also transfers some of the work to the quadriceps.
- Varying the position of the bar on the back (for example, lowering it onto the posterior deltoids) changes the angle to increase the leverage of the back, and this helps you lift heavier weights. This technique is essential for powerlifters.
- The squat can be done in a rack, which keeps you from tilting your torso and lets you focus the work on the quadriceps.

HOW TO POSITION YOUR FEET DURING SQUATS

When doing traditional squats (with the feet approximately shoulder-width apart), you must place your feet properly. They should be parallel or slightly pointed to the outside. However, you must take your unique morphology into consideration and ensure that your feet are in line with your knees. For example, if you naturally walk with your feet pointed out, do your squats with your feet pointed out.

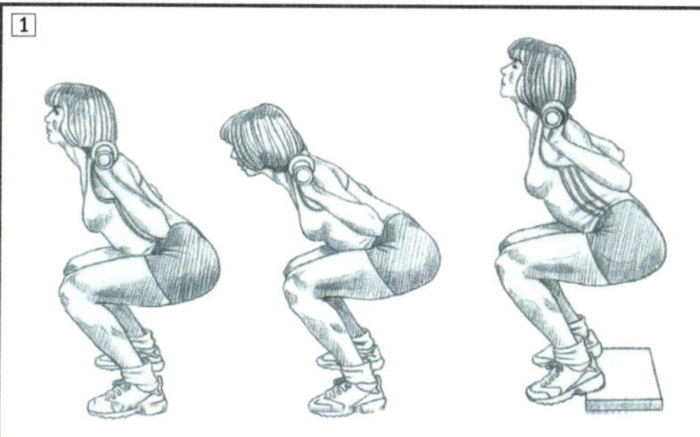
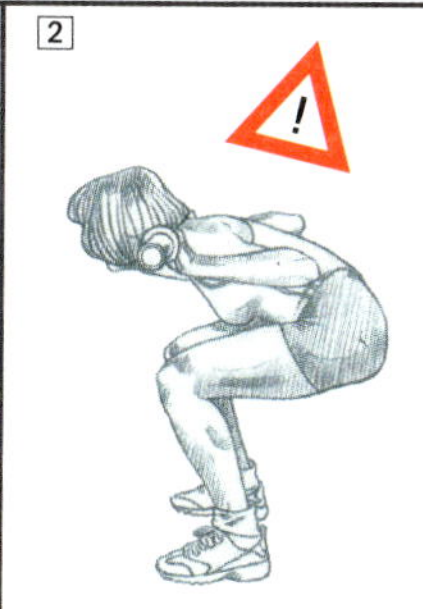

1 Correct positions

When squatting, the back needs to be as straight as possible. Given the variations in each person's morphology (different leg lengths and ankle flexibility) and variations in technique (width of stance, use of heel blocks, barbell higher or lower), the tilt of each person's torso will vary; however, you should lean forward from the hips.

2 Incorrect position

Never round your back when squatting. This mistake is responsible for most lower back injuries, especially herniated discs.

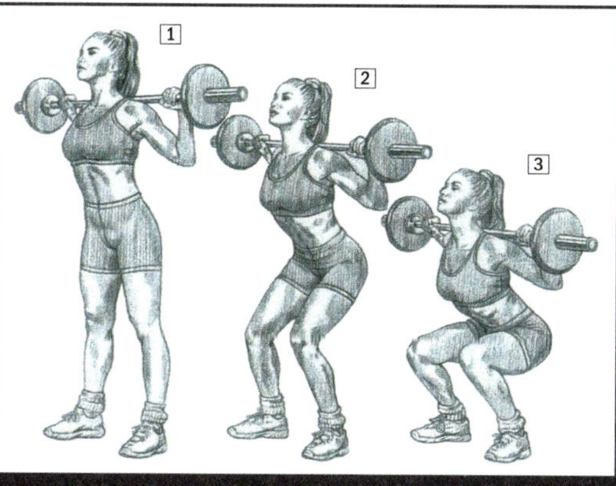

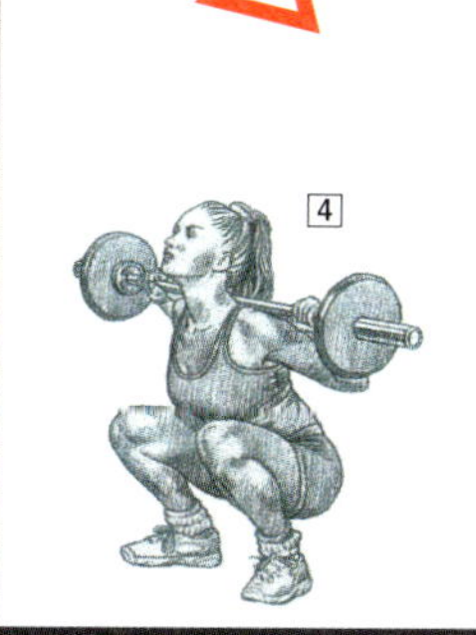

1 2 3 Negative phase
4 Complete squat

To better feel the gluteus muscles working, you can lower your hips below your knees. However, this technique can only be done by people with flexible ankles or short femurs. Moreover, you must do complete squats very carefully, as it can cause you to round the lower back, which can lead to serious injury.

No matter what the exercise, as soon as heavy weights are involved, it is essential to create a block:

1. Expanding the chest by holding a deep breath that fills the lungs will support the rib cage and prevent the torso from leaning forward.
2. Contracting all of the abdominal muscles will support the core and increase intra-abdominal pressure to prevent the torso from slumping forward.
3. Finally, arching the lower back by contracting the lumbar muscles will place the spinal column in extension.

These three actions together are referred to as *blocking*. They will keep you from rounding or bending your back. When lifting heavy weights, rounding the back can cause a herniated disc (see pages 176-177).

SQUAT-SPECIFIC STRETCH

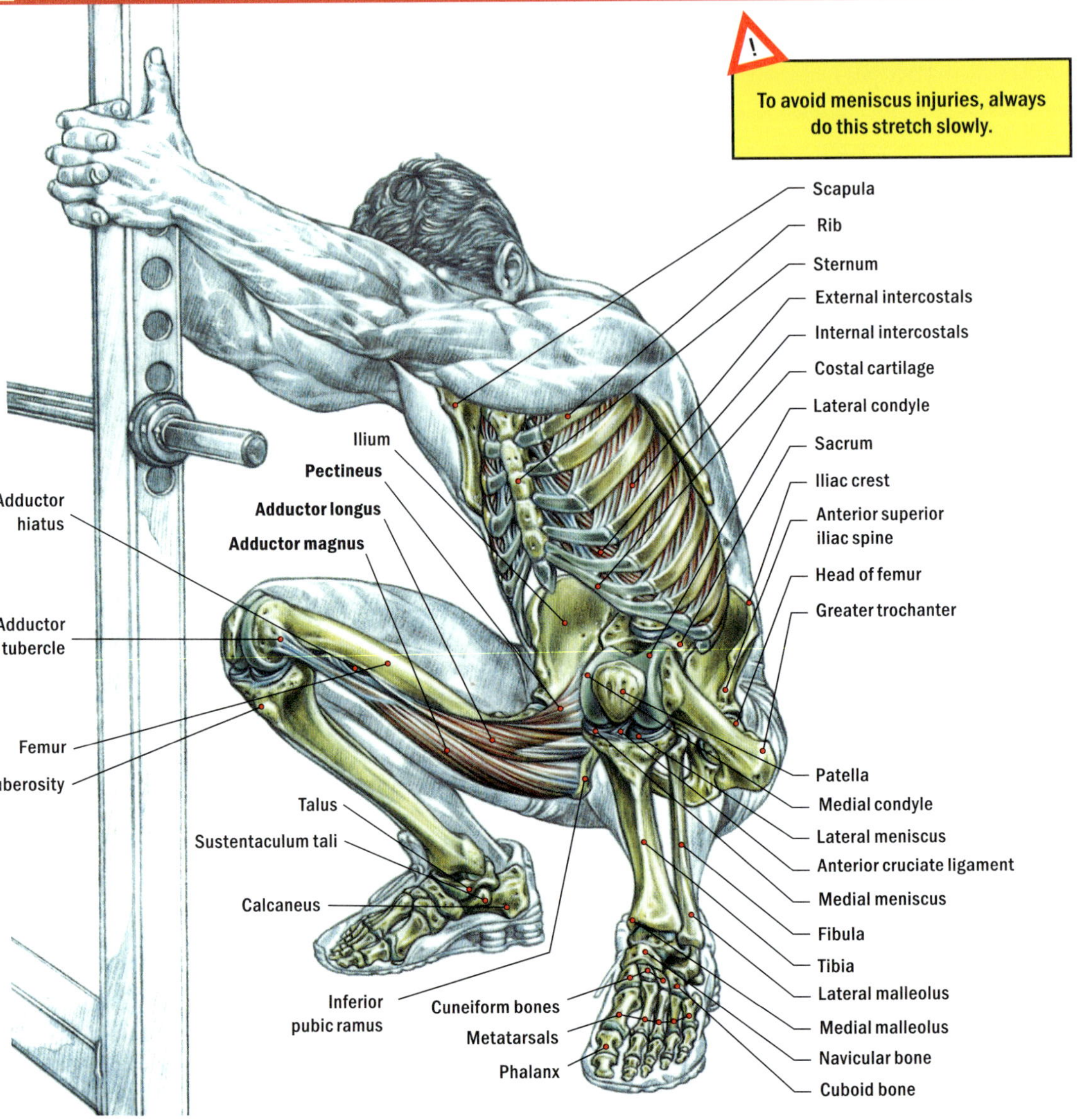

To avoid meniscus injuries, always do this stretch slowly.

To avoid tearing muscles when squatting, you should do some stretching exercises at the beginning of the workout, while warming up, and between the initial sets. One stretching exercise often performed by powerlifters involves crouching slowly while holding onto a stable support such as the pole or frame of a weight training machine.

This exercise corresponds perfectly to the bending action of a squat and helps effectively stretch the adductors, especially the adductor magnus, which is frequently injured during excessive tilting of the torso when using heavy weights. The stretch is good for the quadriceps (except for the rectus femoris); gluteus maximus; and all of the small, deep external rotator muscles of the hip, which also stabilize and slow the forward tilt of the pelvis when crouching.

To properly feel the stretch on the inside of the leg, you can shift your body weight from one leg to the other.

POWER SQUATS 05

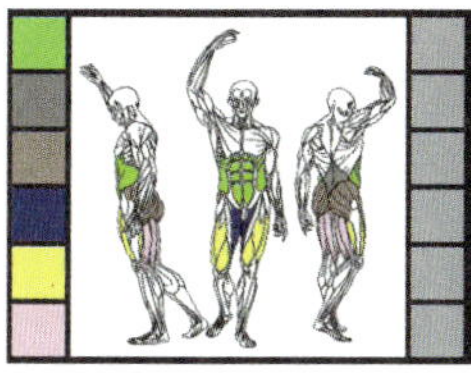

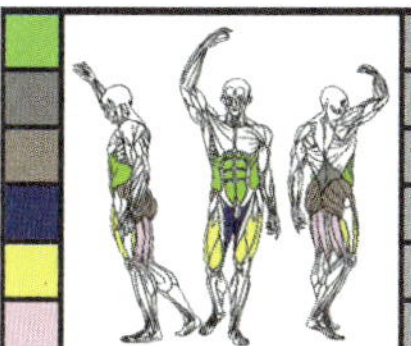

Rectus abdominis (under the aponeurosis)
Internal oblique (under the aponeurosis)
Iliopsoas
Pubic symphysis
Pectineus
Quadriceps
Rectus femoris
Vastus medialis
Adductor longus
Sartorius
Meniscus
Gracilis
Gastrocnemius, medial head
Tibia, medial surface
Soleus
Adductor magnus
Semimembranosus
Semitendinosus
External oblique
Gluteus medius
Anterior superior iliac spine
Tensor fasciae latae
Greater trochanter
Gluteus maximus
Pyramidalis (under the aponeurosis)
Iliotibial band, fasciae latae
Vastus lateralis
Vastus intermedius
Quadriceps
Head of fibula
Patella
Patellar ligament
Peroneus longus
Tibialis anterior
Extensor digitorum longus
Peroneus brevis

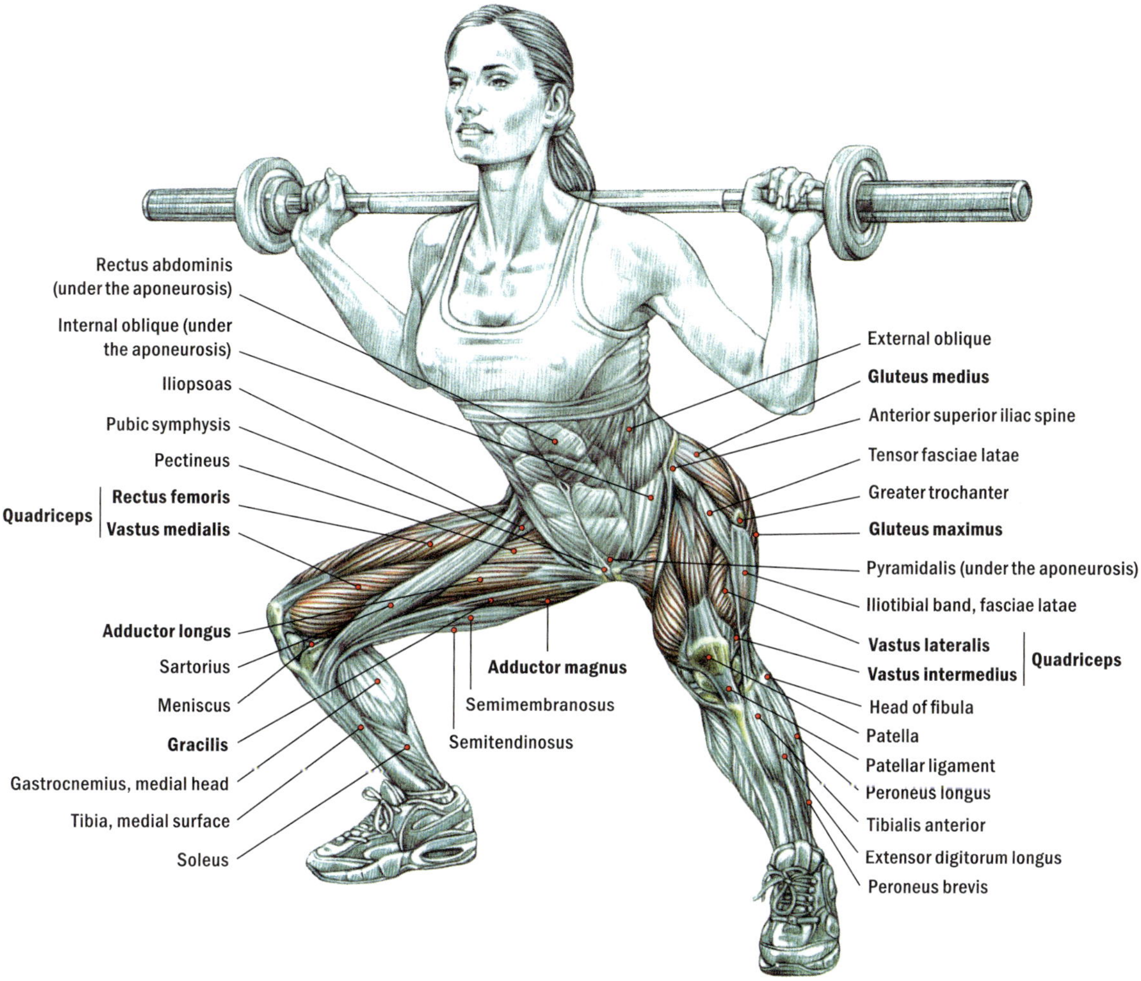

This exercise is performed in the same way as a traditional squat, except that the legs are placed farther apart and the toes point outward, which works the inner thighs intensely. It uses the following muscles:

- Quadriceps
- Adductor muscles (adductor magnus, adductor longus, adductor brevis, adductor pectineus, and gracilis)
- Gluteus muscles
- Hamstrings
- Abdominal muscles
- Lumbosacral muscles

In this squat, where the legs are farther apart, the torso is more upright at the bottom of the movement than in the traditional squat; some powerlifters choose the wide-leg version to reduce stress on the back. However, some powerlifters using heavy weights prefer traditional squats since they relieve pressure on the lower back as the torso rests on the thighs.

THREE POSITIONS FOR THE FEET DURING SQUATS

1
2
3

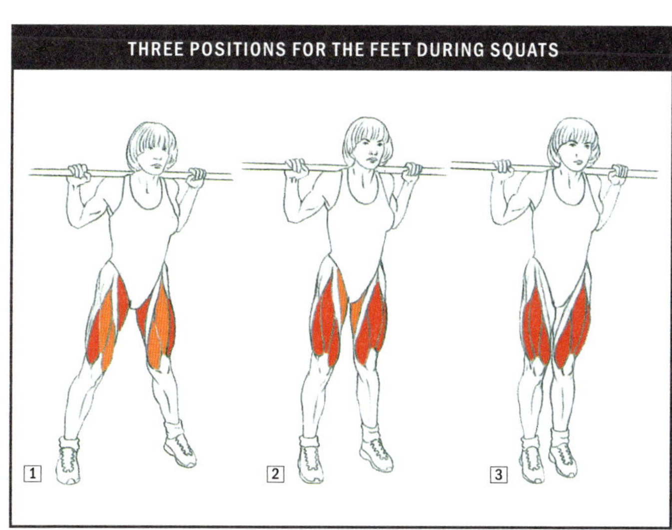

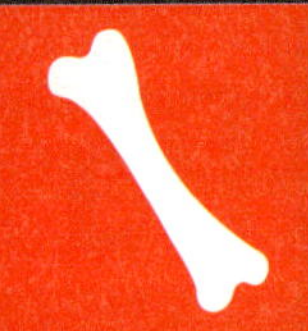

ADAPTING TRAINING TO YOUR MORPHOLOGY

SHORT-LIMBED AND LONG-LIMBED INDIVIDUALS

In strength training, it is important to consider your individual morphology when selecting exercises, particularly the squat and deadlift. Both these exercises work the muscles quite differently in short-limbed and long-limbed people.

A short-limbed individual has a proportionately longer torso and shorter limbs, whereas a long-limbed person has a relatively shorter torso and longer extremities. This has nothing to do with size, muscular development, or fat (a person can be overweight and long-limbed or very thin and short-limbed).

Short-limbed people can do squats more easily. Because of the shortness of the femur, the torso will only tilt a little, limiting the stress on the lower back and the hamstring muscles, allowing the exercise to be performed in relative safety, and focusing almost all the work on the quadriceps. Therefore, it is not surprising that almost all squat champions fall into this morphological category. Extreme examples would be the individuals born with dwarfism who dominate the lighter powerlifting categories.

On the other hand, long-limbed individuals will have more difficulty doing squats. Due to the length of the femurs, the torso will lean far forward. This will place a dangerous amount of stress on the hamstring muscles as well as the adductor magnus and the gracilis. Long-limbed people constantly struggle to avoid losing their balance and falling forward.

People with long limbs must also concentrate on the position of the back to avoid rounding it. Rounding is an error that can lead to severe vertebral injuries, including the all-too-common herniated disc.

When performing the squat, the length of the legs has a huge influence on the tilt of the torso.

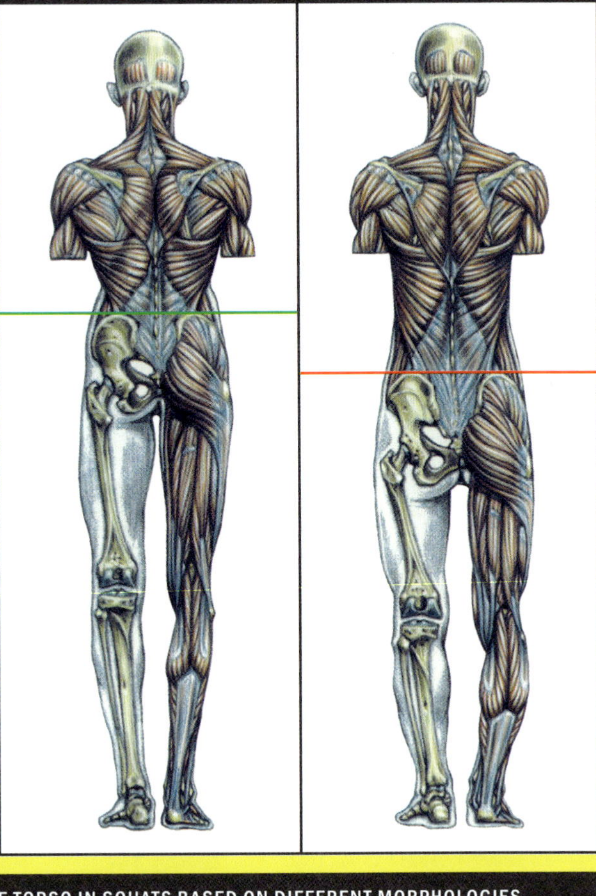

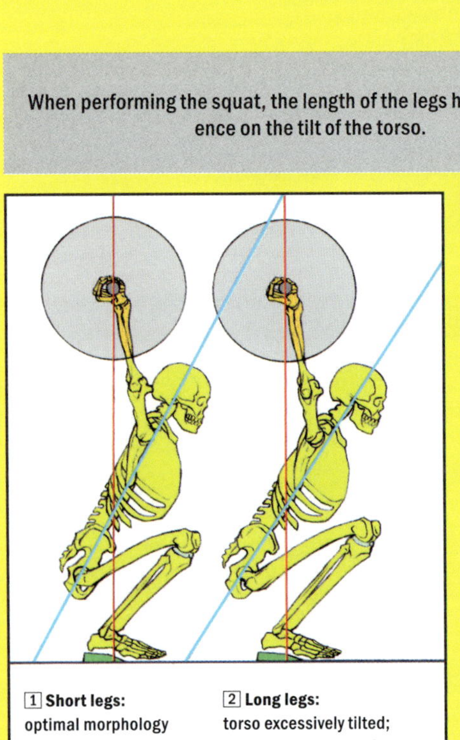

1 **Short legs:**
optimal morphology

2 **Long legs:**
torso excessively tilted; shoulders dangerously stretched backward

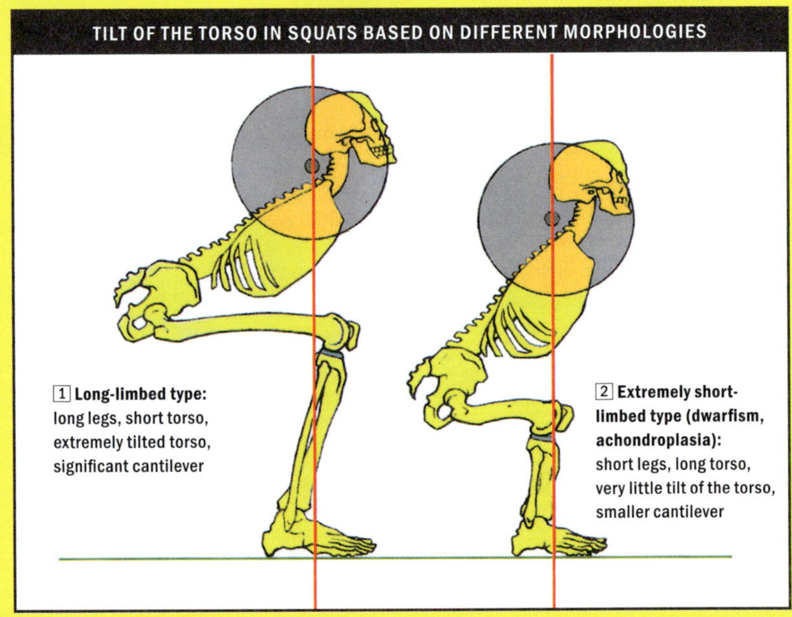

1 **Long-limbed type:**
long legs, short torso, extremely tilted torso, significant cantilever

2 **Extremely short-limbed type (dwarfism, achondroplasia):**
short legs, long torso, very little tilt of the torso, smaller cantilever

People with long limbs leaning forward to squat will work the gluteus maximus muscles intensely, which come into play when straightening the pelvis and the torso. They also work the erector spinae muscles, which battle against the rounding of the back.

The squat is excellent for developing powerful glutes and strong lumbar muscles in long-limbed people, who will, however, need to concentrate on their positioning a great deal. Squats become dangerous when heavier weights are used. Long-limbed people who wish to target the work on the quadriceps should work with machines, especially the hack squat machine (page 182).

Short-limbed people dominate squat competitions, but they have trouble with deadlifts. Because of their shorter extremities, they are forced to bend the legs while grasping the bar on the floor. They must bring their femurs practically parallel to the floor, and initiating the exercise in this position requires an enormous amount of energy.

Long-limbed people, meanwhile, start their deadlifts with the legs partially bent, a position in which the quadriceps can generate the maximum amount of push. Despite a greater forward tilt of the back and more intense work on the gluteus muscles and the erector spinae muscles, their morphology allows them to lift significantly heavier weights than short-limbed people can. This is why deadlift champions are most often long-limbed individuals.

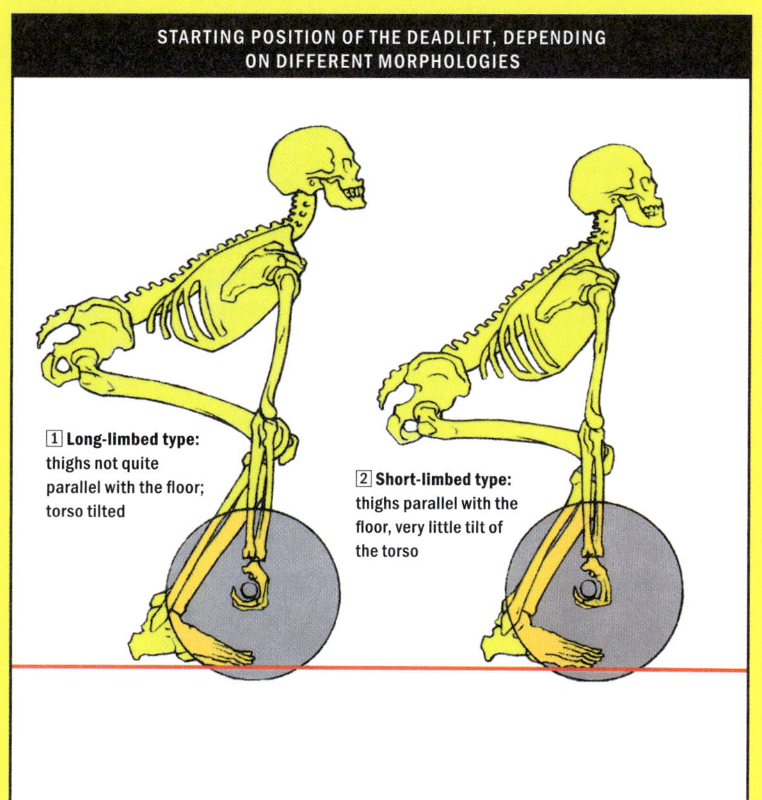

Although the femurs in figures 1 and 2 are parallel to the floor, the bending of the ankles in figure 2 is less than in figure 1.

ANKLE FLEXIBILITY

Ankle flexibility has a big impact on the execution of the squat. Whether it is due to a musculotendinous restriction (such as the retraction of the calves) or bone restriction, when dorsiflexion (raising the front part of the foot) is limited, the squat technique will be profoundly altered. In fact, a lack of flexibility at the ankles limits the forward tilt of the tibias and therefore the forward movement of the knees. This forces the squat to be performed with the gluteus muscles extremely far back and the back tilted very far forward. This works the gluteus muscles and erector spinae muscles intensely.

This type of squat, due to the excessive tilt of the torso, puts a dangerous amount of tension on the posterior muscles of the thigh and on the adductor magnus and gracilis muscles, increasing the risk of muscle tears. In addition, the lowering of the hips below the knees forces the lower back to round, increasing the risk of vertebral injuries. This squat requires enormous concentration to maintain the correct position. Because of its risks, the possibility of using heavier weights is limited.

Notice that, in comparison with the traditional squat, rigid ankles also limit the bending of the legs even though the thighs are parallel to the floor. Finally, the angle, which is larger than in a traditional squat, compels the quadriceps to provide a greater force to straighten the legs.

IMPROVING YOUR SQUAT POSITION

To relieve stress on the lower back and limit stress on the hamstring muscles, it is possible, as powerlifters do, to lower the bar to the posterior deltoids. This technique enables you to reduce the cantilever and increase the power of the lift from the back, which allows you to use heavier weight.

Using a block under your heels or wearing powerlifting shoes with rigid, raised heels reduces the cantilever by limiting the backward movement of your gluteus muscles as your knees move forward, allowing for greater range of motion as your knees bend. This technique enables you to feel the work of your quadriceps muscles while limiting the tilt of your torso and the work of your gluteus maximus muscles and your erector spinae.

The combination of lower bar placement and raised heels allows you to use significantly heavier weight. It is highly recommended for people with long limbs and those with rigid ankles, because it helps to correct their squat position.

FRONT SQUAT TO TARGET THE QUADRICEPS

By limiting the tilt of the torso, the front squat exercise reduces the work of the lower back and limits stress on the hamstrings and adductor magnus muscles.

However, by increasing the cantilever, the front position of the bar forces the quadriceps to work harder to straighten the thigh over the lower leg. This is, therefore, the very best squat for the thighs, but it should always be done with much lower weight than a traditional squat. For greater stability, it is best to always do it with raised heels.

Unfortunately, this squat is difficult for people with long limbs. A more tilted torso makes it harder to hold the bar, which might fall forward out of the hands.

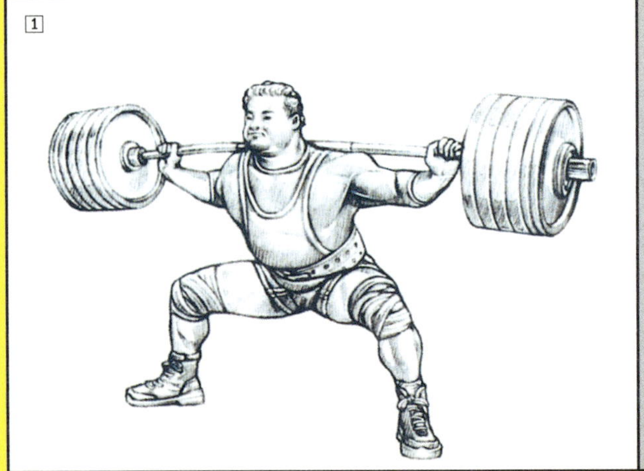

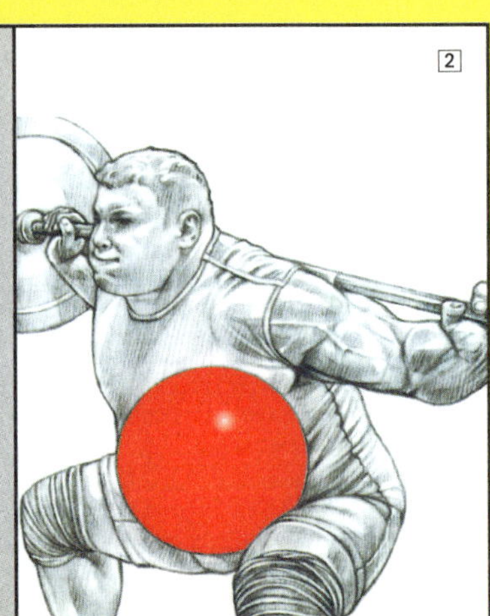

SPREADING THE LEGS TO RAISE THE TORSO

When squatting, to limit excessive and dangerous tilting of the torso, you can spread your legs farther apart by turning your toes out. Certain powerlifters take this technique to the extreme by placing the legs in practically a full split (which also allows them to limit their leg flexion). The squat with an extra-wide stance requires good flexibility in the adductor muscles of the leg and an adequate hip joint structure. Consequently, not everyone can perform this type of squat.

THE ADVANTAGE OF A LARGE BELLY

A large belly presses against the thighs and helps limit flexion of the hips and rounding of the back in the squat and deadlift. It also protects the lower back and limits the risk of a herniated disc. This is why this physical characteristic is common among many powerlifters and weightlifters, who make sure to maintain it through an excessively rich diet.

DIFFERENT TYPES OF KNEES

In strength training, it is important to consider individual morphology variations, especially in the knees. Although being bow-legged (genu varum) does not carry more risk than having normal legs, being knock-kneed (genu valgum) or having hyperextended knees (genu recurvatum) may even be a contraindication to lifting heavy weights.

Genu valgum is generally found in the following:

1. Those who were overweight during their youth. During that time, the bones of the legs are not yet fully developed and still malleable, so they become deformed and develop an *X* shape.
2. Women, who tend to have wider hips due to reproductive functions. This can increase the angle of the femurs.

If the genu valgum is too great, the joint is overused. The medial collateral ligament is overstretched, and the lateral meniscus, along with the joint surfaces covered with cartilage on the lateral condyle of the femur and the lateral external tuberosity of the tibia, are subjected to excessive friction. The excessive friction can lead to overuse injuries.

Genu recurvatum is mainly found in people who are very supple (referred to as hypermobile), especially women, in whom this frequent ligamentous and muscular hyperlaxity is directly related to reproductive functions. Rarely pathological, the recurvatum knee can result in complications such as a pinched meniscus, which occurs when the knee moves rapidly into hyperextension and the menisci do not have the time to slide, or during exercises with heavy weights that force hyperextension of the thigh. For this reason, people who have pathological recurvatum should never completely lock the knees at the end of extension during squats or leg presses.

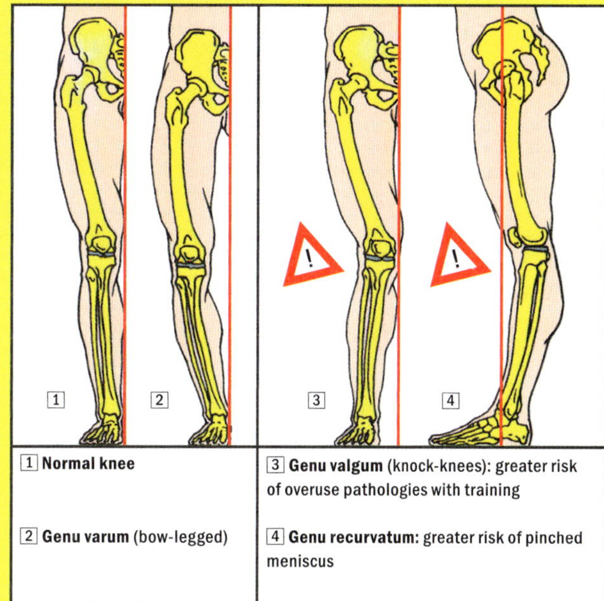

1 **Normal knee**

2 **Genu varum** (bow-legged)

3 **Genu valgum** (knock-knees): greater risk of overuse pathologies with training

4 **Genu recurvatum:** greater risk of pinched meniscus

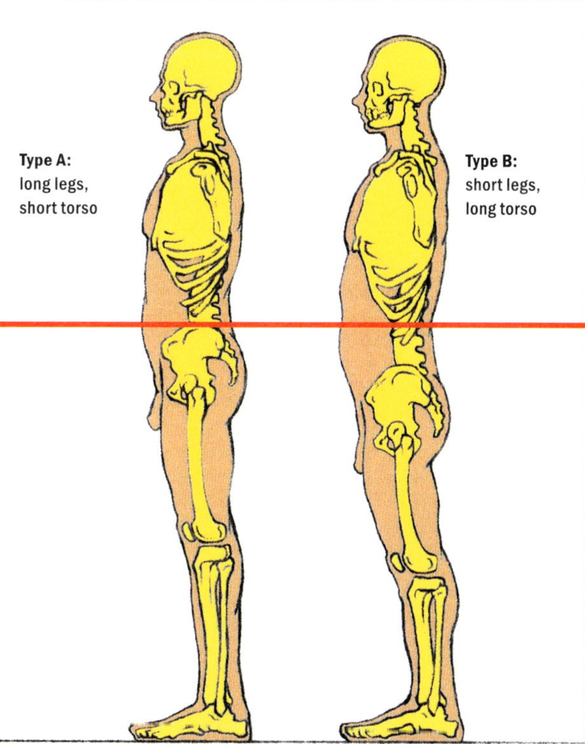

It is important to consider the relationship between the length of the torso and the length of the leg.

Type A: Individuals whose legs are proportionately longer and whose torsos are proportionally shorter will find it harder to squat correctly without leaning the torso too far forward. However, limiting the cantilever helps a person with a short torso do good morning exercises, the traditional deadlift, and the stiff-legged deadlift.

Type B: Individuals whose torsos are proportionately longer and whose legs are proportionally shorter will find it easier to squat safely without leaning too far forward. Therefore, it is not surprising that the greatest powerlifting champions specializing in the squat have this type of morphology.

HERNIATED DISCS

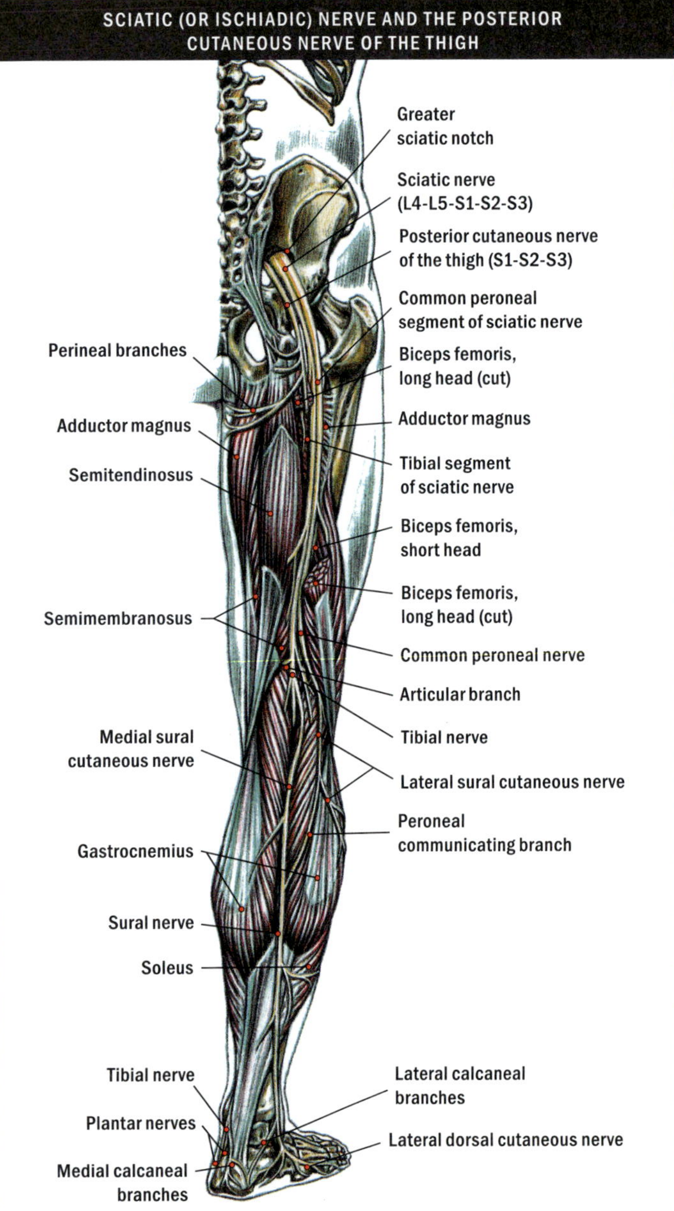

A herniated disc is a relatively frequent injury in strength training. It is most often caused by an incorrect back position during certain exercises such as the squat, deadlift, or bent-over row. When doing these exercises, the classic error is rounding the back (vertebral flexion), which pinches the front of the disc and pushes the back of the disc outward. If the intervertebral disc is cracked or aging, the gelatinous liquid of the nucleus pulposus migrates backward and can compress on the spinal cord or the roots of the spinal nerves. Symptoms depend on the type of injury, the amount of nucleus pulposus pushed out, and the surface that is compressed. The nucleus pulposus can bulge or, worse, explode through the annulus fibrosus that surrounds it and sometimes even tear the posterior ligament that links the vertebrae to each other. Compression of the nerves caused by the tearing of the annulus fibrosus is particularly painful and incapacitating.

In strength training, hernias usually occur in the lumbar area, most often between the third and fourth or between the fourth and fifth lumbar vertebrae. The pain is dull and deep, sometimes accompanied by swelling and tingling. The pain is felt in the middle of the back or more often to one side, radiating to the gluteus muscles, pelvis, pubis, and down the leg, following the path of the sciatic nerve if its root is compressed (hence the name *sciatica* is used to describe this type of pain).

Generally, these hernias are spontaneously reabsorbed, and the pain eventually disappears. But in some cases, the bulge in the disc does not disappear and continues to press painfully against the nerves or a detached piece of intervertebral cartilage compresses the nerves. In both these cases, a surgeon can remove the part that is pressing against the nerves. To prevent a herniated disc, use proper form and technique when performing risky exercises such as the squat, deadlift, good morning, and bent-over row.

After a heavy workout, it is advisable to stretch the back muscles by hanging from a bar and focusing on relaxing the body. This allows the back muscles to relax and rebalances the pressure inside the intervertebral discs.

No matter what the exercise, as soon as heavy weights are involved, it is essential to create a block:

1. Expanding the chest by holding a deep breath that fills the lungs will support the rib cage and prevent the torso from leaning forward.
2. Contracting all of the abdominal muscles will support the core and increase intra-abdominal pressure to prevent the torso from slumping forward.
3. Finally, arching the lower back by contracting the lumbar muscles will place the spinal column in extension.

These three actions together are referred to as *blocking*. They will keep you from rounding or bending your back, a position that, when lifting heavy weights, can cause a herniated disc.

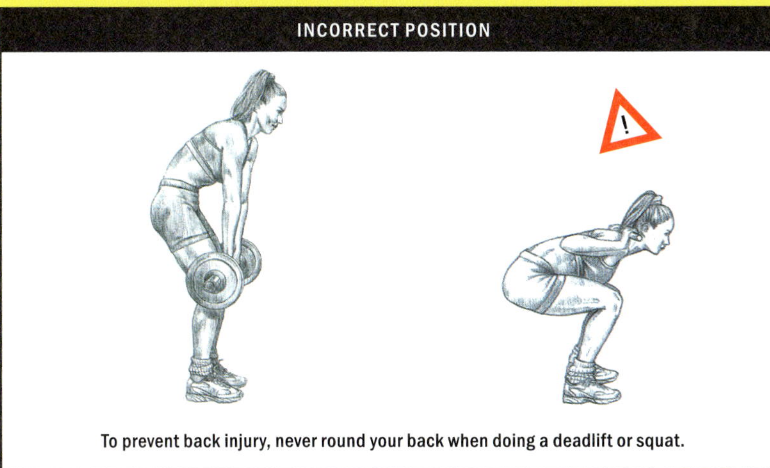

To prevent back injury, never round your back when doing a deadlift or squat.

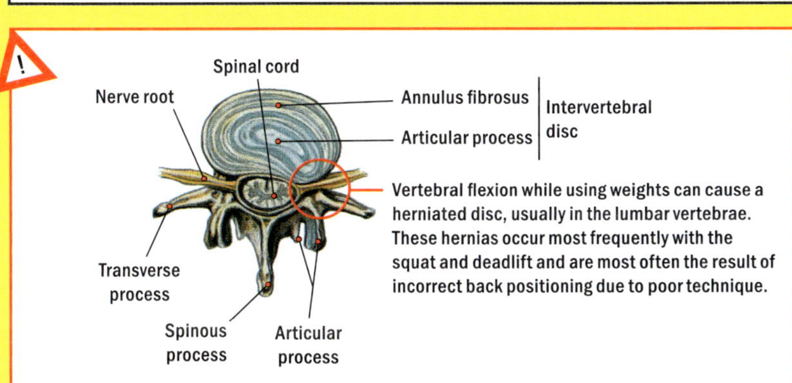

Vertebral flexion while using weights can cause a herniated disc, usually in the lumbar vertebrae. These hernias occur most frequently with the squat and deadlift and are most often the result of incorrect back positioning due to poor technique.

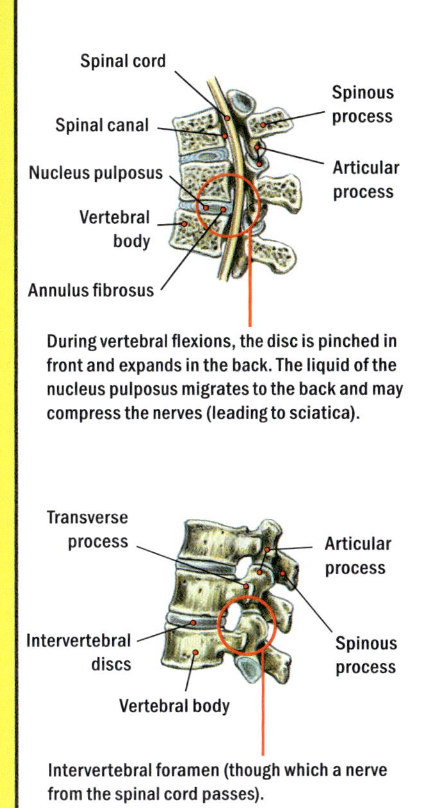

During vertebral flexions, the disc is pinched in front and expands in the back. The liquid of the nucleus pulposus migrates to the back and may compress the nerves (leading to sciatica).

Intervertebral foramen (though which a nerve from the spinal cord passes).

LUMBAR VERTEBRAL SEGMENT: CUTAWAY VIEW

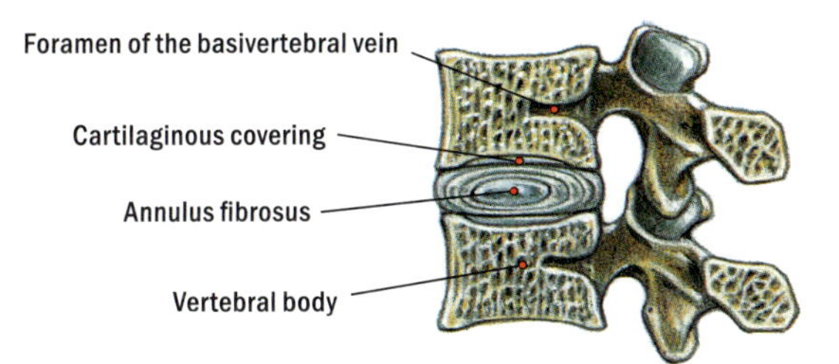

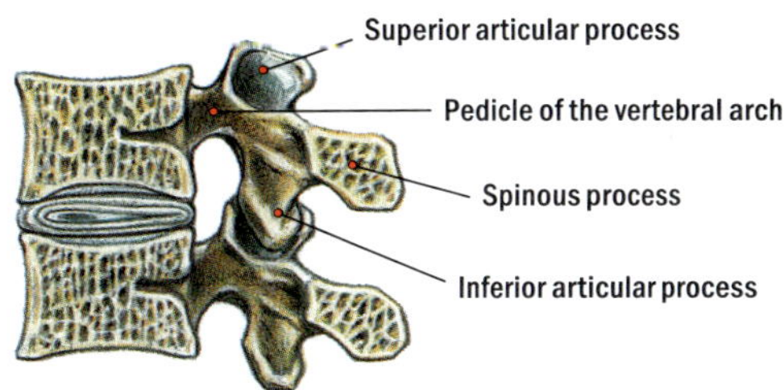

1 Young vertebral segment:
The intervertebral disc is still healthy.

After the age of 30, the intervertebral discs degenerate, and the annulus fibrosus can crack as the nucleus pulposus begins to dehydrate. This means that the discs of older athletes are more rigid and less elastic, limiting the mobility of the spine. On the other hand, as the viscous gel of the nucleus pulposus dehydrates, it becomes smaller and is less likely to be displaced and compress the nerves.

2 Older vertebral segment:
With age, the annulus fibrosus begins to develop fissures, and the viscous gel of the nucleus pulposus gradually starts to dehydrate. The intervertebral disc then collapses, and the vertebral segments lose their mobility.

In comparison, a herniated disc in a young person results in the movement of a greater amount of gelatinous fluid from the nucleus pulposus, causing more compression, pain, and incapacity of the nerves. Herniated discs are much more common in young athletes.

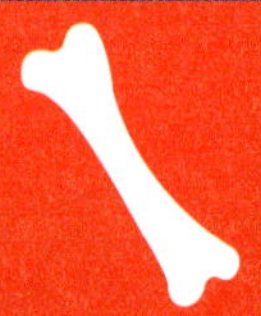

MORPHOLOGY DIFFERENCES BETWEEN WOMEN AND MEN TO CONSIDER FOR TRAINING

DISTINCTIVE FEATURES OF THE LOWER LIMBS IN WOMEN TO CONSIDER DURING TRAINING

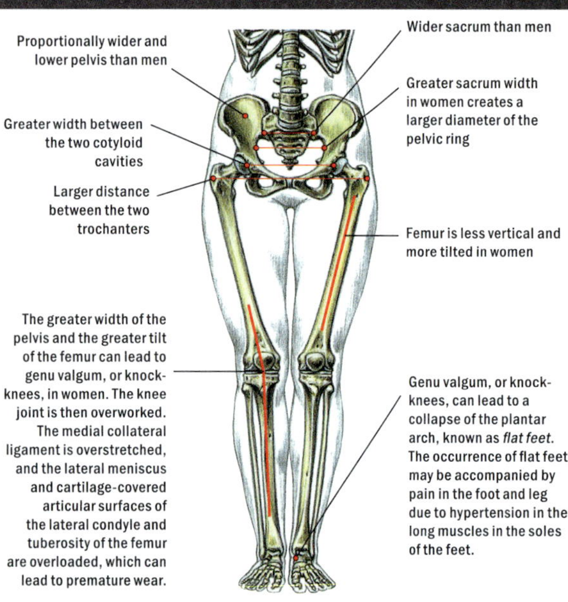

COMPARISON BETWEEN THE MALE AND FEMALE PELVIS, SHOWING THE INFLUENCE OF THE SKELETON ON EXTERNAL SHAPE

COMPARISON BETWEEN THE MALE AND FEMALE PELVIC OUTLET

* The pelvic ring is wider and more circular in women.

The morphological features of women and men are the consequence of differences between the volume and proportions of similar anatomical elements. Generally speaking, the female skeleton differs from the male skeleton in that it has less mass; smoother edges; and less accentuated indentations, depressions, or roughness (these are the consequence of the insertion of muscles or the movement of tendons—as the musculature is generally more developed in men, it marks the skeleton more). The female rib cage is often more circular and smaller than the male rib cage. Proportionally, the skeletal width of the shoulders is the same as that of the man, but greater muscular development in men makes it appear wider.

The lumbar curve is slightly more pronounced in women and the pelvis is tilted farther forward (anteverted), giving the impression that the lumbar arch is more pronounced than it actually is. A woman's waist is thinner because her rib cage is narrower, and her pelvis is generally lower and proportionally wider than a man's.

The most important difference between the male and female skeleton is in the pelvis. The female pelvis is adapted to gestation and childbirth and is therefore lower and proportionally wider than the male pelvis. The female sacrum is wider, and the pelvic ring is more circular to allow a baby to pass through.

Since the pelvic ring is wider in women, the cotyloid cavities (where the heads of the femurs are housed) are farther apart. This increases the distance between the greater trochanters, and the width between the hips is greater. Therefore, in women, the greater width of the hips has a direct influence on the position of the femurs, which are often tilted more inward than in men to follow the central axis of gravity, giving the legs a slightly *X*-shaped appearance.

A wide pelvis and a significant tilting of the femurs can be the cause of a pathological genu valgum, further accentuated by hyperlaxity related to the female reproductive function. The legs then take on a typically knock-kneed appearance. The knee joint is excessively stressed; the medial collateral ligament is too tight; and the lateral meniscus, the cartilage-covered articular surfaces of the lateral condyle of the femur, and the tuberosity of the tibia are subjected to excessive stresses that can lead to premature wear.

Sometimes a pathological genu valgum is accompanied by an internal collapse of the ankle and the disappearance of the plantar arch (flat feet). This can cause pain due to the overstretching of certain muscles, ligaments, and fascia in the soles of the feet.

Thus, it is very important to consider individual morphologies and gender variations and to remember that women are more often subject to problems related to genu valgum, while men are more frequently bowlegged (genu varum), a morphology that only rarely causes complications in this specific area.

People with a very pronounced genu valgum must work cautiously, avoiding weights that are too heavy when bending the knees, such as in squats or leg presses. One should always control the movement during these exercises, taking care not to tighten the knees when bending the them to avoid accentuating any knee problems and collapsing the ankles due to genu valgum.

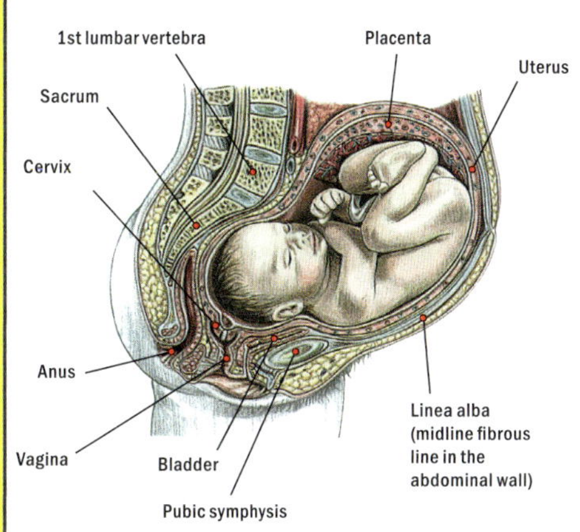

MEDIAL SECTION OF A PREGNANT WOMAN'S BELLY

The forward-tilting (anteverted) position of the woman's pelvis allows the weight of the baby to be partly transferred to the abdominal muscles. In this case, the abdominal muscles are like a hammock.

COMPARISON OF PELVIC TILT IN MEN AND WOMEN

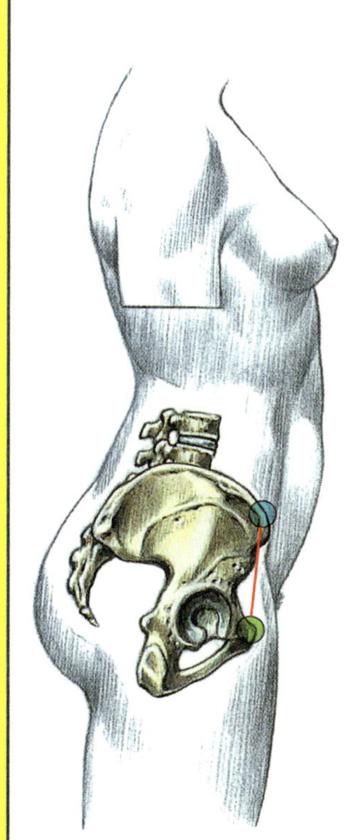

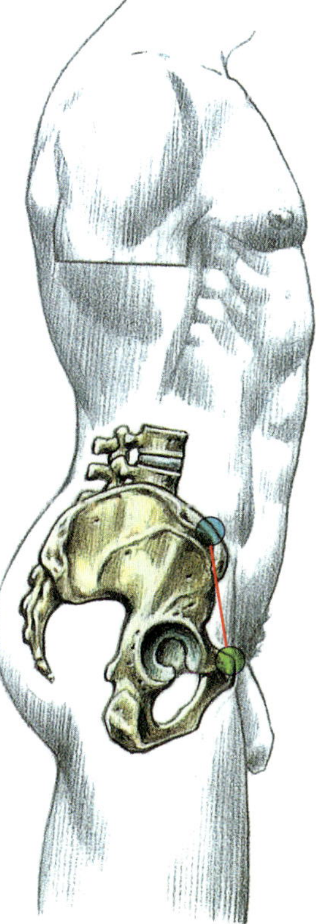

Compared to men, women generally have a slightly more forward-tilting pelvis. This anteversion results in the buttocks being farther out and the pubis being farther in between the thighs. This gives the impression that the lower abdomen is slightly bulging. This typically feminine small belly contrasts with the vertical abdominal wall that is more common in men, in whom the pelvis tends to be less tilted.

When a woman is pregnant, the position of her pelvis helps prevent the fetus from compressing the viscera excessively, due to the fact that part of the weight of the fetus is transferred to the abdominal muscles.

179

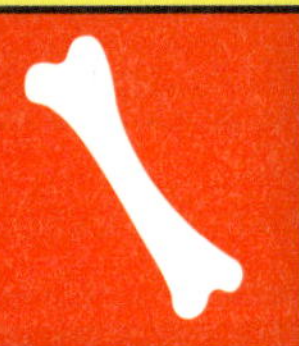

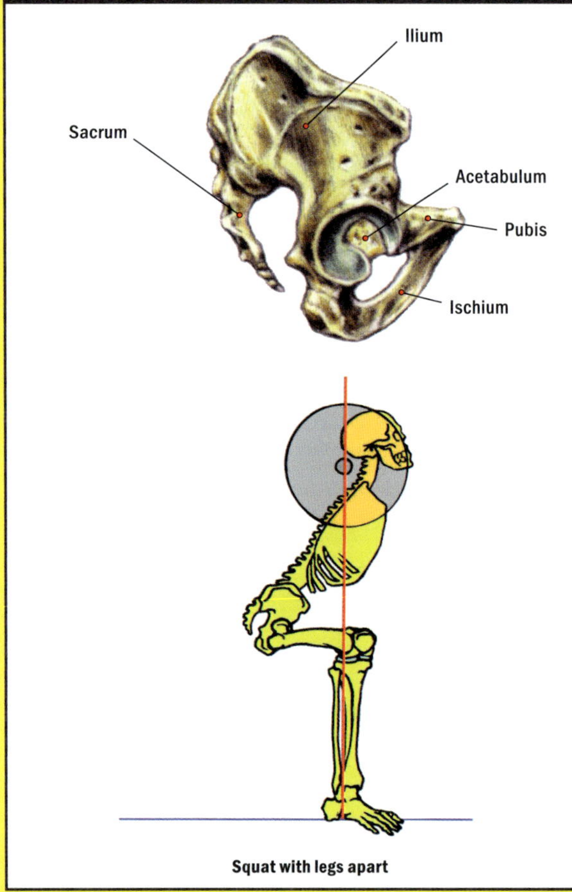

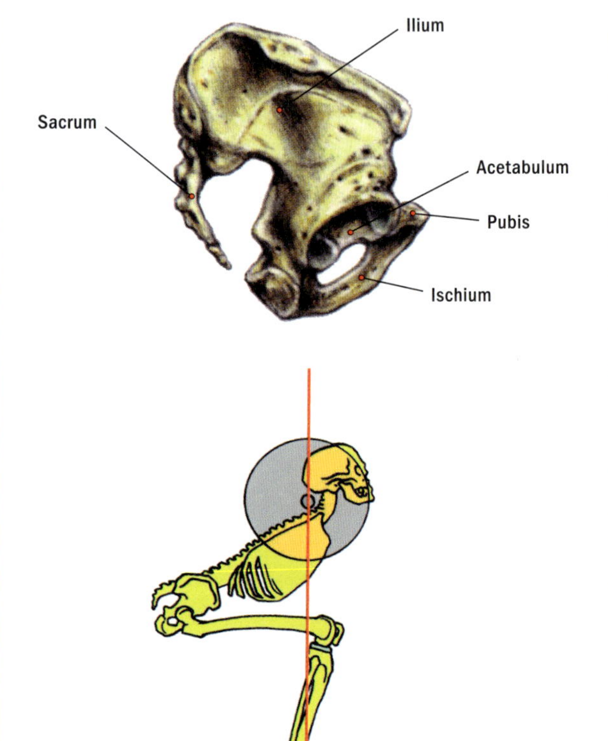

In the squat, for long-limbed individuals or people with less mobile ankles, it is advisable to turn the toes of the feet outward. This limits the tilting of the torso. If the weight is substantial, tilting of the torso can lead to a frontal imbalance and a rounding of the lumbar spine that increases the risk of a herniated disc.

But this technique, often used by powerlifters to optimize their lifting power in the squat, can only be done by people with suitable hip joint bone structure. In fact, only people with an outward-facing acetabulum and a relatively vertical neck of the femur will be able to spread their legs wide enough to do this type of squat.

Other people (those with a front-facing acetabulum and a relatively horizontal neck of the femur) will only be able to perform traditional squats with the thighs parallel or very slightly apart. It is not appropriate to ask someone with the wrong bone structure to do a squat with their legs apart. Forcing the hip to open with an unsuitable morphology creates a long-term risk of generating excessive friction that can lead to progressive deterioration of the hip, manifesting in arthritis that is particularly painful and incapacitating.

In addition to their greater flexibility, women often find it easier to place their feet farther apart than men, as their lower weight does not cause the neck of femur to sag during growth, which is often the case with men. Regardless of gender, however, with age and sometimes with bone calcification, the necks of the femurs tend to sag anyway, causing a loss of mobility when opening the thighs outward.

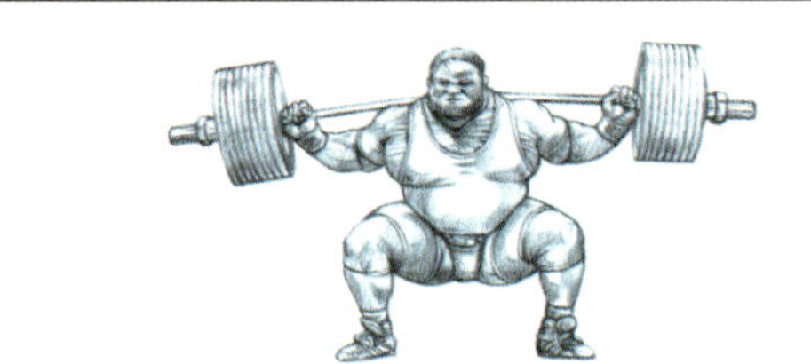

Opening up the thighs in the squat limits the tilt of the torso, but this technique can only be performed by individuals who have the appropriate hip bone structure.

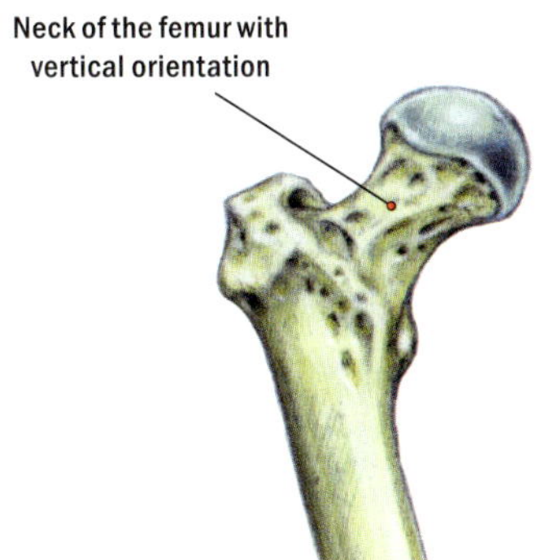

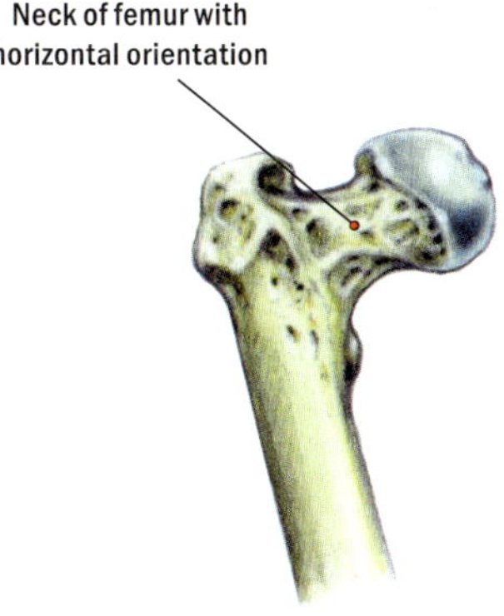

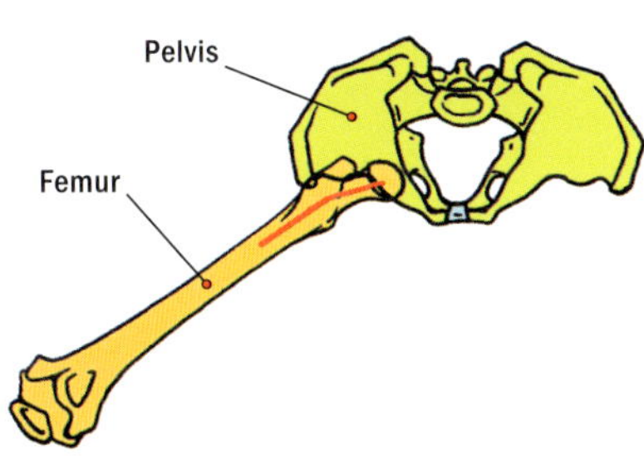

A vertical neck of the femur enables the
legs to be opened more widely.

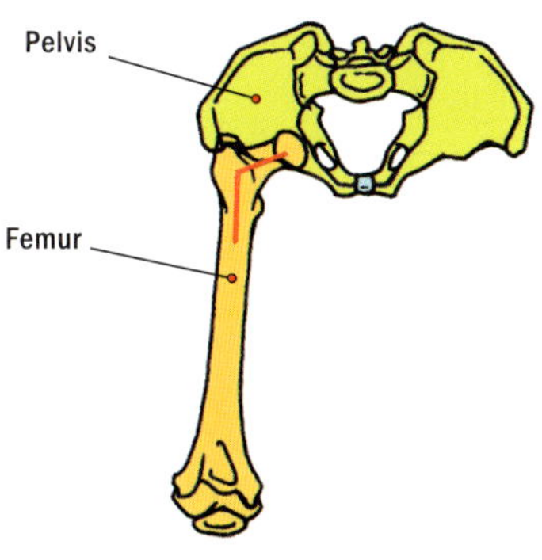

A horizontal neck of the femur prevents
the legs from being opened widely.

OSTEOARTHRITIS OF THE HIP

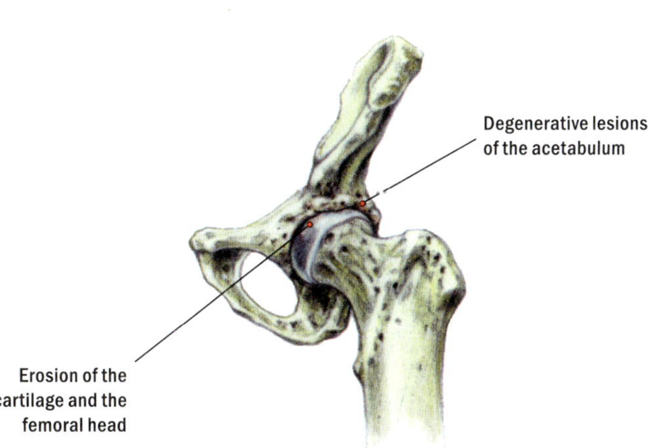

Excessive mobility in hip movements can lead to long-term cartilage and bone damage.

06 HACK SQUATS

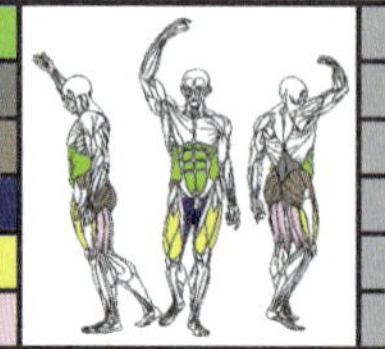

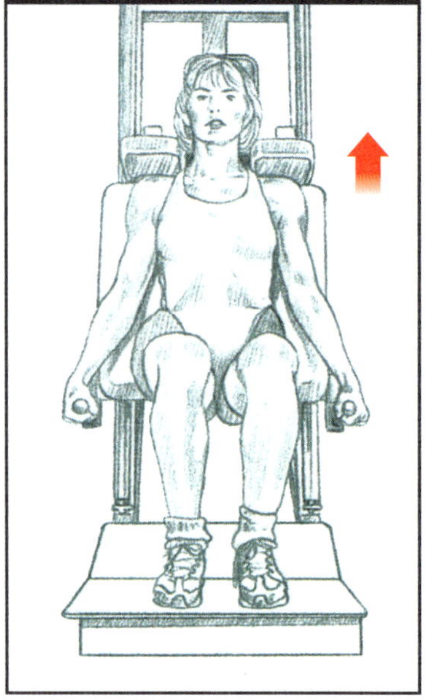

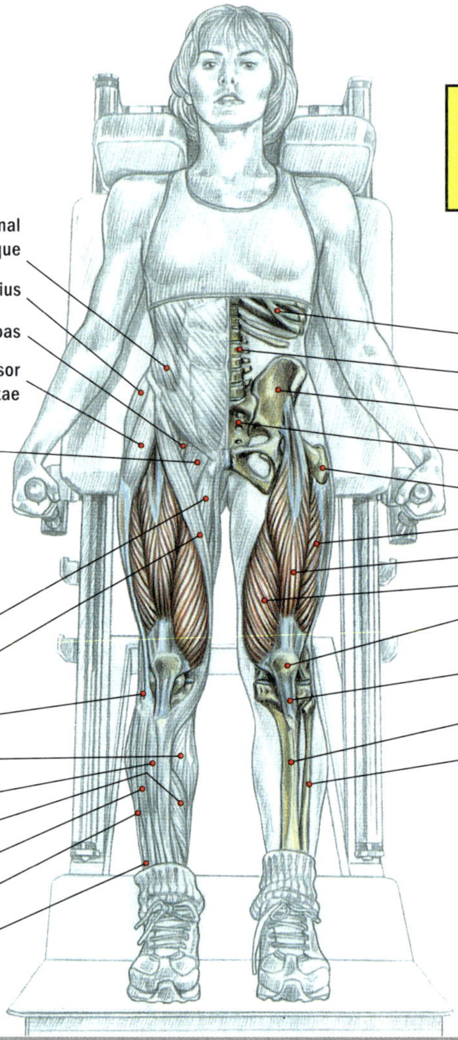

To protect the back, it is important to contract the core, which eliminates any lateral movement of the pelvis or spine.

External oblique

Gluteus medius

Iliopsoas

Tensor fasciae latae

Pectineus

Rib

Vertebra

Hip bone

Sacrum

Femur

Vastus lateralis

Rectus femoris | Quadriceps

Vastus medialis

Patella

Patellar ligament

Adductor longus

Sartorius

Biceps femoris

Gastrocnemius, medial head

Tibialis anterior

Soleus

Extensor digitorum longus

Peroneus longus

Peroneus brevis

Tibia

Fibula

Stand with your legs straight and feet slightly apart, your back against the back pad, and your shoulders positioned under the shoulder pads. *Hack* refers to a yoke—the pads are reminiscent of the collar placed around the neck of draft animals, thus the name of the exercise:

- Inhale, release the safety catch, and bend your knees.
- Return to the starting position and exhale at the end of the exercise.

This exercise focuses the effort on the quadriceps. Placing the feet farther forward works the gluteus muscles more, and placing the feet farther apart works the adductors more.

ADAPTING TO WALK ON TWO LEGS

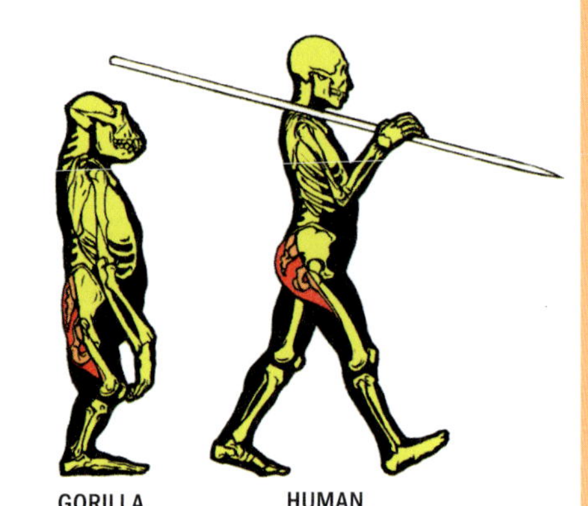

In the gorilla, one of our closest relatives, the well-developed torso, combined with an underdeveloped gluteus maximus, makes raising the trunk and standing erect difficult and causes an awkward bipedal gait. The human is the only primate who has completely adapted to walking upright on two legs. Besides the well-developed gluteus maximus muscle, the entire human structure has adapted to walk on two legs. The torso is relatively small, which makes it easier to stay upright, and, unlike the gorilla or chimpanzee, humans can lock the knee joint when it is extended, which makes standing much less tiring.

INCLINE LEG PRESSES 07

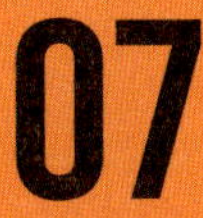

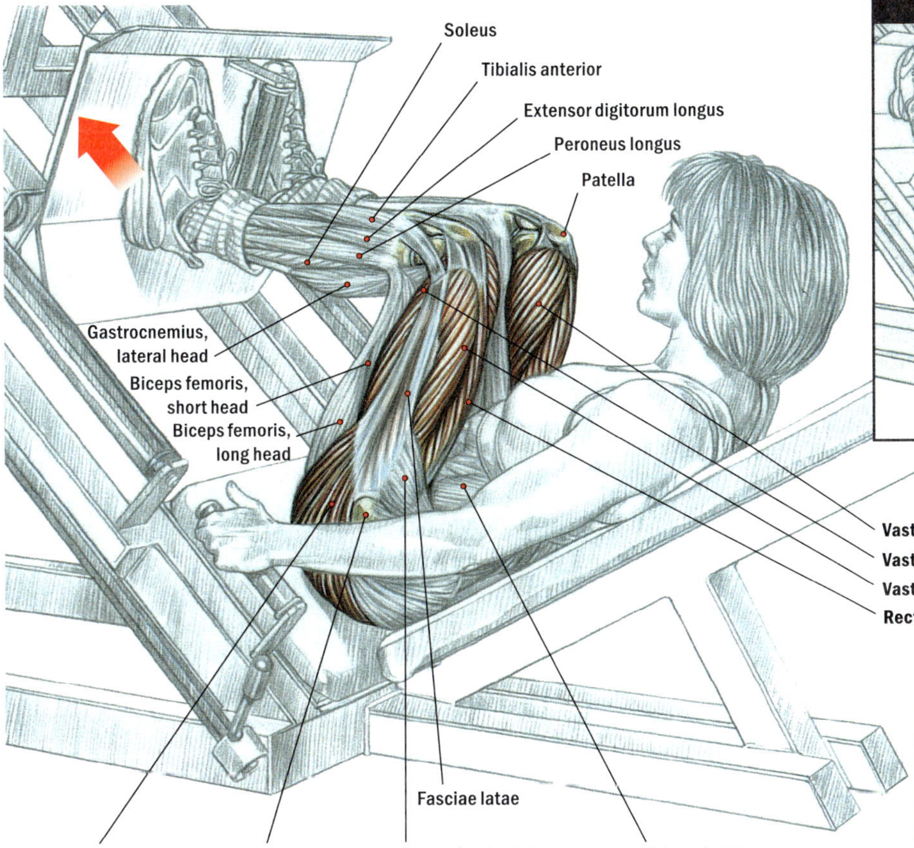

Soleus
Tibialis anterior
Extensor digitorum longus
Peroneus longus
Patella
Gastrocnemius, lateral head
Biceps femoris, short head
Biceps femoris, long head
Vastus medialis
Vastus intermedius
Vastus lateralis
Rectus femoris
Quadriceps
Gluteus maximus
Greater trochanter
Fasciae latae
Tensor fasciae latae
External oblique

STARTING POSITION

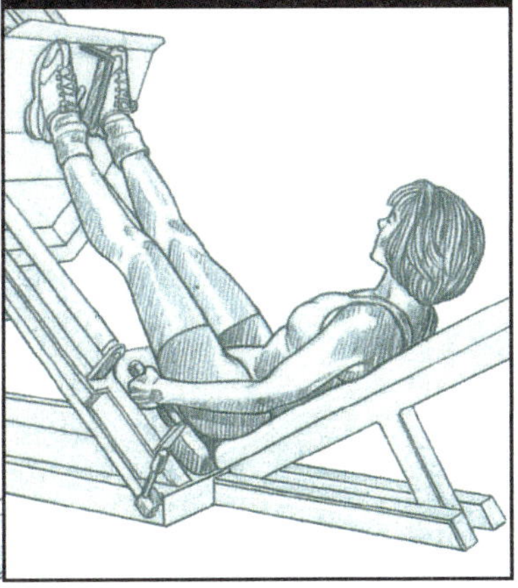

Using the press with heavy weights can cause sacroiliac joint dysfunction in some people. This can induce very painful muscle spasms.

Position your back firmly against the backrest on the machine, with your feet slightly apart:

- Inhale, release the safety, and then bend your knees completely to bring your thighs to your rib cage.
- Return to the starting position and exhale at the end of the exercise.

Placing the feet low against the foot plate focuses the work on the quadriceps, but placing the feet higher on the foot plate works the gluteus muscles and the hamstrings more. Placing the feet farther apart focuses the work on the adductors.

People with back pain who cannot do squats can do this exercise; however, they must never lift the buttocks off the seat.

DIFFERENT FOOT POSITIONS

Feet high on the foot plate

Works the **gluteus muscles and hamstrings**

Feet low on the foot plate

Works the **quadriceps**

Feet apart

Works the **adductors**

Feet close together

Works the **quadriceps**

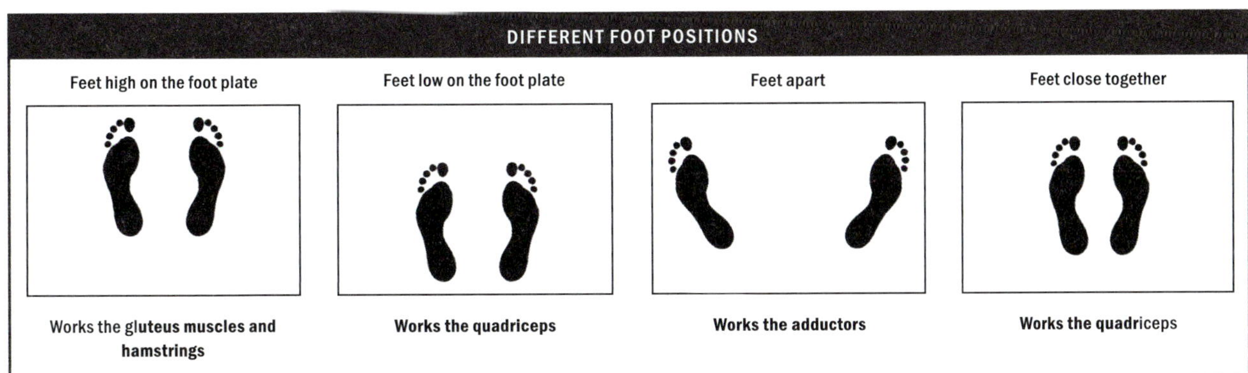

THE MAIN CAUSE OF HERNIATED DISCS IN STRENGTH TRAINING

THE INFLUENCE OF HIP MOBILITY ON THE RISK OF HERNIATED DISCS WHEN SQUATTING

1 The hip joint is not very mobile in terms of frontal movement, and this limits the tilt of the pelvis. When you are squatting, if your torso leans too far forward, your body compensates by rounding your lower back, which could lead to vertebral pathologies such as a very painful, incapacitating herniated disc (see pages 176-177).

2 The hip joint is very mobile in terms of frontal movement. If your torso leans too far forward when you are squatting, it allows an anterior tilt of your pelvis, and this protects your lumbar region and preserves the integrity of your intervertebral discs.

The root cause of herniated discs is the premature degeneration of an intervertebral disc. However, using poor form in any exercise can result in rounding the back, which puts pressure on the front of the disc, forces the back of the disc to protrude, and then compresses the nerves. This means that the aggravating factor in strength training is, first and foremost, a morphological issue.

In fact, if the bone structure of the hip joint does not allow for a great deal of flexion of the thigh toward the torso, the risks of herniated discs during squats or incline leg presses are much greater, and perhaps almost inevitable in the long term if the anterior hip flexion limitation is not diagnosed. If the flexion of the thigh toward the torso is limited by the bone morphology of the hip joint, then the descent in squats will be restricted by the lack of hip mobility without the individual feeling it. This forces those doing the exercises to round the lower back dangerously at the end of the flexion to maintain the bar in the axis of gravity and avoid tipping forward. Worse still, if the person is unbalanced and tips forward at the end of thigh flexion during a squat, the pelvis will not tilt onto the necks of the femurs during the fall but will be blocked at hip level. This will entail a catastrophic rounding of the lumbar spine that will almost certainly cause an injury to the intervertebral discs.

Similarly, if the hip joint is limited in frontal movement, an overly fast descent of the foot plate during incline leg presses will inevitably involve, by compensation, a rounding of the lower back, which can cause deterioration of the intervertebral discs in the lumbar region.

To avoid herniated discs, it is very important to consider your hip bone morphology by verifying that your thighs have good frontal mobility. If

BONE ANATOMY

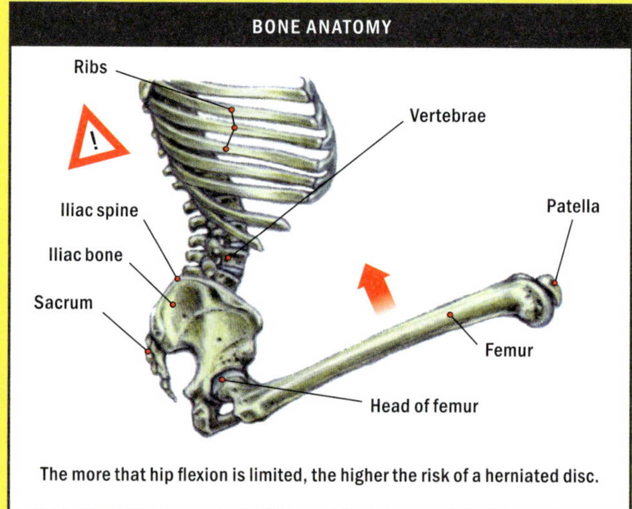

The more that hip flexion is limited, the higher the risk of a herniated disc.

your bone morphology limits the anterior flexion of your thighs, then you must be careful not to lower too far when squatting. You can do half-squats instead of full squats, and, in the event of a frontal imbalance, you should drop the bar and let it slide backward so that you are not dragged forward and forced to round your lower back dangerously.

THE INFLUENCE OF HIP MOBILITY ON THE RISK OF HERNIATED DISCS IN INCLINE LEG PRESSES

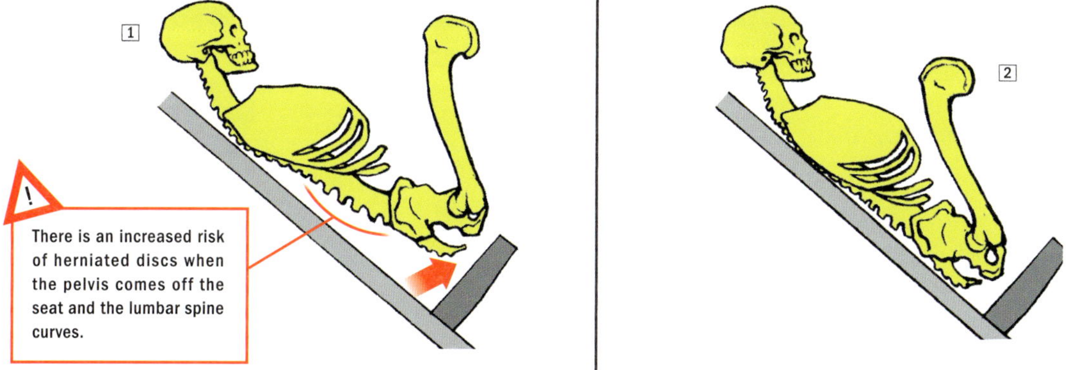

1 Hip joint with limited frontal flexion mobility and limited flexion of the femur toward the torso.

2 Hip joint with good frontal flexion mobility and substantial flexion of the femur toward the torso.

Finally, to avoid excessive rounding of the lumbar spine in the incline leg press, you must learn how to limit the descent of the foot plate before the hip joint locks and causes the lower back to round. Ensure that the backrest of the press is in an optimal position so as to avoid excessive bending of the hip.

BACKREST POSITIONING ON THE INCLINE LEG PRESS AND HIP BONE MORPHOLOGY

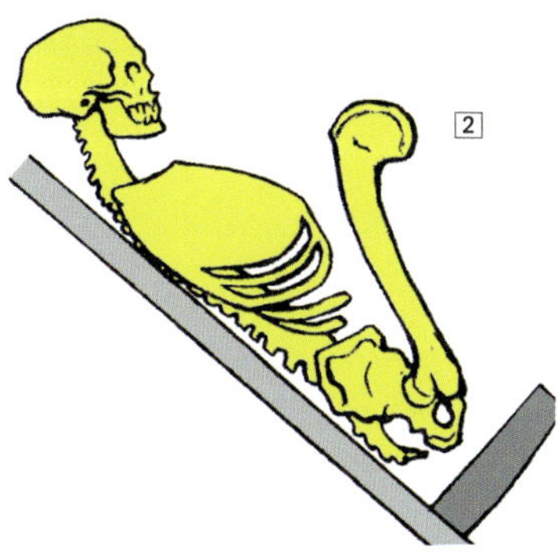

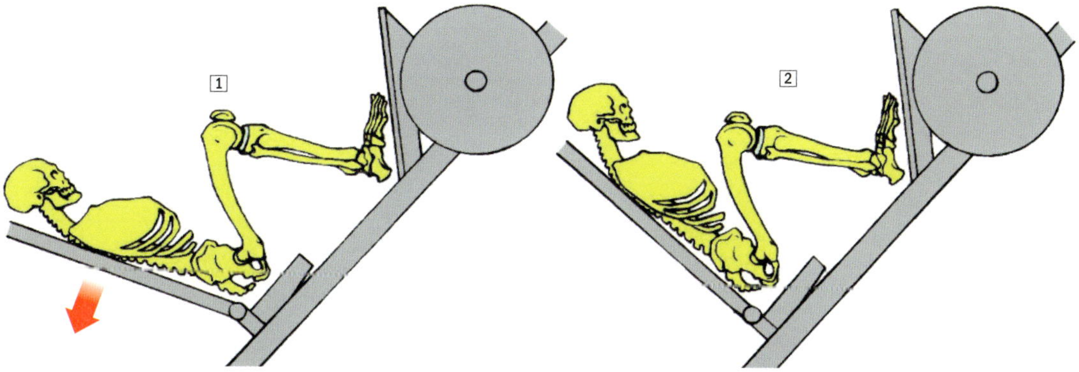

1 For individuals with a hip bone structure that limits flexion, it is best to lower the backrest of the leg press to avoid excessive rounding of the lumbar spine and to decrease the risk of a herniated disc.

2 The angle of the backrest on the incline press must be considered to avoid injury to the lumbar spine. In fact, only people with the appropriate hip bone structure that facilitates thigh flexion can do this exercise with the backrest raised without the risk of rounding the lumbar spine and potentially causing herniated discs.

1 Starting position.

2 Sit on the bench. Keep the thighs relaxed, arch your back slightly, and lean forward.

The box squat is primarily used by powerlifters to get stronger at squats. This technique involves performing a squat by sitting on a bench for 1 or 2 seconds before standing. In a traditional squat, tension accumulates in the muscles during the negative (lowering) phase, much like a rubber band being stretched, and is released during the positive (standing up) phase. Sitting on a bench during the box squat relaxes the muscles of the thighs so that they cannot use accumulated energy from the descent during the positive phase of standing up.

For this reason, given the same amount of weight, the effort put in by the quadriceps is more intense in the box squat than in the traditional squat. It is therefore a very good exercise for focusing the work on the thighs.

This exercise can be included in a program for long-legged athletes who have difficulty feeling the quadriceps working during a squat. Moreover, initiating a squat from a sitting position helps develop the automatic pushing reflex in the traditional squat, making the positive standing phase quicker and more powerful.

Although the box squat is an excellent exercise, you must do it very carefully, always controlling the descent and sitting gently on the bench. If the lowering phase is too rapid and the buttocks slam down on the bench, the shock and the excessive pressure on the vertebral joints can cause serious injury.

There are special benches whose height can be adjusted to adapt to individual morphologies. Their cushioned seats minimize the shock of the lowering phase and limit the risk of vertebral injury by compression. To do this exercise properly, always keep your back slightly leaning forward. If your back is too straight when you stand up from the bench, it will be impossible to do the exercise.

LEG EXTENSIONS 09

PERFORMING THE EXERCISE

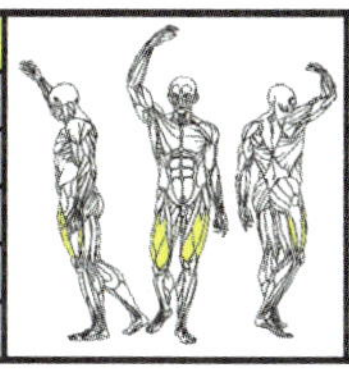

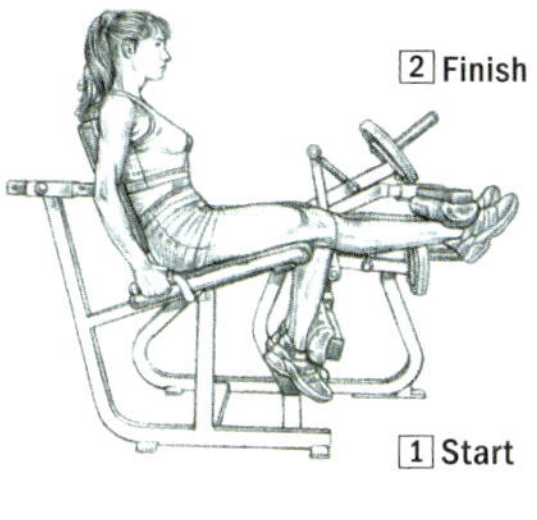

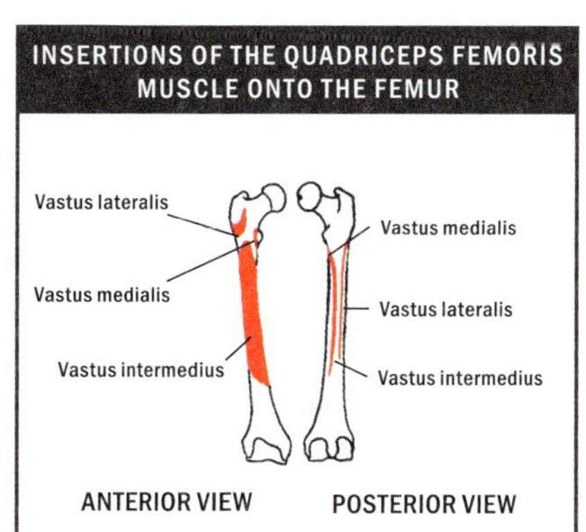

Sit at the machine and grasp the handles or the seat to hold your torso still. Bend your knees and place your ankles under the ankle pads.

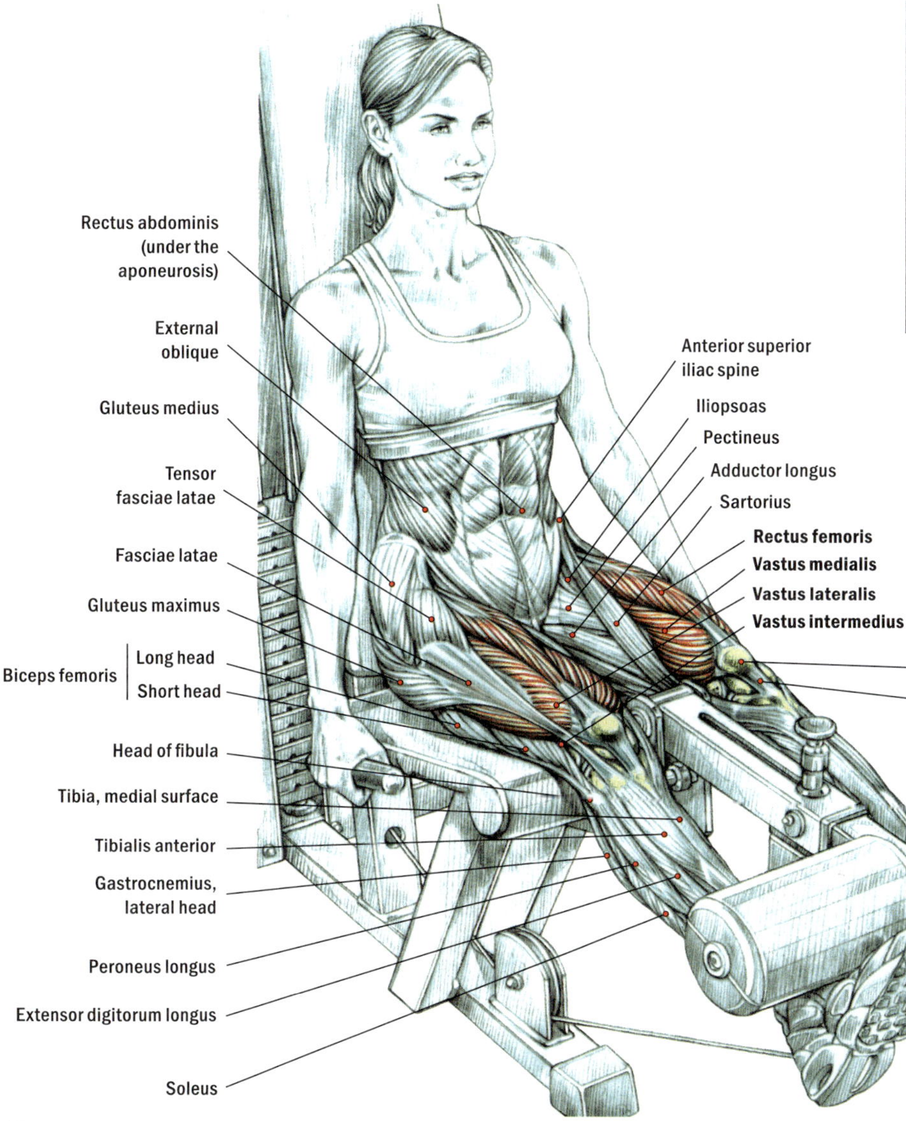

- Inhale and raise your legs to a horizontal position.
- Exhale at the end of the exercise.

This is the best exercise for isolating the quadriceps. The greater the angle of the backrest, the farther backward the pelvis will tilt, and that will stretch the rectus femoris (the midline biarticular portion of the quadriceps), which will work harder to straighten the legs. This exercise is recommended for beginners so that they can develop enough strength to move on to more technically demanding exercises.

INSERTIONS OF THE QUADRICEPS FEMORIS MUSCLE ONTO THE FEMUR

QUADRICEPS FEMORIS MUSCLE

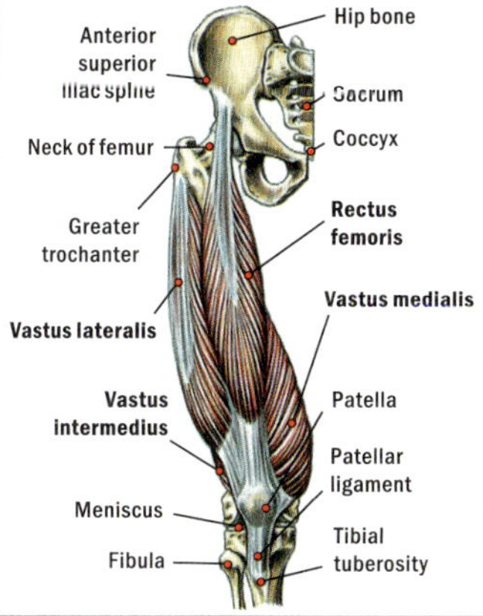

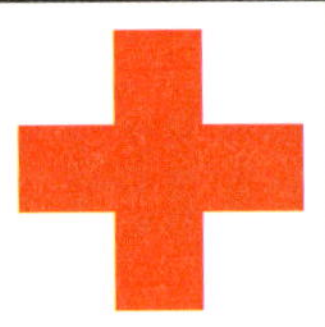

LIGAMENT HYPERLAXITY

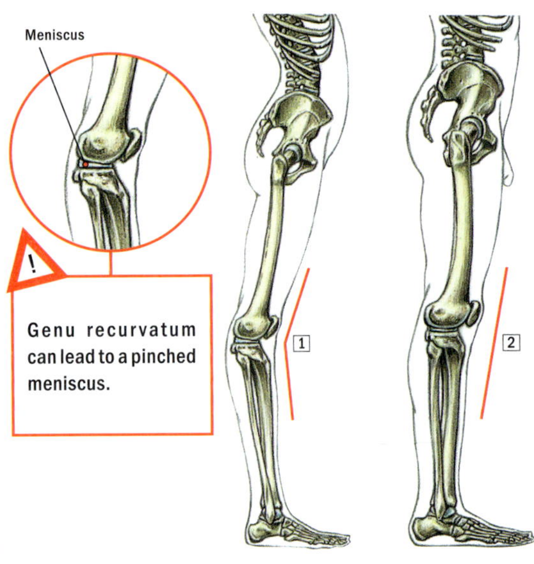

In women, ligament hyperlaxity can allow small movements of the less mobile joints of the pelvis (sacroiliac and pubic), which help the baby to pass through during childbirth. This hyperlaxity can lead to some morphological peculiarities such as genu recurvatum (locking of the knee joint in extension, which makes it look like the leg is bent slightly backward).

Though it rarely causes problems, genu recurvatum can nevertheless cause complications such as a pinched meniscus in some individuals. This can happen when the knees are extended very quickly and the meniscus has not had time to slide, or during leg exercises with heavy weights. For these reasons, it is common in group exercise classes for instructors to recommend doing the exercises without ever fully extending the knees and, in exercises with additional weight such as leg presses or squats, to recommend that participants never lock the knees in extension.

It is important to remember that this cautionary advice only applies to people with pathological genu recurvatum, as most individuals can lock their knees in extension without risk since the joints stack upon each other like a column.

1 Typical female leg with genu recurvatum
2 Typical male leg with the joints stacked in a column

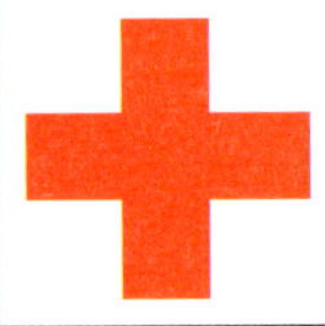

DISLOCATED KNEECAP

The quadriceps muscle pulls the kneecap (patella) in the direction of the femur (diagonally outward). The patella tends to move laterally outward, but the more prominent lateral condyle of the femur prevents it from popping out, and the lower vastus medialis (quadriceps) pulls it back inward.

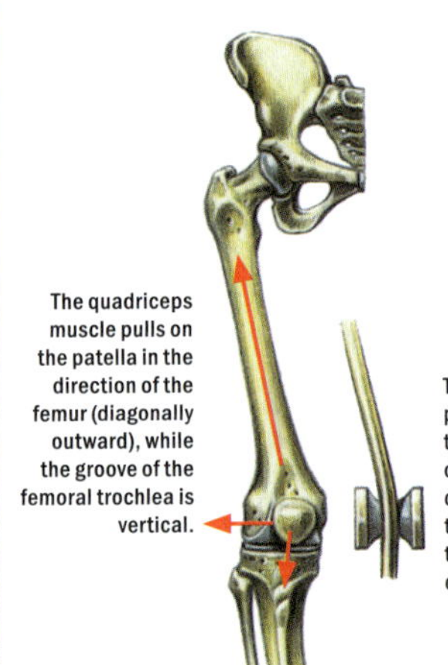

In women, the more oblique nature of the femurs, coupled with a smaller protrusion of the lateral condyles, greater ligament laxity, and an occasional lack of tone in the lower part of the vastus lateralis and vastus medialis of the quadriceps contribute to a greater frequency of lateral external kneecap dislocations. To prevent this kind of dislocation, leg extensions (see page 187) are excellent, because these strengthen the lower part of the quadriceps—especially the vastus medialis.

Ligament laxity in women varies during the menstrual cycle, reaching its peak during ovulation. This is when the risk of knee injury is greatest.

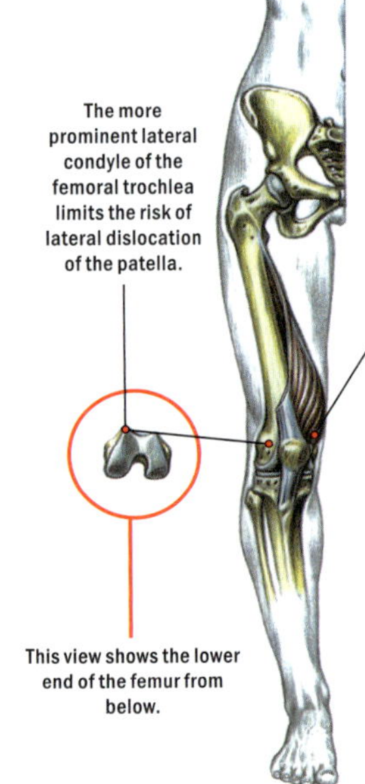

STRETCHING THE QUADRICEPS

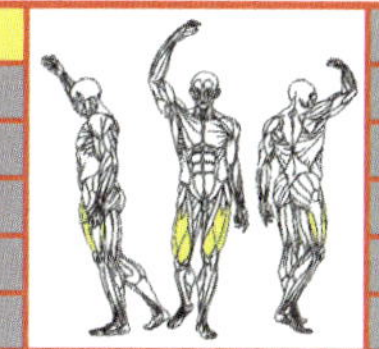

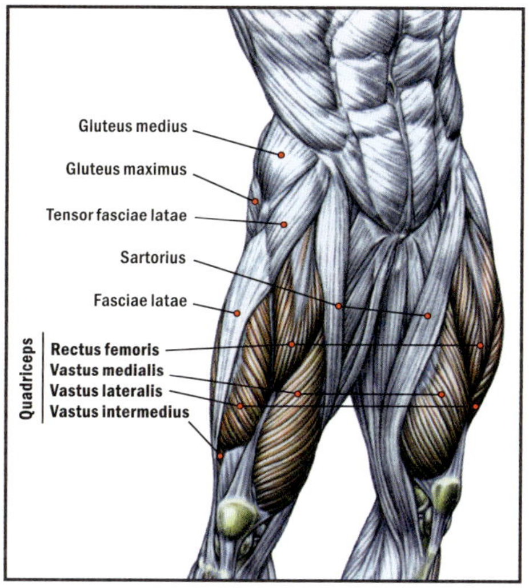

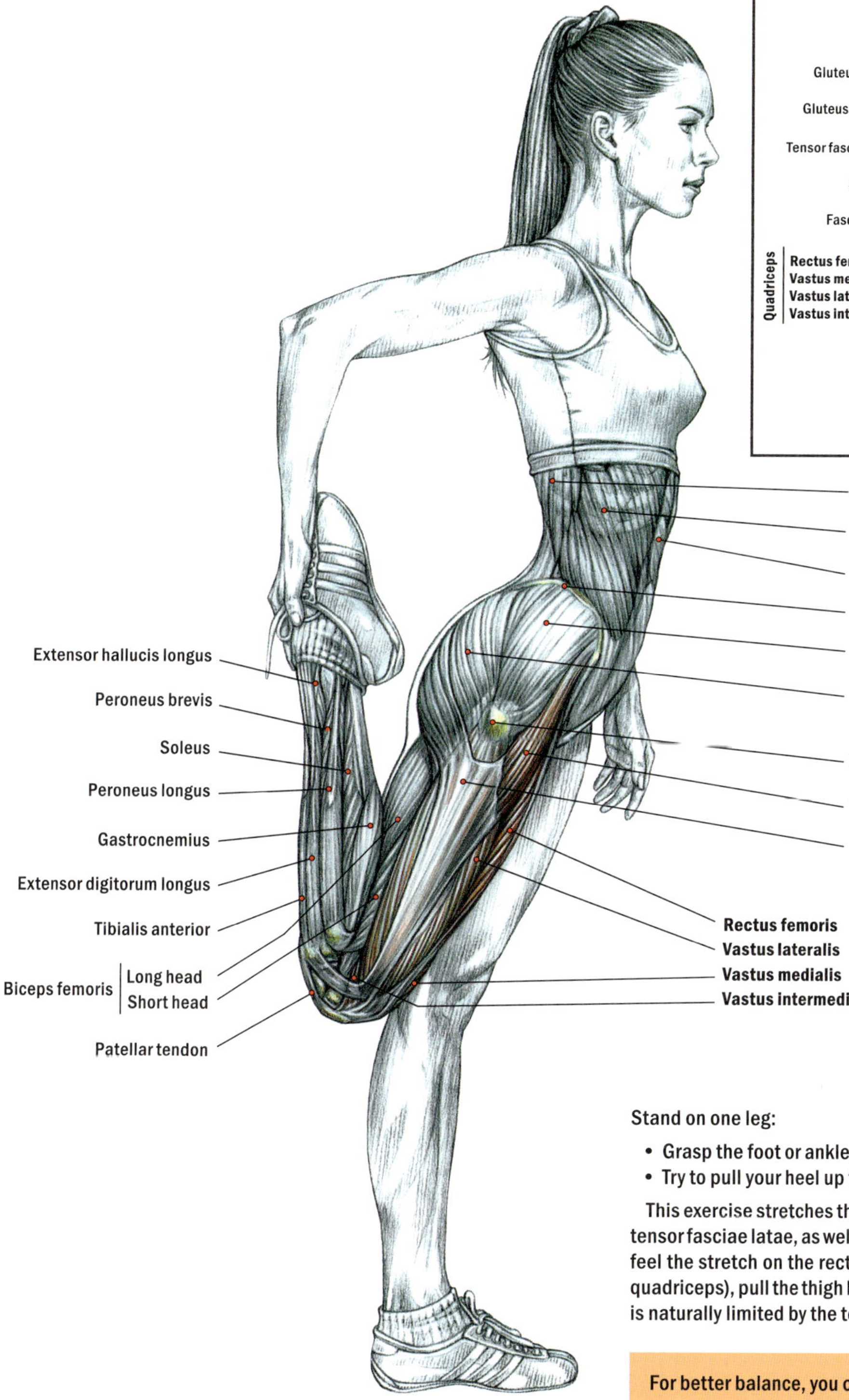

Stand on one leg:

- Grasp the foot or ankle of the other leg.
- Try to pull your heel up to your buttocks.

This exercise stretches the quadriceps and, to a lesser degree, the tensor fasciae latae, as well as the deeper iliopsoas muscle. To really feel the stretch on the rectus femoris (the biarticular portion of the quadriceps), pull the thigh backward as far as possible. Its extension is naturally limited by the tension of the iliofemoral ligament.

For better balance, you can use your other arm to support yourself against a wall or a stable object.

LYING LEG CURLS

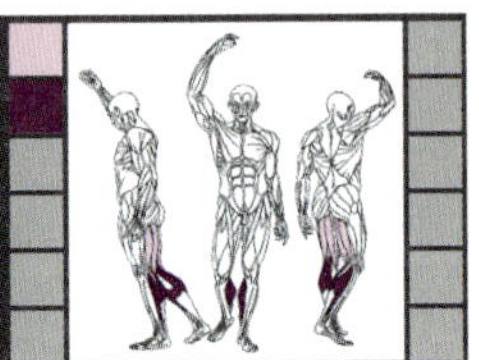

PERFORMING THE EXERCISE

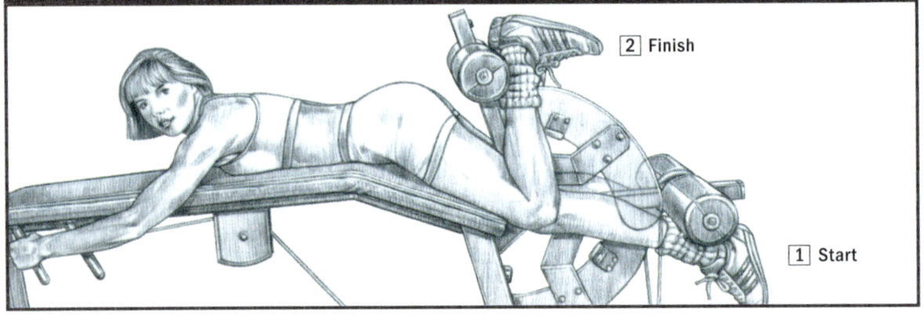

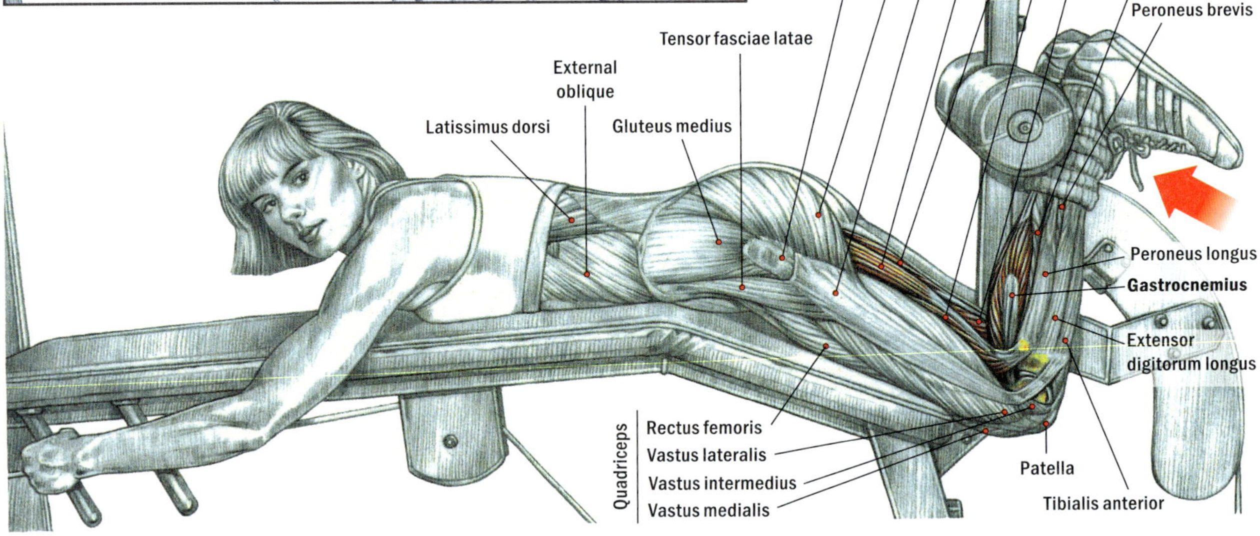

Lie facedown on the machine. Grasp the handles, extend both legs, and position your ankles under the ankle pads:

- Inhale and bend both legs at the same time, trying to touch your heels to your buttocks. Exhale at the end of the exercise.
- Return to the starting position while controlling your movement carefully.

This exercise works the hamstrings and gastrocnemius, as well as the deeper popliteus muscle. In theory, during flexion, it is possible to target the semitendinosus and semimembranosus by internally rotating the feet or to target the long and short heads of the biceps femoris by externally rotating the feet. But in practice, this can be difficult, and only the following variations can be easily done:

- Point your toes (plantar flexion) to work the hamstrings.
- Flex your feet (dorsiflexion) to work the gastrocnemius.

Variations

- This exercise may be done by alternating legs.
- Without a machine, the exercise can be done with a dumbbell.

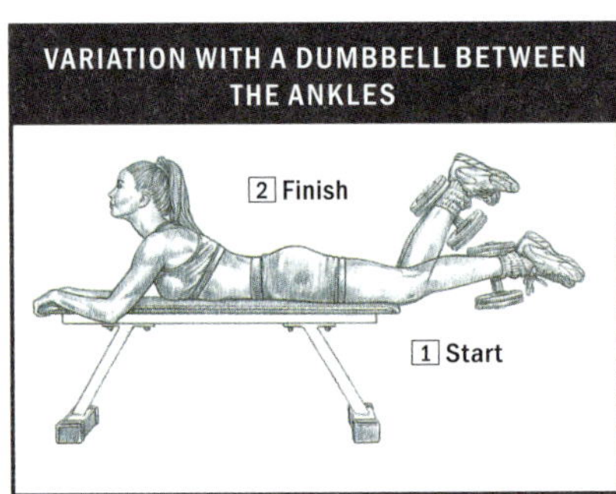

VARIATION WITH A DUMBBELL BETWEEN THE ANKLES

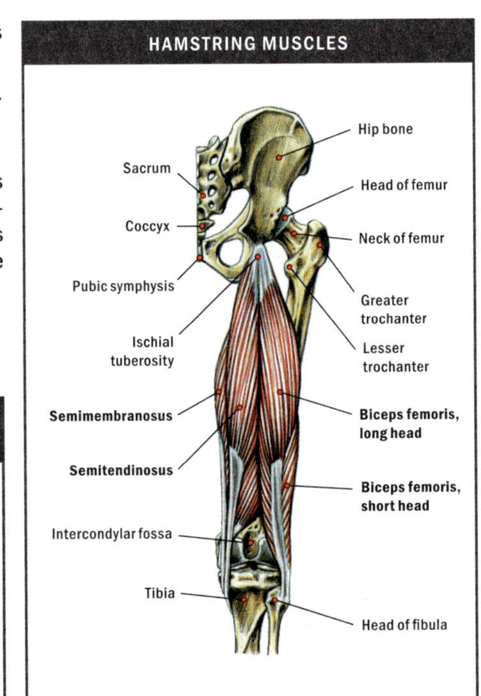

HAMSTRING MUSCLES

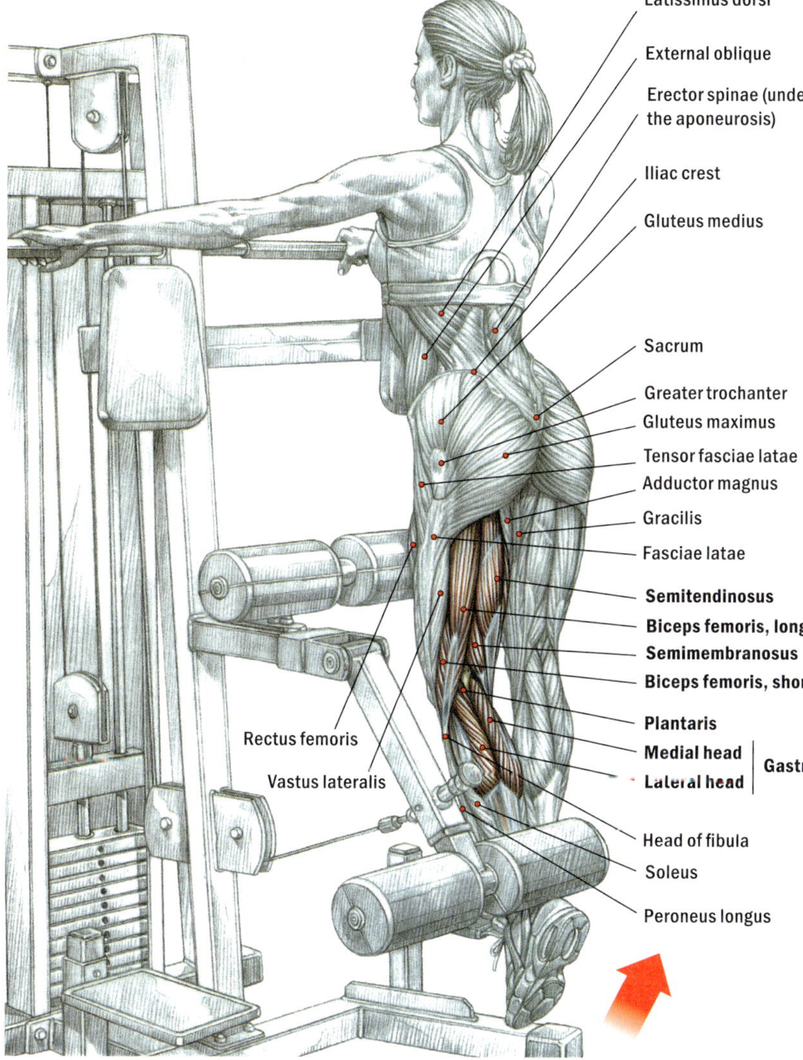

PERFORMING THE EXERCISE

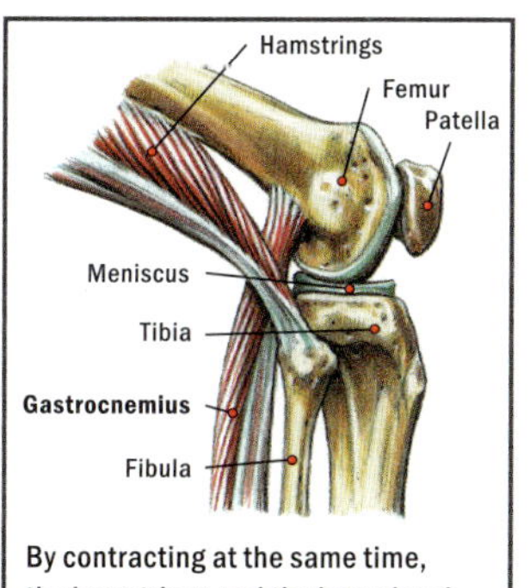

By contracting at the same time, the hamstrings and the lateral and medial heads of the gastrocnemius flex the knee joint.

Stand with your torso resting against the pad, with your knee straight and your ankle under the ankle roll:

- Inhale and bend your knee.
- Exhale at the end of the exercise.

This exercise uses the hamstrings (semitendinosus, semi-membranosus, and the long and short heads of the biceps femoris) and, to a lesser extent, the gastrocnemius. To work the gastrocnemius more intensely, simply bend your ankle when bending your knee. To decrease its participation, which is often the goal, simply point your toes.

SHORT HEAD OF THE BICEPS FEMORIS

Of all the flexor muscles, only the short head of the biceps femoris works across just one joint. Its function is to bend the knee.

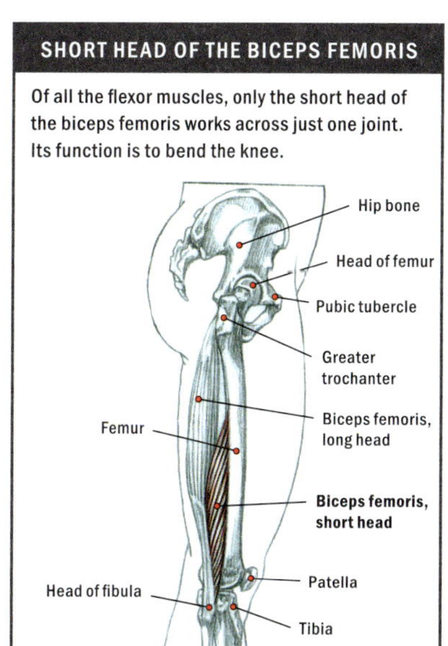

12 SEATED LEG CURLS

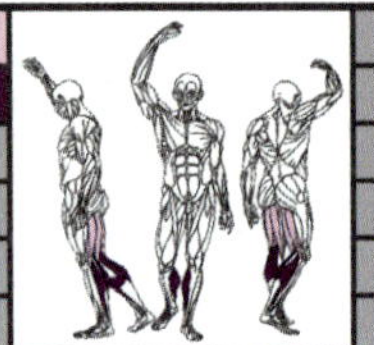

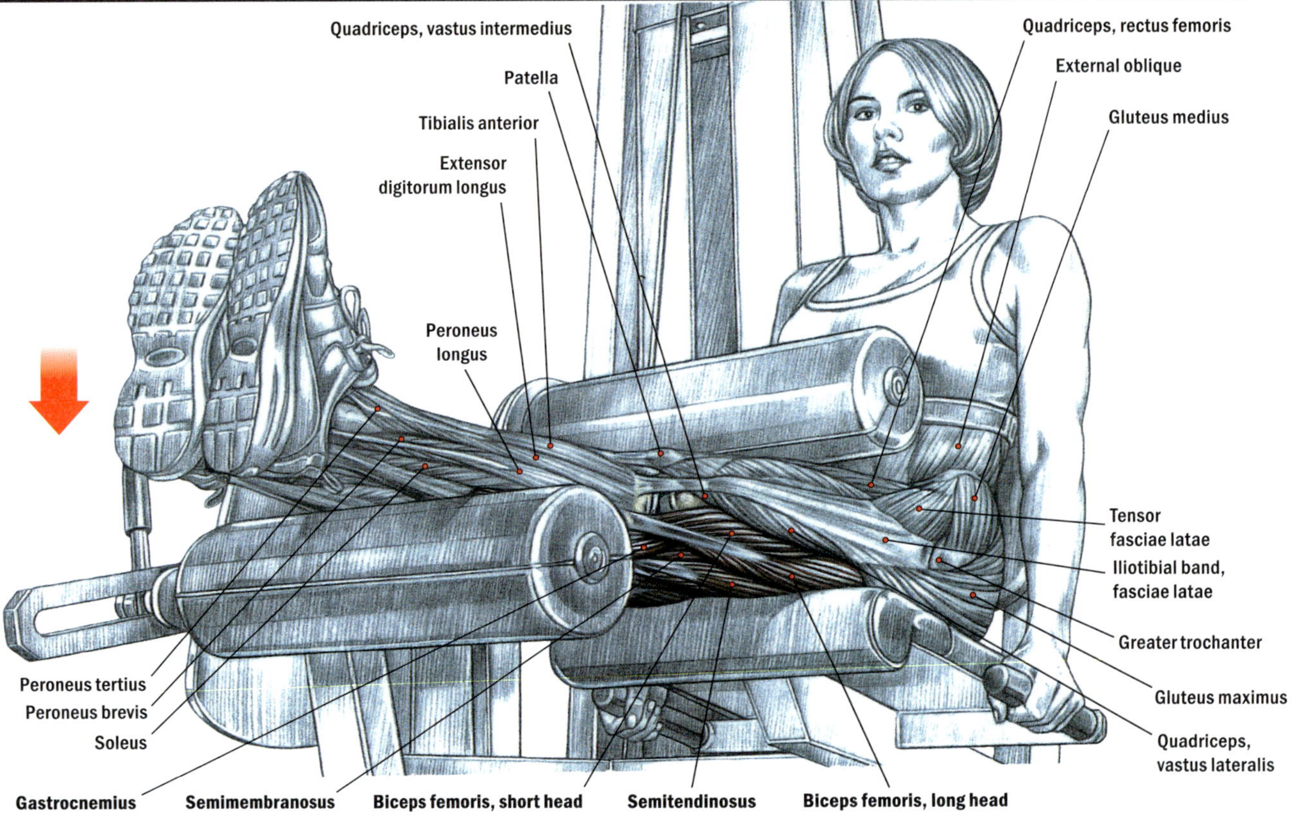

Quadriceps, vastus intermedius
Patella
Tibialis anterior
Extensor digitorum longus
Peroneus longus
Quadriceps, rectus femoris
External oblique
Gluteus medius
Tensor fasciae latae
Iliotibial band, fasciae latae
Greater trochanter
Gluteus maximus
Quadriceps, vastus lateralis
Peroneus tertius
Peroneus brevis
Soleus
Gastrocnemius
Semimembranosus
Biceps femoris, short head
Semitendinosus
Biceps femoris, long head

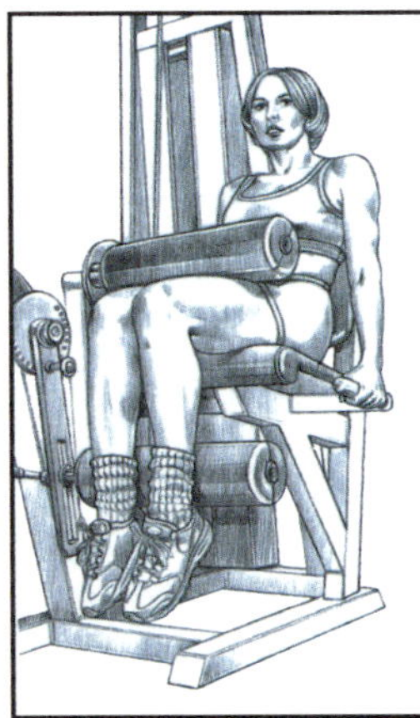

END OF THE EXERCISE

Sit at the machine with your legs extended, ankles resting on the ankle pad, and thighs wedged in place. Grasp the handles:

- Inhale and bend your knees.
- Exhale at the end of the exercise.

This exercise works the hamstring muscles and the deeper popliteus. To a lesser extent, it also works the gastrocnemius.

Variations

- Do this exercise with your feet flexed to increase the work of your gastrocnemius muscles.
- Do this exercise with your feet pointed to focus the effort on your hamstrings.

A seated position with the pelvis in a forward tilt stretches the semimembranosus, the semitendinosus, and the long head of the biceps femoris, allowing you to really focus the work on these muscles.

POPLITEUS MUSCLE

Femur
Condyles
Popliteus
Fibula
Tibia

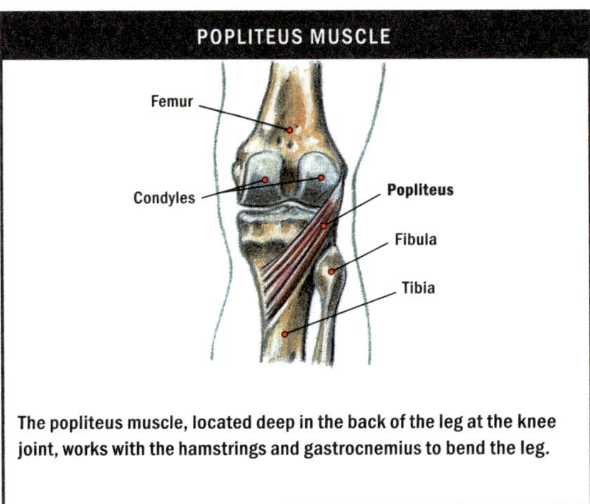

The popliteus muscle, located deep in the back of the leg at the knee joint, works with the hamstrings and gastrocnemius to bend the leg.

MUSCLES USED

Biceps femoris, long head
Semitendinosus
Semimembranosus
Biceps femoris, short head
Gastrocnemius, medial head
Gastrocnemius, lateral head

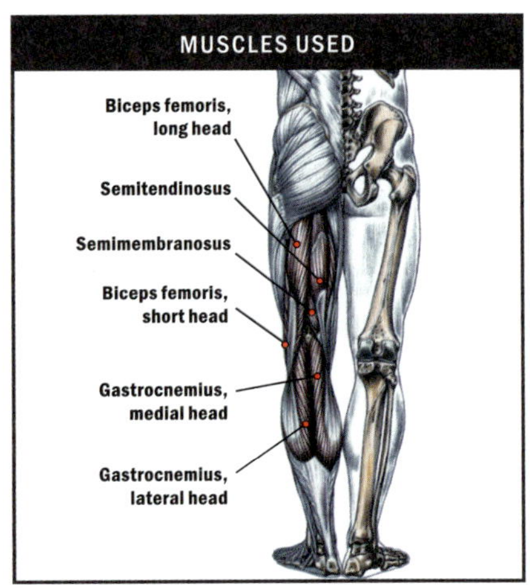

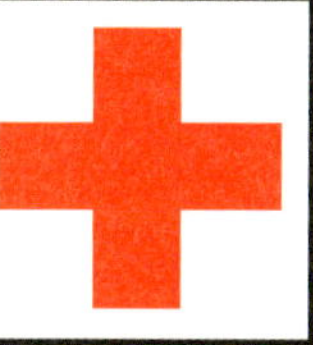

ACTION OF THE HAMSTRINGS DURING A SQUAT

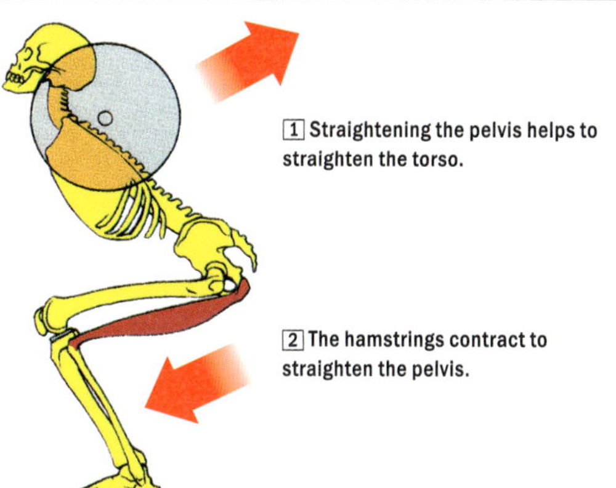

During the squat, the hamstrings contract to straighten the pelvis and to prevent the torso from tilting too far forward, as long as the pelvis aligns with the torso via a contraction of the abdominal and lumbar muscles.

HAMSTRING MUSCLES

HAMSTRING TEARS

In strength training, hamstring tears occur frequently. This injury occurs most often during the squat when the torso is too far forward. The hamstrings—with the exception of the short head of the biceps femoris, which is in an extremely stretched position—contract forcefully to straighten the pelvis. This can lead to tearing, most often at the high or middle portion of the muscle group.

Hamstring tears can also occur when using heavy weights on a leg curl machine. This most often happens at the beginning of the exercise when the legs are extended and the muscles are stretched.

In general, hamstring tears are not extensive and not serious (it is rare to see a significant tear in the muscle or its tendinous insertion), but they are always painful and prone to complications. In fact, fibrous scarring frequently occurs after a tear in this muscle group. This creates friction that is especially painful and incapacitating during athletic activity. Moreover, this scar tissue is not flexible and can also tear during intense effort.

PREVENTING HAMSTRING TEARS

To prevent muscle tears, it is important to do specific hamstring stretches as part of a stretching workout or to incorporate hamstring stretches between sets of squats, deadlifts, and exercises for the back of the thigh.

Certain exercises, such as good mornings, stiff-legged deadlifts, and Romanian deadlifts, are the best protection for the hamstrings because of their combined action of muscle strengthening and stretching.

AFTER A HAMSTRING TEAR

To prevent the formation of fibrous scar tissue in the hamstrings, it is essential to reeducate the muscles as soon as possible. A week after a tear, you must perform gentle stretches for the back of the thighs. The goal here is to stretch the injured muscles and, most importantly, to soften the scar so that it doesn't tear when you resume training.

A massage therapist can also treat fibrous scars by using massage or mechanical techniques to soften the lesion.

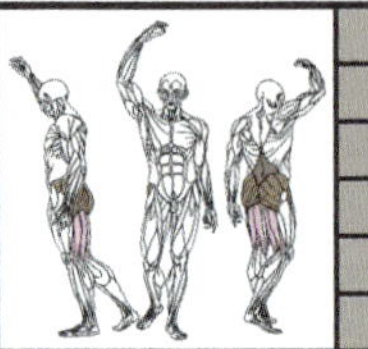

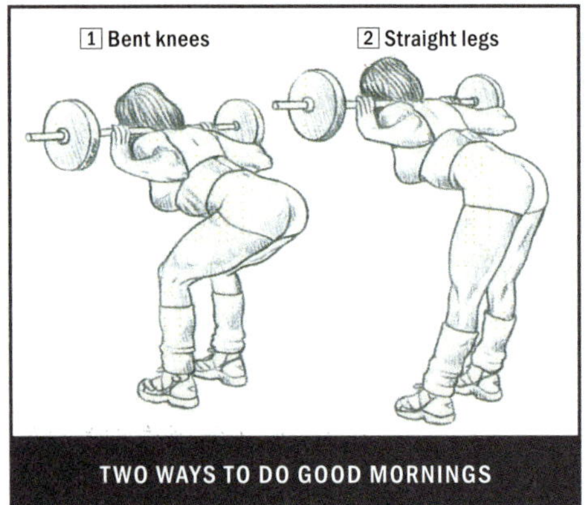

TWO WAYS TO DO GOOD MORNINGS

Stand with your feet slightly apart and the bar resting on your trapezius or a little lower on your posterior deltoids:

- Inhale and bend your torso forward, keeping your back very straight. The axis of rotation should pass through your hips.
- Return to the starting position and exhale.

To make the exercise easier, bend slightly at your knees.

This exercise, which works the gluteus maximus and the spinal muscles, is especially noteworthy for its work on the hamstrings (except the short head of the biceps femoris, which only flexes the knee).

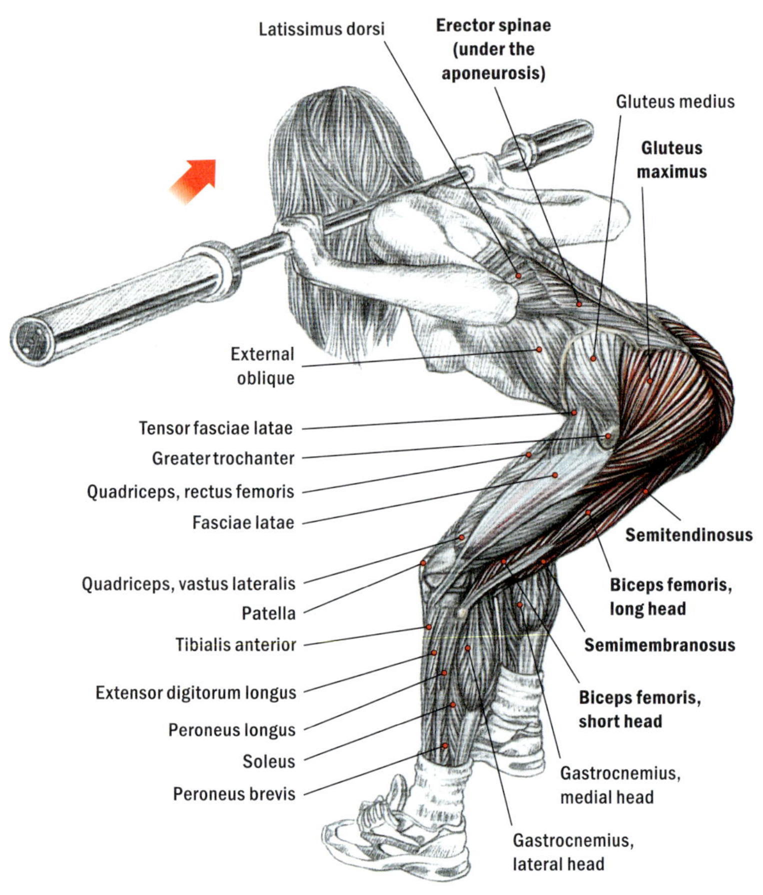

TIGHT HAMSTRINGS

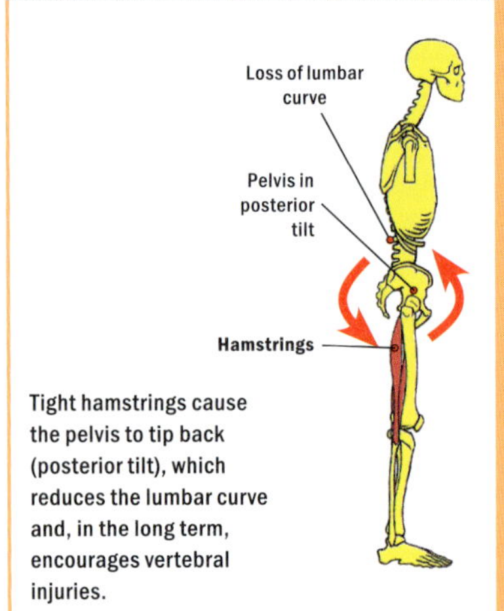

Tight hamstrings cause the pelvis to tip back (posterior tilt), which reduces the lumbar curve and, in the long term, encourages vertebral injuries.

In today's modern world, sitting for long periods during the day can lead to tight hamstrings. These tight muscles on the back of the thigh tip the pelvis back, causing poor spine position. The spine can lose its normal curvature. This causes the person to adopt poor posture with the pelvis tucked under and the back rounded, which can, over time, lead to vertebral injuries. To limit the relatively frequent occurrence of tight hamstrings, it is important to do exercises that stretch the thigh, such good mornings with light weight and straight legs, as well as the stiff-legged deadlift (see page 138). Additionally, hamstring stretches after a hamstring workout are also recommended (see page 196).

LEG POSITION

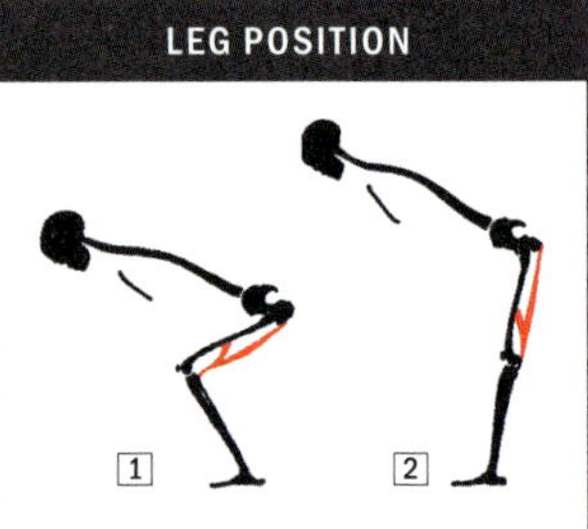

1 Bending your knees while tilting forward allows your hamstrings to relax, which facilitates hip flexion.

2 Straightening your legs while tilting forward lengthens your hamstrings, helping you to feel them working more as you straighten your torso.

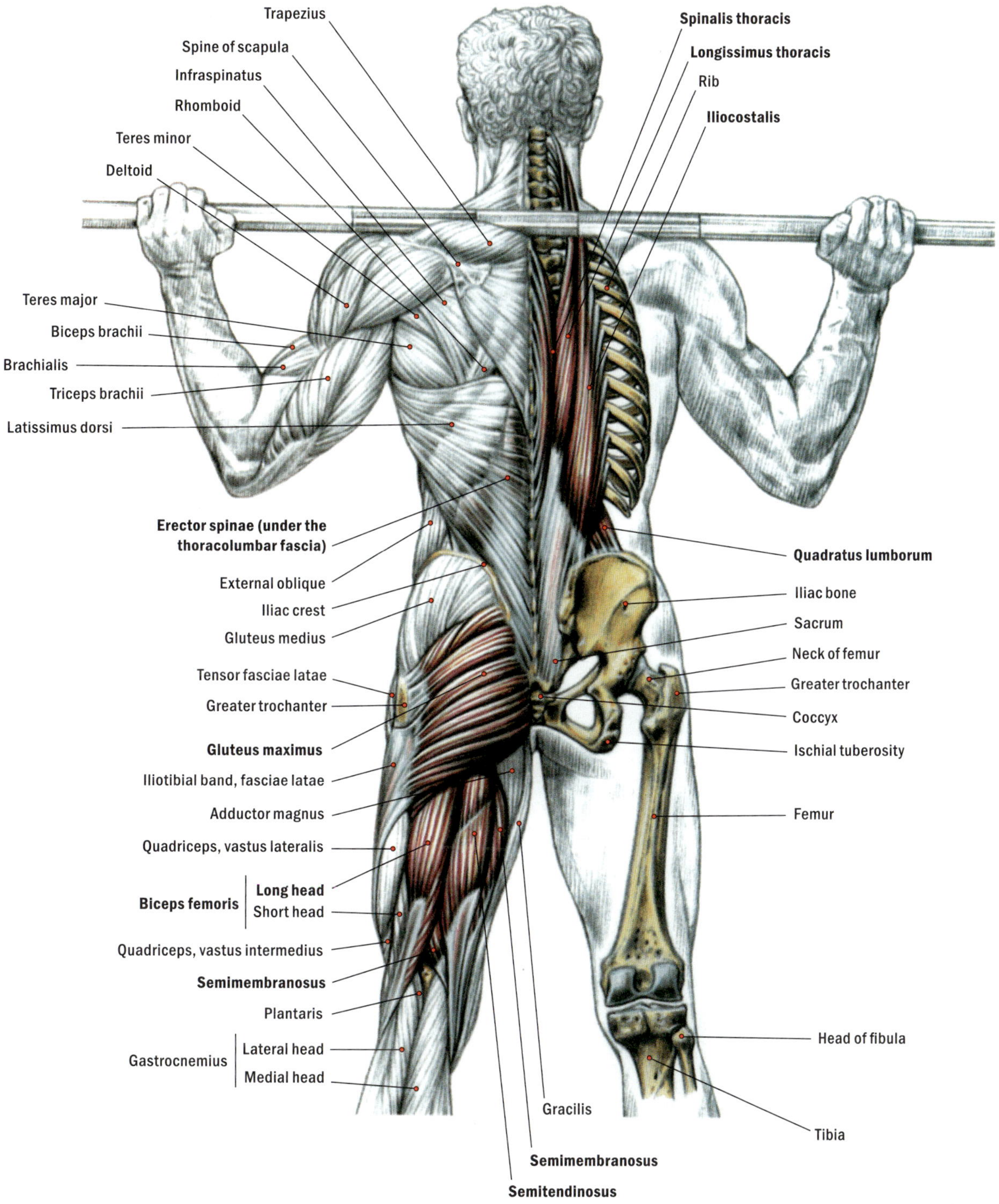

Trapezius
Spine of scapula
Infraspinatus
Rhomboid
Teres minor
Deltoid
Teres major
Biceps brachii
Brachialis
Triceps brachii
Latissimus dorsi
Erector spinae (under the thoracolumbar fascia)
External oblique
Iliac crest
Gluteus medius
Tensor fasciae latae
Greater trochanter
Gluteus maximus
Iliotibial band, fasciae latae
Adductor magnus
Quadriceps, vastus lateralis
Biceps femoris
Long head
Short head
Quadriceps, vastus intermedius
Semimembranosus
Plantaris
Gastrocnemius
Lateral head
Medial head
Gracilis
Semimembranosus
Semitendinosus
Spinalis thoracis
Longissimus thoracis
Rib
Iliocostalis
Quadratus lumborum
Iliac bone
Sacrum
Neck of femur
Greater trochanter
Coccyx
Ischial tuberosity
Femur
Head of fibula
Tibia

Besides knee flexion, the main function of the hamstrings is to tip the pelvis back (posterior rotation) and straighten the torso when the pelvis locks to the torso through isometric contraction of the core muscles and the lumbosacral muscle group. To feel the hamstrings working more, avoid working with heavy weights.

In the negative phase, the good morning exercise is excellent for stretching the back of the thighs. When done regularly, it helps prevent injury during heavy squats.

1
2
3

1 Pelvis, posterior tilt
2 Pelvis, neutral position
3 Pelvis, forward tilt

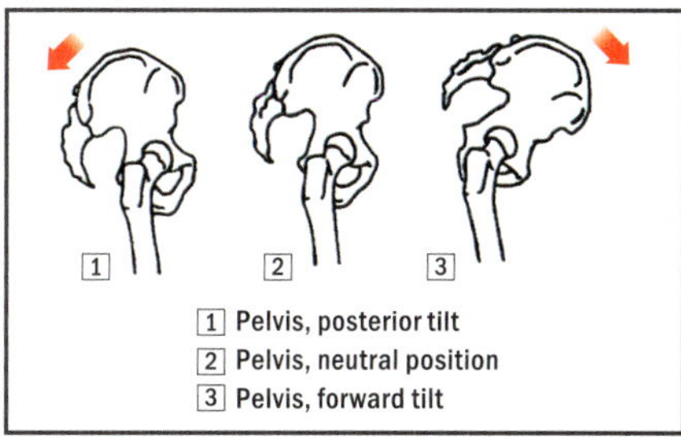

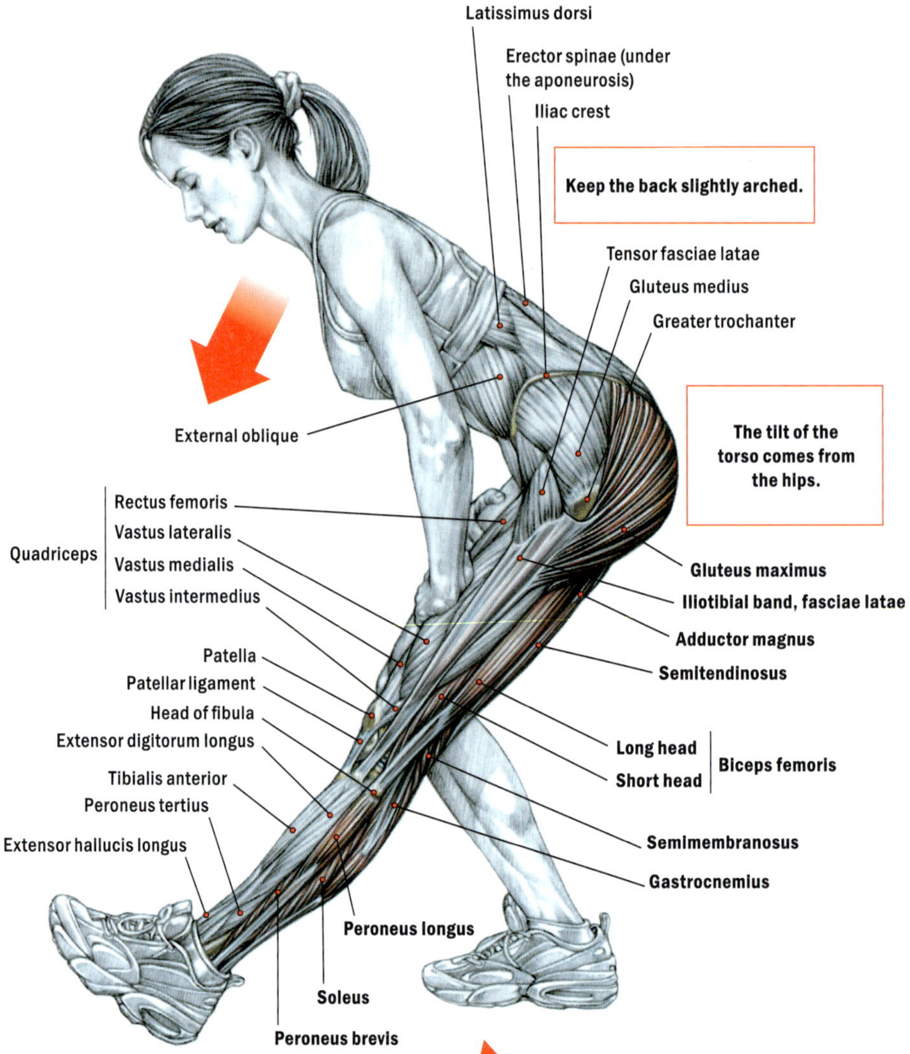

Stand on one leg, slightly bending at your knee. Extend your other leg with your foot in dorsiflexion:

- Place your hands on your thighs and slightly arch your back. Slowly bend your torso forward, concentrating on the stretching feeling at the back of your thigh. The tilt occurs at your pelvis.
- Hold this position for 20 seconds. Return slowly to the starting position and then change sides.

This exercise mainly stretches the hamstrings and the adductor magnus, as well as the gastrocnemius, soleus, and, to a lesser degree, the gluteus maximus.

To avoid injury during squats and deadlifts, it is best to practice this stretch at the beginning of a workout by incorporating it into the first few sets.

In strength training, the main function of stretching exercises is to equalize the muscle fiber tension inside the muscle and limit the risk of injury.

With heavy weights, if the muscle fiber tension is not homogeneous, the tightest fibers are the ones at risk of tearing. At the beginning of the workout, between each warm-up set, you should do a few stretching exercises that are specifically for the muscle groups about to be worked.

Always stretch gently and in moderation to protect the joints and to avoid excessive stretching of the ligaments, which can destabilize the joints and cause pathological inflammation.

FORWARD FOLD HAMSTRING STRETCH

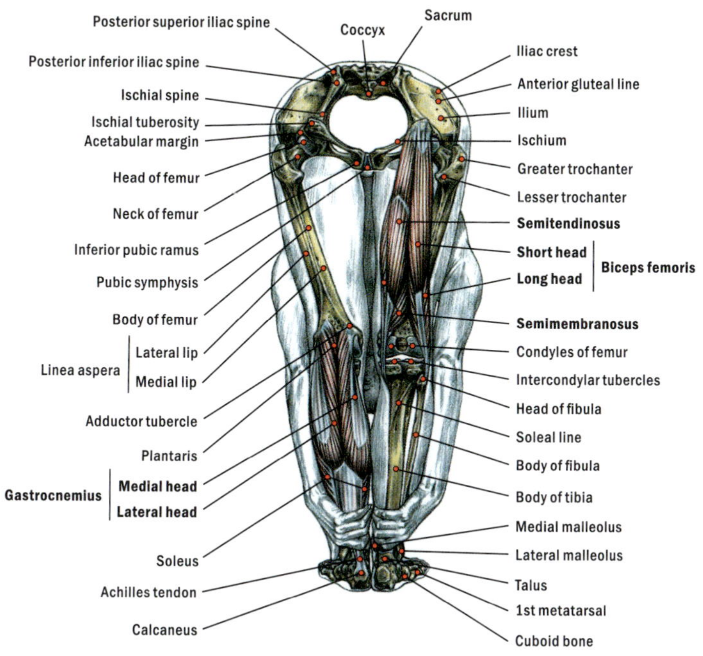

When the pelvis tilts forward, the hamstring muscles are stretched.

VARIATION WITH A BENCH

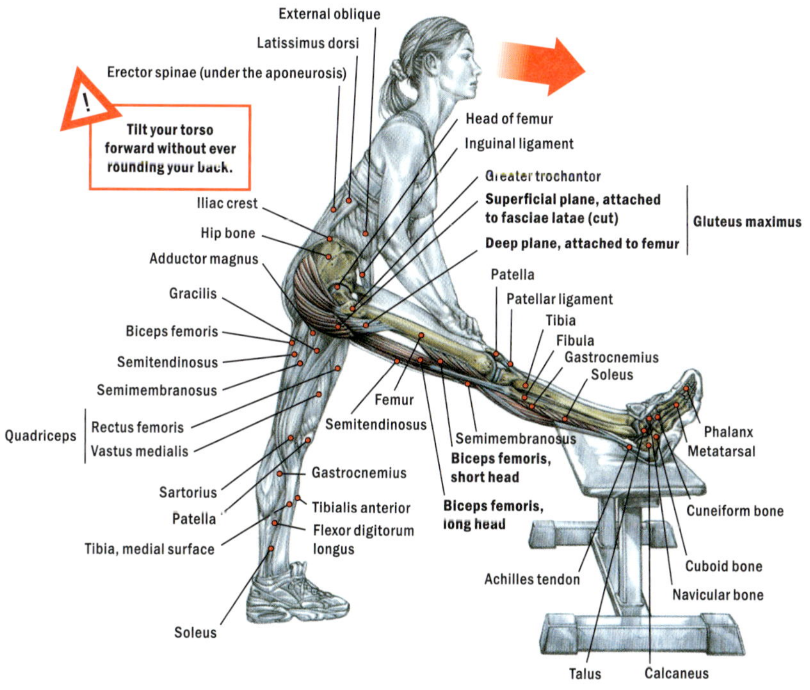

Variations

Stand on one leg with the other leg extended and resting on a bench with the foot flexed:

- Place your hands on the thigh of the extended leg. Slightly arch your back and slowly lean your torso forward, focusing on the stretching feeling at the back of your thigh. The tilt occurs at your pelvis.
- Hold the stretch for 20 seconds.
- Return slowly to the starting position and change sides.

To better focus on the stretching of the hamstrings, relax your calf muscles by pointing your front foot.

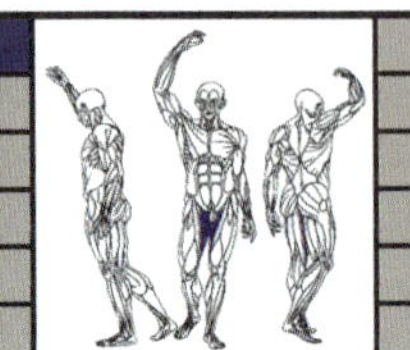

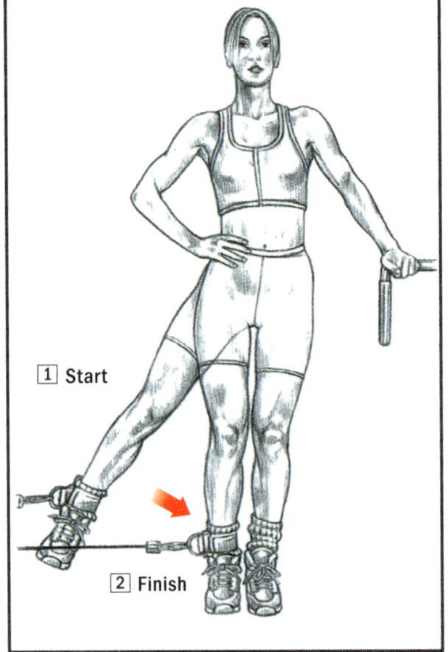

PERFORMING THE EXERCISE

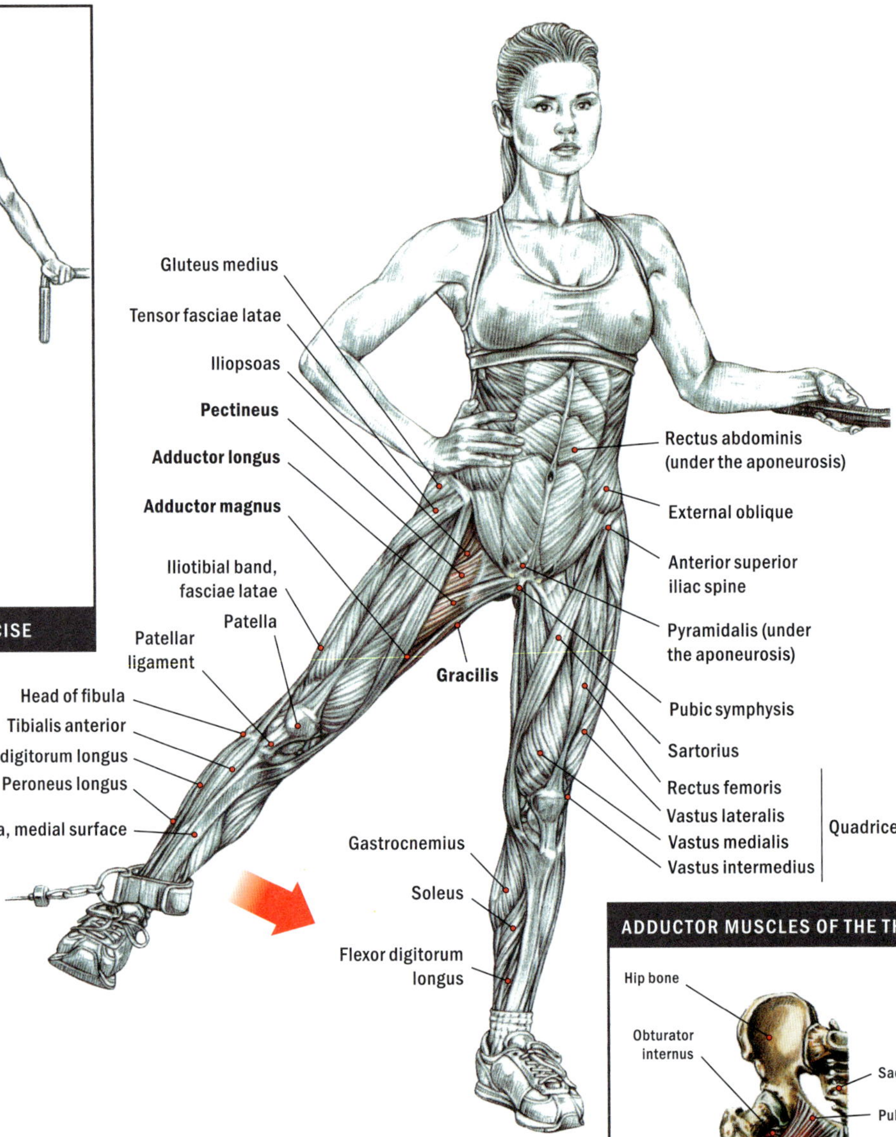

1 Start

2 Finish

Gluteus medius

Tensor fasciae latae

Iliopsoas

Pectineus

Adductor longus

Adductor magnus

Iliotibial band, fasciae latae

Patella

Patellar ligament

Head of fibula

Tibialis anterior

Extensor digitorum longus

Peroneus longus

Tibia, medial surface

Gracilis

Rectus abdominis (under the aponeurosis)

External oblique

Anterior superior iliac spine

Pyramidalis (under the aponeurosis)

Pubic symphysis

Sartorius

Rectus femoris

Vastus lateralis

Vastus medialis

Vastus intermedius

Quadriceps

Gastrocnemius

Soleus

Flexor digitorum longus

ADDUCTOR MUSCLES OF THE THIGHS

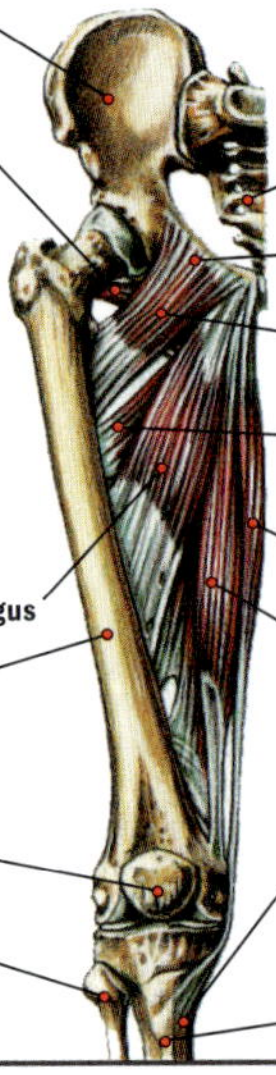

Hip bone

Obturator internus

Sacrum

Pubis

Pectineus

Adductor brevis

Gracilis

Adductor longus

Adductor magnus

Femur

Common insertion

Patella

Fibula

Tibia

Stand on one leg, with the other leg in the ankle cuff and with the hand on the supporting leg side holding onto the frame of the machine or some other support:

- Pull the working leg to the supporting leg or pull it in front of and across the supporting leg.

This exercise works all of the adductors (pectineus, adductor brevis, adductor longus, adductor magnus, and gracilis). It is excellent for developing definition of the inside of the thighs; to achieve this, you should perform long sets.

SEATED MACHINE HIP ADDUCTIONS 15

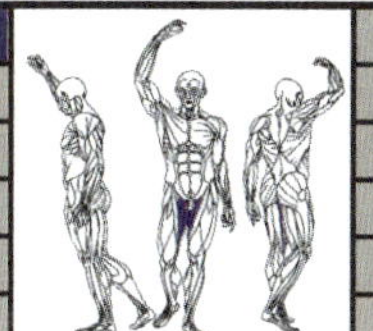

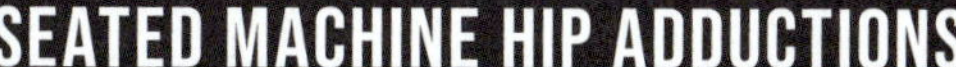

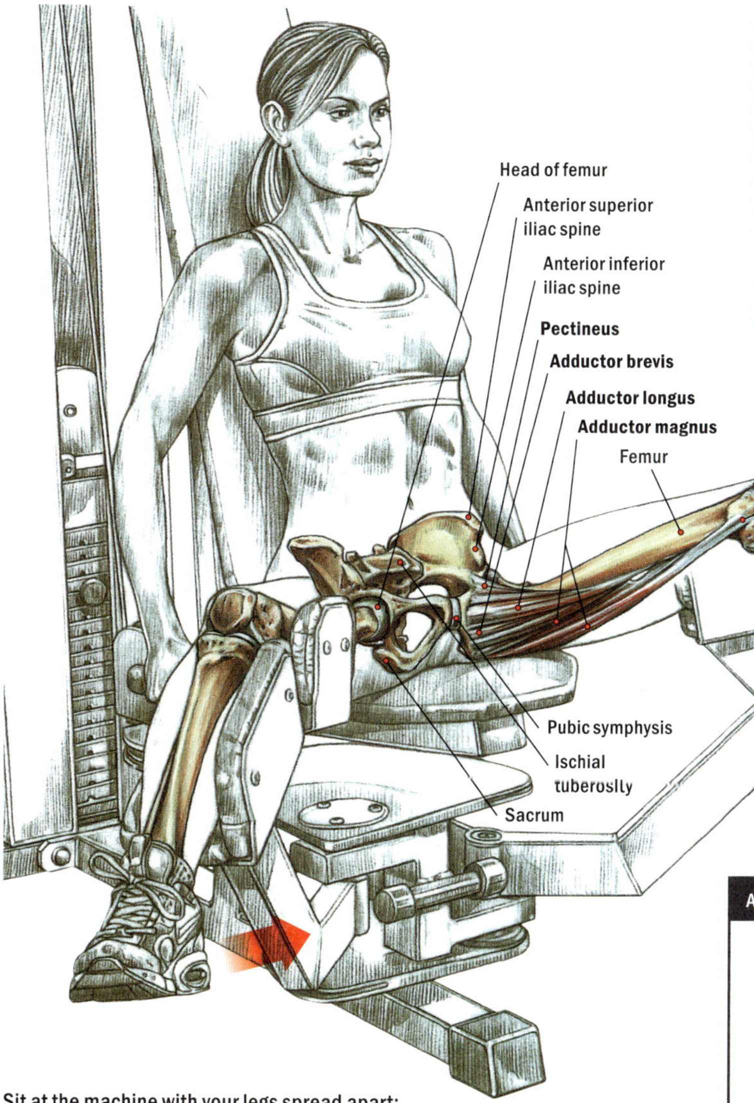

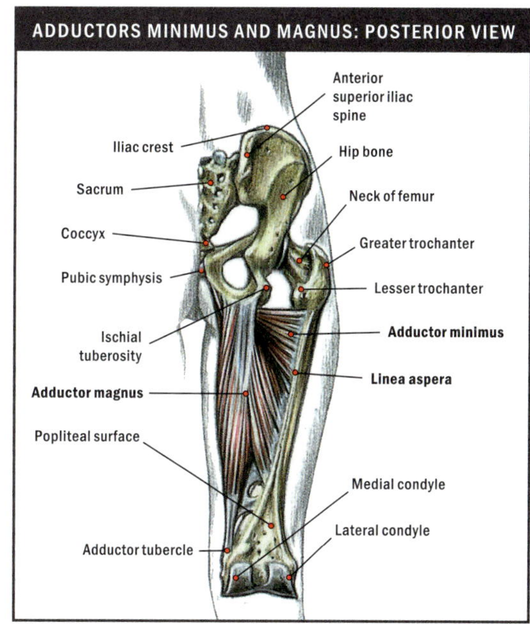

Head of femur
Anterior superior iliac spine
Anterior inferior iliac spine
Pectineus
Adductor brevis
Adductor longus
Adductor magnus
Femur
Patella
Adductor tubercle
Medial meniscus
Tibial tuberosity
Tibia, subcutaneous medial surface
Metatarsals
Proximal phalanx
Distal phalanx
Pubic symphysis
Ischial tuberosity
Sacrum
Calcaneus
Sustentaculum tali
Talus
Navicular bone
Cuneiform bones

1 Start
2 Finish

PERFORMING THE EXERCISE

Sit at the machine with your legs spread apart:

- Contract your thighs to bring your legs together.
- Return to the starting position with control.

This exercise works all of the adductor muscles of the thigh (pectineus, adductor minimus, adductor magnus, adductor longus, adductor brevis, and gracilis) and allows you to use heavier weights than you can with cable hip adductions. However, you do so with a decreased range of motion. Best results are achieved in long sets until you feel a burn.

This exercise can be used to strengthen the adductors, as this muscle group is often injured during intense exertion. It is best to increase the weights gradually in heavy sets and to do specific adductor muscle stretches at the end of the workout.

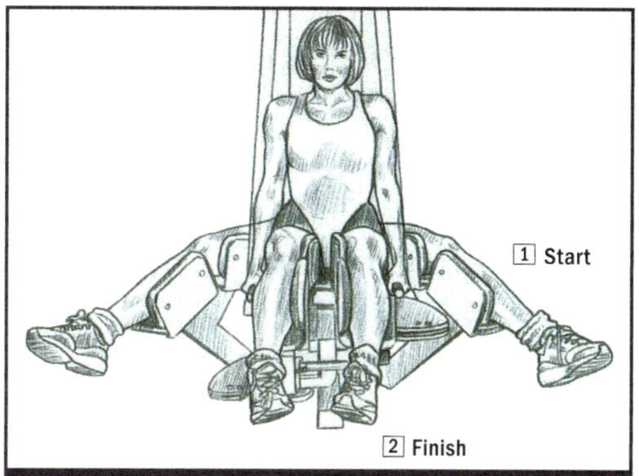

ADDUCTORS MINIMUS AND MAGNUS: POSTERIOR VIEW

Anterior superior iliac spine
Iliac crest
Hip bone
Sacrum
Neck of femur
Coccyx
Greater trochanter
Pubic symphysis
Lesser trochanter
Ischial tuberosity
Adductor minimus
Linea aspera
Adductor magnus
Popliteal surface
Medial condyle
Lateral condyle
Adductor tubercle

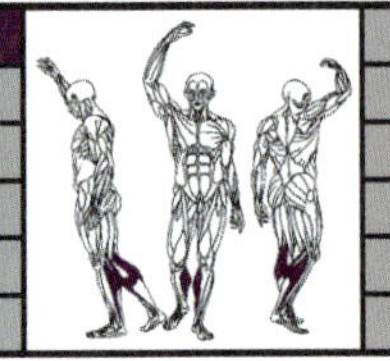

16 STANDING CALF RAISES

5th lumbar vertebra
Iliac crest
Sacrum
Coccyx
Pubic symphysis
Iliac spine
Neck of femur
Ischial tuberosity
Greater trochanter
Lesser trochanter
Body of femur
Linea aspera
Medial condyle
Lateral condyle
Gastrocnemius
Lateral head
Medial head
Line of the soleus muscle
The space between the tibia and fibula is filled with an interosseous membrane. This creates a sufficiently large, flat surface where the calf muscles attach.
Fibula
Tibia
Tibialis posterior
Flexor hallucis longus
Flexor digitorum longus
Calcaneal tuberosity
Talus
Sustentaculum tali
Quadratus plantae
Flexor digitorum longus, tendon
Flexor hallucis longus, tendon
Abductor hallucis
Flexor digitorum brevis
Abductor digiti minimi
Trapezius
Deltoid
Teres minor
Infraspinatus
Teres major
Triceps
Latissimus dorsi
External oblique
Gluteus medius
Gluteus maximus
Greater trochanter
Adductor magnus
Semitendinosus
Gracilis
Quadriceps, vastus lateralis
Long head
Short head
Biceps femoris
Semimembranosus
Adductor tubercle
Plantaris
Femur
Head of fibula
Soleus
Gastrocnemius (cut)
Soleus
Peroneus longus
Peroneus brevis
Achilles tendon
Medial malleolus
Lateral malleolus
Calcaneus
Navicular bone
Cuboid bone
Cuneiform bone
Metatarsals

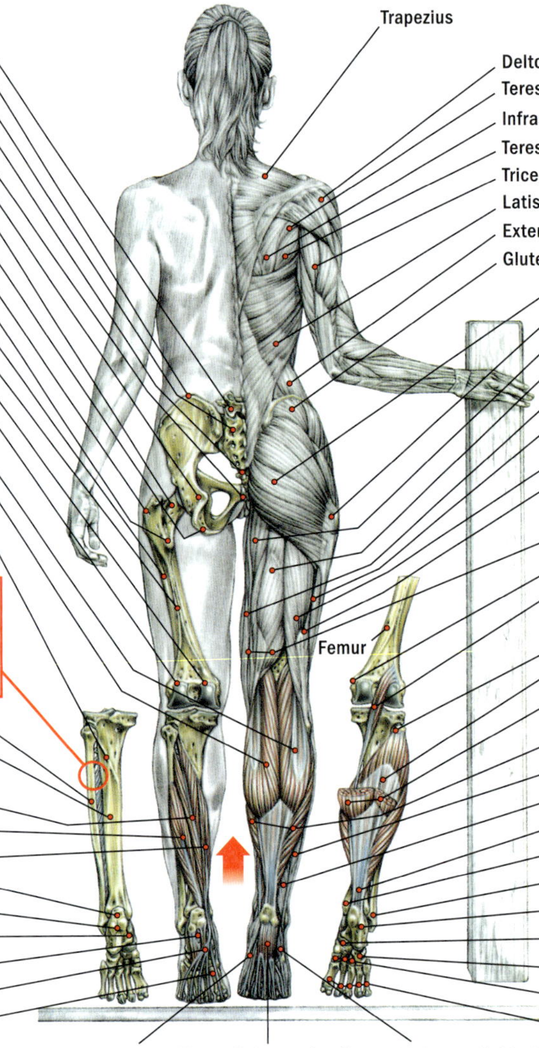

Stand on a step with one hand holding a wall or railing for stability:

- Slowly lower your heels to get a good stretch in your calves.
- Rise up on your toes while keeping your knees extended or slightly bent.

Perform this exercise slowly in long sets until you feel a burn. The combined action of muscle contraction and stretching makes this exercise ideal as a warm-up at the beginning of a training session for the calves to help avoid injury. It is also ideal at the end of a workout to really feel the muscle contraction.

This exercise mainly works the triceps surae (made up of the two gastrocnemius and the soleus), as well as the flexor hallucis longus, tibialis posterior, and flexor digitorum longus (these last three muscles are deeper).

This exercise is also excellent for stretching the muscles of the plantar surface of the foot, such as the flexor digitorum brevis and the quadratus plantae, and for making the plantar aponeurosis more flexible.

PERFORMING THE EXERCISE

1 Extension 2 Flexion

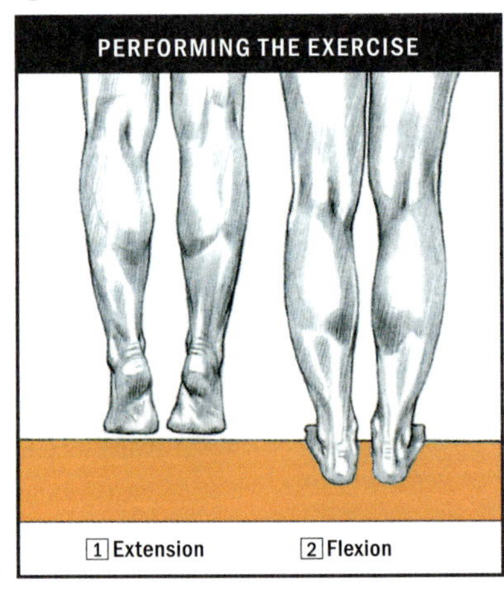

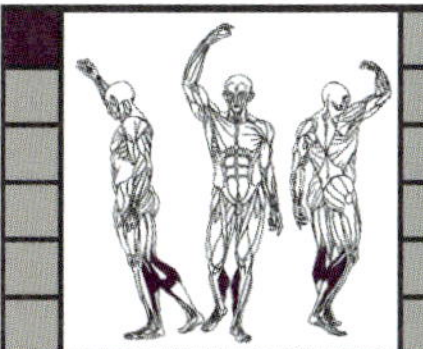

PERFORMING THE EXERCISE

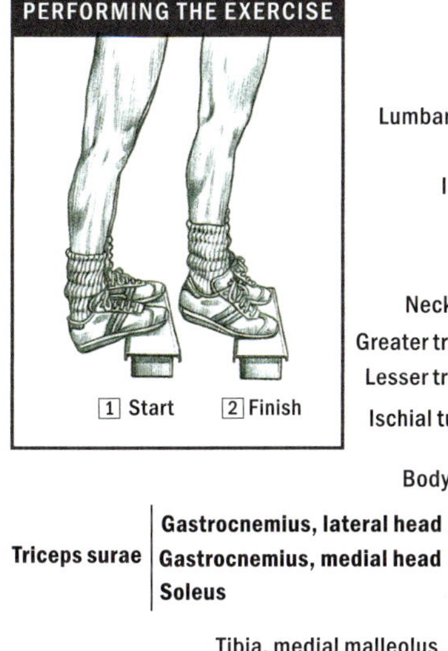

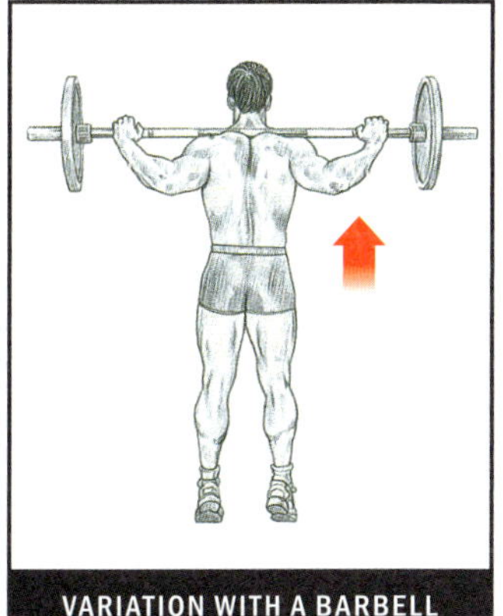

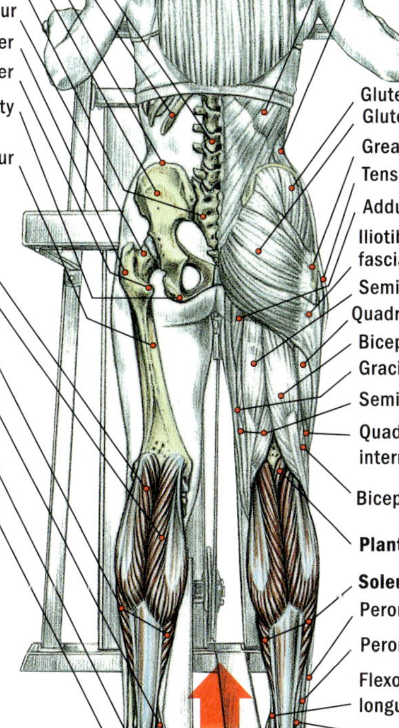

GASTROCNEMIUS MUSCLES, MEDIAL HEADS

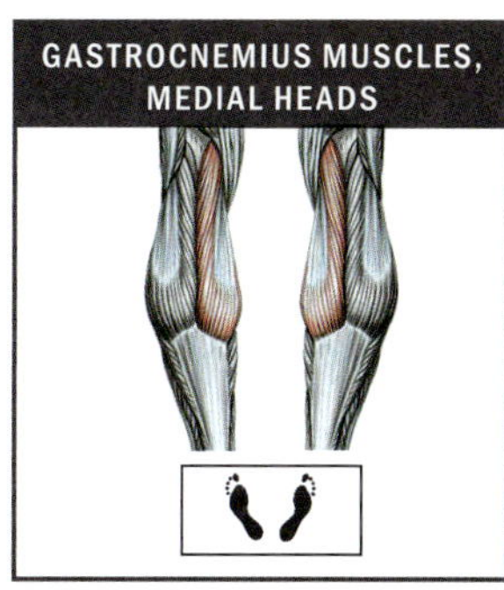

GASTROCNEMIUS MUSCLES, LATERAL HEADS

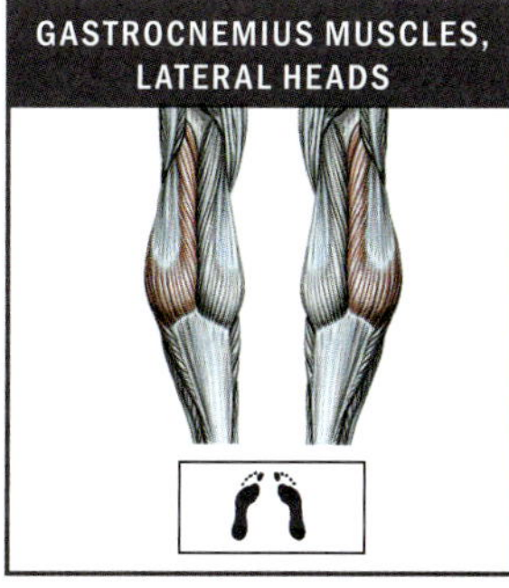

VARIATION ON AN INCLINE MACHINE

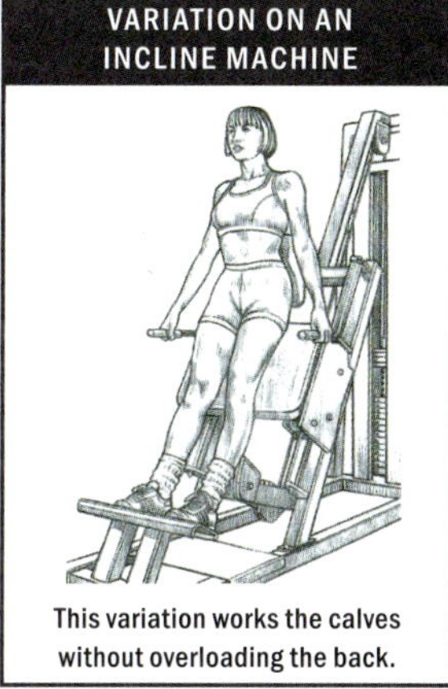

This variation works the calves without overloading the back.

Stand at the machine with a straight back, shoulders under the pads, and the balls of your feet on the foot plate, with your heels hanging down:

- Rise up by extending your feet (plantar flexion), keeping your legs straight.

This exercise works the triceps surae (made up of the soleus and the lateral and medial heads of the gastrocnemius). Move your feet through the complete range of motion with each repetition in order to stretch the muscles properly. In theory, it is possible to isolate the medial gastrocnemius by pointing the toes out and to isolate the lateral gastrocnemius by pointing the toes in, but in practice this is difficult to achieve. Only separating the work of the soleus and gastrocnemius is easy to achieve: This is done by bending the knees to relax the gastrocnemius, which transfers part of the effort onto the soleus.

<u>Variations</u>

- Do the exercise using a rack with a wedge under your feet or using a barbell without a wedge for more balance; however, this decreases the range of motion.
- The exercise can also be done on an incline machine, which helps to work the calves without overloading the back.

The triceps surae is an extremely powerful and tough muscle group that lifts the entire weight of the body thousands of times a day when we walk. Don't hesitate to work it with heavy weights.

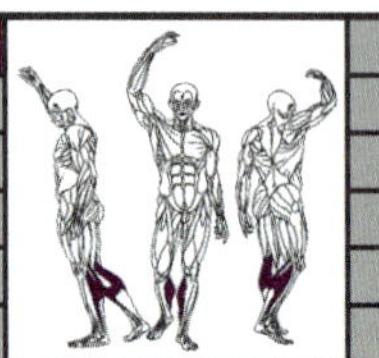

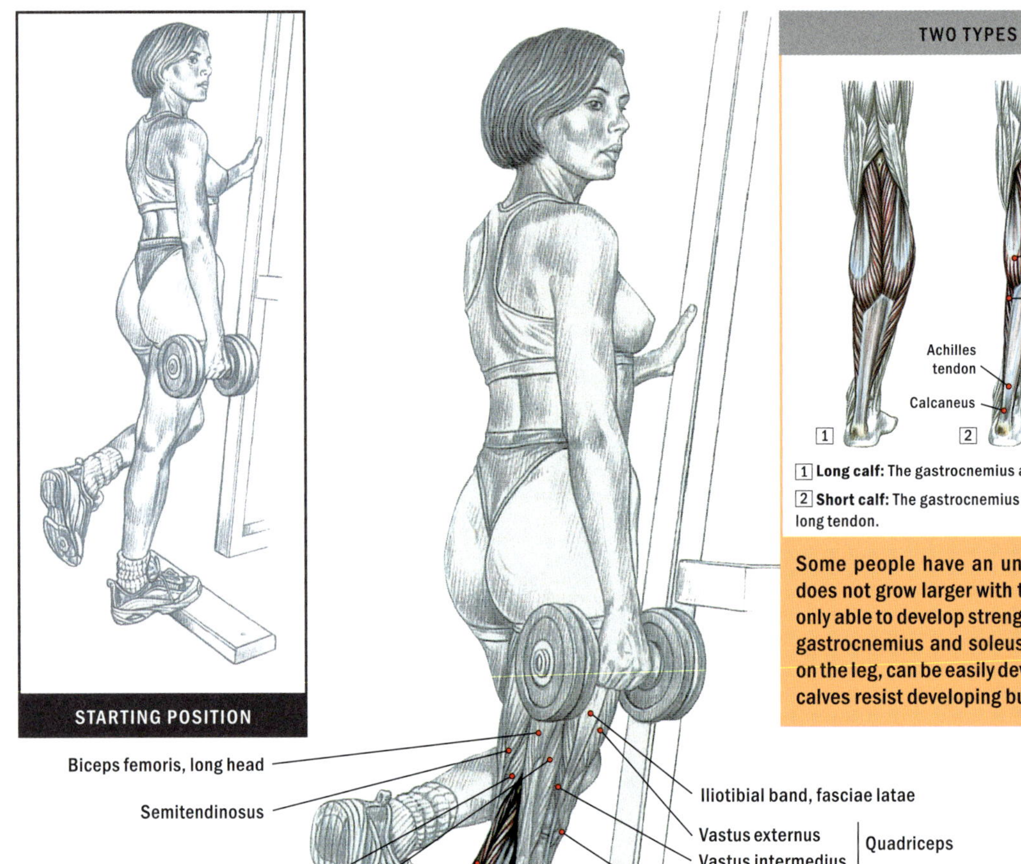

TWO TYPES OF CALVES

1 **Long calf:** The gastrocnemius and soleus descend low on the leg.

2 **Short calf:** The gastrocnemius and soleus are higher up with a long tendon.

Some people have an unusual triceps surae that does not grow larger with training. These people are only able to develop strength. Long calves, where the gastrocnemius and soleus muscles come down low on the leg, can be easily developed. Conversely, short calves resist developing bulk.

TRICEPS SURAE MUSCLE

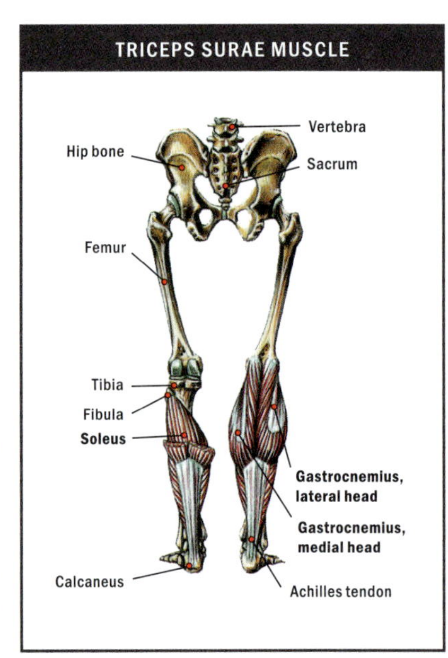

Stand on one leg with the front of your foot on the foot plate and hold a dumbbell in one hand. Use the other hand for support and balance:

- Rise up on your toes (plantar flexion), keeping your knee joint straight or slightly flexed.
- Return to the starting position.

This exercise works the triceps surae (made up of the soleus and the lateral and medial heads of the gastrocnemius). Completely flex your foot with each repetition to stretch the triceps surae properly. Optimal results are obtained through long sets until you feel a burn.

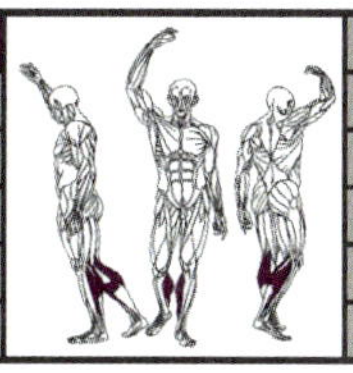

Iliotibial band, fasciae latae

Quadriceps
- Vastus medialis
- Vastus lateralis

Biceps femoris, short head

Patella

Head of fibula

Triceps surae
- **Gastrocnemius, lateral head**
- **Gastrocnemius, medial head**
- **Soleus**

Peroneus longus

Extensor digitorum longus

Tibialis anterior

Flexor digitorum longus

Extensor hallucis longus

Lateral malleolus

Extensor retinaculum

Triceps surae
- **Gastrocnemius, medial head**
- **Soleus**

Tibia, medial surface

Medial malleolus

Peroneal retinaculum

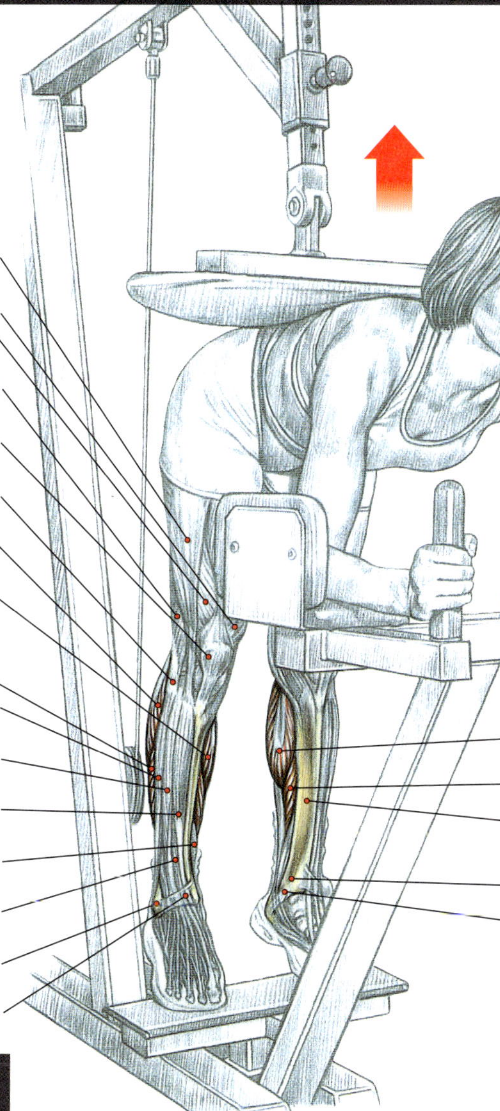

TRICEPS SURAE INSERTIONS

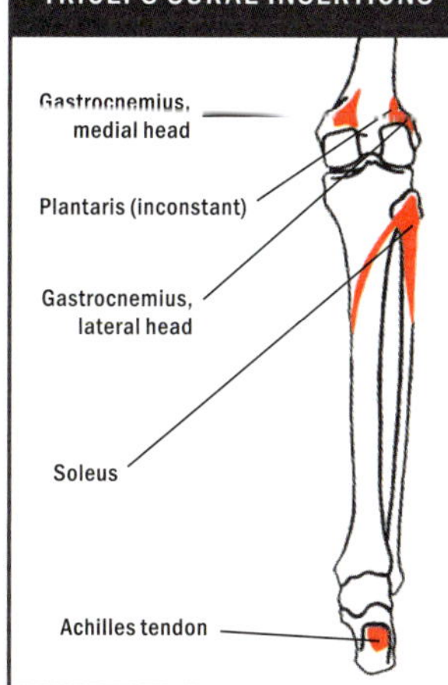

Stand with your legs relaxed and extended, toes on the foot plate, torso leaning forward, forearms resting on the front support, and the padded plate of the machine resting on the back of your hips:

- Rise up onto your toes (plantar flexion).

This exercise focuses on the triceps surae, especially the gastrocnemius muscles.

Variation

If there is no machine for this exercise, put a block under your feet, bend forward, rest the forearms on a support, and do this exercise with someone sitting on your hips.

TRICEPS SURAE ACTION

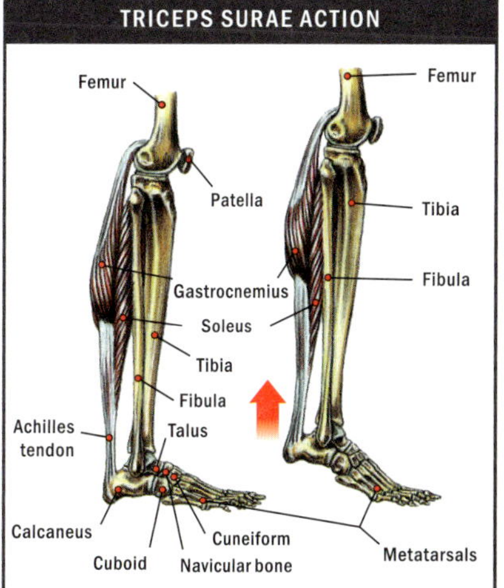

20 SEATED MACHINE CALF RAISES

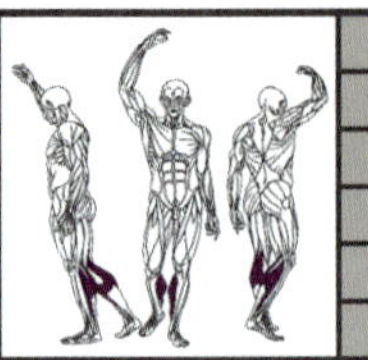

VARIATION WITH A BARBELL RESTING ON THE KNEES

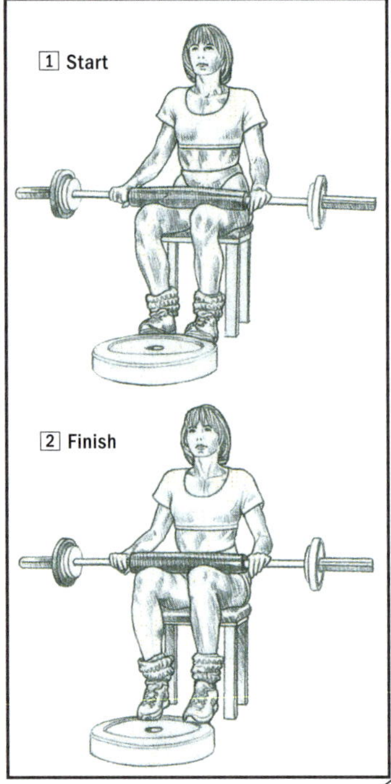

1 Start
2 Finish

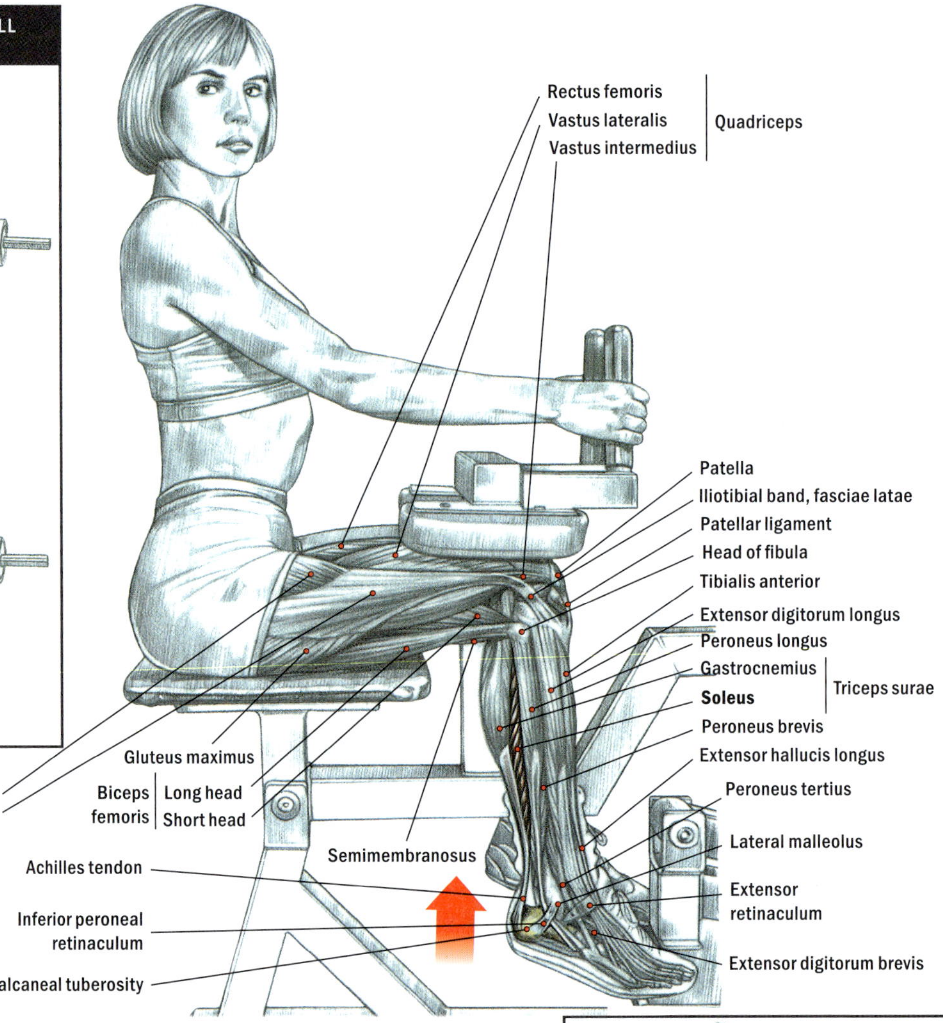

Rectus femoris
Vastus lateralis
Vastus intermedius
Quadriceps
Patella
Iliotibial band, fasciae latae
Patellar ligament
Head of fibula
Tibialis anterior
Extensor digitorum longus
Peroneus longus
Gastrocnemius
Soleus
Triceps surae
Peroneus brevis
Extensor hallucis longus
Peroneus tertius
Lateral malleolus
Extensor retinaculum
Extensor digitorum brevis
Gluteus maximus
Tensor fasciae latae
Iliotibial band, fasciae latae
Biceps femoris
Long head
Short head
Semimembranosus
Achilles tendon
Inferior peroneal retinaculum
Calcaneal tuberosity

Sit at a machine with your knees positioned under the pads, your toes on the foot bar, and your ankles relaxed:

- Extend your feet and point your toes (plantar flexion).

This exercise isolates the soleus, the name of which is derived from its resemblance to a flatfish—the sole. (This muscle inserts at the top at the tibia and fibula under the knee joint and attaches at the bottom to the calcaneus by the Achilles tendon. Its purpose is to extend the feet at the ankles.) Bending at the knees relaxes the gastrocnemius, which attaches above the knee joint and, at the bottom, to the Achilles tendon. In this position, it can only contribute weakly to ankle extension.

Vertebra
Sacrum
Hip bone
Femur
Patella
Peroneus longus*
Fibula
Tibia
Tibialis posterior*
Flexor digitorum longus*
Flexor hallucis longus*
Peroneus brevis*

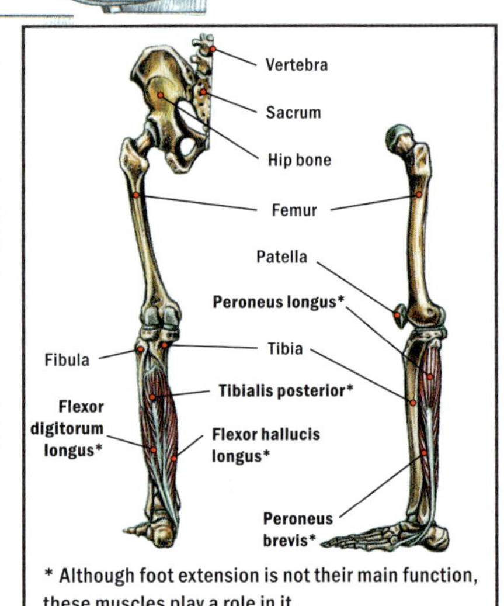

* Although foot extension is not their main function, these muscles play a role in it.

Variation

You can also do this exercise by sitting on a bench with a wedge under your feet and a barbell resting on your thighs. You should cushion the bar with a rubber pad or place a folded towel on your thighs to make the exercise more comfortable.

SEATED BARBELL CALF RAISES 21

STARTING POSITION

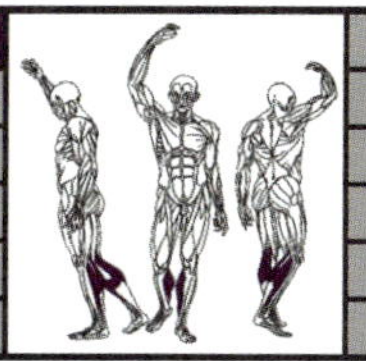

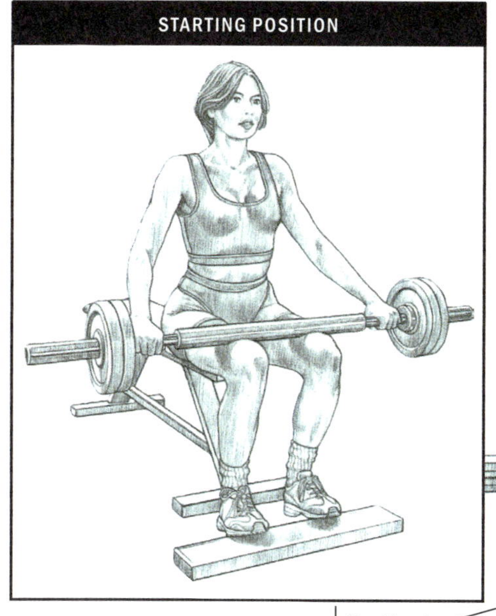

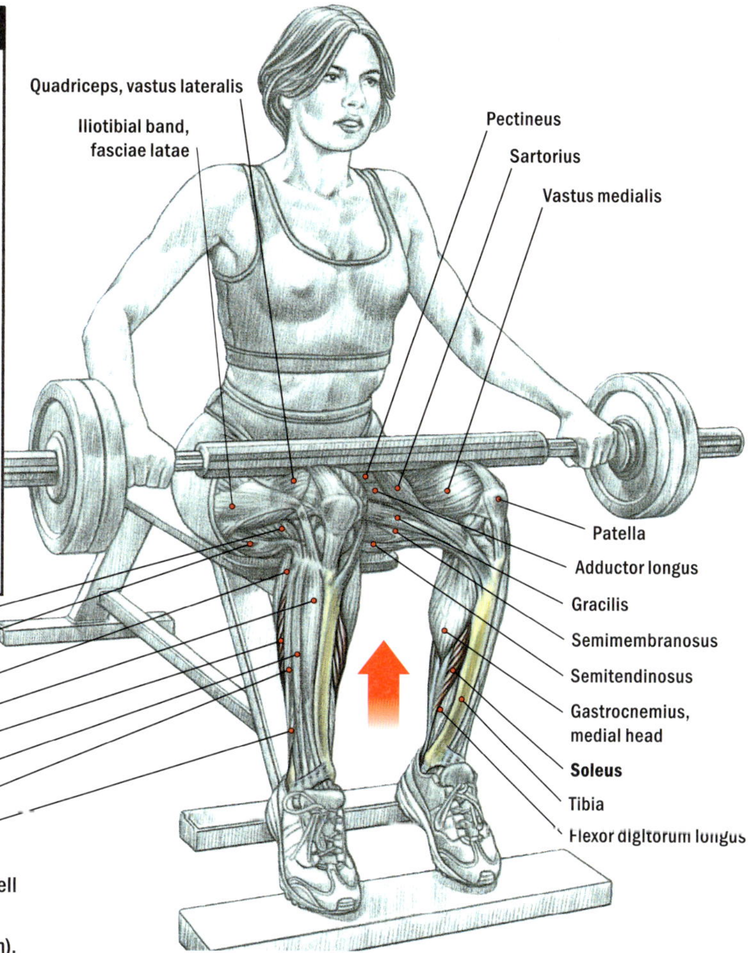

Sit on a bench with a wedge under your toes and a barbell resting on your thighs:

- Extend your feet and point your toes (plantar flexion).

This exercise mainly works the soleus. This muscle, which is part of the triceps surae group, inserts at the top below the knee joint on the tibia and fibula. At the bottom, it attaches to the calcaneus via the Achilles tendon. Its function is to extend the feet at the ankles.

Unlike seated machine calf raises, which allow you to work with heavy weights, this exercise does not allow heavy weights because of the awkwardness of the bar position. For best results, work in sets of a minimum of 15 to 20 reps.

Variation

You can also do this exercise without additional weights while sitting on a chair or bench. In this case, work in very long sets until you feel a burn.

It is advisable to cushion the bar on the thighs with a rubber pad or a folded towel to make the exercise more comfortable.

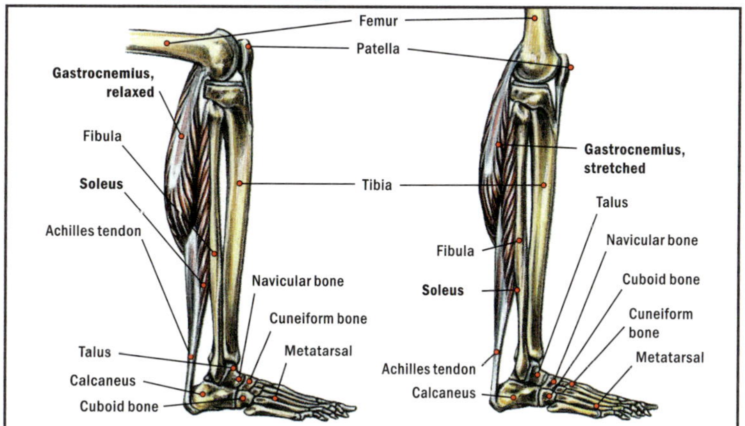

1 When the knees are bent, the gastrocnemius muscle, which attaches above the knee, is relaxed. In this position, it only slightly assists ankle extension because most of the work is done by the soleus.

2 Conversely, when the knee is straight, the gastrocnemius is stretched. In this position, it actively participates in ankle extension and completes the action of the soleus.

STRETCHING THE CALF

INSERTION OF THE ACHILLES TENDON

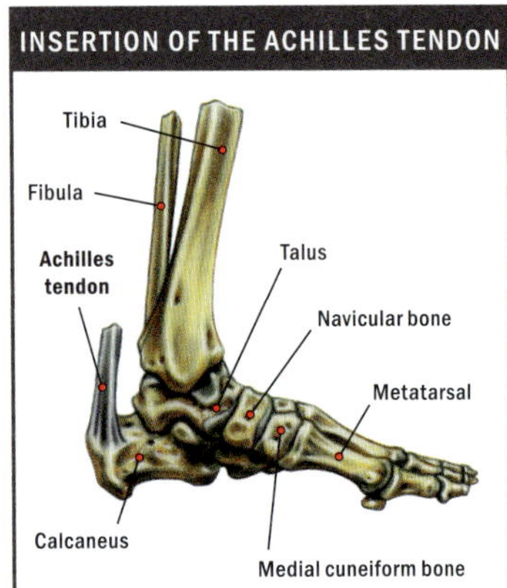

Stand with your hands on your hips, with one leg forward in a lunge stance, with your knees straight, and with your feet in line with your knees:

- Bend the forward knee by pushing your pelvis forward, being careful to always keep the back leg extended with the heel on the ground.
- Hold this position until you feel the stretch on the back leg.

This exercise stretches the triceps surae, which is made up of the gastrocnemius and the soleus, as well as the flexor digitorum muscles and the tibialis posterior, located deeper underneath the triceps surae. It also stretches, to a lesser degree, the peroneus longus and brevis muscles.

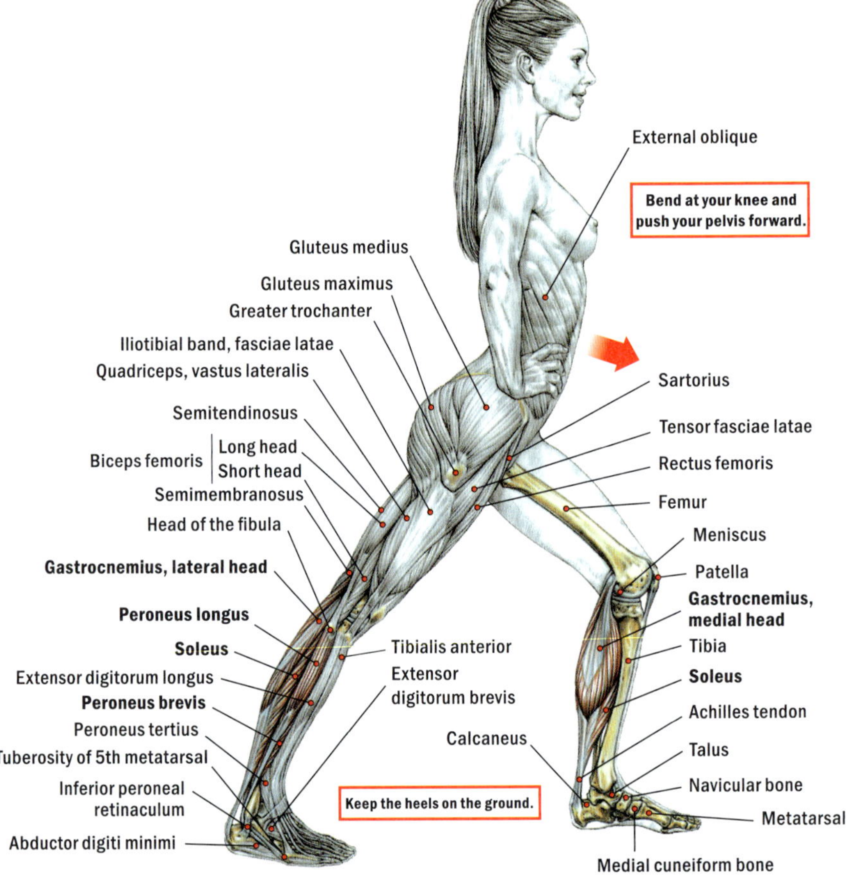

LONG CALF, SHORT CALF

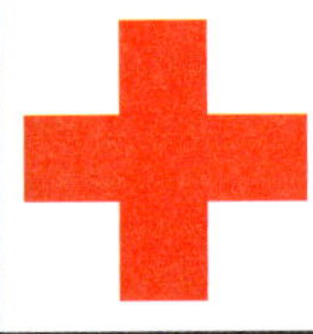

[1] Long calves, which are not very tendinous, are not the most suitable for running, due to their heaviness, even though they are powerful and can grow large through training.

[2] Short calves, which tend to be tendinous, generally accumulate a lot of kinetic energy during movement due to the stretching of tendons and release it like a spring during the propulsive phase. These thin, light calves are the most suitable for running. On the other hand, it is more difficult to add bulk to them through training.

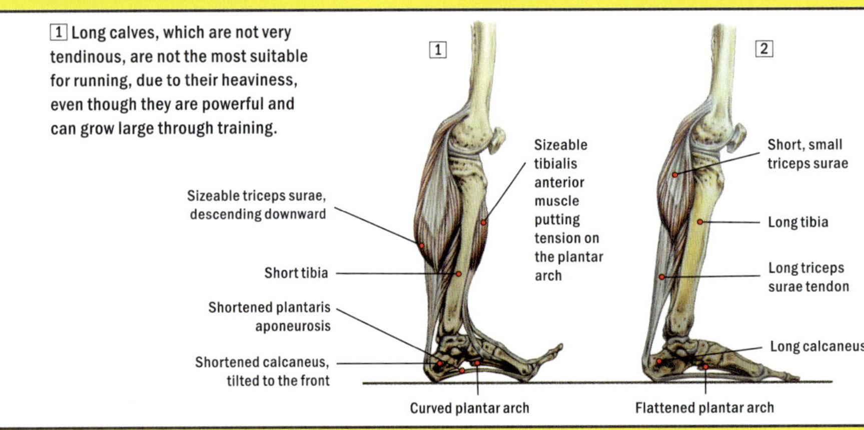

ANALYSIS OF HUMAN RUNNING

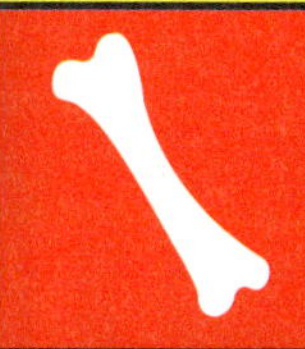

PROPULSIVE PHASE WITH MUSCLE CONTRACTION

CONTRACTION

MAXIMUM CONTRACTION

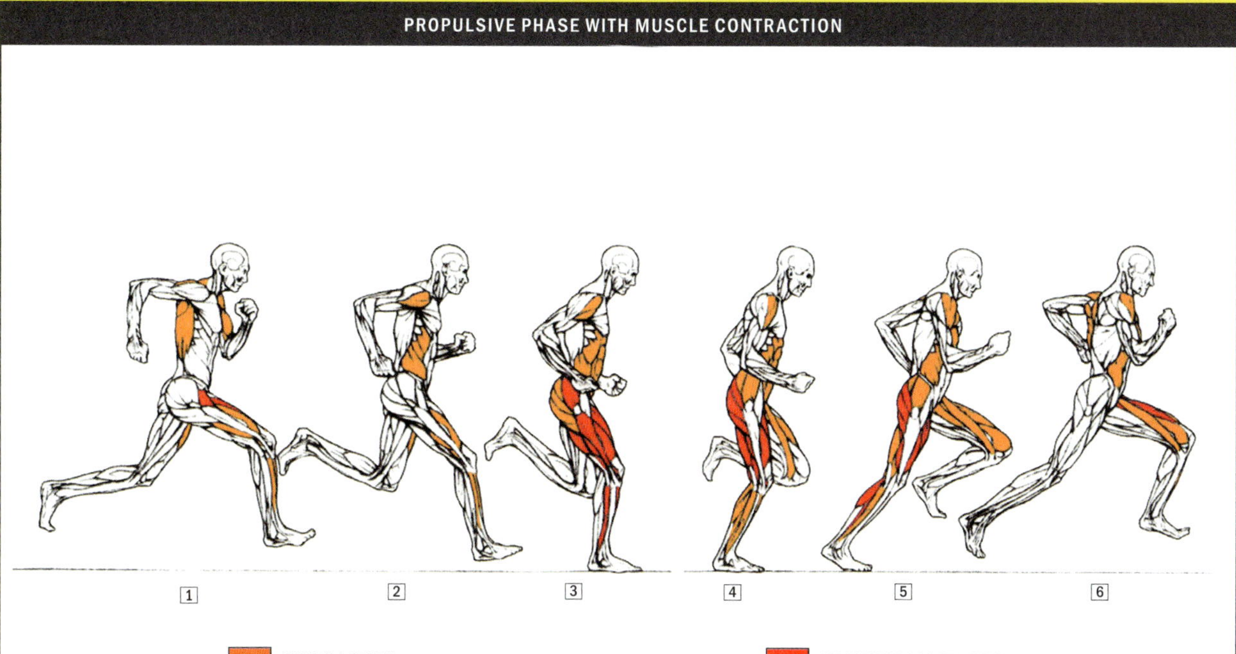

KINETIC ENERGY ACCUMULATION PHASE

STRETCHING

MAXIMUM STRETCHING

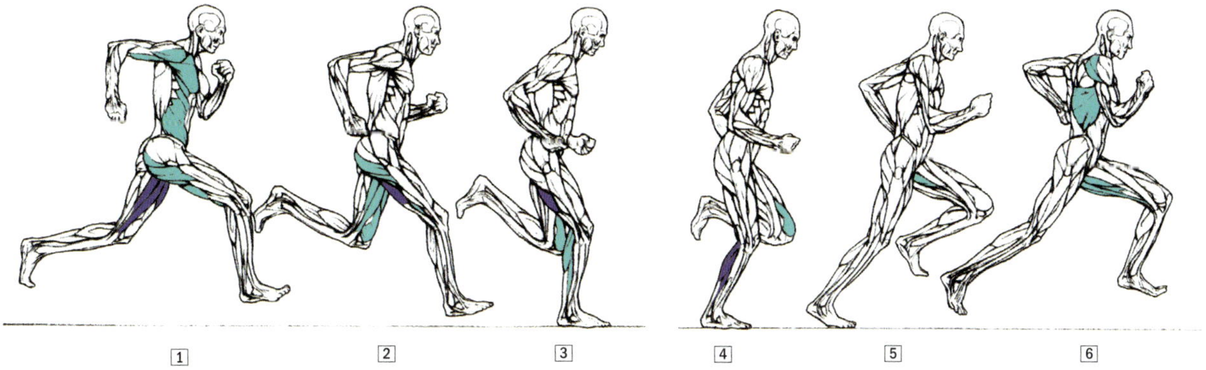

When the muscles are stretched, energy is released during the propulsive phase.

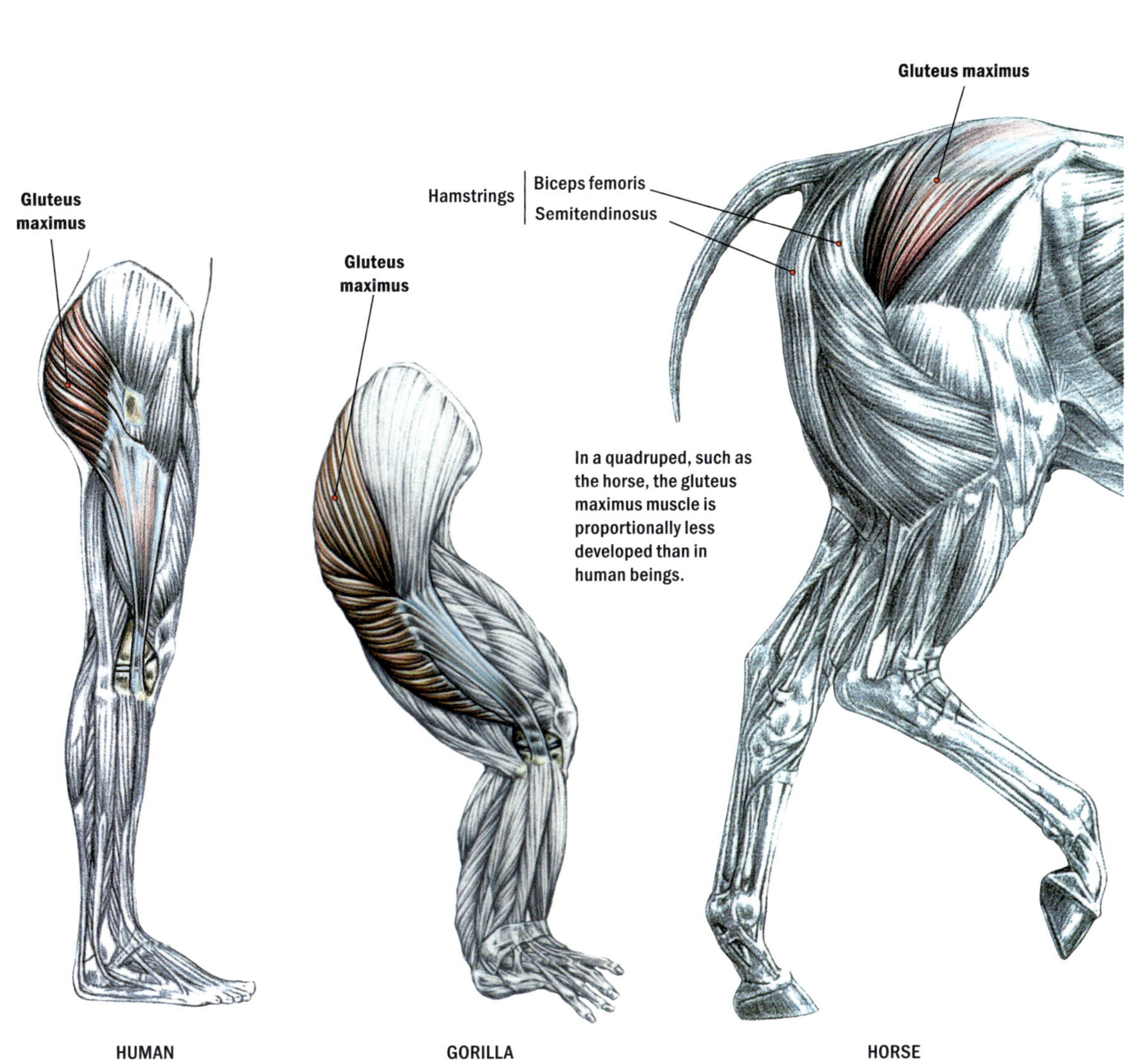

THE GLUTEUS MUSCLES, A HUMAN CHARACTERISTIC

Although some of the larger primates do occasionally walk, humans are the only primates and one of the few mammals that have completely adapted to two-legged locomotion. One of the structural features directly related to this way of moving around is the significant development of the gluteus maximus muscle, which has become the biggest and most powerful muscle in the human body.

The development of the gluteal muscles is uniquely human. In comparison, the gluteal muscles in quadrupeds are proportionately underdeveloped, and the hindquarters of the horse, which some consider as typical for animals, are in fact made up of the hamstrings (the back of the thigh in humans).

In humans, the gluteus maximus, which extends the hip, does not play an important role in walking. Instead, the hamstrings play the major role in straightening the pelvis (hip extension) with each stride. You just have to put your hand on your buttocks while walking, and you can feel that they do not contract very much. However, as soon as the effort becomes significant, such as when walking uphill, walking quickly, or running, the gluteus muscles begin to work to extend the hip and straighten the torso.

These biomechanical points help explain why, in exercises for the gluteus muscles and the hamstrings, such as good mornings (see page 194) and stiff-legged deadlifts (see page 138), as the weights get heavier, the gluteus muscles work more, and the hamstrings work less.

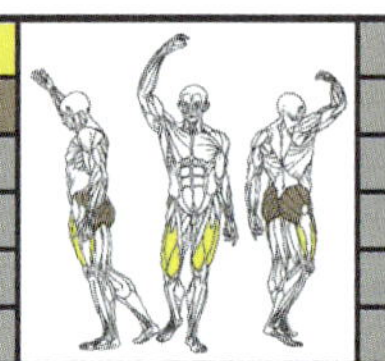

Muscle anatomy diagram labels:

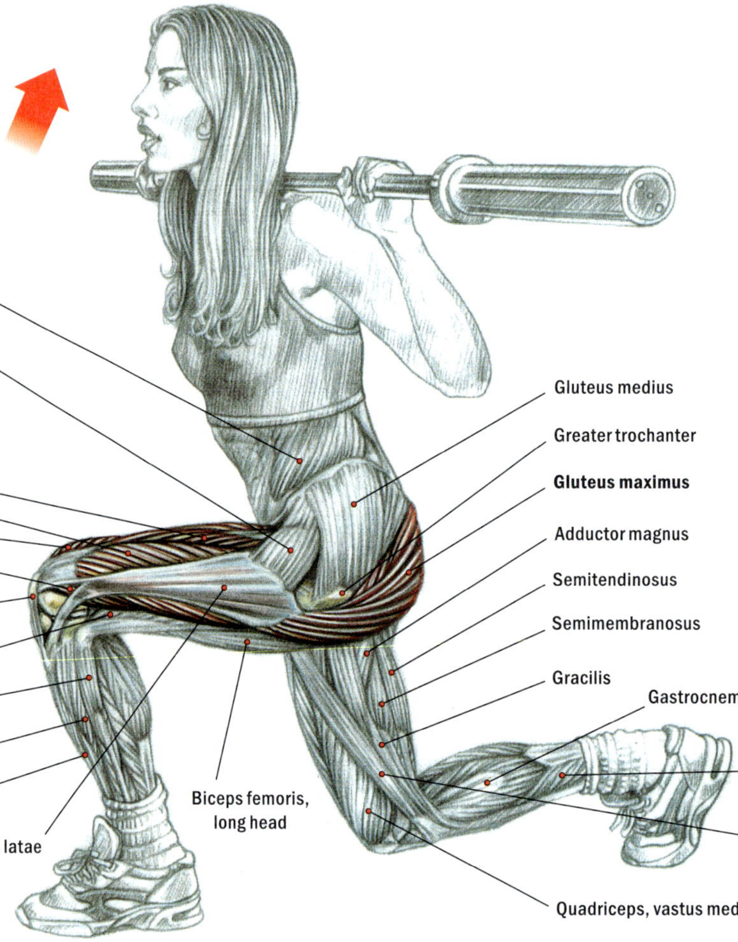

Stand with your legs slightly apart and the bar behind your neck resting on your trapezius muscles:

- Inhale and take a big step forward, keeping your torso as straight as possible. Perform a lunge so that the front thigh is parallel to the floor or your knee is slightly above hip level.
- Exhale and return to the starting position.

This exercise, which works the gluteus maximus intensely, can be performed two different ways: either by taking a small step (which isolates the quadriceps) or a big step (which isolates the hamstrings and gluteus maximus and stretches the rectus femoris and iliopsoas of the back leg).

Because the front leg must support almost all of the weight in the lunge position and the exercise requires a good sense of balance, it is best to begin with very light weights.

DIFFERENT WAYS TO DO THE EXERCISE

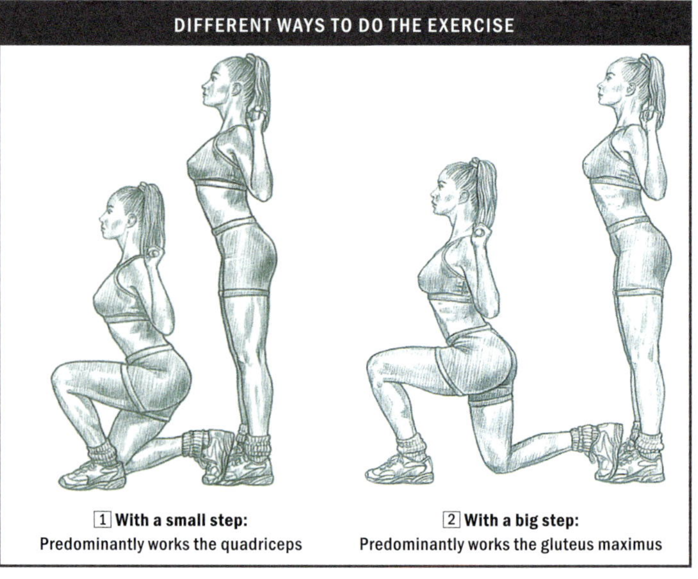

1 With a small step:
Predominantly works the quadriceps

2 With a big step:
Predominantly works the gluteus maximus

DUMBBELL FORWARD LUNGES 02

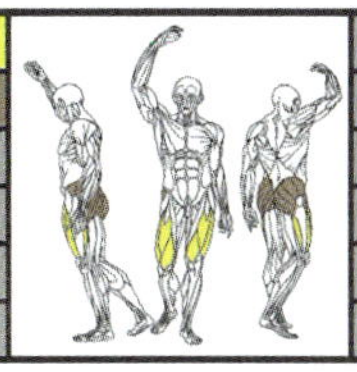

External oblique
Tensor fasciae latae
Quadriceps
Rectus femoris
Vastus lateralis
Vastus medialis
Vastus intermedius
Patella
Biceps femoris
Short head
Long head
Semitendinosus
Gastrocnemius
Peroneus longus
Extensor digitorum longus
Tibialis anterior
Soleus
Peroneus brevis
Iliotibial band, fasciae latae
Quadriceps, vastus medialis
Gluteus medius
Gluteus maximus
Adductor magnus
Semitendinosus
Semimembranosus
Gracilis
Sartorius
Gastrocnemius
Soleus

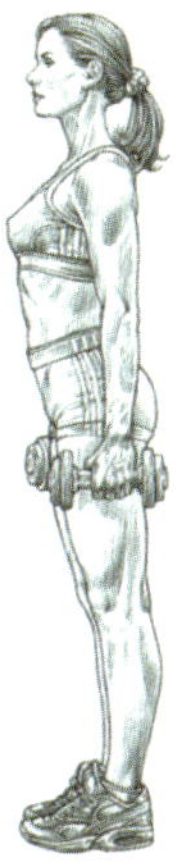

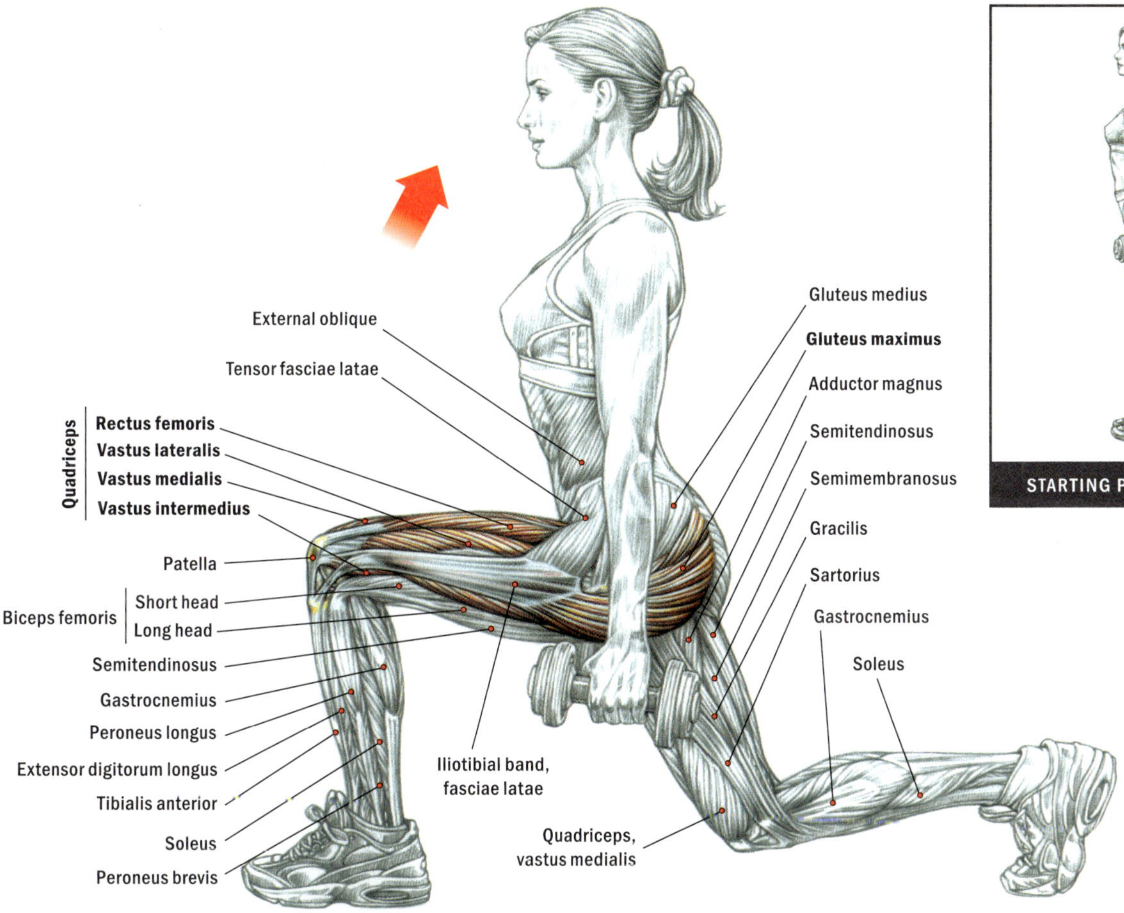

STARTING POSITION

Stand with your legs slightly apart and hold a dumbbell in each hand:

- Inhale and take a big step forward, keeping your torso as straight as possible.
- When the front thigh is parallel to the floor or your knee is slightly above hip level, push through your foot to return to the starting position.
- Exhale at the end of the exercise.

This exercise mainly works the gluteus maximus and quadriceps. The bigger the step, the more the gluteus maximus of the front leg is used and the iliopsoas and rectus femoris of the back leg are stretched. A smaller step isolates the quadriceps of the forward leg. You can perform a complete set on one side and then the other, or you can work your legs alternately during the same set.

Because all of the weight is supported by the front leg in the lunge position and the exercise requires a good sense of balance, it is best to work with light weights to protect the knees.

ANATOMY OF THE BUTTOCKS

Latissimus dorsi
Iliac crest
External oblique
Gluteus medius
Erector spinae (under the thoracolumbar fascia)
Gluteus maximus
Tensor fasciae latae
Coccyx
Greater trochanter
Iliotibial band, fasciae latae
Adductor magnus
Biceps femoris, long head
Semitendinosus
Semimembranosus
Gracilis
Quadriceps, vastus lateralis

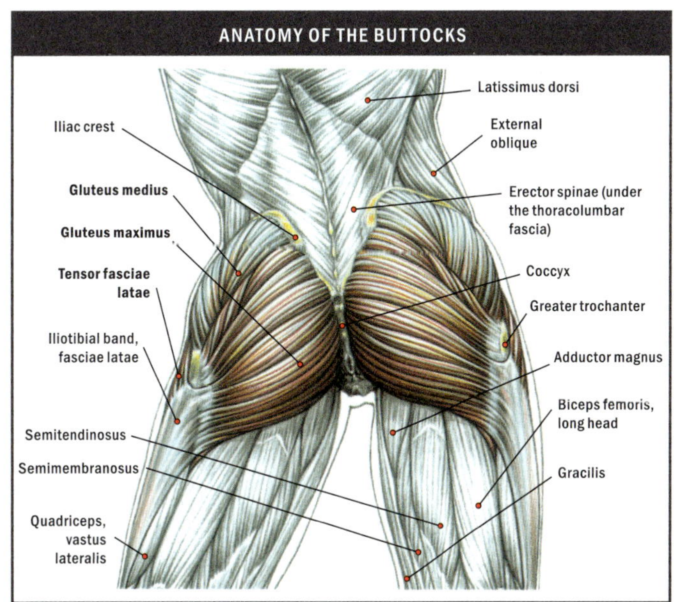

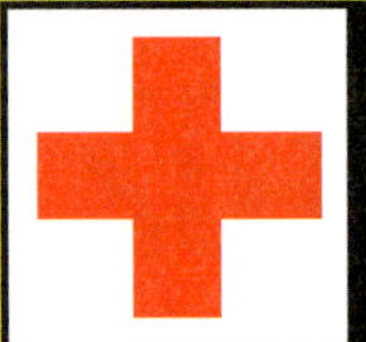

KNEE INSTABILITY

When the knee is extended, the medial and lateral collateral ligaments are stretched and prevent rotation of the joint. When a person is standing on one leg, the knee locks in extension, and there is no need for muscle tension to stabilize the joint.

When the knee is bent, the medial and lateral collateral ligaments are relaxed. In this position, the joint is only stabilized by muscle tension.

When the knee flexes and rotates, the meniscus travels forward to the side that is rotating. If the subsequent extension is not controlled properly, the meniscus may not return to its normal position fast enough. It can then become pinched between the condyles, which can tear the meniscus. If a piece of the meniscus is severed when it is pinched, surgery may be necessary to remove it. With asymmetrical exercises such as forward lunges (see pages 210 and 211), it is important to control the speed and the form of the movement to protect the knee from injury.

KNEE POSITION AND JOINT STABILITY

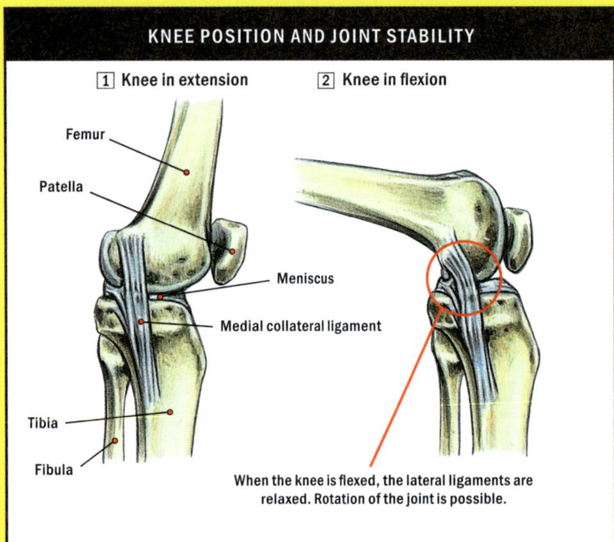

MENISCUS ACTION

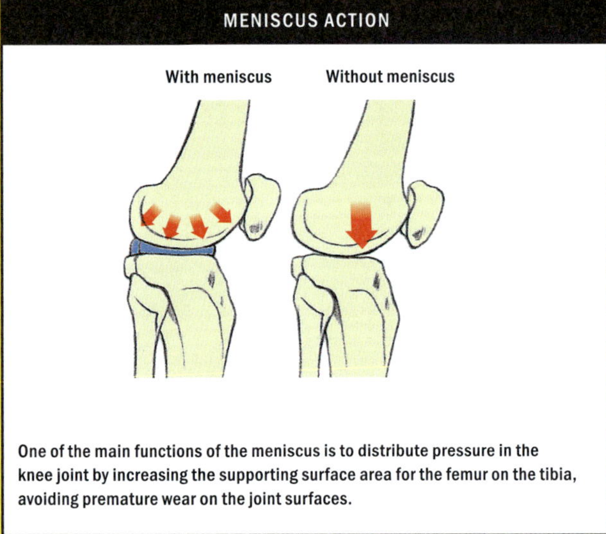

One of the main functions of the meniscus is to distribute pressure in the knee joint by increasing the supporting surface area for the femur on the tibia, avoiding premature wear on the joint surfaces.

DIAGRAM OF THE MENISCUS AND KNEE LIGAMENTS

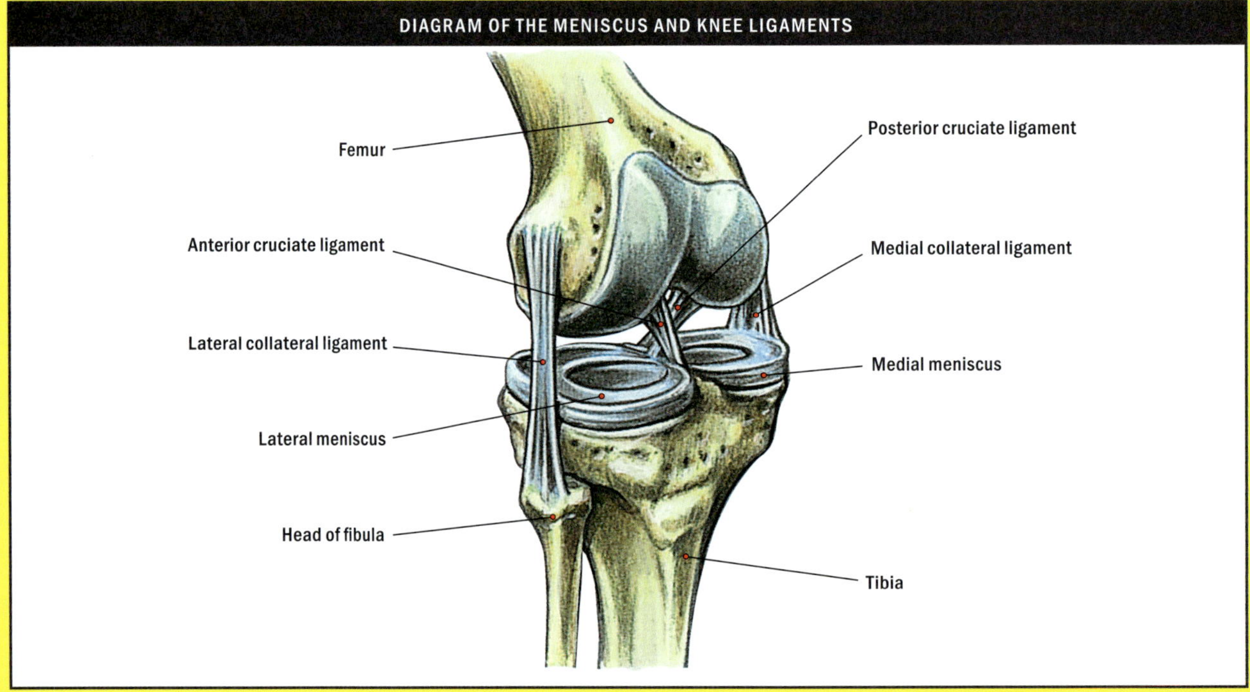

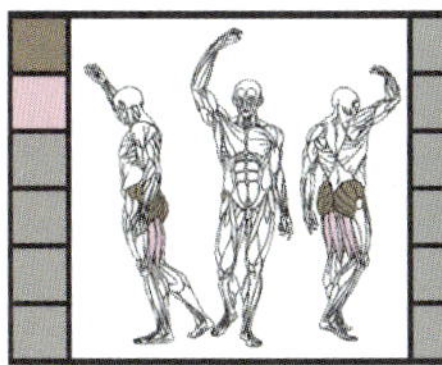

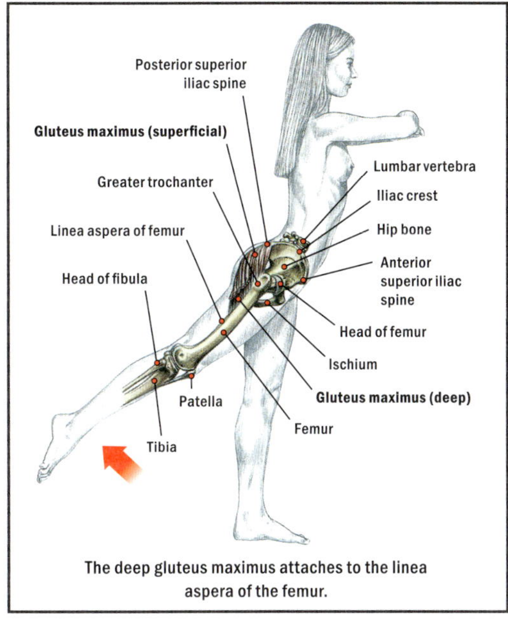

The deep gluteus maximus attaches to the linea aspera of the femur.

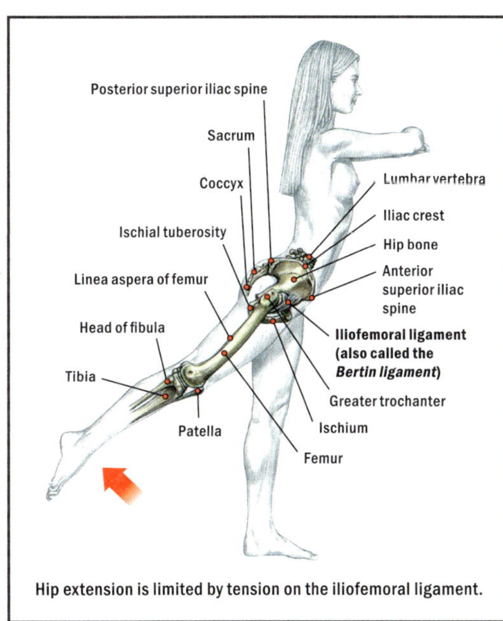

Hip extension is limited by tension on the iliofemoral ligament.

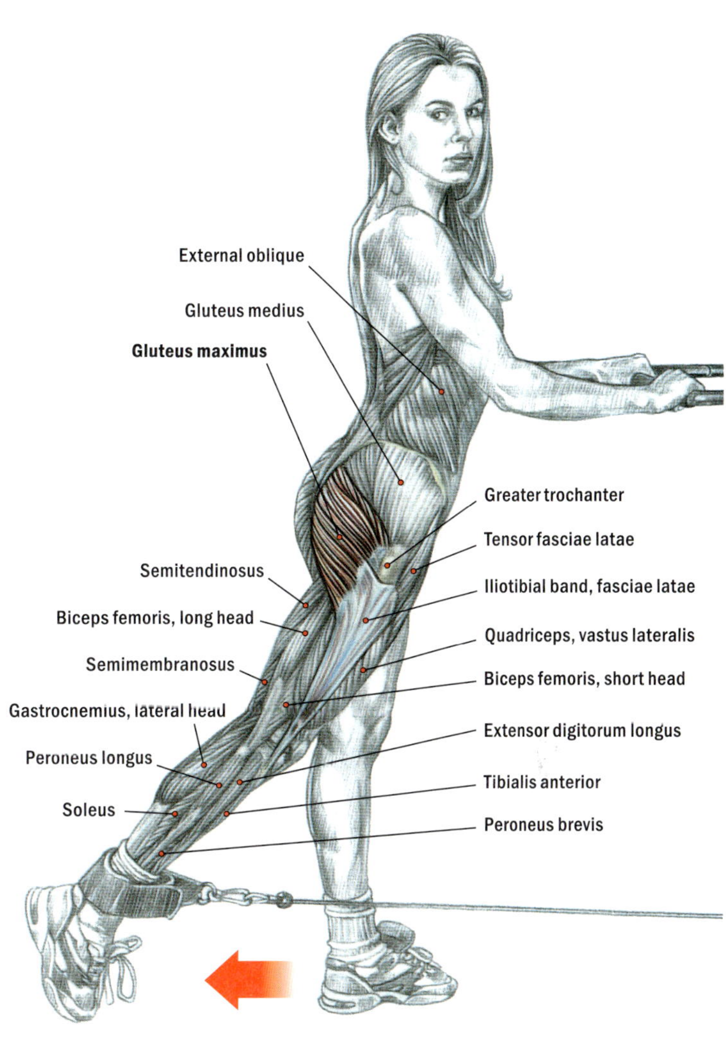

Stand on one leg facing the machine, with the other leg in the ankle strap of a low pulley and your pelvis tilted forward. Grasp the handle with both hands:

- Extend your hip and pull your leg back. Hip extension is limited by the tension on the iliofemoral ligament, also known as the *Bertin ligament*.

This exercise mainly works the gluteus maximus and, to a lesser extent, the hamstrings (except for the short head of the biceps femoris). It helps develop nice curves while firming up the gluteal region.

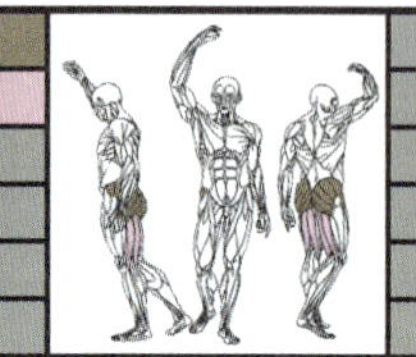

ILIOFEMORAL LIGAMENT

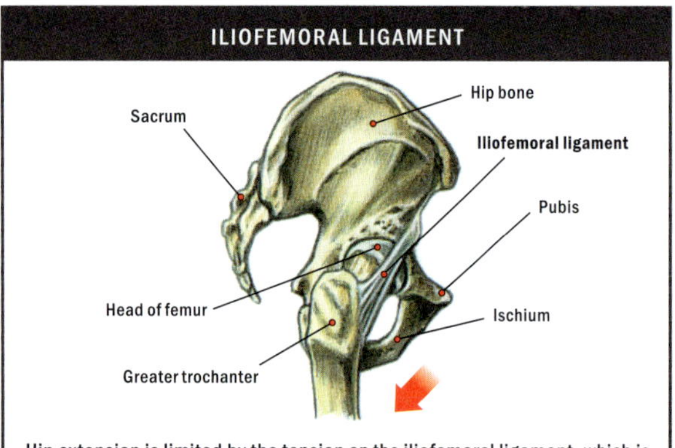

Hip extension is limited by the tension on the iliofemoral ligament, which is actually a thickening of the joint capsule.

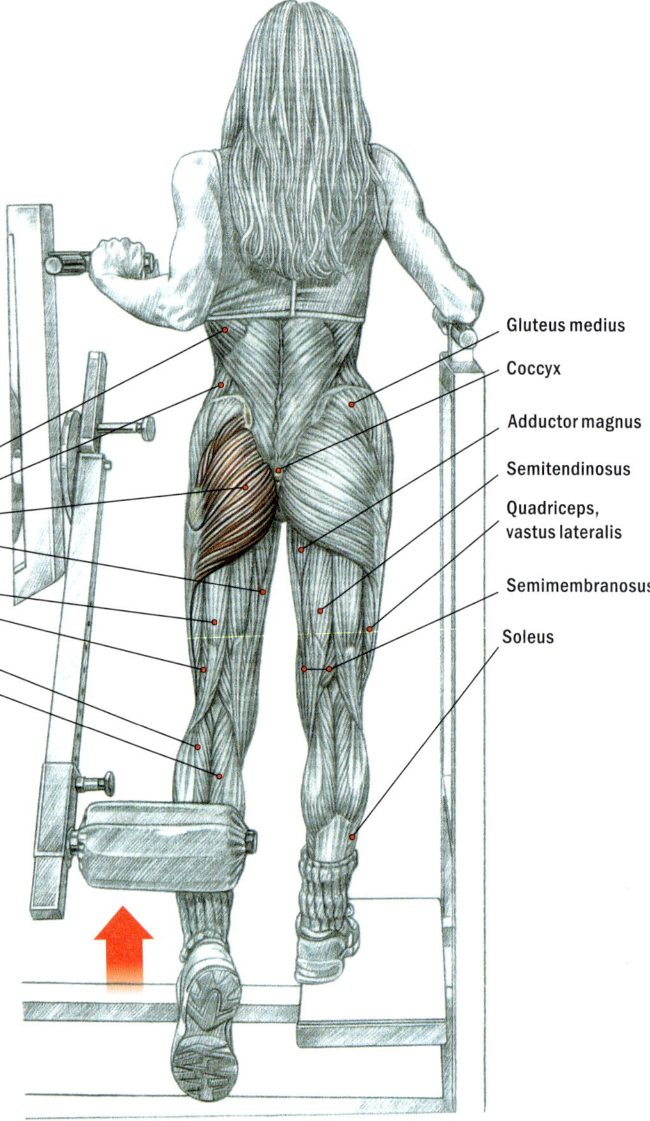

MUSCLES WORKED: POSTERIOR VIEW

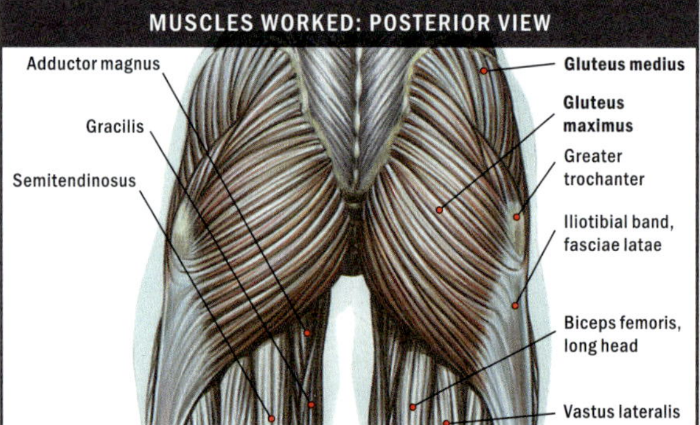

MUSCLES WORKED: THREE-QUARTERS VIEW

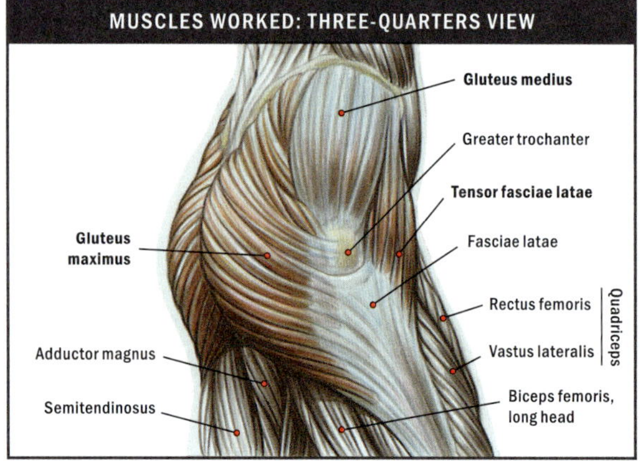

Stand on one leg with the other slightly forward and position the pad against your calf halfway between your knee and your ankle. Lean your torso forward slightly and grasp the handles:

- Inhale and push your thigh back until your hip is hyperextended.
- Hold the position in an isometric contraction for a couple of seconds and return to the starting position. Exhale at the end of the extension.

This exercise mainly works the gluteus maximus and, to a lesser extent, the semitendinosus, semimembranosus, and long head of the biceps femoris.

HIP EXTENSIONS USING THE ASSISTED PULL-UPS AND DIPS MACHINE 05

END OF THE EXERCISE

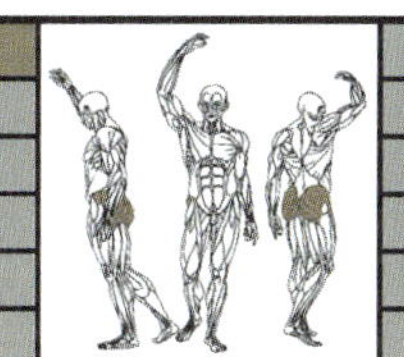

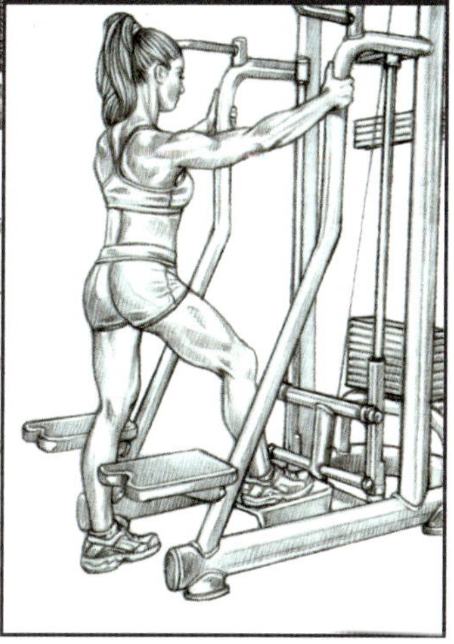

This type of hip extension is done using the assisted pull-ups and dips machine, but it is done in a nontraditional way. Stand with one foot on the ground and the other foot on the machine plate. Bend your leg and hold the machine firmly:

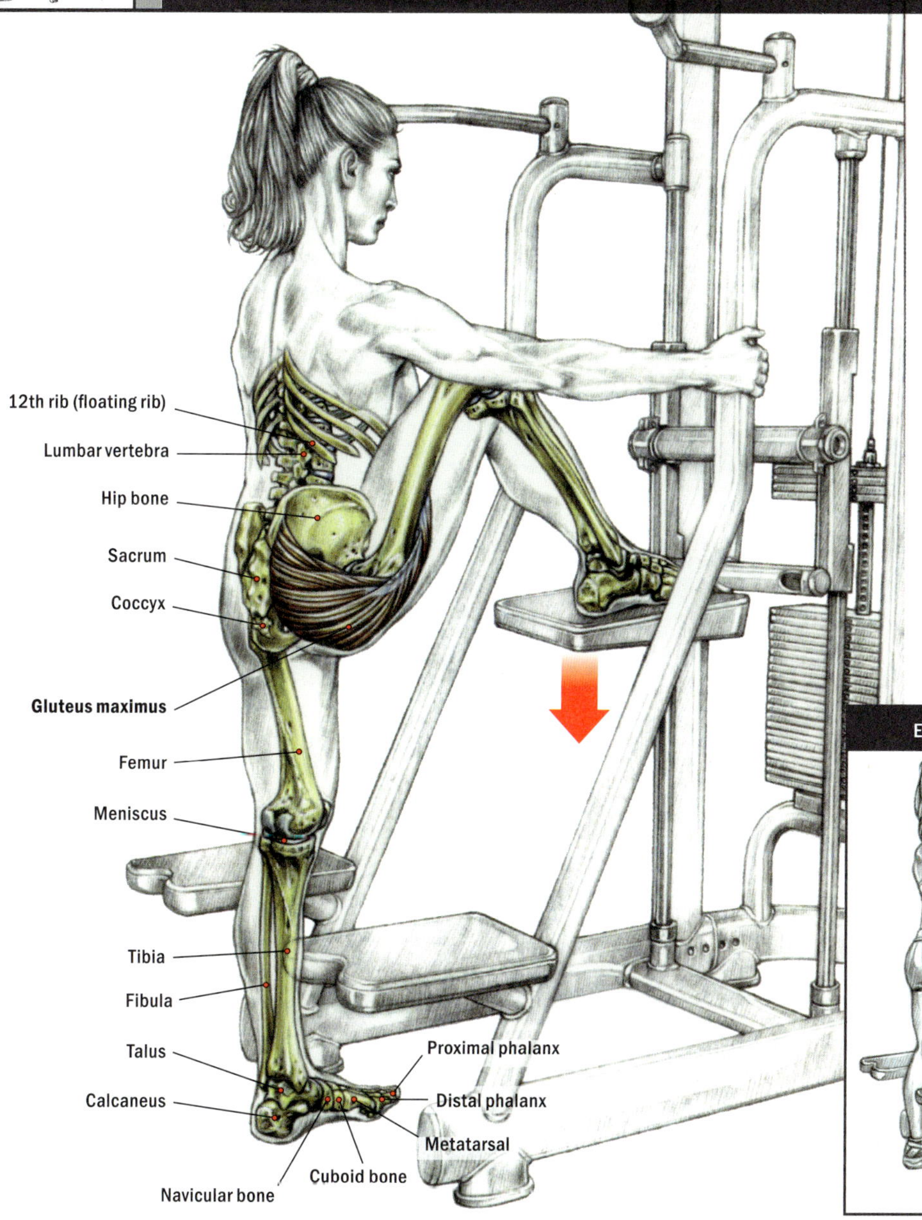

- Inhale, hold your breath, and straighten your leg. Exhale at the end of the exercise.
- Return to the starting position while controlling your movement.

This exercise mainly works the gluteus maximus and, to a lesser degree, the quadriceps, while stretching the adductor magnus. What makes this exercise interesting is that it stretches the gluteus maximus favorably when the thigh is flexed, and this makes it possible to feel and target the work on this muscle. For individuals whose buttocks are a weak point, this is one of those rare exercises that lets them feel the muscle working and to catch up on its development.

Sets of 10 to 20 reps provide the best results.

For additional stability, when using heavier weight, lean your torso farther forward, and grip the machine tighter.

06 FLOOR HIP EXTENSIONS

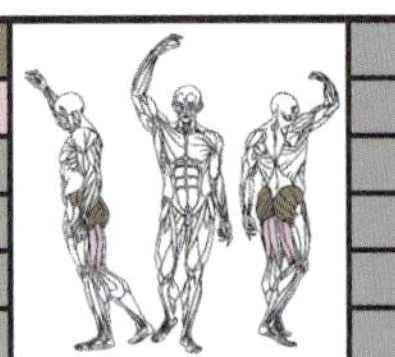

Soleus
Gastrocnemius, lateral head
Peroneus longus
Biceps femoris, short head
Semimembranosus
Biceps femoris, long head
Semitendinosus
Gluteus maximus
Gluteus medius
Tibialis anterior
Extensor digitorum longus
Fasciae latae
Quadriceps
Vastus lateralis
Rectus femoris
Tensor fasciae latae
Greater trochanter
External oblique

2 Finish
1 Start

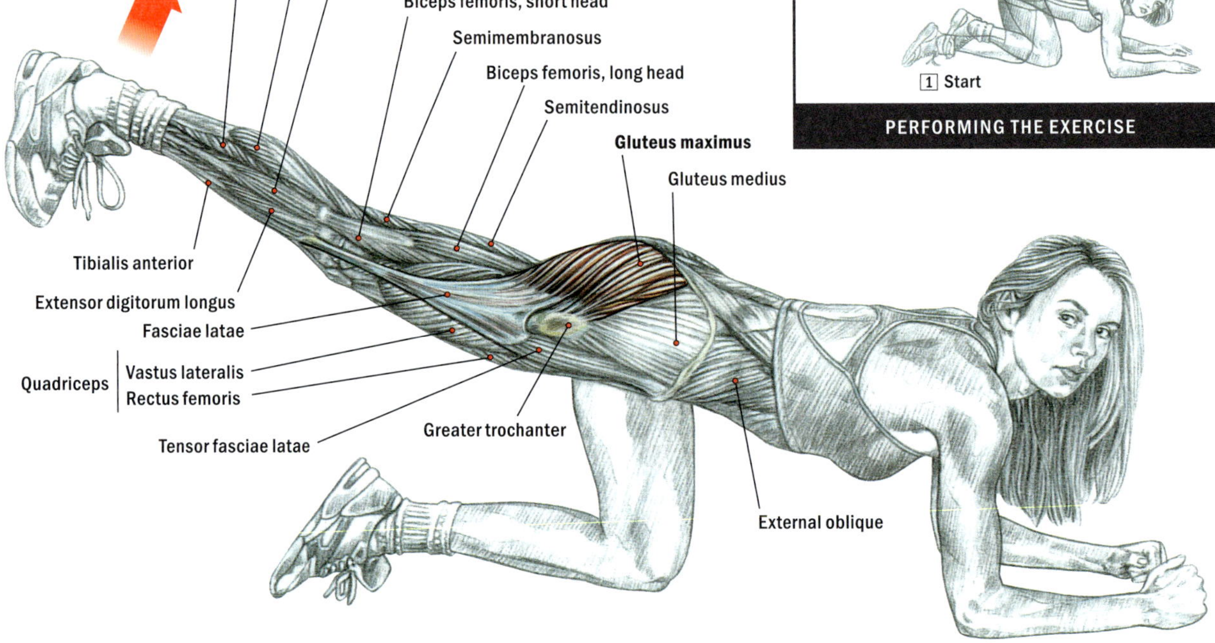

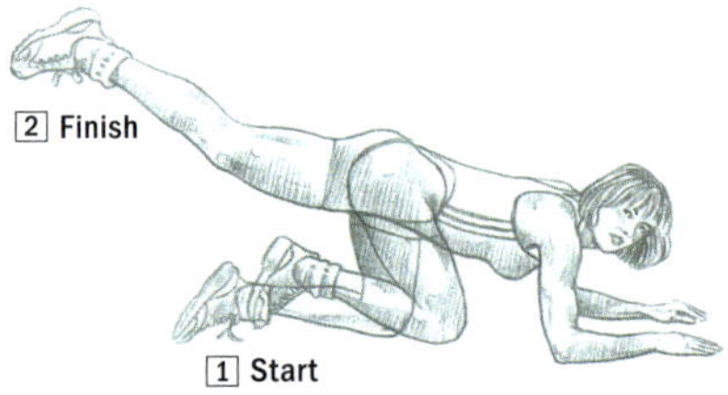

PERFORMING THE EXERCISE

Kneel on one leg and bring the other knee up to your chest while supporting your body on your elbows or on your hands with your arms extended:

- Extend the bent leg back with complete hip extension.

With your leg extended, this exercise works the hamstrings and gluteus maximus. With the knee bent, only the gluteus maximus is used, and it is less intense. This exercise can be done with a wide range of motion or with a smaller range of motion during the last part of the extension. You can hold an isometric contraction for 1 or 2 seconds at the end of the exercise. To increase the intensity, use ankle weights. Its ease of execution and effectiveness have made this exercise very popular, and it is frequently used in group classes.

VARIATION ON A BENCH

1 Start
2 Finish

VARIATION WITH BENT KNEE

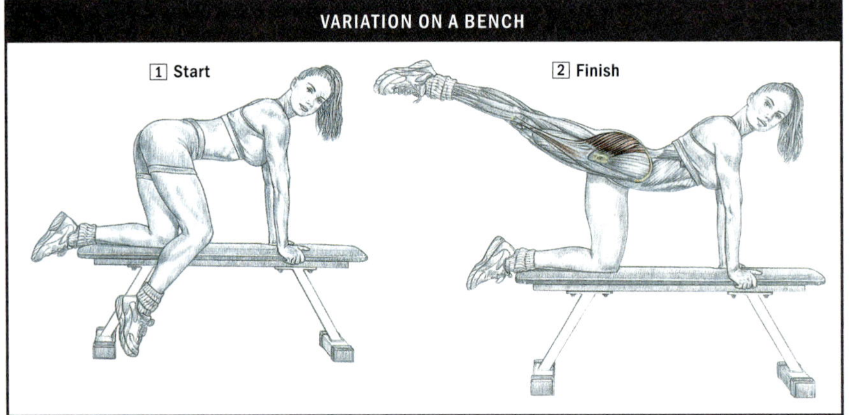

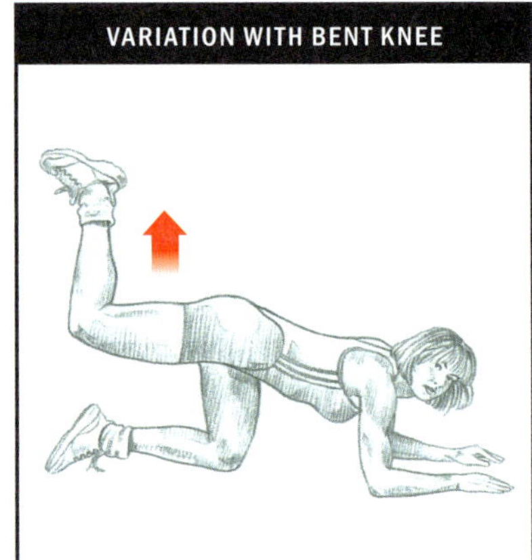

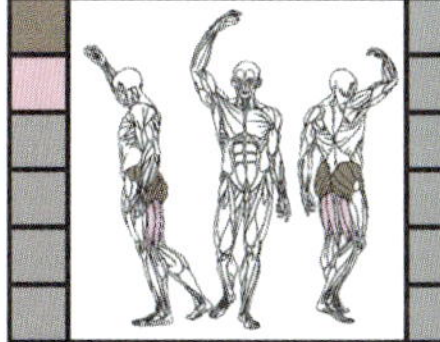

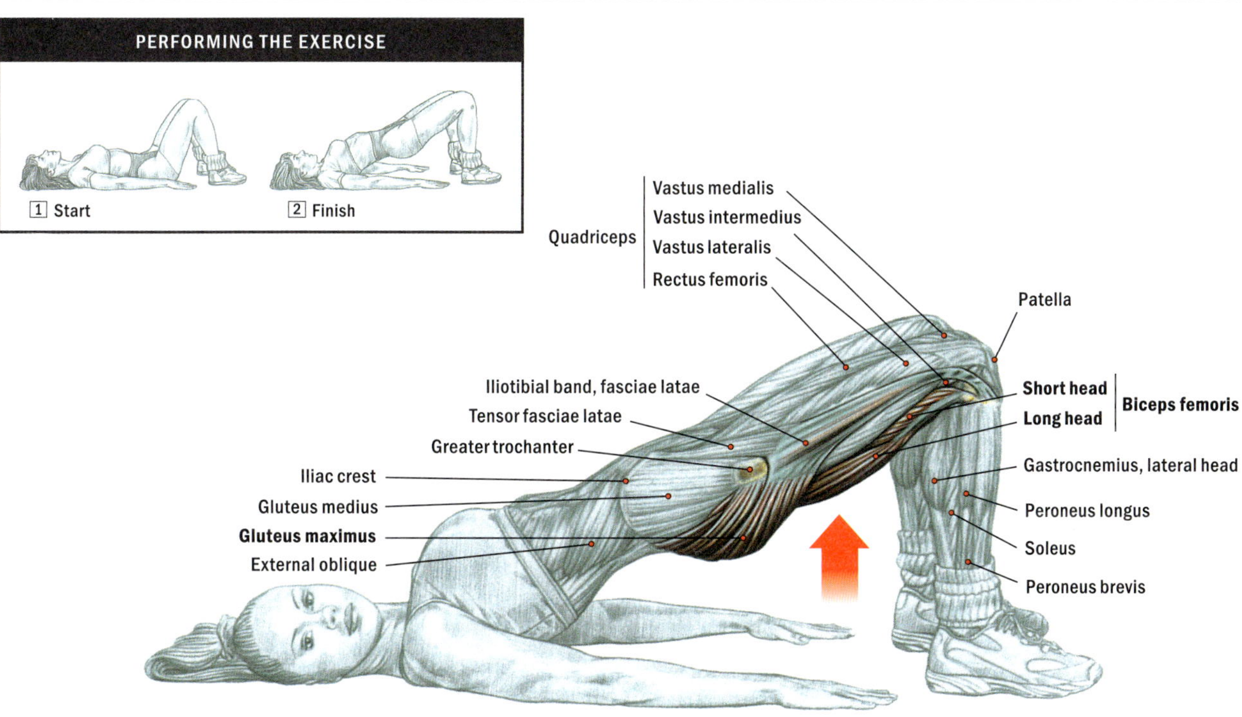

Lie on your back with your hands flat on the ground, your arms alongside your body, and your knees bent:

- Inhale and lift your buttocks off the ground, pushing down through your feet.
- Hold the position for a couple of seconds and lower your pelvis without letting your buttocks touch the ground.
- Exhale and repeat.

This exercise mainly works the hamstrings and gluteus maximus.

Do this exercise in long sets, making sure to contract the muscles at the top of the lift, when your pelvis is off the ground.

It is possible to do this exercise with a small range of motion, without lowering your pelvis too close to the floor until you feel the burn.

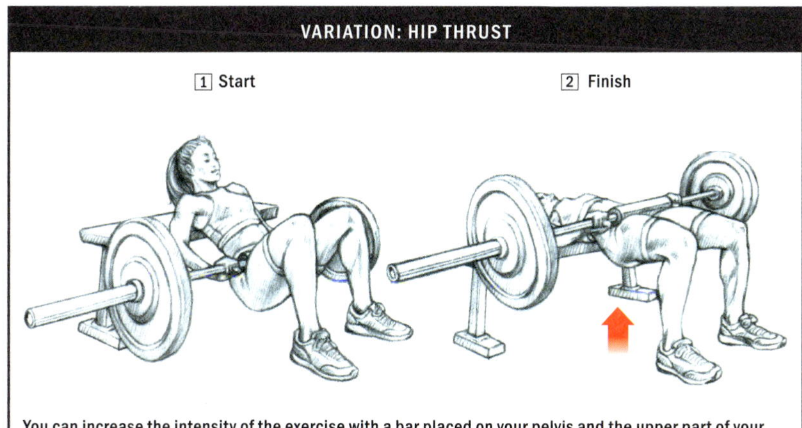

You can increase the intensity of the exercise with a bar placed on your pelvis and the upper part of your torso supported on a bench. In this variation, it is best to place a rubber pad around the bar so that it does not press down painfully on the pelvis and thighs.

Because it is easy and effective, bridges have become part of most group exercise classes.

It is important to note, however, that bridges are, in reality, a type of hip extension.

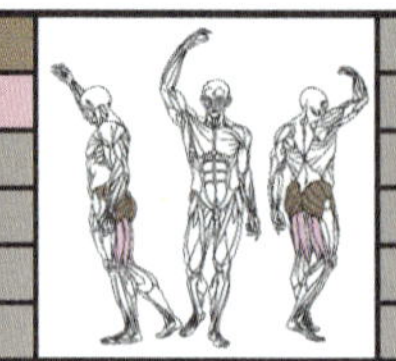

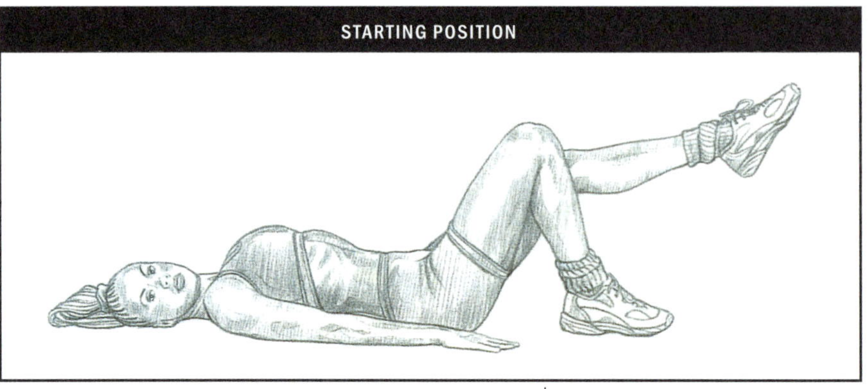

STARTING POSITION

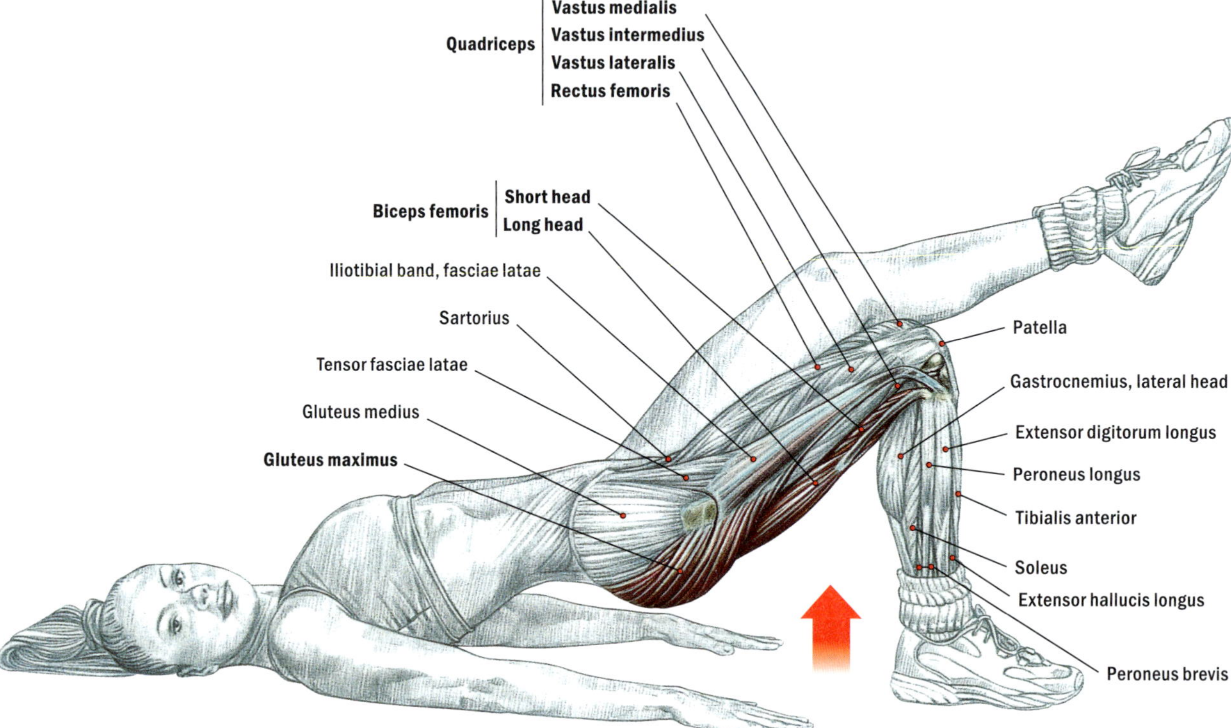

Lie on your back with your hands flat on the ground, arms alongside your body, one knee bent with your foot flat on the floor, and the other leg extended up off the floor:

- Inhale and lift your buttocks off the ground, pushing down as hard as you can through the foot on the floor.
- Hold the position for a couple of seconds and lower your pelvis without letting your buttocks touch the ground.
- Exhale and repeat.

This exercise mainly works the hamstring muscles (semitendinosus, semimembranosus, and biceps femoris) and the gluteus maximus. It should be performed using high-repetition sets, making sure that you feel the contraction of the muscles at the top of the pelvic lift.

You can do a full set on one side and then on the other, or you can alternate legs during the same set by resting your back on the ground after each repetition.

BRIDGES WITH BOTH FEET RAISED 09

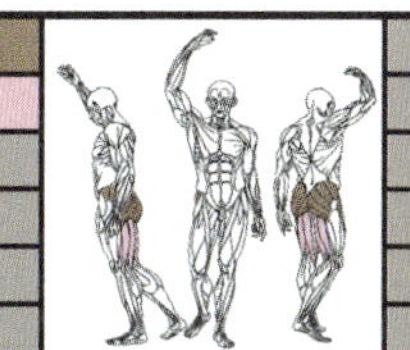

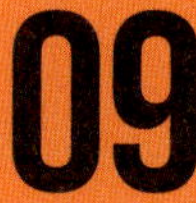

STARTING POSITION

Rectus femoris
Vastus lateralis
Vastus medialis
Vastus intermedius
Quadriceps
Patella
Gastrocnemius, lateral head
Peroneus longus
Soleus
Peroneus brevis
Iliotibial band, fasciae latae
Greater trochanter
Tensor fasciae latae
Gluteus maximus
Gluteus medius
Iliac crest
External oblique
Short head
Long head
Biceps femoris

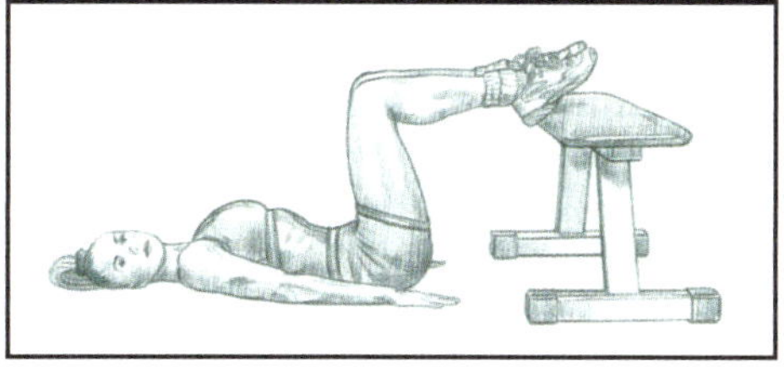

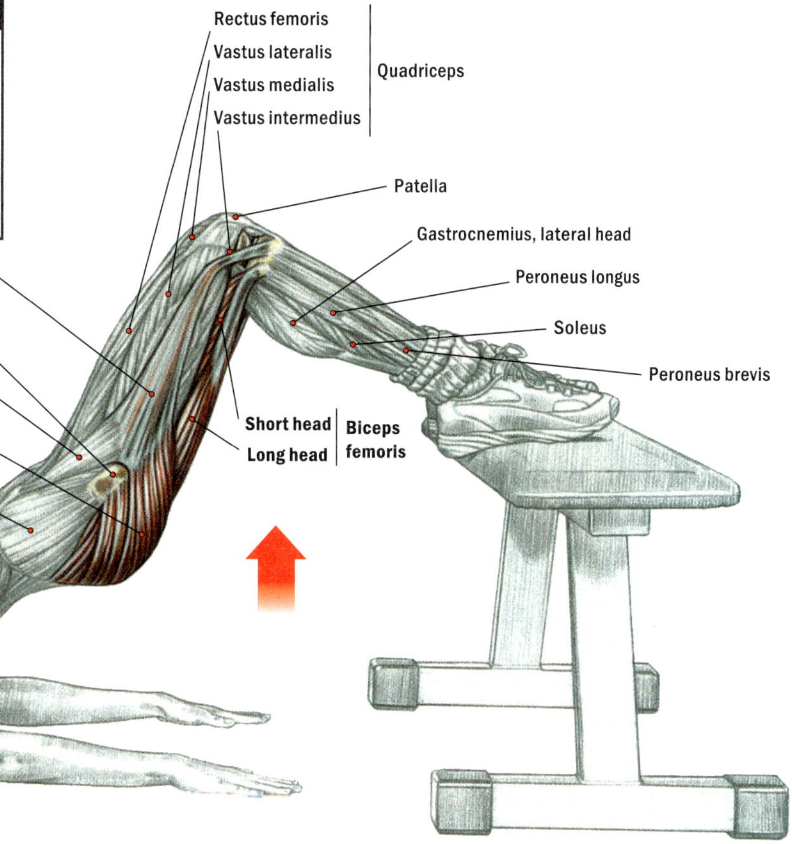

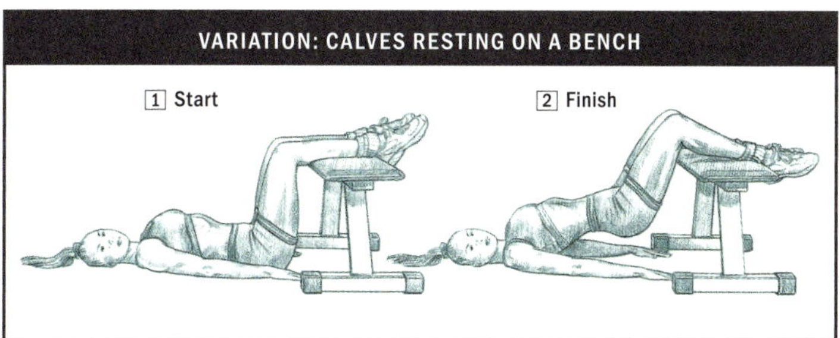

VARIATION: CALVES RESTING ON A BENCH

1 Start
2 Finish

Lie on your back with your hands flat at your sides, your arms alongside your body, your thighs vertical, and your feet resting on a bench:

- Inhale and raise your buttocks off the ground.
- Hold the position for a couple of seconds and lower your pelvis without letting your buttocks touch the ground.
- Exhale and repeat.

This exercise works the gluteus maximus. It also puts special emphasis on the hamstrings. The hamstrings are used more in this exercise than when bridging from the ground. Do this exercise slowly, focusing on the muscle contraction. Sets of 10 to 15 reps provide the best results.

Variations

- Limit the range of motion by not lowering your pelvis as far toward the ground and keep going until you feel the burn.
- Bridging with the calves resting on a bench works the hamstrings even more intensely and also requires a strong contribution from the gastrocnemius muscles.

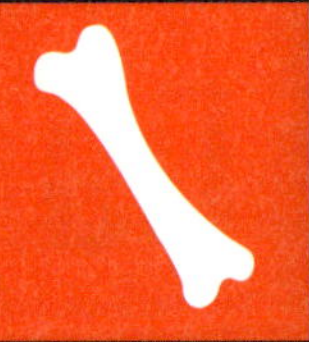

FAT DEPOSITS IN MEN AND WOMEN

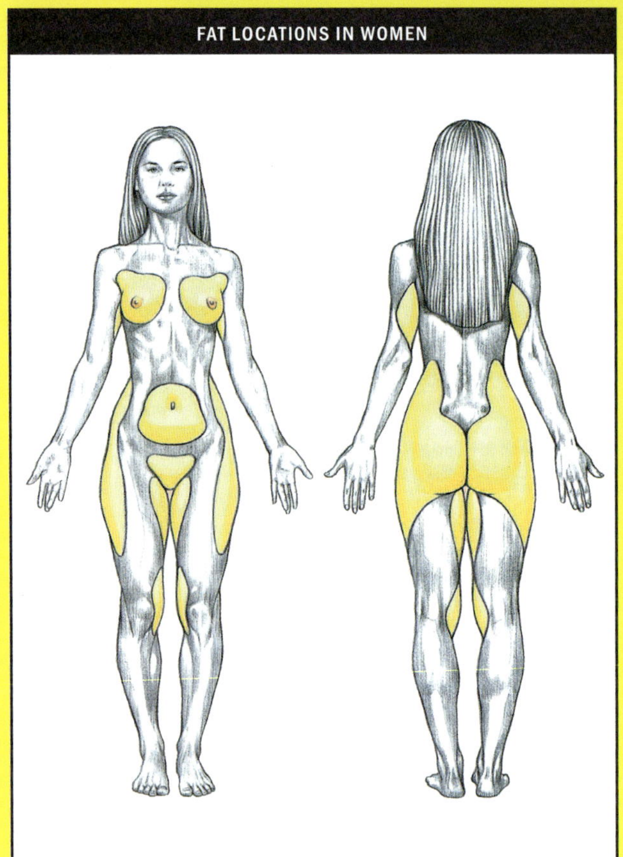

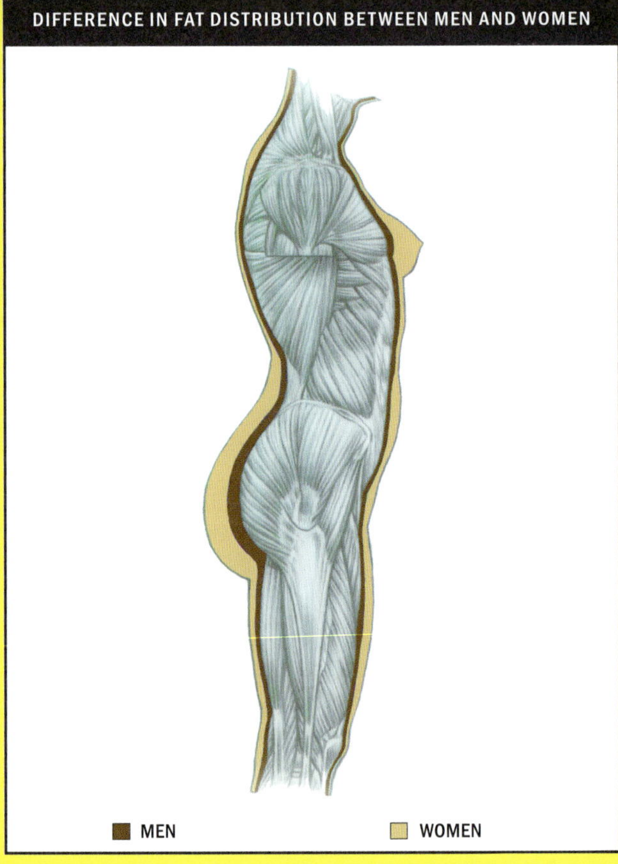

One of the main morphological differences between men and women is the greater amount of fat in the female body, which softens the muscular contours, hides the bony protrusions, and rounds out surfaces.

In the average woman, fat makes up between 18 and 25 percent of the body weight, whereas in the average man, it generally represents only 10 to 15 percent. This difference is because the woman will, at some point in her life, be able to nourish a fetus; she must, therefore, store energy in the form of fat for possible future pregnancies (and periods of scarcity). It is important to point out that every healthy person has a reserve of fat necessary for the proper functioning of his or her body, and the obsessive fear of obesity or the need to identify with unhealthy aesthetics should not lead to its total disappearance. In fact, the near total disappearance of fat can lead to serious hormonal problems, such as the lack of menstrual periods (amenorrhea) and the temporary absence of ovulation.

In addition to this difference in mass, the location of fat also differs between men and women. Fat in women is more likely to be found around the hips, while in men it can be found in the abdominal area. The reason for this is both hormonal and related to reproduction. Since a woman carries her child in the abdominal region during pregnancy, it would be a hindrance for fat to be stored in this area. Her energy reserves tend to be located near the center of gravity so as not to hinder walking and movement; thus, it is generally located subcutaneously on the buttocks, hips, and upper thighs.

In men, on the other hand, fat tends to accumulate less in the subcutaneous area and more in between the viscera, in the belly—closer to the center of gravity. Fat located at the core of the body has the advantage of being easily accessible to provide energy quickly, unlike subcutaneous fat, which is more difficult to metabolize since it is compressed by the fibers connecting the skin to the muscle fascia or the bones.

These stores are an asset in the event of an immediate and major energy requirement such as running or strength work. However, unfortunately, with our sedentary lifestyle and our unfettered access to food, they have become a disadvantage and even a danger. This is because, in overweight individuals, the unused visceral fat is associated with vascular problems or degenerative diseases such as diabetes.

STRETCHING THE GLUTEUS MAXIMUS AND HAMSTRINGS

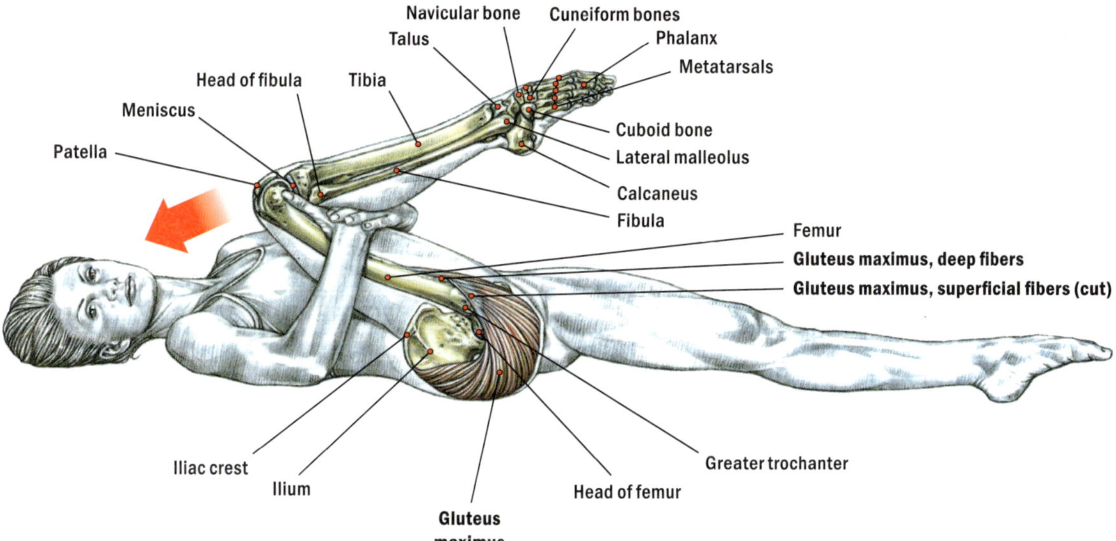

Lie on your back with your legs extended on the floor:

- Gently guide one leg with your knee bent (to relax your hamstring muscles) up to your chest with your hands.
- Hold the stretch, breathing slowly and trying to feel the stretch in your gluteus maximus muscle.
- Return to the starting position and then change legs and repeat.

Variation

You can do this stretch by bringing the straight leg toward your chest. In this case, the stretch will be more intense on the hamstrings but less so on the gluteus maximus. Note that tension on the hamstring muscles may severely restrict bending at the hip for certain individuals.

VARIATION WITH A STRAIGHT LEG

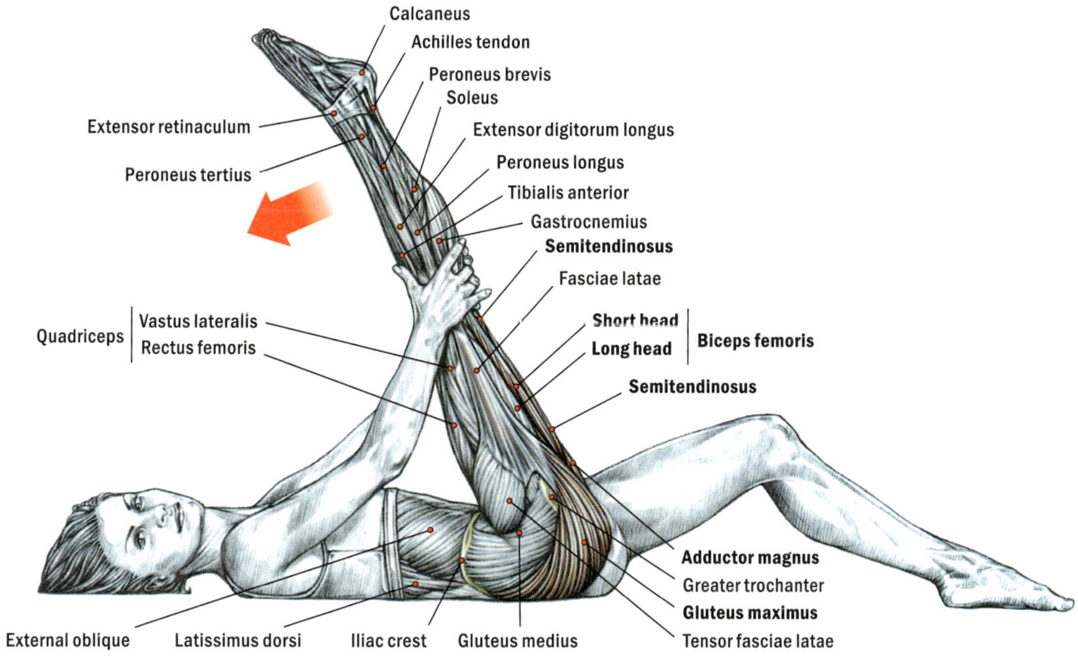

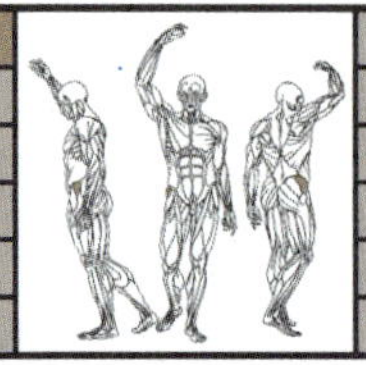

GLUTEAL INSERTIONS ON THE HIP BONE

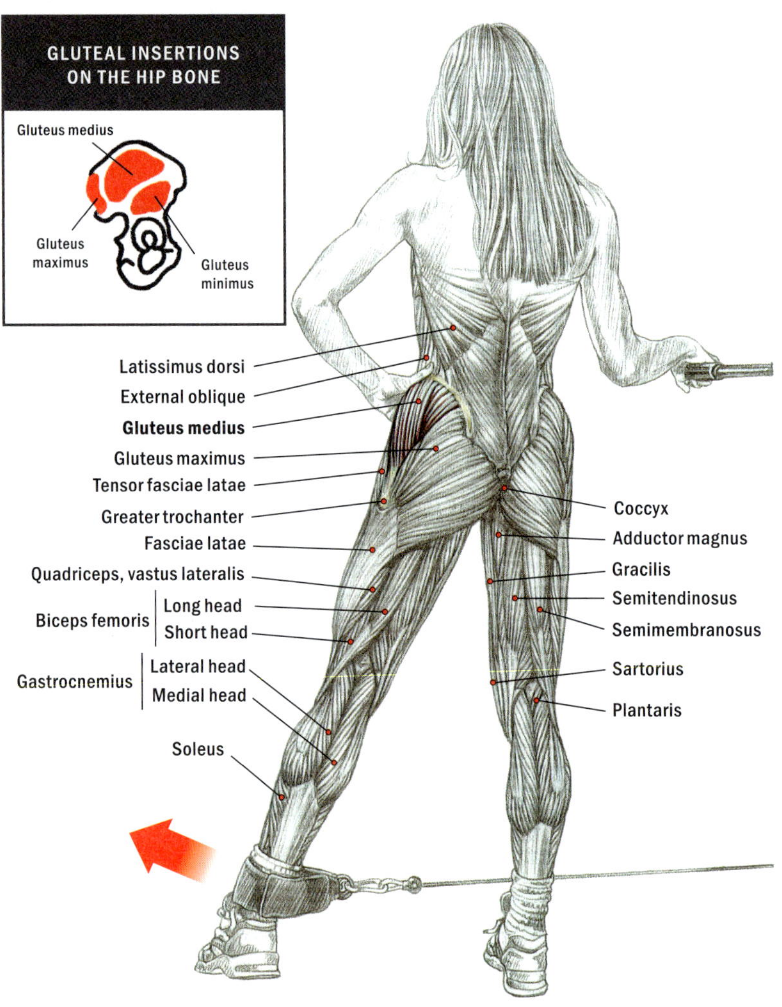

SECTION OF A FEMALE HIP SHOWING THE GLUTEUS MEDIUS AND THE GLUTEUS MINIMUS

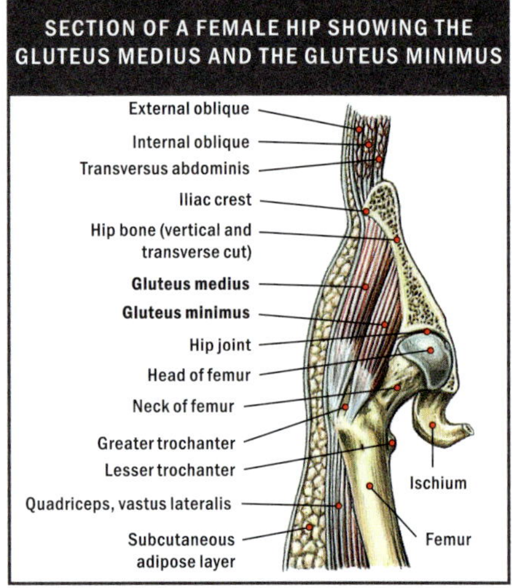

GLUTEAL "DELTOID"

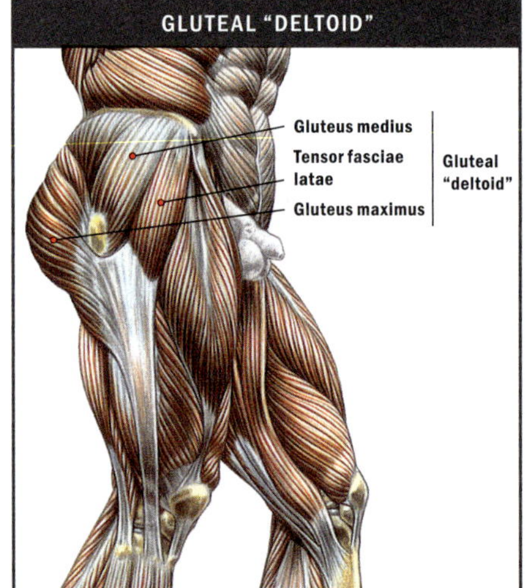

GLUTEUS MINIMUS MUSCLE

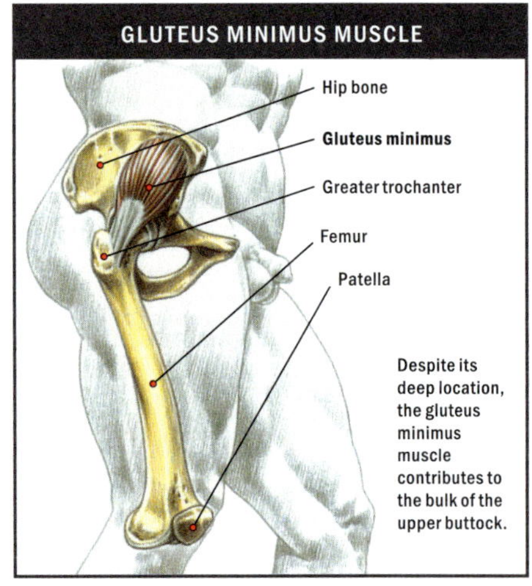

Despite its deep location, the gluteus minimus muscle contributes to the bulk of the upper buttock.

Stand on one leg with a pulley attached to the other ankle, using the opposite hand for support to keep your body steady:

- Raise your leg to the side as high as possible.

This exercise mainly works the gluteus medius and the deeper gluteus minimus muscle. To make this exercise most effective, do long sets until you feel a burn.

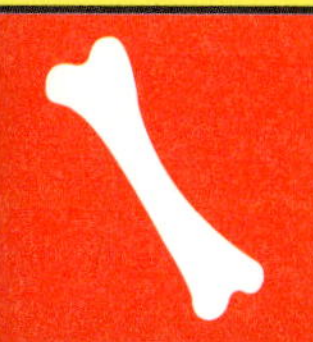

Regardless of individual muscle flexibility and tension in the ligaments, the shape of the bones of the hip joint is primarily responsible for variations in hip mobility. Bone structure plays a crucial role in the range of motion possible in hip abduction.

Examples

- When the neck of the femur is almost horizontal (coxa vara) and associated with a well-developed superior rim of the acetabulum covering the head of the femur, abduction movements are limited.
- When the neck of the femur is close to a vertical position (coxa valga) and associated with an undeveloped superior acetabular rim, abduction movements are easier.

So it is pointless to try to raise the leg high laterally if your hip joint does not lend itself to the movement.

If hip abduction is forced, the neck of the femur will hit the rim of the acetabulum, and the pelvis will tilt onto the head of the opposite femur to compensate for the lateral extension of the leg. For some individuals, performing sets of forced abductions may lead to microtraumas over time, and these may lead to excessive development of the superior rim of the acetabulum, limiting hip mobility and risking painful inflammation.

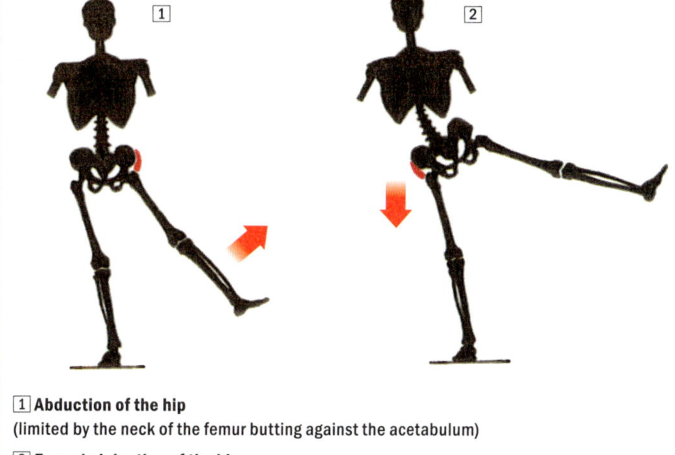

1 **Abduction of the hip**
(limited by the neck of the femur butting against the acetabulum)

2 **Forced abduction of the hip**
(tilting the pelvis onto the head of the opposite femur)

HIP JOINT

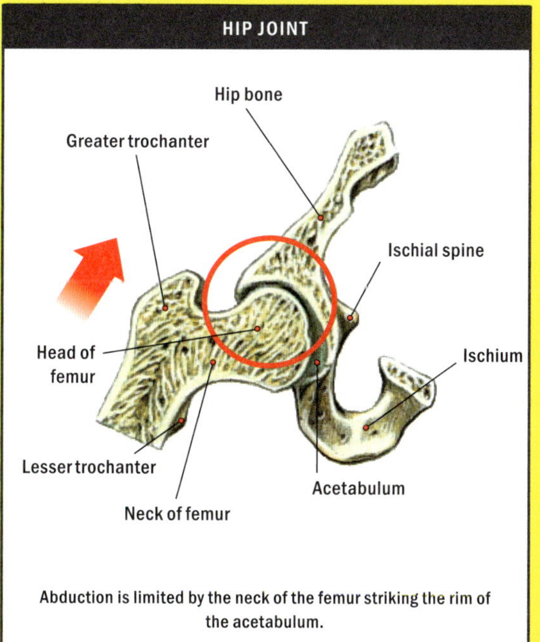

Abduction is limited by the neck of the femur striking the rim of the acetabulum.

DIFFERENT HIP BONE MORPHOLOGIES

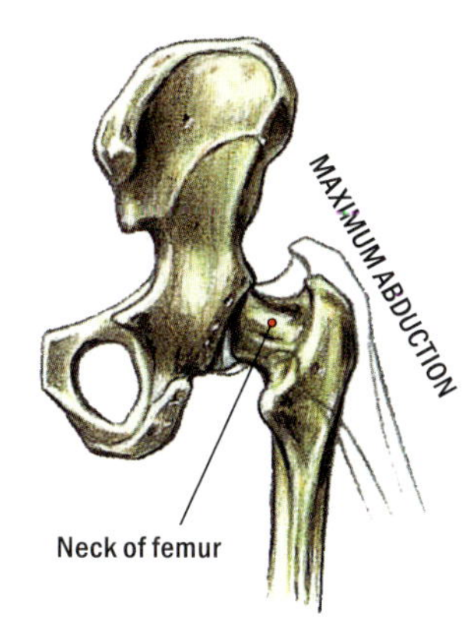

An almost horizontal neck of the femur is called *coxa vara*. It limits abduction movements because it strikes the rim of the acetabulum more quickly.

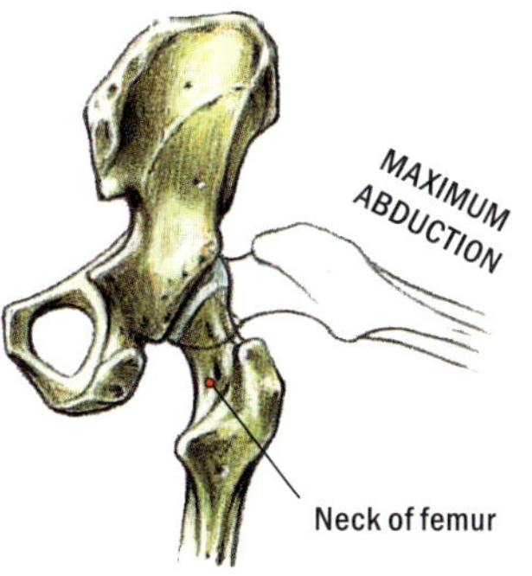

An almost vertical neck of the femur is called *coxa valga*. It allows greater abduction movements.

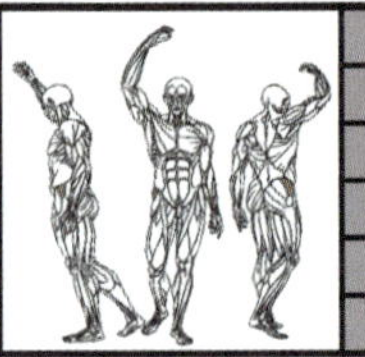

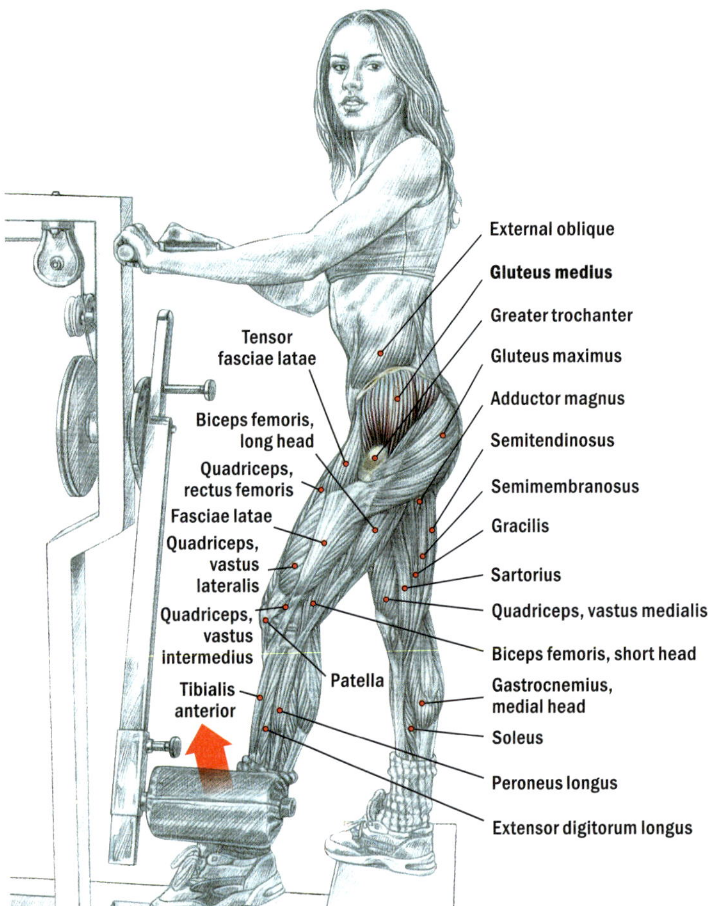

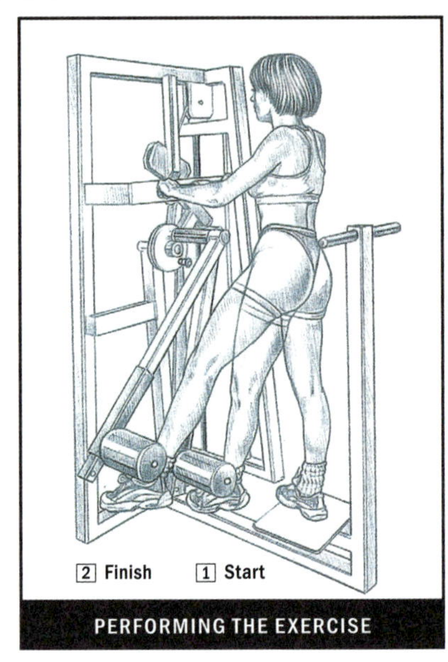

Stand on one leg at the machine and place the outside of your other leg against the pad, above your ankle joint:

- Slowly raise your leg as high as possible and then slowly return to the starting position.

Abduction is limited by the fact that the neck of the femur quickly strikes the rim of the acetabulum.

This exercise is excellent for developing the gluteus medius. It also develops the deeper gluteus minimus, whose function is identical to the anterior fibers of the gluteus medius. For best results, work in long sets.

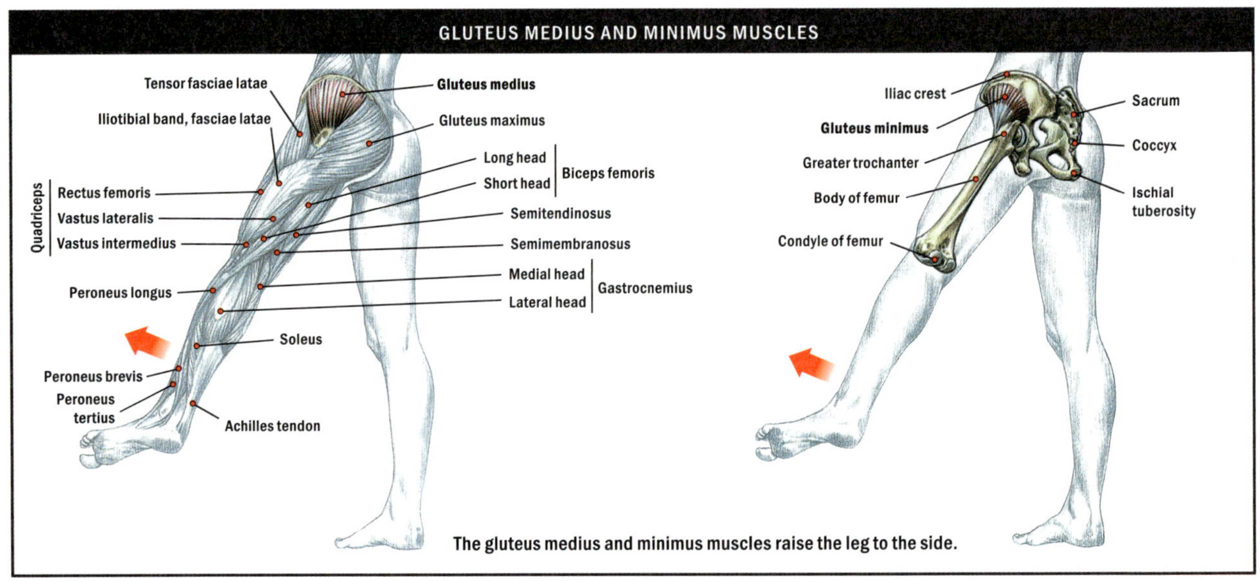

The gluteus medius and minimus muscles raise the leg to the side.

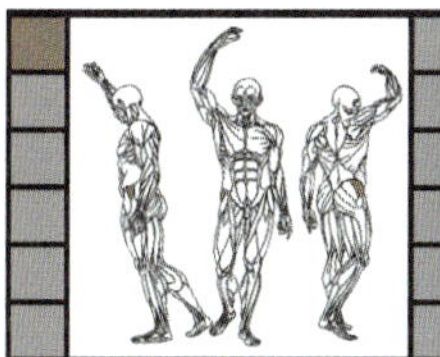

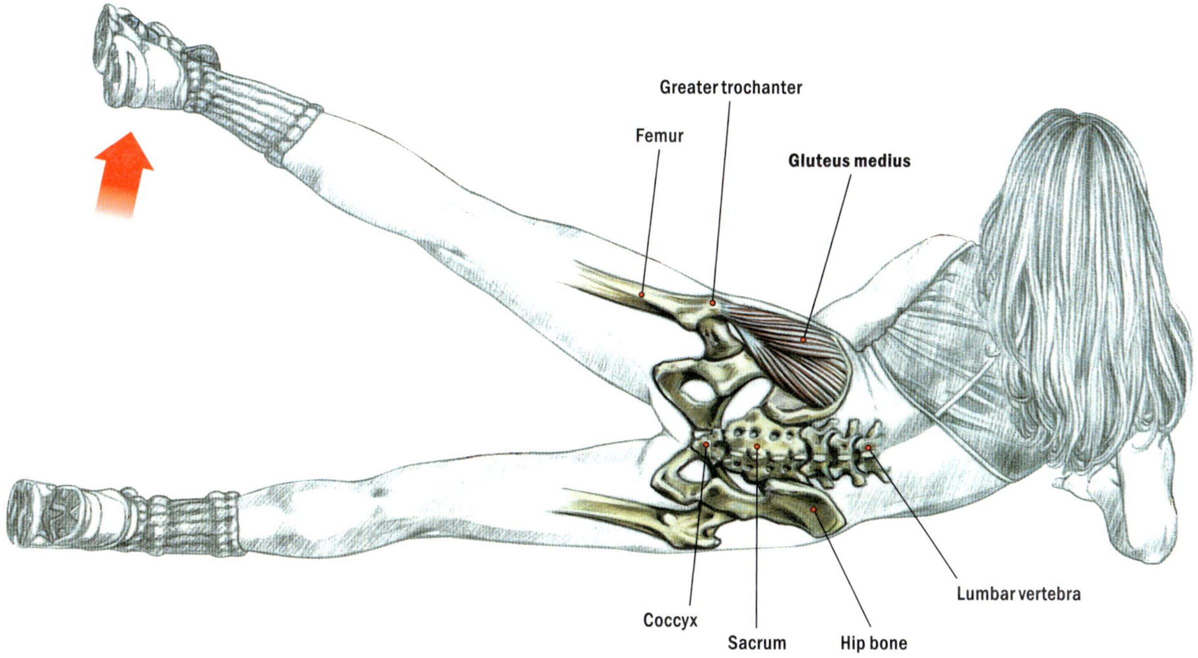

PERFORMING THE EXERCISE

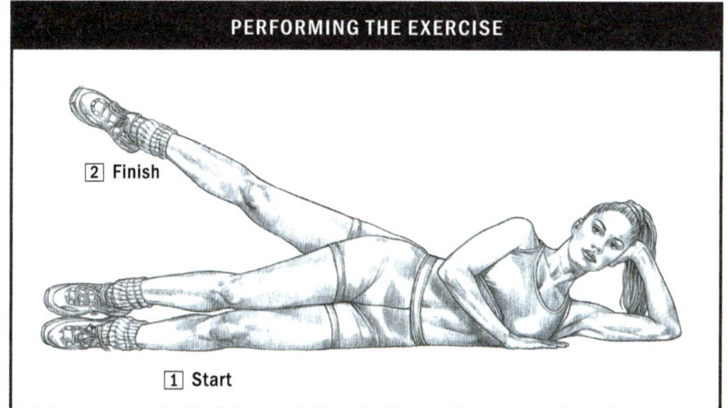

Lie on one side and support the upper body with your forearm:

- Raise your leg up no more than 70 degrees, keeping your knee straight.

This exercise works the gluteus medius and minimus. You can change how high you raise your leg. Hold your leg at the height of the abduction for a few seconds with an isometric contraction. You can raise your leg slightly to the front or the back or just raise it vertically. For increased effectiveness, you can use ankle weights, an elastic band, or a low pulley.

THREE WAYS TO RAISE THE LEG

AREAS RECRUITED

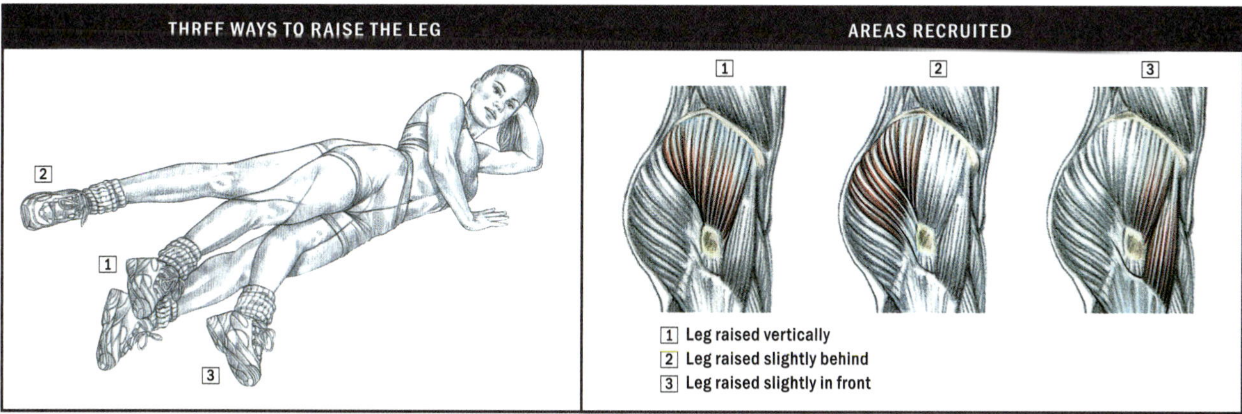

1 Leg raised vertically
2 Leg raised slightly behind
3 Leg raised slightly in front

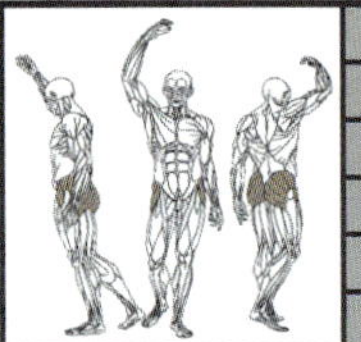

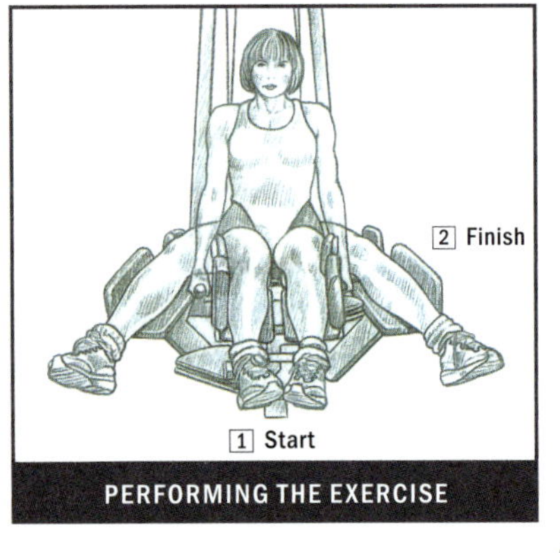

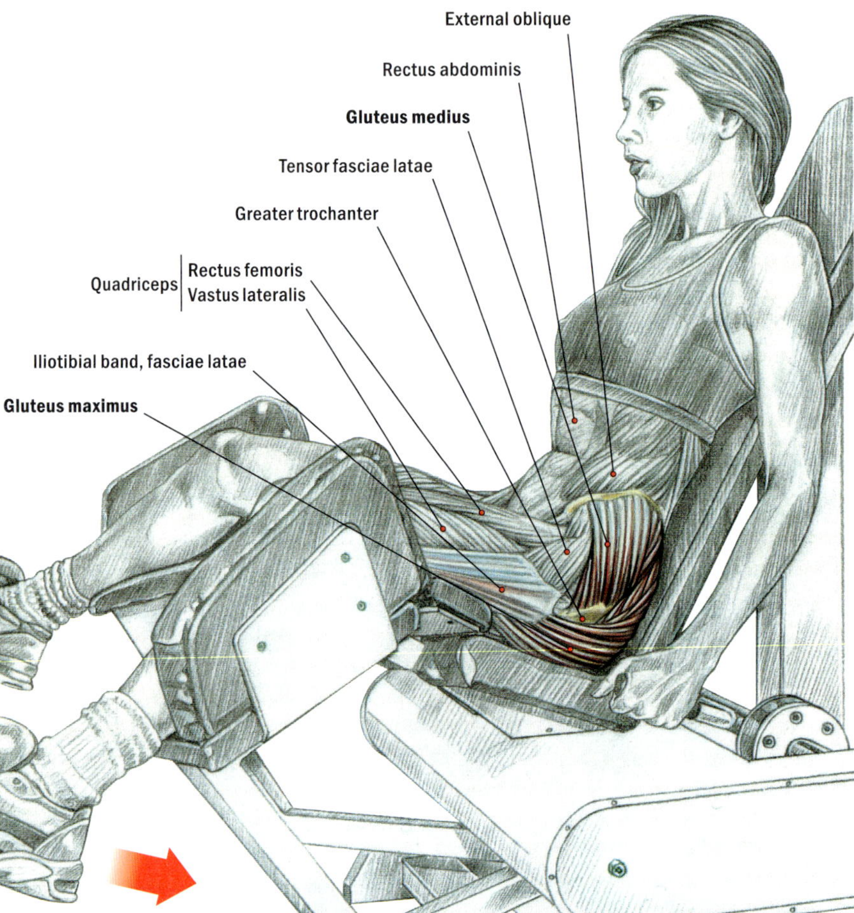

Sit at the machine:

- Spread your legs as wide as possible.

The more inclined the backrest is, the more the gluteus medius will work. The more vertical the backrest is, the more the upper part of the gluteus maximus will work. Ideally, you should change the angle of your torso during a set by leaning forward. You could, for example, do 10 reps with your torso resting against the backrest and 10 reps with your torso leaning forward. This exercise is excellent for women, as it sculpts and firms the top of the hip, which makes the waistline look narrower.

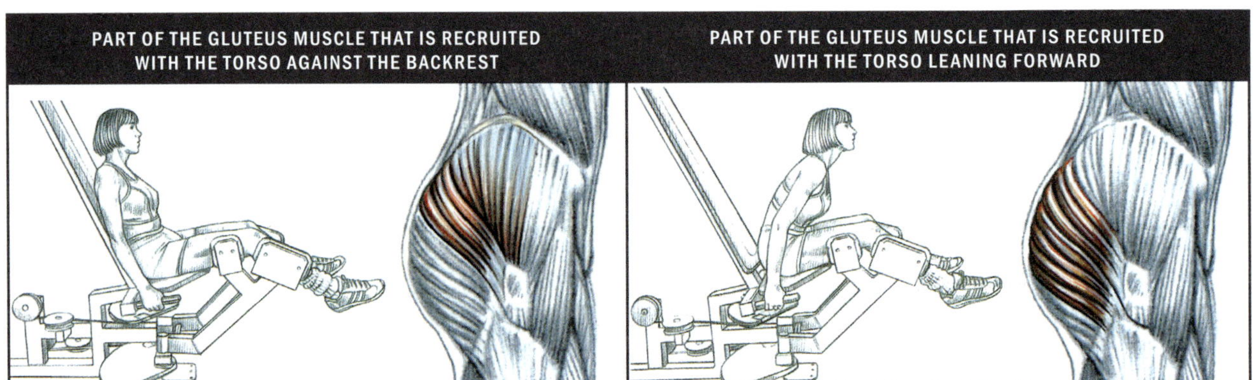

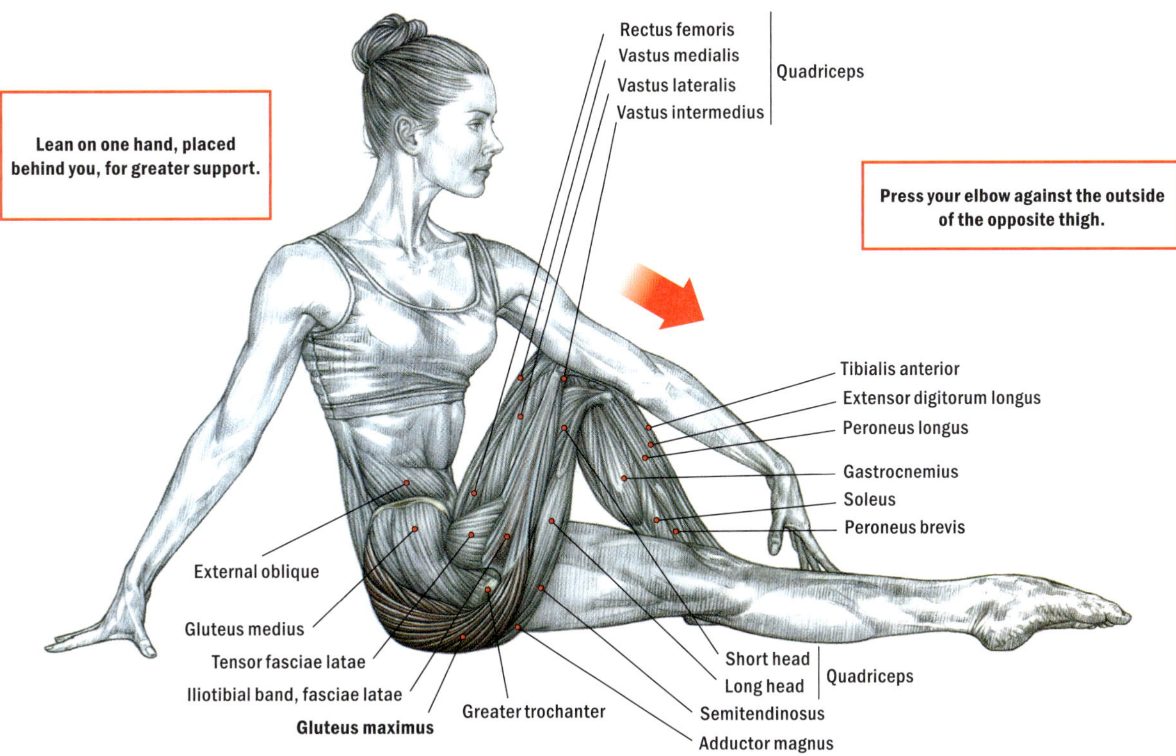

VARIATION TO ACCENTUATE THE STRETCH IN THE LUMBAR REGION

This variation stretches the internal oblique, erector spinae, and splenius capitis on the side of the leg that is on the floor. It also stretches the external oblique, rotators, multifidus of the neck, and sternocleidomastoid on the side of the bent leg.

Sit on the floor with one leg extended and the other bent with your foot on the floor to the outside of the extended leg:

- Put pressure on the knee of the bent leg with the opposite elbow.

This stretch is primarily for the gluteus maximus muscle and, on a deeper level, the rotator muscles of the hip (pyramidalis, gastrocnemius, quadratus femoris, and obturator internus and externus).

Variation

Rather than use your elbow to put pressure against your knee, you can use both hands.

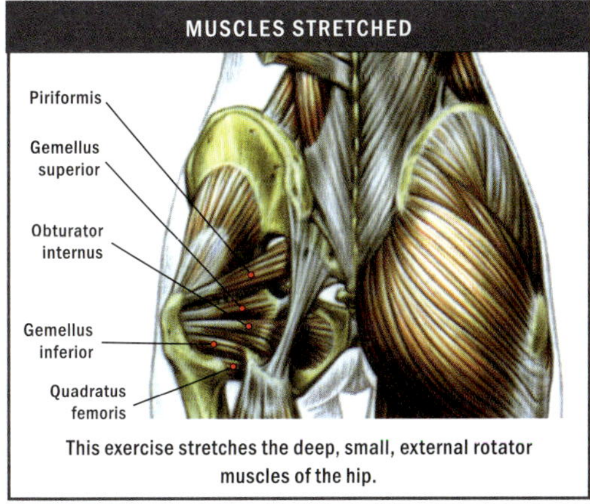

MUSCLES STRETCHED

This exercise stretches the deep, small, external rotator muscles of the hip.

07 ABDOMEN

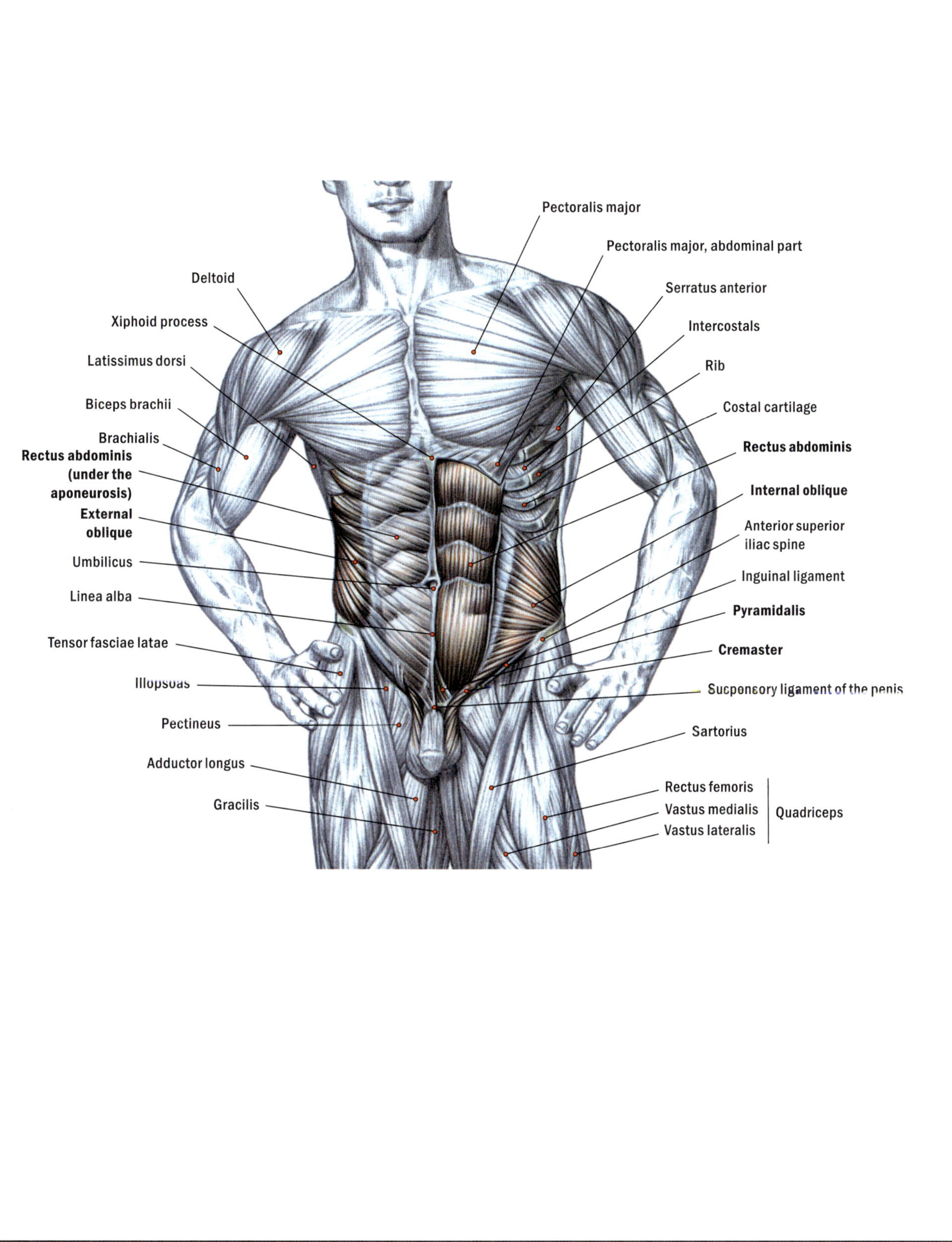

Deltoid
Xiphoid process
Latissimus dorsi
Biceps brachii
Brachialis
Rectus abdominis (under the aponeurosis)
External oblique
Umbilicus
Linea alba
Tensor fasciae latae
Iliopsoas
Pectineus
Adductor longus
Gracilis
Pectoralis major
Pectoralis major, abdominal part
Serratus anterior
Intercostals
Rib
Costal cartilage
Rectus abdominis
Internal oblique
Anterior superior iliac spine
Inguinal ligament
Pyramidalis
Cremaster
Suspensory ligament of the penis
Sartorius
Rectus femoris
Vastus medialis
Vastus lateralis
Quadriceps

01 CRUNCHES

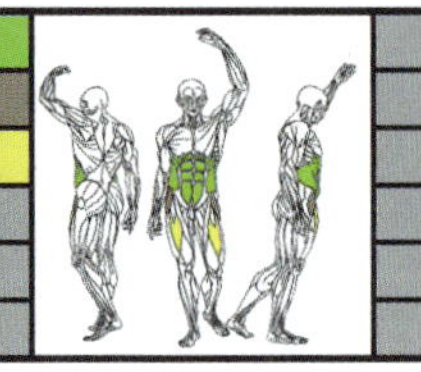

Tibialis anterior
Extensor digitorum longus
Gastrocnemius, lateral head
Quadriceps, vastus intermedius
Patella
Quadriceps, vastus medialis
Rectus abdominis
External oblique
Pectoralis major
Peroneus longus
Soleus
Biceps femoris, short head
Quadriceps, vastus lateralis
Biceps femoris, long head
Fasciae latae
Quadriceps, rectus femoris
Greater trochanter
Gluteus maximus
Gluteus medius
Tensor fasciae latae
Serratus anterior
Latissimus dorsi
Teres major

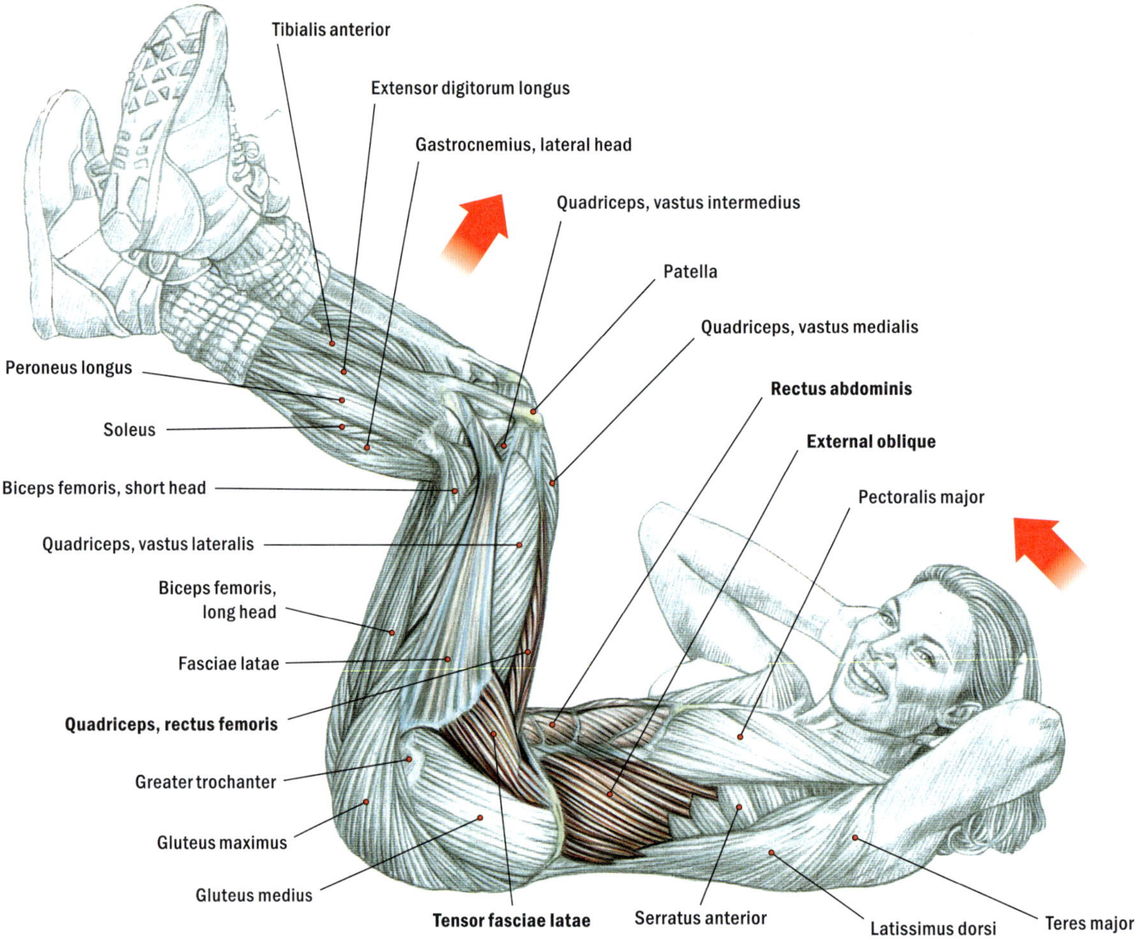

Lie on your back with your hands close to your ears with your legs in the air, thighs vertical, and knees bent:

- Inhale and raise your shoulders off the ground. Bring your head toward your knees by rounding your back and rolling your spine up.
- Exhale at the end of the exercise.

This exercise mainly works the rectus abdominis. To work the obliques more intensely, bring your right elbow to your left knee and then your left elbow to your right knee alternately with each crunch.

Rounding the back and rolling the spine up, which brings the pubis and sternum toward each other through voluntary contraction, is known as a *crunch* in strength training jargon.

PERFORMING THE EXERCISE

1 Start
2 Finish

VARIATION: SEATED CRUNCH ON A BENCH

1 Start
2 Finish

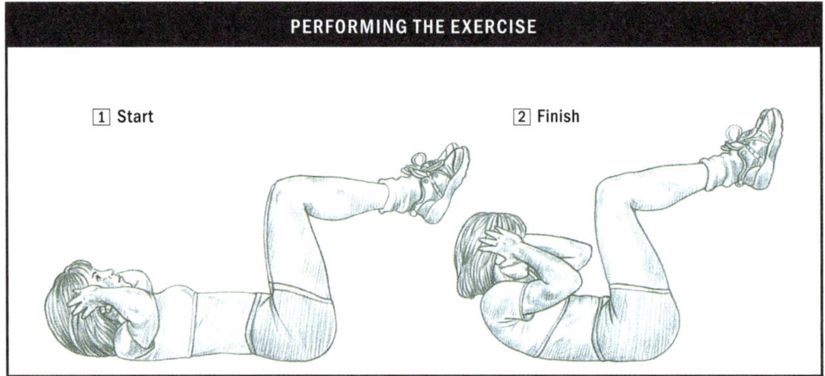

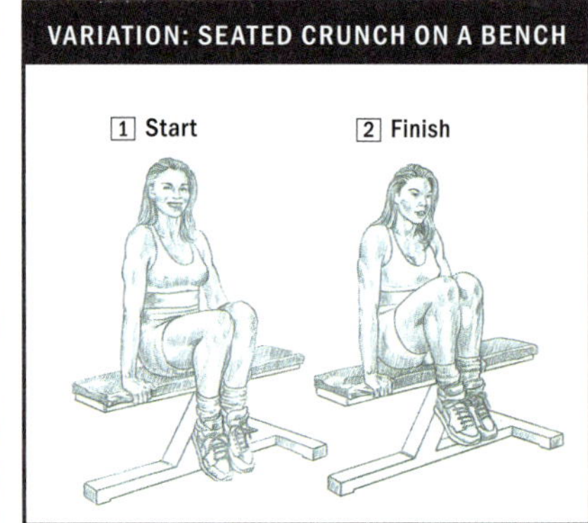

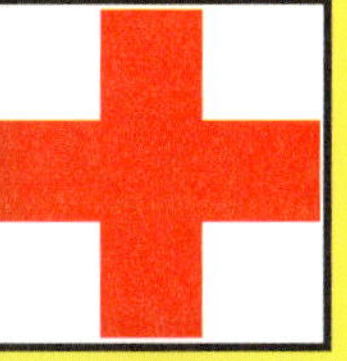

ACTION OF THE PSOAS MAJOR ON THE LUMBAR CURVE

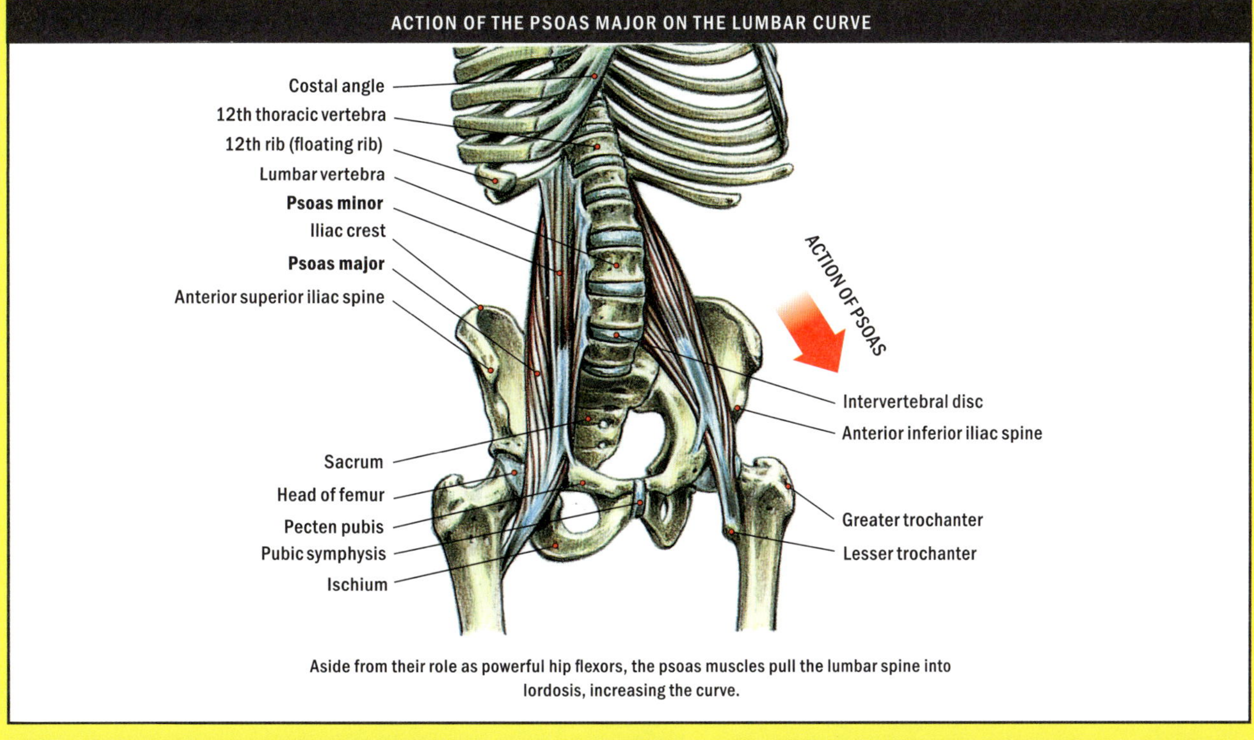

Aside from their role as powerful hip flexors, the psoas muscles pull the lumbar spine into lordosis, increasing the curve.

CORRECT POSITION, ROUNDED BACK — INCORRECT POSITION, ARCHED BACK

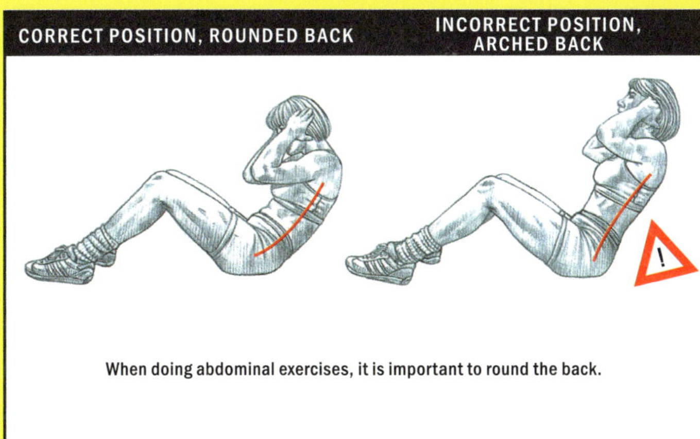

When doing abdominal exercises, it is important to round the back.

INCORRECT POSITION, ARCHED BACK

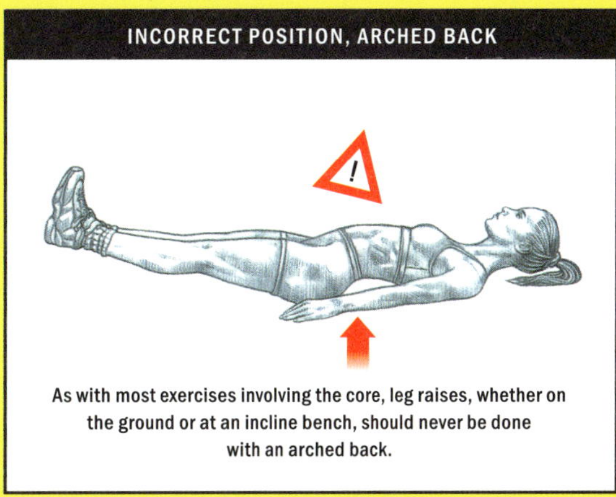

As with most exercises involving the core, leg raises, whether on the ground or at an incline bench, should never be done with an arched back.

Unlike other muscle-strengthening exercises, abdominal exercises, especially those for the rectus abdominis, should always be done with a rounded back (rolling up the spine). When doing exercises that roll the spine up off the floor, as in sit-ups, you hold the spine differently than when performing squats, deadlifts, or other standing exercises.

During squats, deadlifts, good mornings, or other exercises with additional weight, if the spine is not arched at the lumbar area, vertical pressure combined with rounding of the back will push the nucleus pulposus of the intervertebral disc to the back, which can compress the nerves and cause sciatica or a herniated disc.

On the other hand, during specific exercises for the abdominal muscles, if you forget to round the back by intensely contracting the rectus abdominis and the obliques, the powerful psoas hip flexors will increase the lumbar curve, forcing the intervertebral discs forward since they are not stabilized by vertical pressure. This causes increased pressure at the back of the vertebral joints in the lumbar region, which can cause lower back pain or, even more seriously, joint deterioration through compression and shearing.

02 SIT-UPS

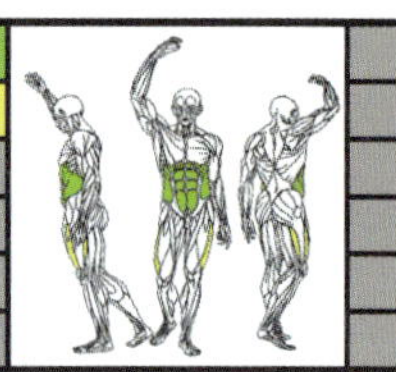

PERFORMING THE EXERCISE

2 Finish
1 Start

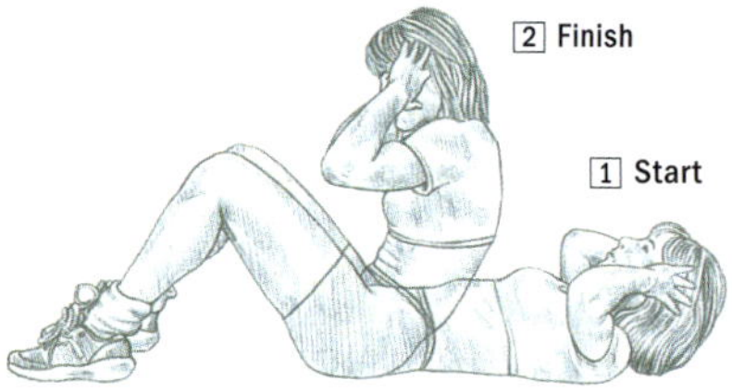

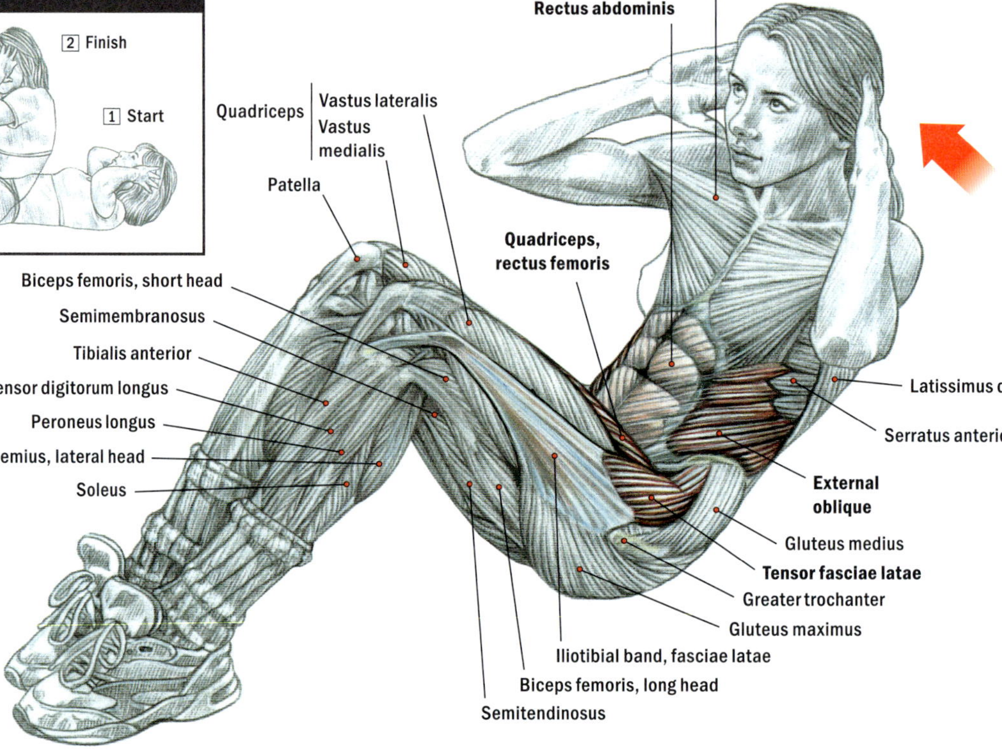

Pectoralis major
Rectus abdominis
Quadriceps
Vastus lateralis
Vastus medialis
Patella
Quadriceps, rectus femoris
Biceps femoris, short head
Semimembranosus
Tibialis anterior
Extensor digitorum longus
Peroneus longus
Gastrocnemius, lateral head
Soleus
Latissimus dorsi
Serratus anterior
External oblique
Gluteus medius
Tensor fasciae latae
Greater trochanter
Gluteus maximus
Iliotibial band, fasciae latae
Biceps femoris, long head
Semitendinosus

Lie on your back with knees bent, feet flat on the ground, and hands close to your ears:

- Inhale and raise your torso by rounding your back.
- Exhale at the end of the exercise.
- Return to the starting position without touching the ground.
- Continue until you feel a burn in your abdominal muscles.

This exercise works the hip flexors as well as the obliques, but it mainly targets the rectus abdominis.

Since women generally have a less bulky torso and proportionally bigger legs than men, it is typically easier for women to do sit-ups without lifting their feet off the ground.

Variations

- Having a partner hold the feet makes the exercise easier.
- Extending the arms forward makes the exercise easier, especially for beginners.
- Working on an incline bench makes the exercise harder.

VARIATION WITH ARMS EXTENDED

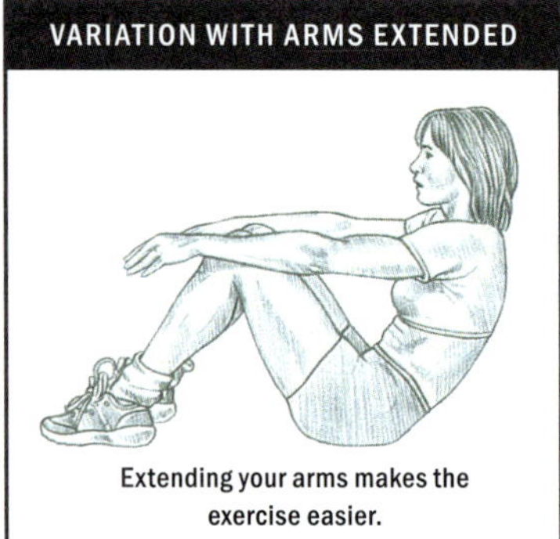

Extending your arms makes the exercise easier.

VARIATION WITH A PARTNER HOLDING THE FEET

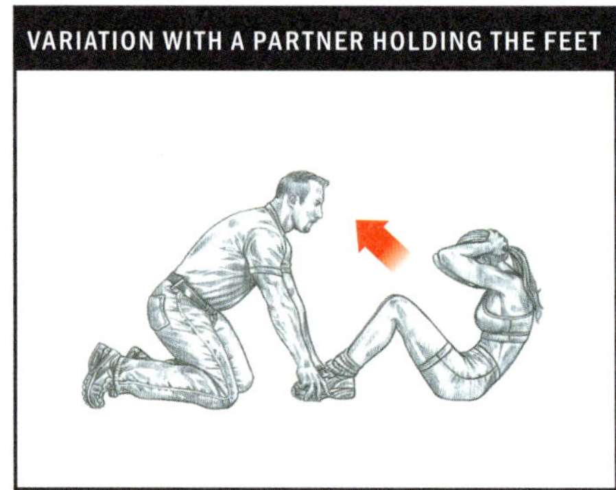

VARIATION ON AN INCLINE BENCH

2 Finish
1 Start

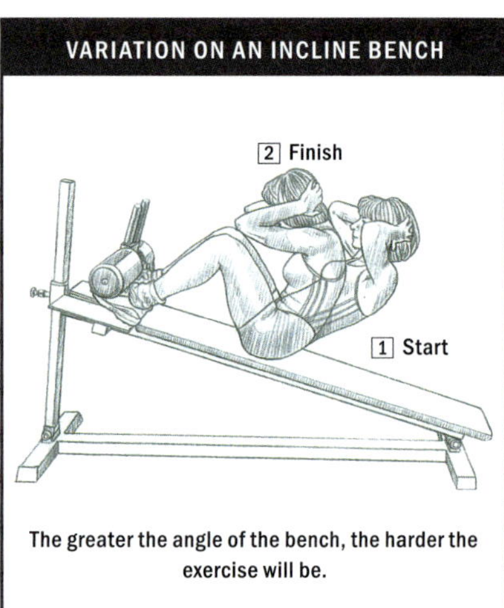

The greater the angle of the bench, the harder the exercise will be.

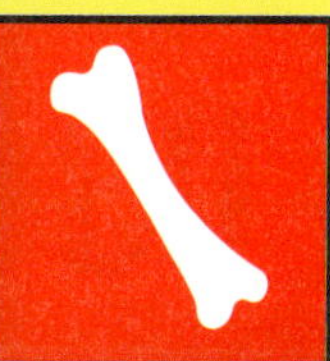

HIP FLEXORS

Iliopsoas action

Rectus femoris action

Tensor fasciae latae action

ABDOMINAL MUSCLES THAT BRING THE STERNUM TOWARD THE PUBIS

Rectus abdominis action

External oblique action

Internal oblique action

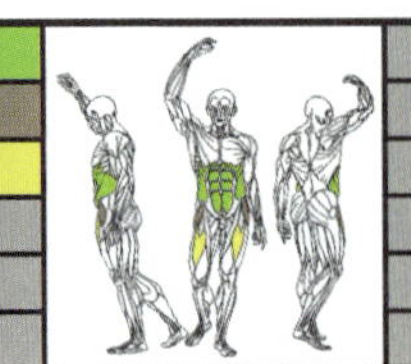

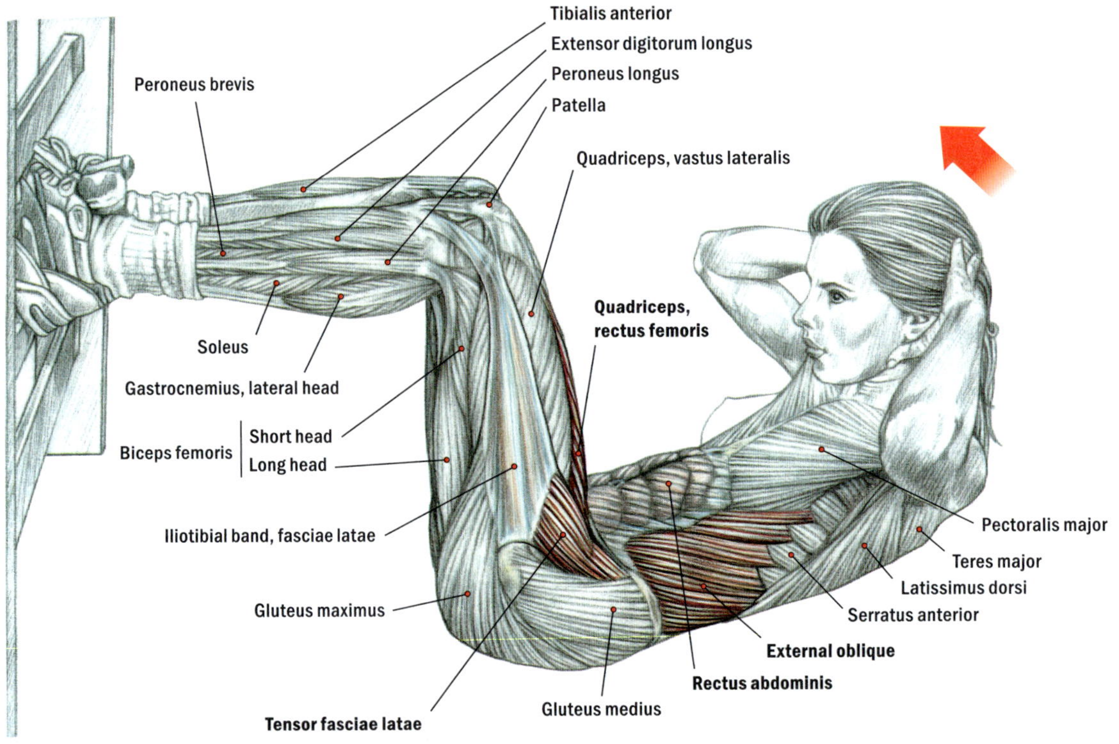

Lie on the ground and hook your feet between two bars in the ladder with your thighs vertical and your hands close to your ears:

- Inhale and raise your torso as high as possible, rounding your spine.
- Exhale at the end of the exercise.

This exercise works the rectus abdominis and, to a lesser degree, the external obliques.

By increasing the distance between your torso and the ladder (by positioning your feet lower on the ladder), you increase the mobility of your pelvis, which works the flexor muscles of your hip (iliopsoas, rectus femoris, and tensor fasciae latae).

ABDOMINAL MUSCLES: CROSS-SECTIONAL VIEW

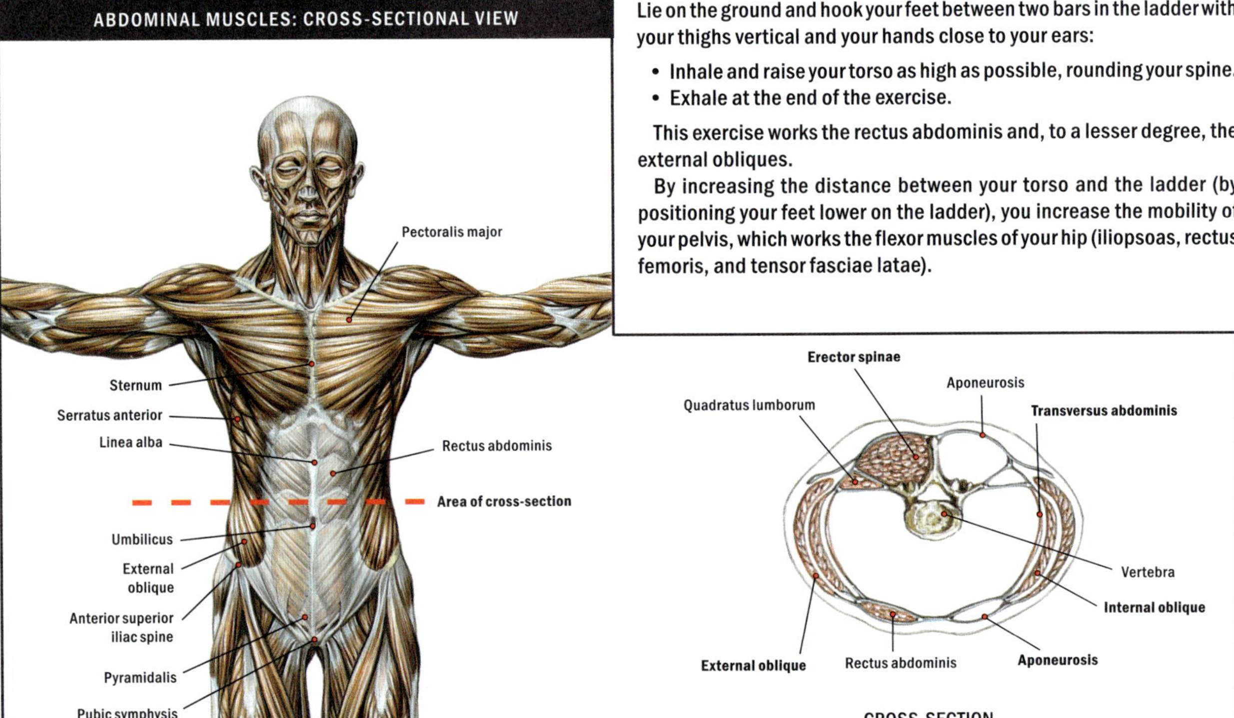

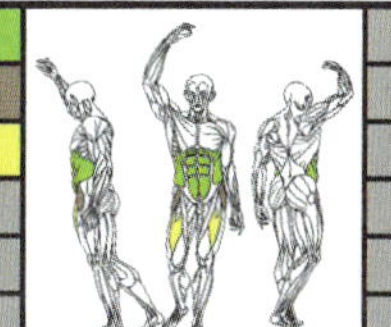

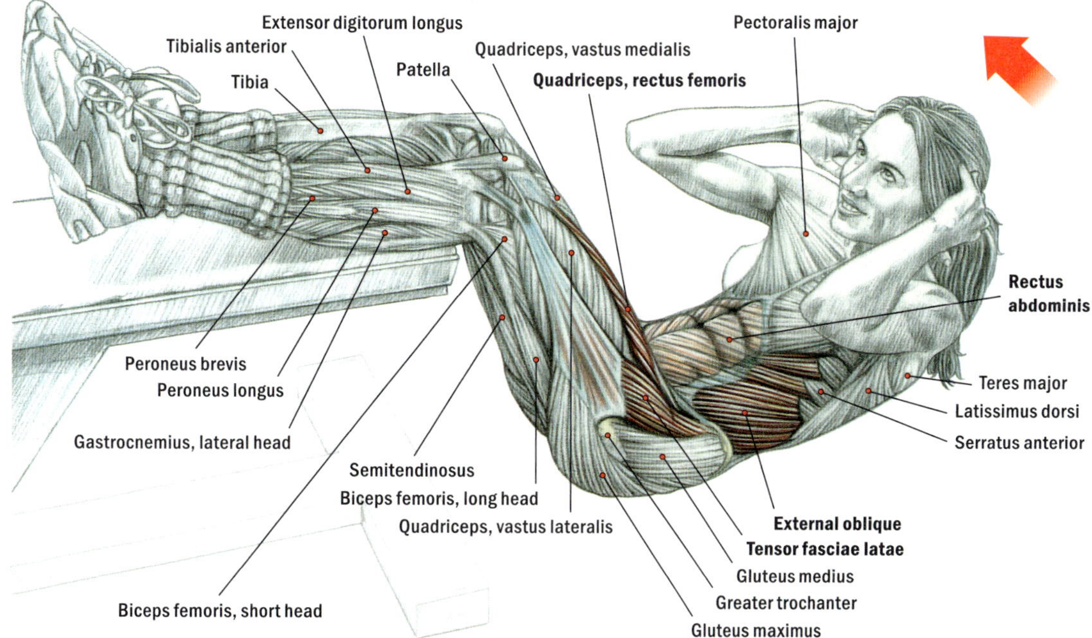

Lie on your back with your legs resting on a bench. Place your hands close to your ears:

- Inhale and lift your shoulders off the floor, rounding your back and trying to touch your head to your knees.
- Exhale at the end of the exercise.

This exercise focuses on the rectus abdominis, particularly above the navel. By increasing the distance between the bench and your torso, you increase pelvic mobility, which enables you to lift your torso by flexing your hips, achieved by contracting the iliopsoas, tensor fasciae latae, and rectus femoris.

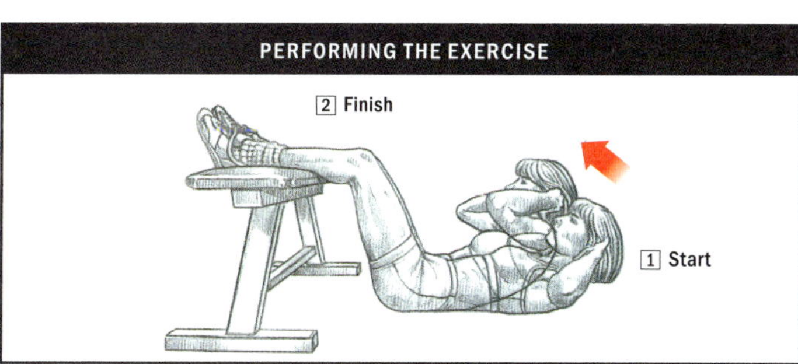

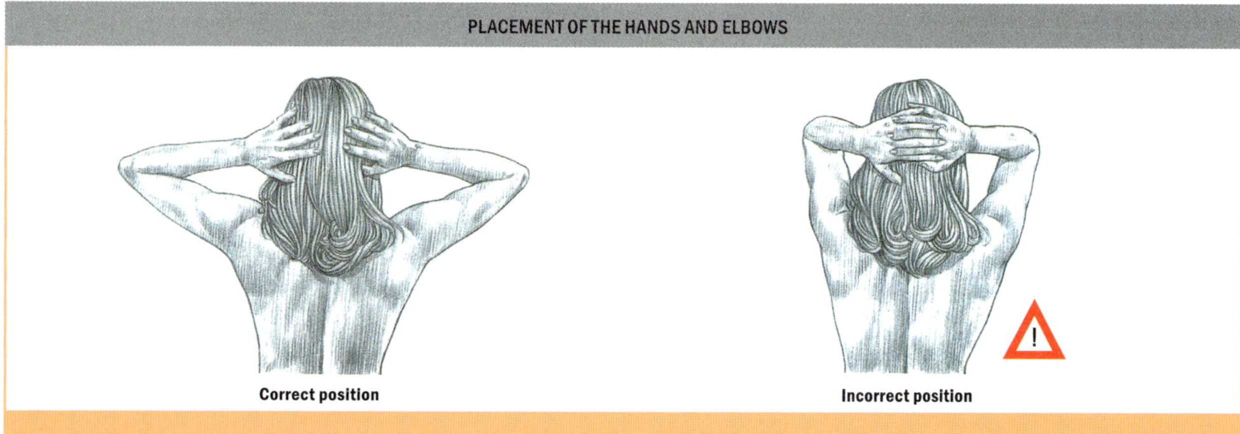

To keep from pulling excessively on your neck, place your hands behind your ears rather than at the back of your head. The wider apart your elbows are, the more difficult the exercise becomes. Conversely, the closer together and more forward your elbows are, the easier it is.

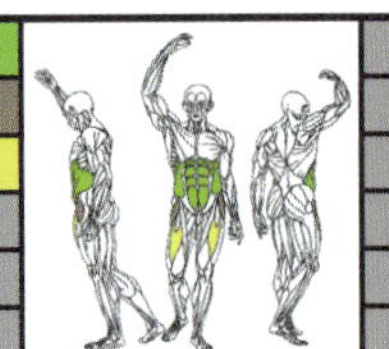

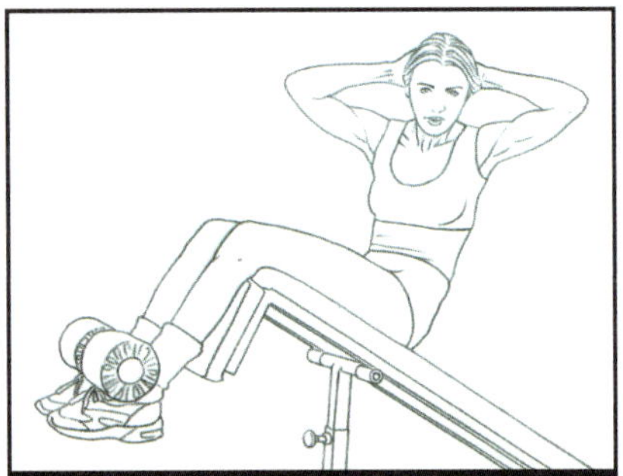

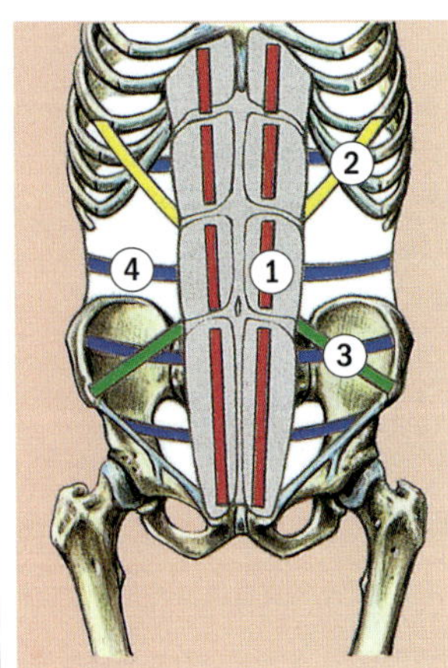

VARIATION WITH TORSO ROTATION

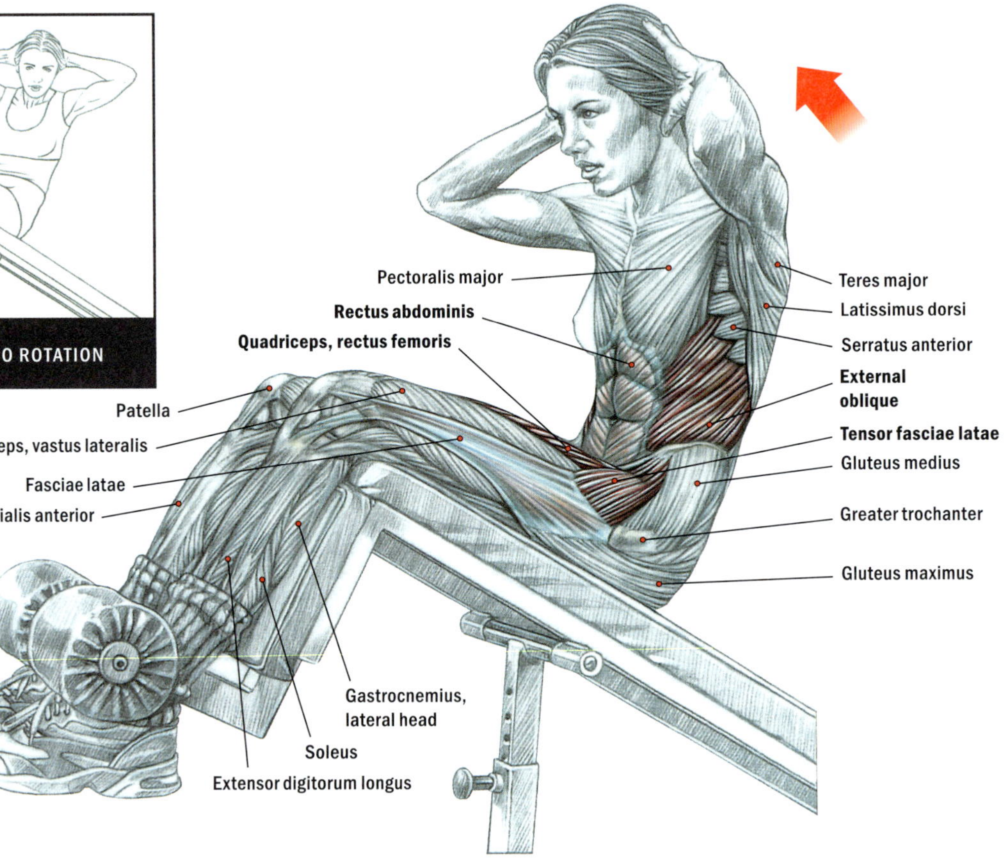

Pectoralis major

Rectus abdominis

Quadriceps, rectus femoris

Patella

Quadriceps, vastus lateralis

Fasciae latae

Tibialis anterior

Teres major

Latissimus dorsi

Serratus anterior

External oblique

Tensor fasciae latae

Gluteus medius

Greater trochanter

Gluteus maximus

Gastrocnemius, lateral head

Soleus

Extensor digitorum longus

THE ABDOMINAL MUSCLES THAT SUPPORT THE INTERNAL ORGANS

1. Rectus abdominis
2. External oblique
3. Internal oblique
4. Transversus abdominis

In quadrupeds, the muscles of the abdomen form a hammocklike structure that passively supports the internal organs; these muscles are not very involved in movement. As humans shifted to bipedal locomotion, the muscles of the abdomen grew stronger to align the pelvis with the trunk in a vertical position and to prevent the torso from swaying too much during walking or running. These muscles have developed into a powerful system that actively supports the internal organs.

Sit on a bench with your feet positioned under the pads and hands behind your neck. Inhale and lean back without going beyond a 20-degree angle in relation to the bench:

- Raise your torso while slightly rounding your back to better focus on your rectus abdominis.
- Exhale at the end of the exercise.

Do this exercise in long sets. It works the entire core as well as the iliopsoas, tensor fasciae latae, and rectus femoris of the quadriceps; the latter three muscles tilt the pelvis forward.

Variation

Rotating the torso on the way up focuses some of the effort on the internal and external obliques. For example, rotating to the left works the right external oblique, the left internal oblique, and the right side of the rectus abdominis more intensely. You can do rotations by alternating sides on each repetition or by doing alternating sets. In either case, concentrate on feeling the muscles contract. There is no point in inclining the bench too steeply.

HANGING SIT-UPS 06

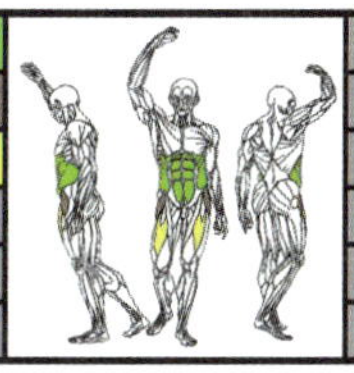

Tibialis anterior
Extensor digitorum longus
Peroneus longus
Patella
Quadriceps, vastus intermedius
Rectus abdominis
External oblique
Tensor fasciae latae
Gluteus medius
Peroneus brevis
Soleus
Gastrocnemius, lateral head
Quadriceps, vastus lateralis
Quadriceps, rectus femoris
Iliotibial band, fasciae latae
Greater trochanter
Gluteus maximus

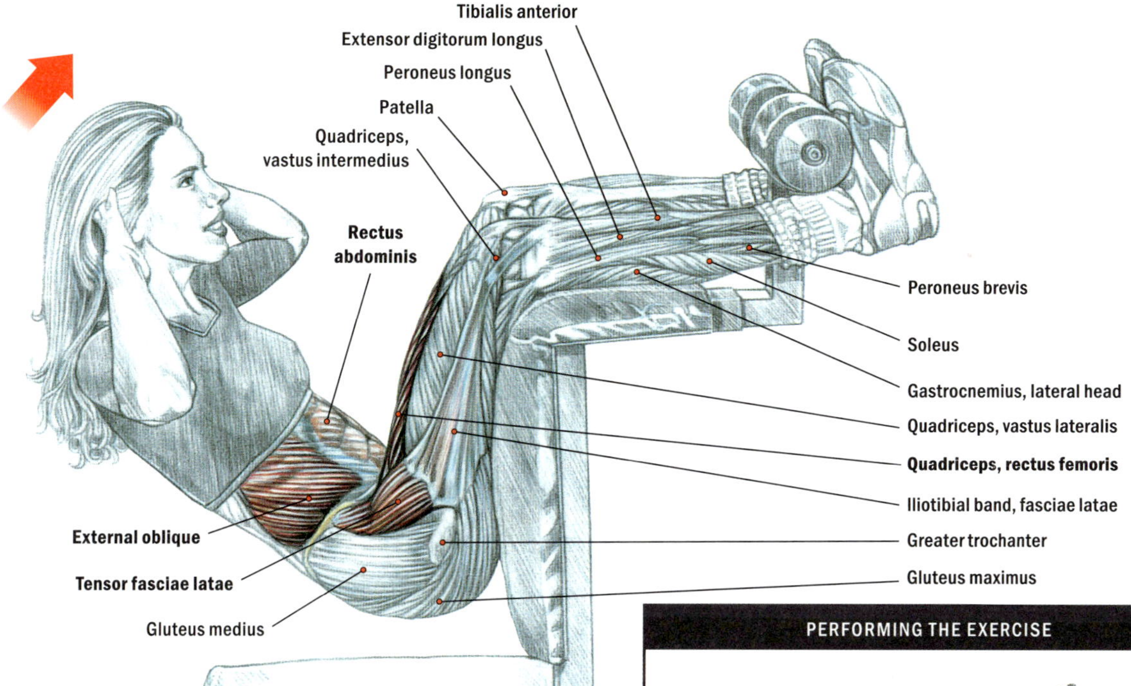

PERFORMING THE EXERCISE

2 Finish
1 Start

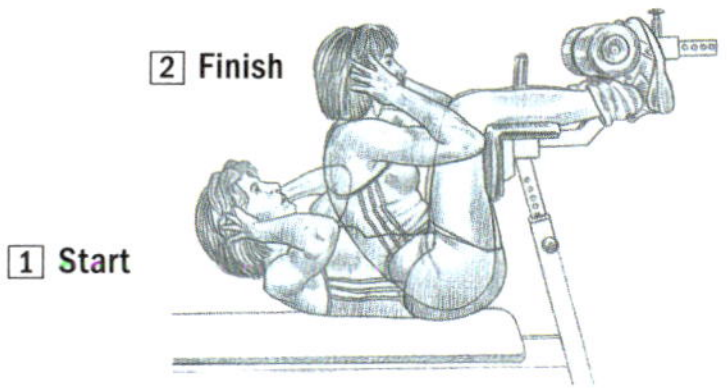

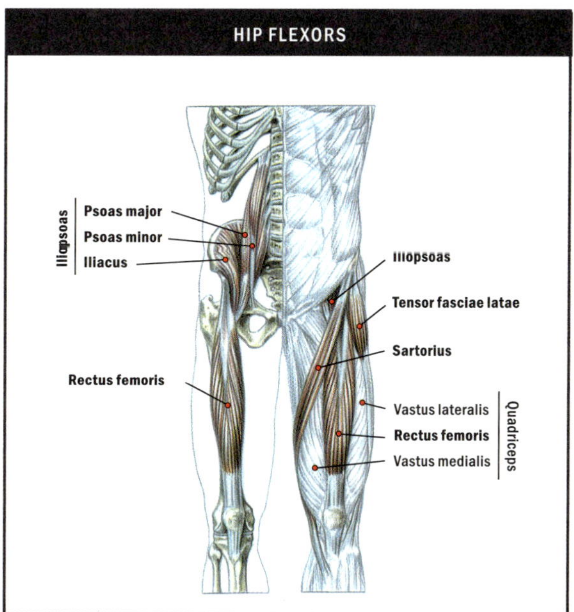

Position your feet under the pads with your torso in midair and your hands behind your ears:

- Inhale and lift your torso, trying to bring your head up to your knees while rounding your spine.
- Exhale at the end of the exercise.

This exercise is excellent for developing the rectus abdominis. It also works the obliques, but less intensely. Because of the forward tilt of the pelvis, the rectus abdominis, iliopsoas, and tensor fasciae latae are worked intensely.

This exercise requires a fair amount of strength, which you can build through other, easier exercises.

HIP FLEXORS

Iliopsoas
Psoas major
Psoas minor
Iliacus
Rectus femoris
Iliopsoas
Tensor fasciae latae
Sartorius
Vastus lateralis
Rectus femoris
Vastus medialis
Quadriceps

VARIATION WITH ARMS EXTENDED

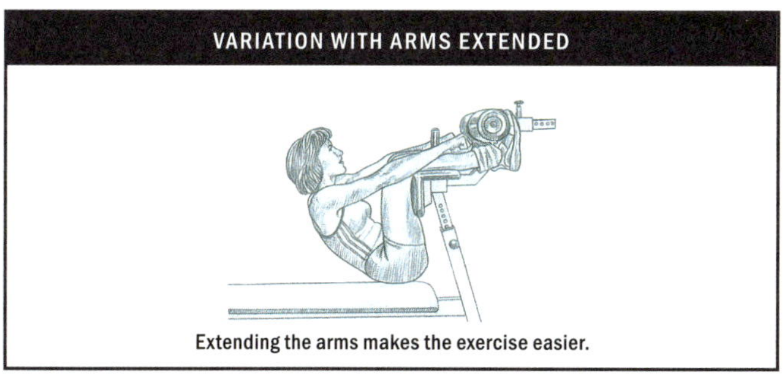

Extending the arms makes the exercise easier.

07 HIGH-PULLEY CRUNCHES

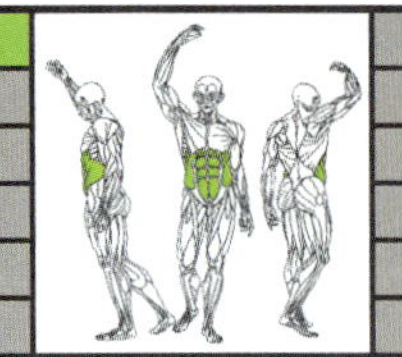

Pectoralis major
Serratus anterior
Latissimus dorsi
External oblique
Rectus abdominis
Iliac crest
Gluteus medius
Pyramidalis
Iliopsoas
Tensor fasciae latae
Pectineus
Quadriceps, rectus femoris
Sartorius
Greater trochanter
Gluteus maximus
Iliotibial band, fasciae latae

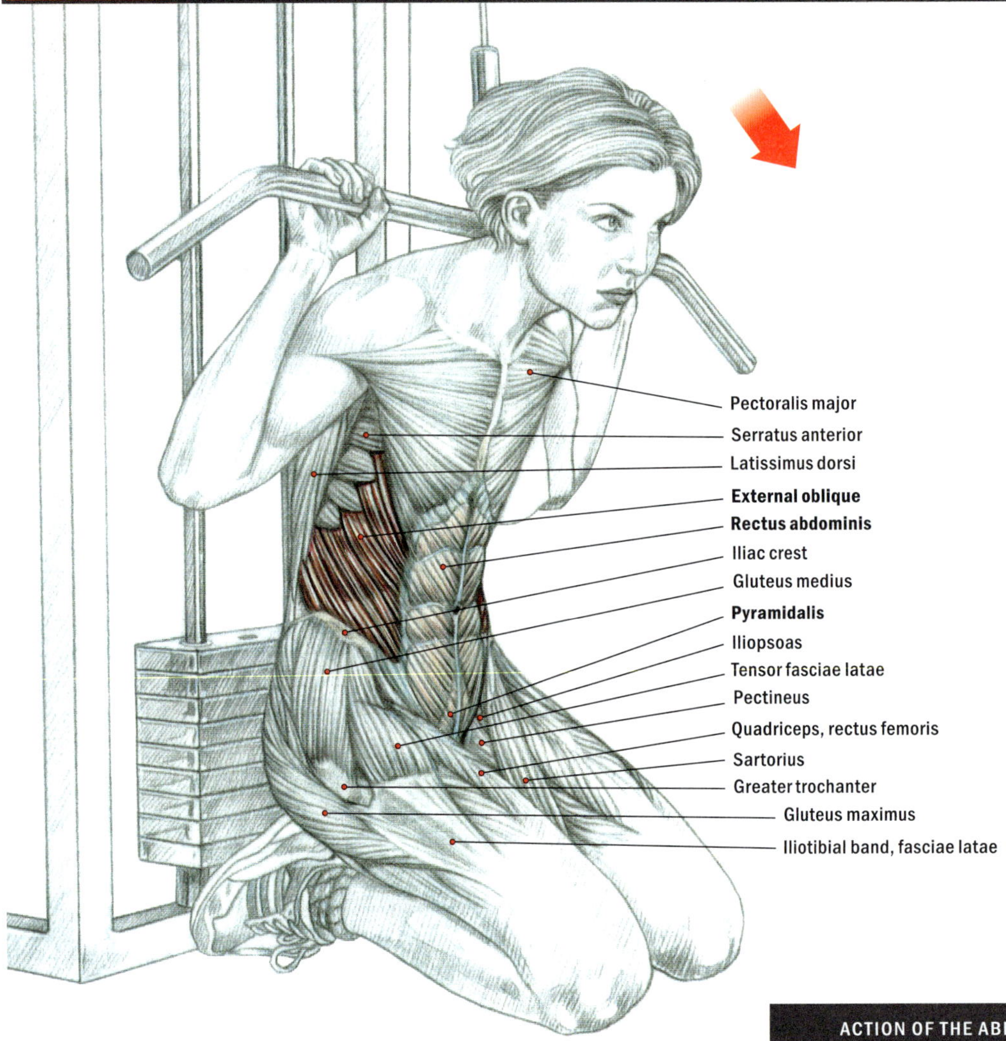

Kneel with your back to the machine and hold the handle behind your neck:

- Inhale and roll your spine to lower your sternum toward your pubis.
- Exhale at the end of the exercise.

This exercise is never done with heavy weights. The key here is to concentrate on feeling the muscles contract in order to focus the work on the core, especially the rectus abdominis.

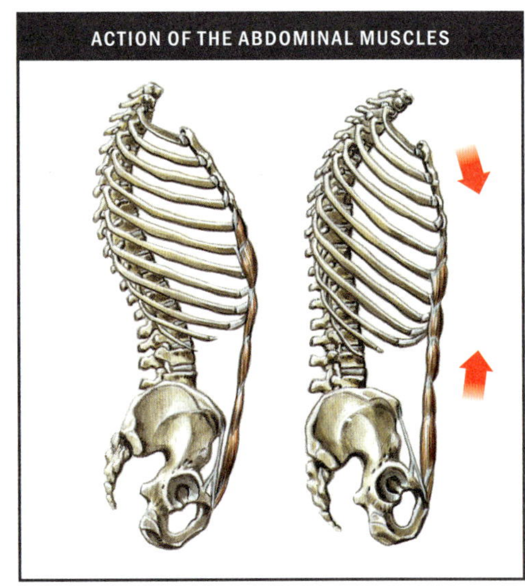

ACTION OF THE ABDOMINAL MUSCLES

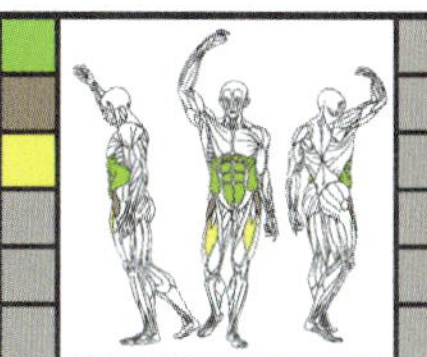

RECTUS ABDOMINIS MUSCLE

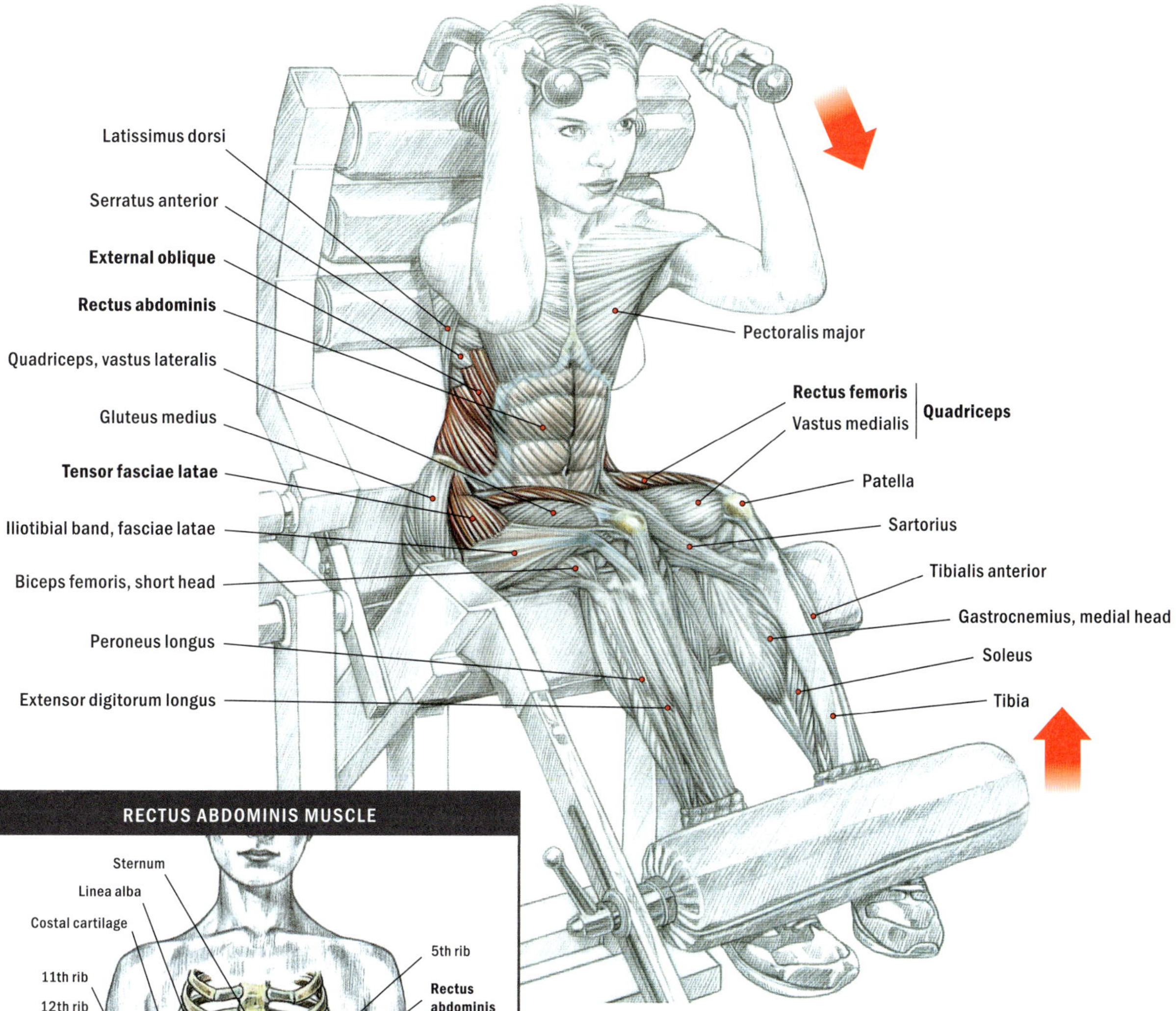

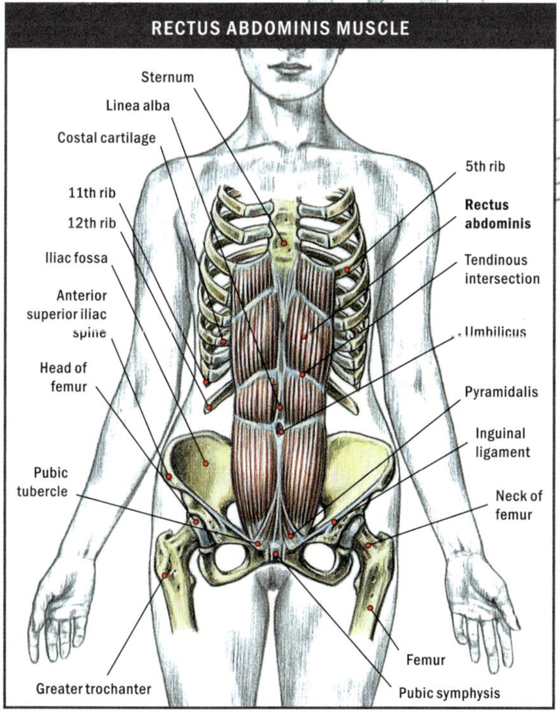

Sit at the machine, grasp the handles, and position your feet under the pad:

- Inhale and roll your spine forward to bring your sternum as close as possible to your pubis.
- Exhale at the end of the exercise.

This excellent exercise allows you to adjust the weight according to your ability. Beginners can use light weights, while experienced athletes can use heavier weights with no risk.

09 INCLINE LEG RAISES

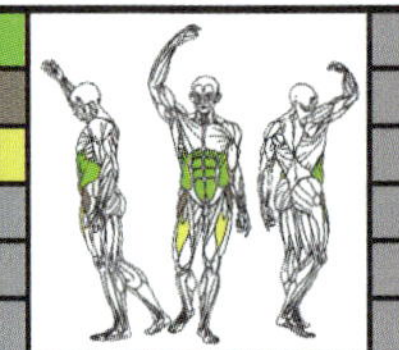

Soleus
Gastrocnemius, medial head
Biceps femoris, short head
Semimembranosus
Biceps femoris, long head
Quadriceps, vastus lateralis
Semitendinosus
Iliotibial band, fasciae latae
Quadriceps, rectus femoris
Tensor fasciae latae
Adductor magnus
Gluteus maximus
Extensor digitorum longus
Peroneus longus
Tibialis anterior
Greater trochanter
Rectus abdominis
External oblique
Gluteus medius
Latissimus dorsi

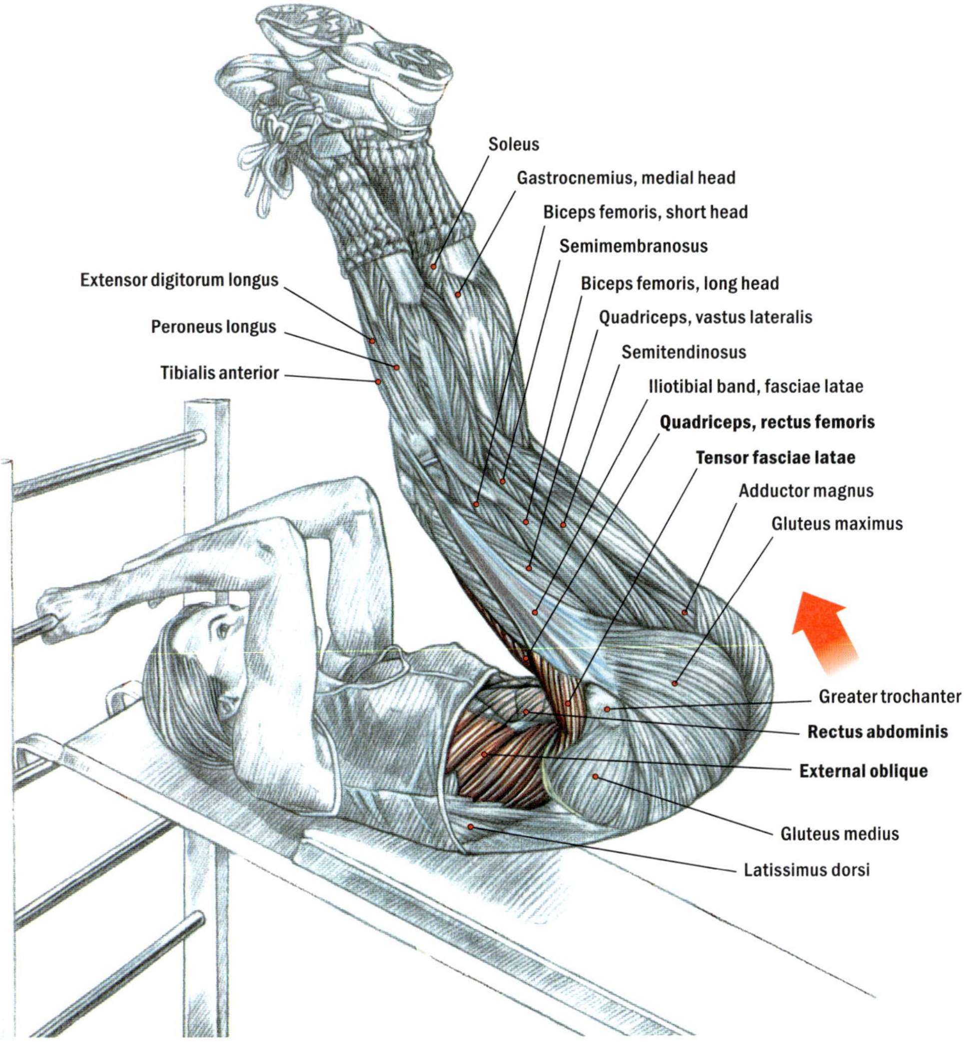

Lie on an incline bench and grip the bars or handles:

- Raise your legs to a horizontal position.
- Lift your pelvis off the bench by rolling your spine up and try to touch your head with your knees.

This exercise first works the iliopsoas, tensor fasciae latae, and rectus femoris of the quadriceps when raising the legs. Then, as the pelvis is raised and the spine rolls up, it works the core, especially the part of the rectus abdominis below the belly button.

This exercise is recommended for individuals having trouble feeling the effort of the lower abdominal muscles.

Given the difficulty of this exercise, beginners should start with the bench only slightly inclined.

2 Finish
1 Start

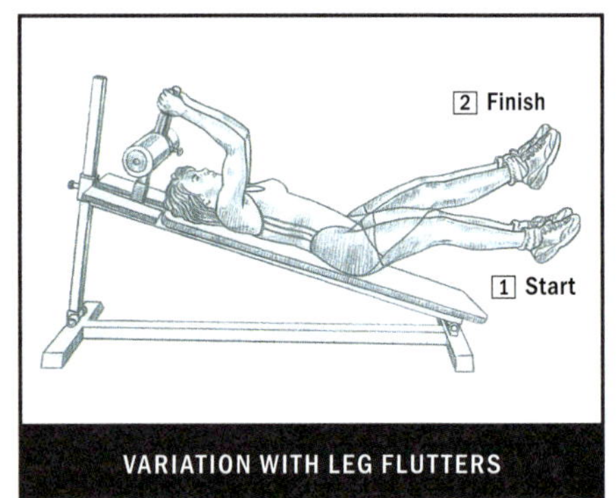

VARIATION WITH LEG FLUTTERS

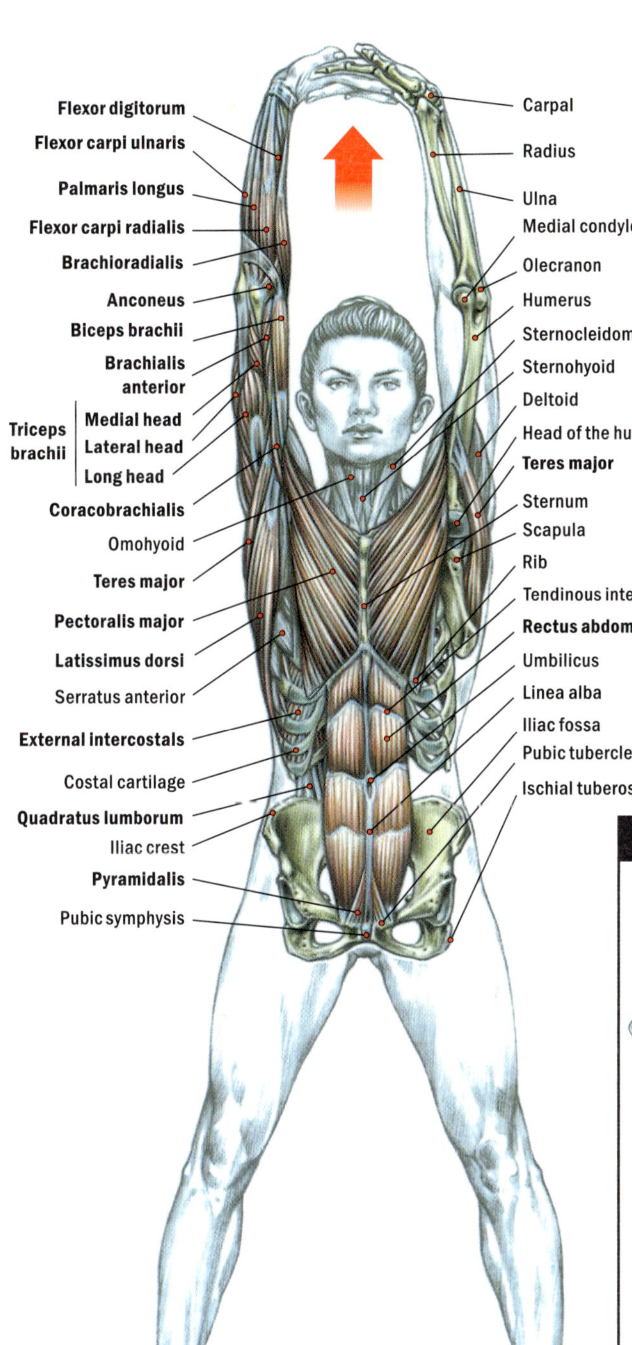

Stand with your legs wider apart than your pelvis and with your back extremely straight:

- Extend your arms vertically, hands clasped together with your fingers interlocked, and your palms facing the ceiling.
- Inhale and expand your chest, stretching your intercostal muscles and trying to push up. Keep your back and head as straight as you can.
- Relax, exhaling slowly, and repeat.

This is a general stretch for the upper body and particularly for the intercostal muscles, rectus abdominis, latissimus dorsi, teres major, and the long portion of the triceps.

Bending to the side increases the stretch of the external and internal obliques of the abdomen, quadratus lumborum, and the inferior and middle erector spinae muscles.

This stretch is ideal for relaxing and returning to a state of calm after an intense session of leg presses, squats, or deadlifts when the rib cage and spine have been compressed. It can, from time to time, replace or complement the stretch at a pull-up bar to rebalance the pressure and tension on the intervertebral joints.

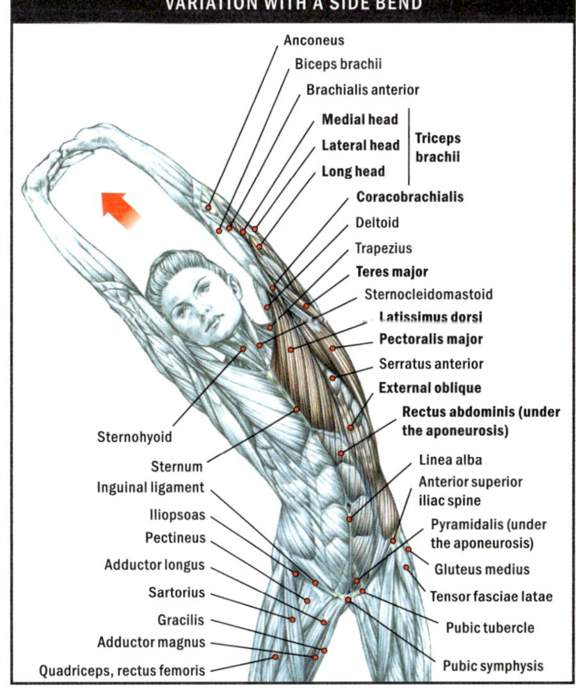

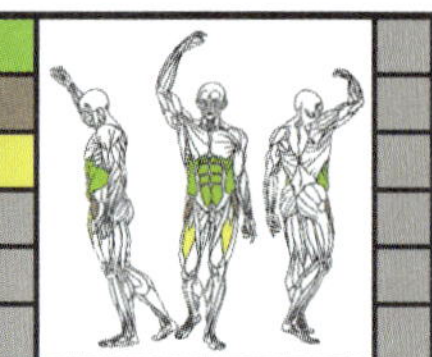

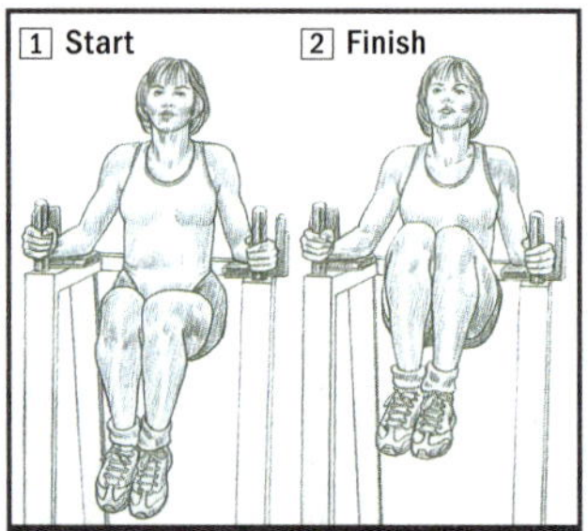

PERFORMING THE EXERCISE

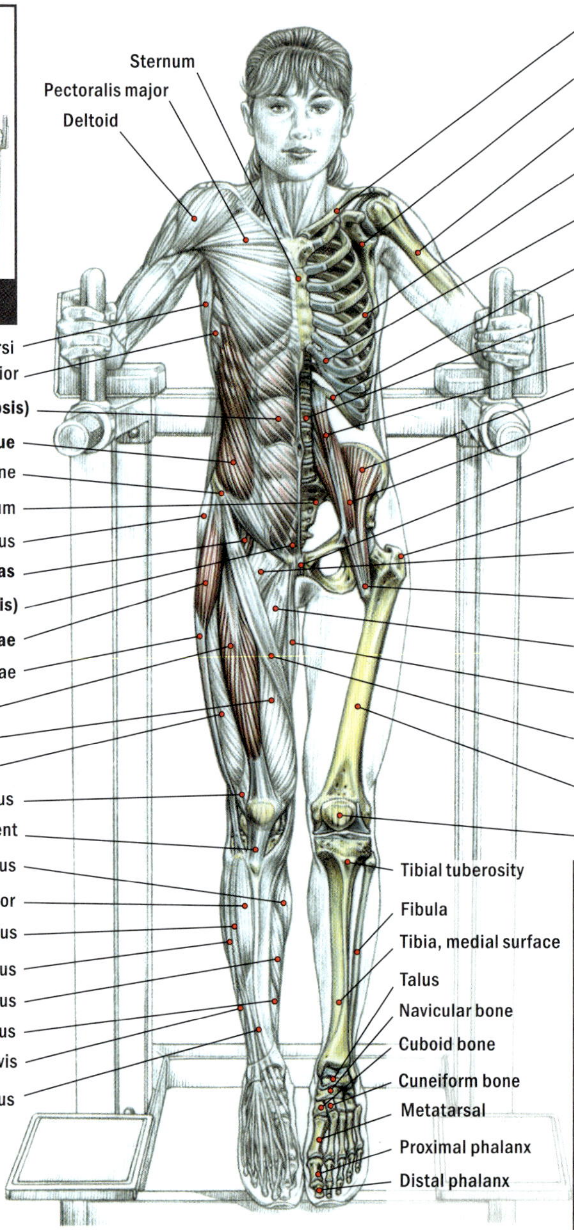

1 Start   2 Finish

Sternum
Pectoralis major
Deltoid
Latissimus dorsi
Serratus anterior
Rectus abdominis (under the aponeurosis)
External oblique
Anterior superior iliac spine
Sacrum
Gluteus medius
Iliopsoas
Pyramidalis (under the aponeurosis)
Tensor fasciae latae
Iliotibial band, fasciae latae
Rectus femoris
Quadriceps
Vastus medialis
Vastus lateralis
Vastus intermedius
Patellar ligament
Gastrocnemius
Tibialis anterior
Extensor digitorum longus
Peroneus longus
Soleus
Flexor digitorum longus
Peroneus brevis
Extensor hallucis longus

Clavicle
Scapula
Humerus
Rib
Costal cartilage
12th rib
Vertebra
Psoas minor
Iliacus   **Iliopsoas**
Psoas major
Pubic symphysis
Greater trochanter
Pectineus
Lesser trochanter
Adductor longus
Gracilis
Sartorius
Femur
Patella
Tibial tuberosity
Fibula
Tibia, medial surface
Talus
Navicular bone
Cuboid bone
Cuneiform bone
Metatarsal
Proximal phalanx
Distal phalanx

ACTION OF THE ILIOPSOAS

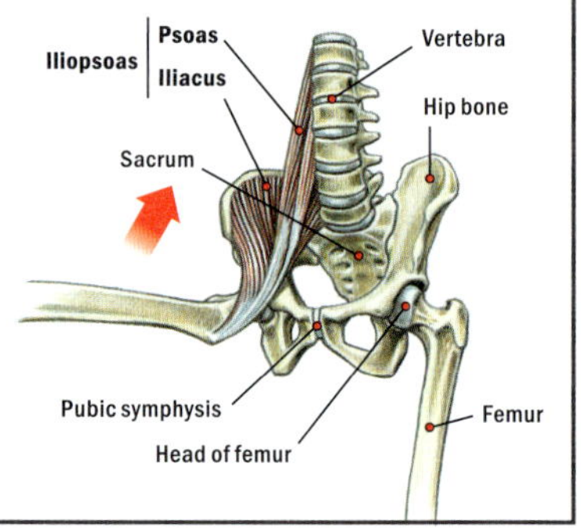

Iliopsoas
Psoas
Iliacus
Vertebra
Hip bone
Sacrum
Pubic symphysis
Head of femur
Femur

Support your body by resting your elbows on the pads. Position your back firmly against the back support:

- Inhale and pull your knees to your chest, rounding your back to firmly contract the core.
- Exhale at the end of the exercise.

This exercise works the hip flexors—mainly the iliopsoas—as well as the obliques and the rectus abdominis. The lower part of the rectus abdominis is worked intensely.

Variations

- To target the abdominal muscles, do small flutters with your legs when rolling up the spine, without dropping your knees below your hips.
- To make the exercise more intense, you can do the exercise with straight legs; however, this requires flexible hamstrings.
- You can hold your knees to your chest with an isometric contraction for several seconds.

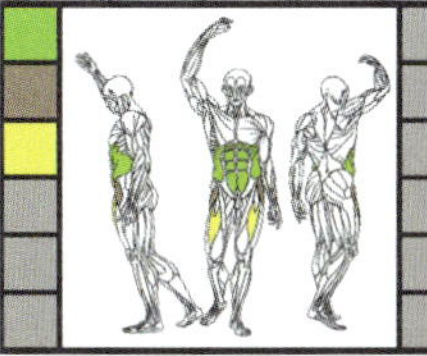

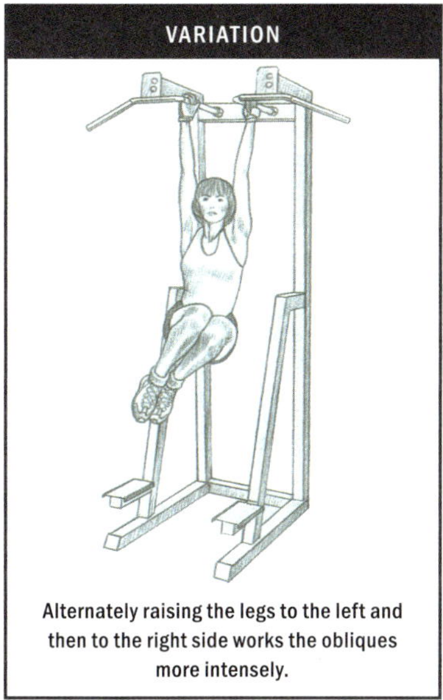

Alternately raising the legs to the left and then to the right side works the obliques more intensely.

Hang from a pull-up bar:

- Inhale and raise your knees as high as possible by rolling up your spine and bringing your pubis toward the sternum.
- Exhale at the end of the exercise.

This exercise works the iliopsoas, rectus femoris, and tensor fasciae latae when you raise your legs and your rectus abdominis and, to a lesser degree, the obliques when you bring your pubis toward your sternum.

Small leg flutters without lowering your knees below the hips will focus the effort on your abdomen.

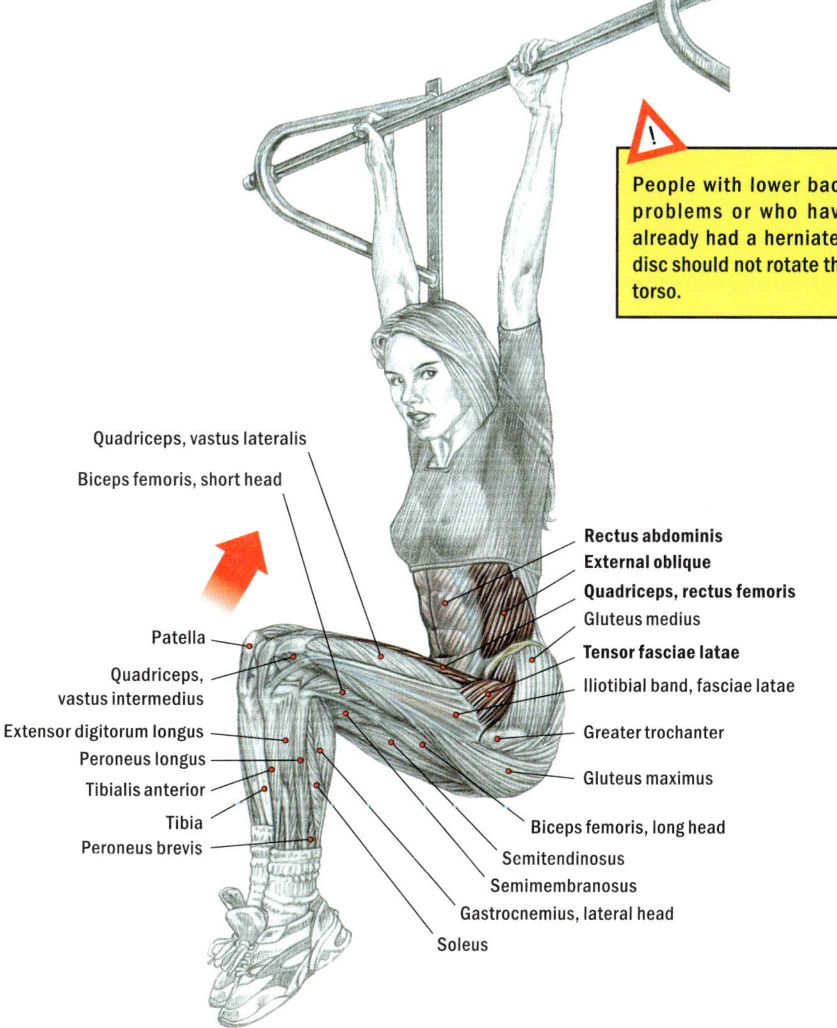

ABDOMINAL–LUMBAR EQUILIBRIUM

It is important to balance the work between the abdominal muscles and the erector spinae muscles. Hypotonicity or hypertonicity of either of these muscle groups can lead to poor posture, which can cause injury over time.

For example: Hypertonicity of the lower part of the erector spinae muscles (lumbosacral mass) associated with hypotonicity of the abdominal muscles leads to hyperlordosis with abdominal ptosis (bulging). Sometimes, if this postural flaw is addressed with exercises to strengthen the core in time, it can be corrected.

Conversely, hypertonic abdominal muscles, coupled with weak erector spinae muscles, especially in the upper part of the back (spinalis thoracis, longissimus thoracis, iliocostalis thoracis), will lead to kyphosis (rounding of the upper back) with loss of the lumbar curve. This postural flaw can be corrected with exercises to strengthen the erector spinae muscles.

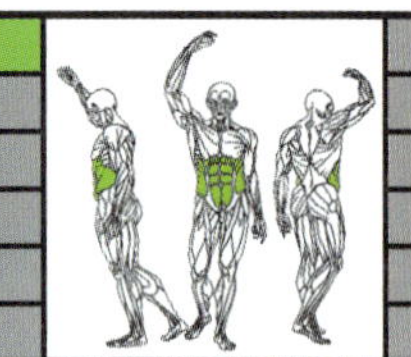

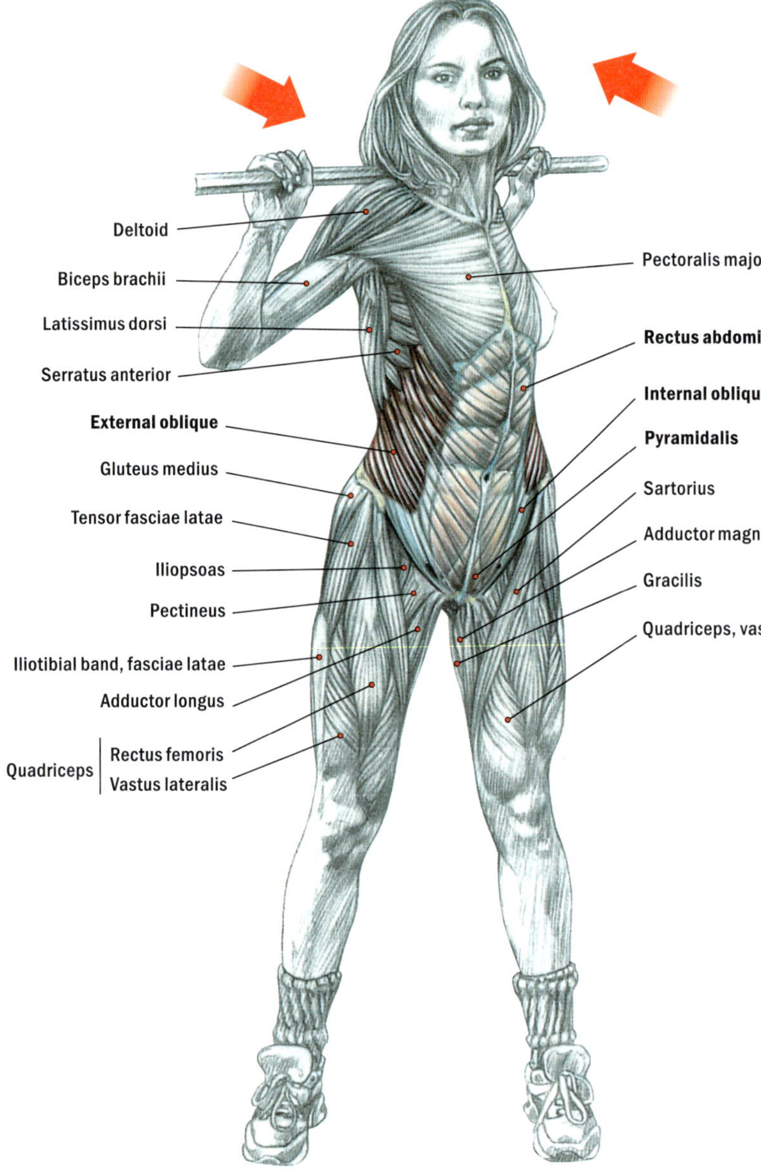

> ! People with lower back problems or who have already had a herniated disc should not do torso rotations because they may aggravate or cause a recurrence of this lumbar pathology.

Stand with your legs apart. Hold a short pole across your trapezius above your posterior deltoids, and rest your hands on it without exerting any pressure:

- Rotate your torso to one side and then the other, keeping your pelvis stable through isometric contraction of the gluteus muscles.

When the right shoulder is forward, this exercise works the right external oblique and, at a deeper level, the left internal oblique. To a lesser degree, it works the rectus abdominis, quadratus lumborum, and the extensor muscles of the spine on the left side.

To increase the intensity, round your back slightly.

Best results are obtained with sets that last for several minutes.

Variation

You can also do this exercise while seated, which helps keep your pelvis stable so that you can focus the effort on your abdominal muscles.

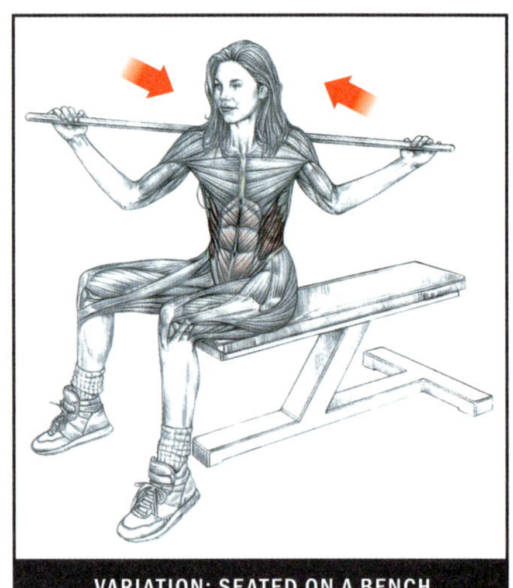

VARIATION: SEATED ON A BENCH

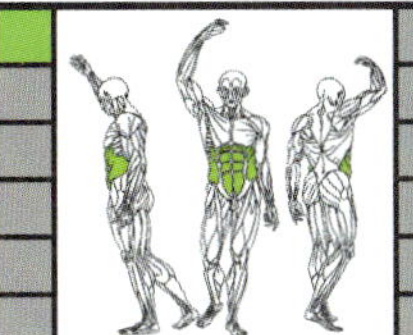

Sternum

Rib

Xiphoid process

Lumbar vertebra

Hip bone

Sacrum

Pyramidalis

Pubic symphysis

Costal cartilage

Rectus abdominis

External oblique

Rectus abdominis (under the aponeurosis)

Internal oblique (under the aponeurosis)

Femur

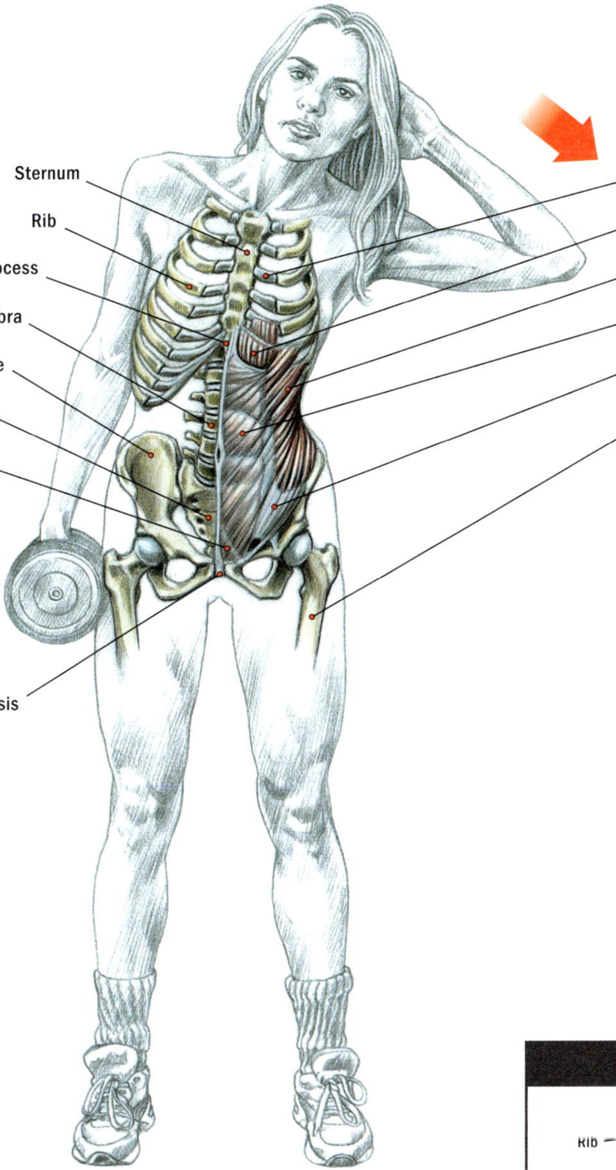

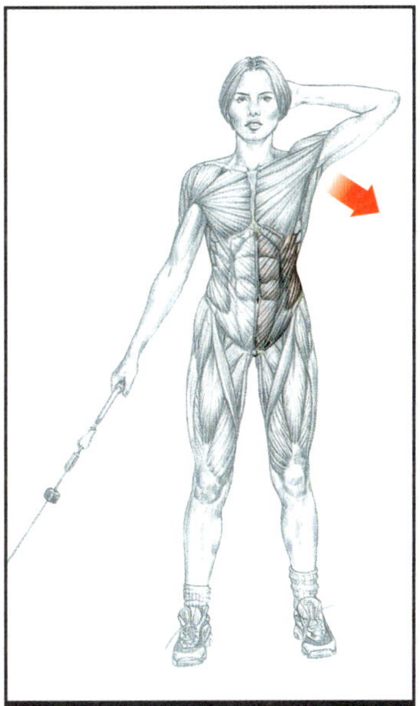

VARIATION WITH A LOW PULLEY

QUADRATUS LUMBORUM MUSCLE

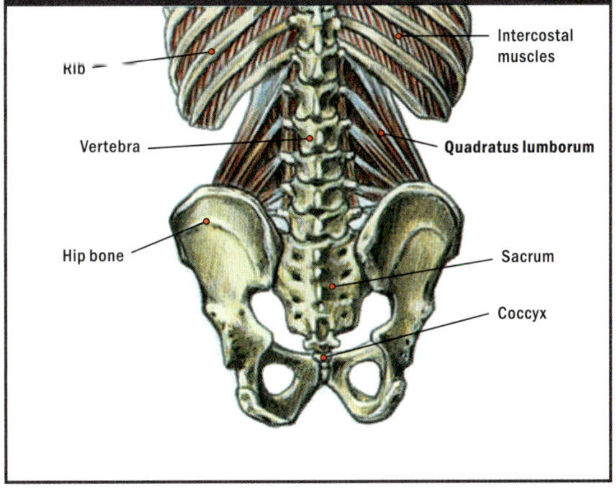

Rib

Vertebra

Hip bone

Intercostal muscles

Quadratus lumborum

Sacrum

Coccyx

Stand with your legs slightly apart and one hand behind your ear. Hold a dumbbell in the other hand:

- Bend your torso to the side opposite the dumbbell.
- Return to the starting position (or beyond, with passive flexion of your torso).
- Alternate sets, switching the dumbbell to your other hand without resting.

This exercise mainly works the obliques on the side that bends. It works these muscles less intensely: the rectus abdominis, the deep muscles of the back, and the quadratus lumborum (a back muscle that inserts on the 12th rib, the transverse processes of the lumbar vertebrae, and the iliac crest).

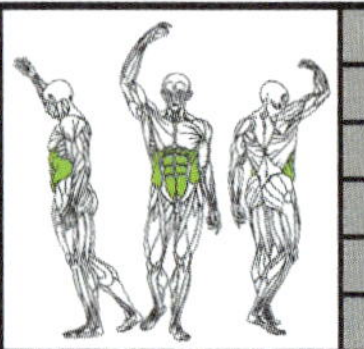

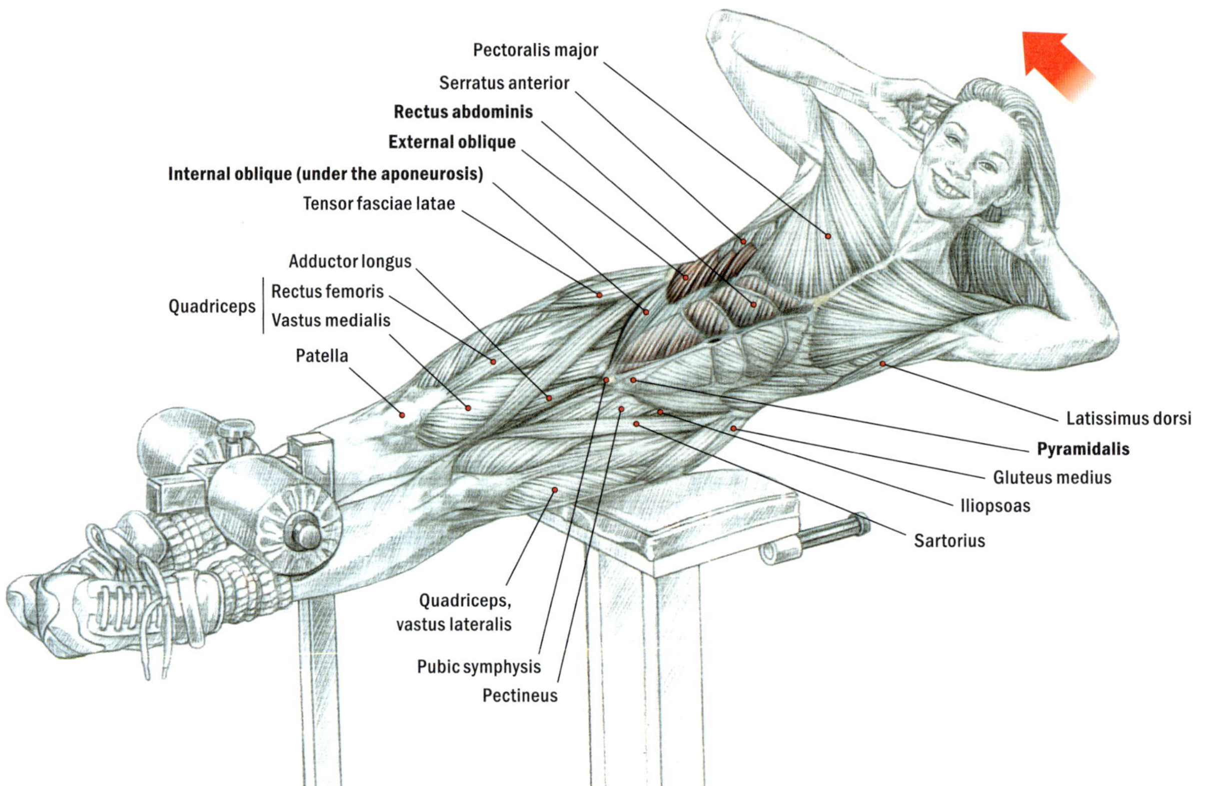

This exercise is performed on a Roman chair, originally designed for lumbar extensions. Lie on your side with your hip on the bench, torso in the air, hands by your ears or on your chest, and feet positioned under the pads:

- Raise your torso toward the ceiling.

This exercise mainly works the obliques and rectus abdominis on the side that is bending, but the obliques and rectus abdominis on the opposite side are also used in an isometric contraction to prevent the torso from lowering too far.

> **The quadratus lumborum muscle is always used when bending the torso to the side.**

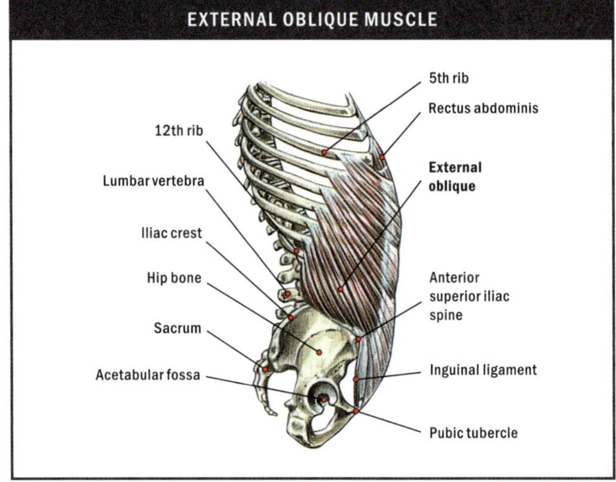

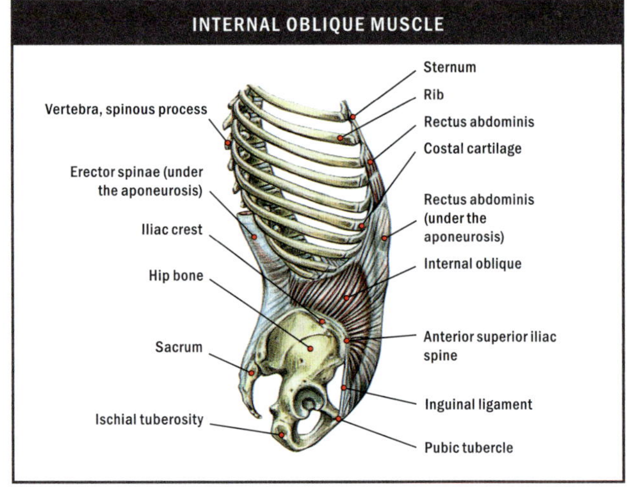

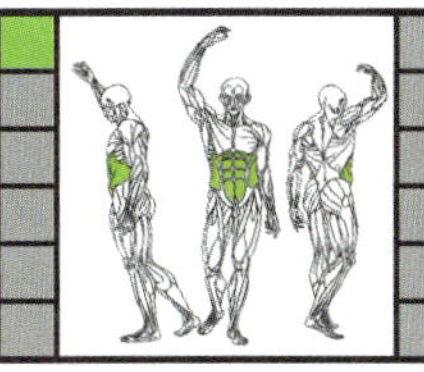

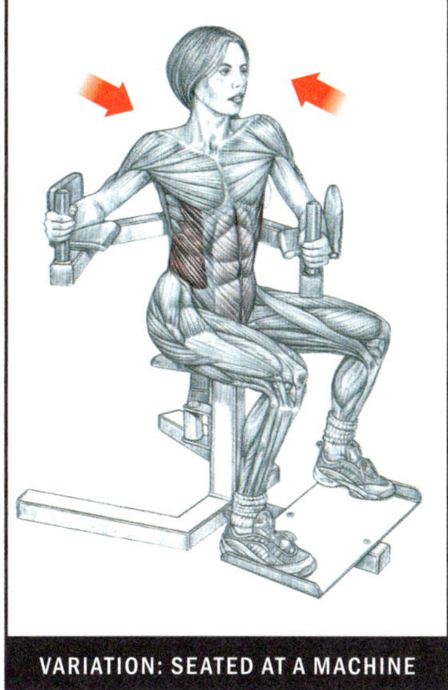

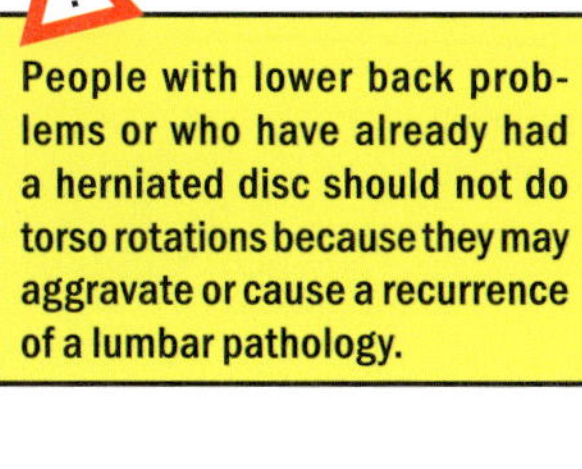

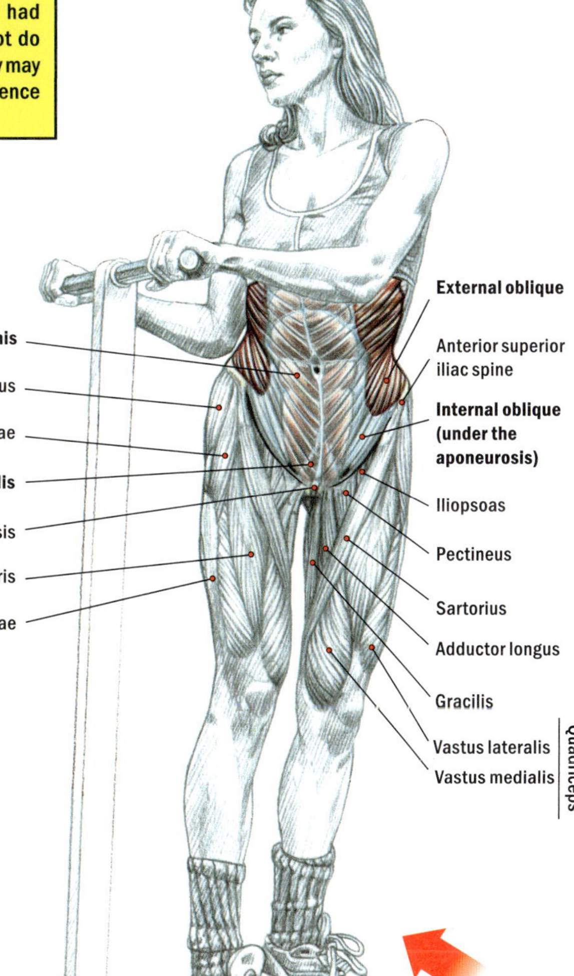

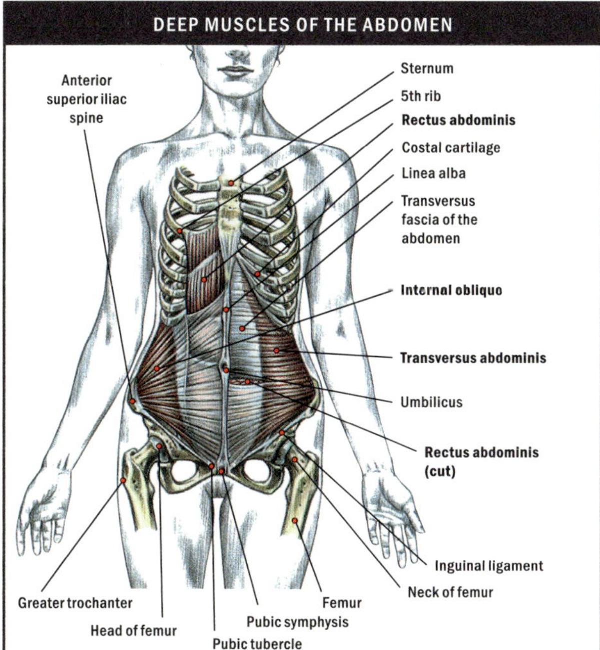

Stand on the swivel plate and grasp the handle:

- Rotate your pelvis to one side and then to the other, keeping your shoulders steady. Your knees should be slightly bent to avoid any stretching of the ligaments, and the exercise must be done with control.

This exercise mainly works the external and internal obliques and, to a lesser degree, the rectus abdominis. To feel the effort more intensely on the obliques, round your back slightly. The best results are obtained with very long sets.

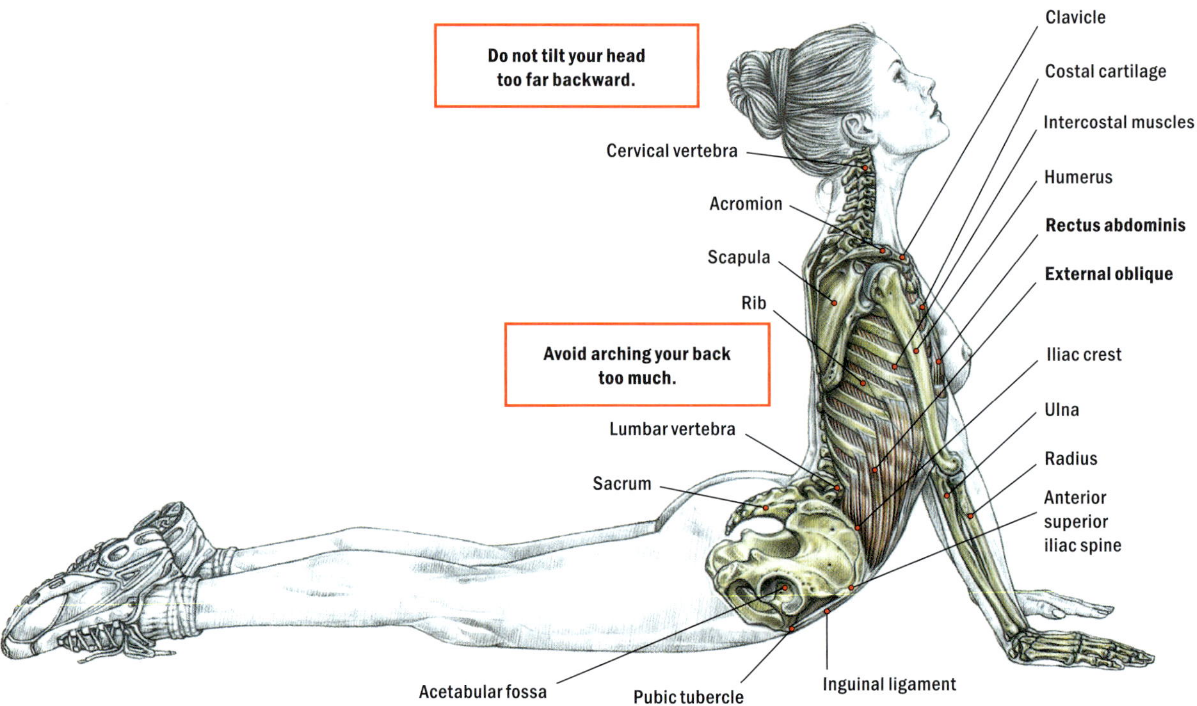

Lie on your belly, supporting yourself on your hands with your arms extended:

- Slowly raise your torso, tilting your head back slightly.
- Hold the stretch for a few moments, breathing slowly to really feel the stretch in the anterior part of your abdomen.

Abdominal stretches are not recommended for those with lower back issues.

Variations

You can stretch the abdominal muscles with your hands resting on a bench. You could also do the exercise with your feet on the floor, or you can lie with your back on an exercise ball.

Stretching the abdominal muscles is recommended in certain sports, such as throwing events in track and field, especially the javelin, where good flexibility and good abdominal range of motion are essential for executing throws perfectly.

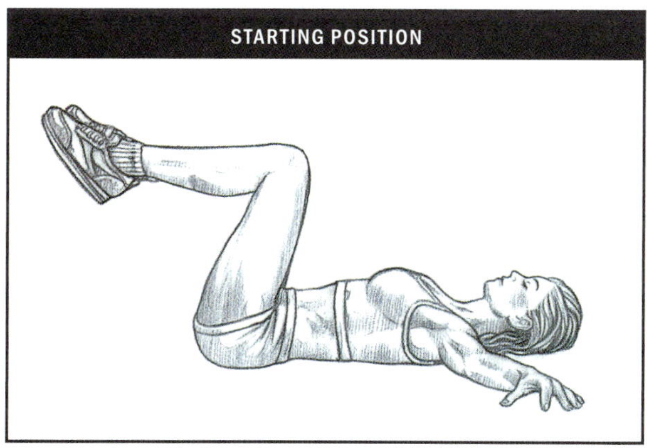

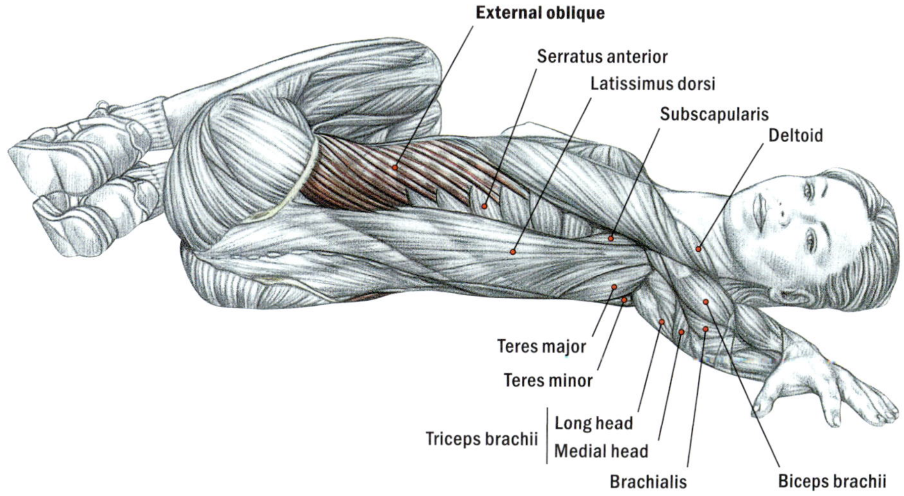

Lie on your back with your arms stretched into a *T* position, with your knees bent and your thighs vertical:

- Exhale as you slowly bring your knees to the floor.
- Inhale and return to the starting position.
- Repeat on the other side.

Although the hip flexor muscles are used in a static way, this exercise mainly works the external and internal obliques and the part of the rectus abdominis below the belly button.

Sets of 20 to 30 reps performed slowly provide the best results.

Variations

- If you have flexible hamstrings, you can increase the intensity of the stretch by doing this exercise with straight legs.
- To stretch the oblique muscles a little more, turn your head with each rotation of your pelvis. For example, when your knees drop to the right, turn your head to the left. This last variation is also a stretch for the obliques and the lumbar region.

To do this stretch properly and effectively, stretch the obliques each time you drop your knees. It is important to keep your head and shoulders on the ground.

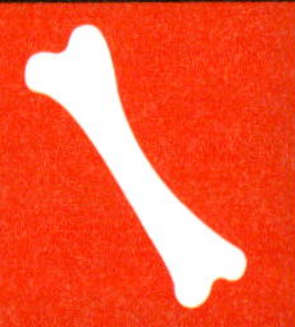

MORPHOLOGICAL VARIATIONS OF THE ABDOMEN

It is generally considered that an abdomen with low subcutaneous fat equates to a toned stomach. However, there can be several different morphological types of abdominal walls that can affect appearance.

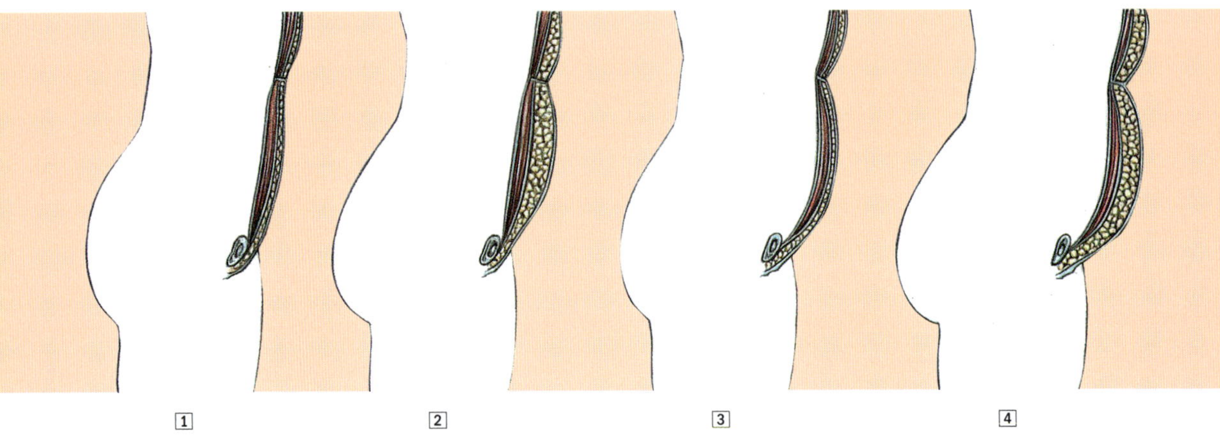

1 Normal abdominal wall, with toned muscles
2 Normal abdominal wall, with toned muscles and extra subcutaneous fat that gives the impression of ptosis (Sinking of an organ is most often caused by the loosening of the structures holding it in place; when the abdominal wall is weak, it can no longer hold in the abdominal viscera; the belly sags and forms a pocket where the small intestines rest.)

3 Protruding abdominal wall due to lack of muscle tone, without excess fat
4 Protruding abdominal wall due to lack of muscle tone, with excess fat

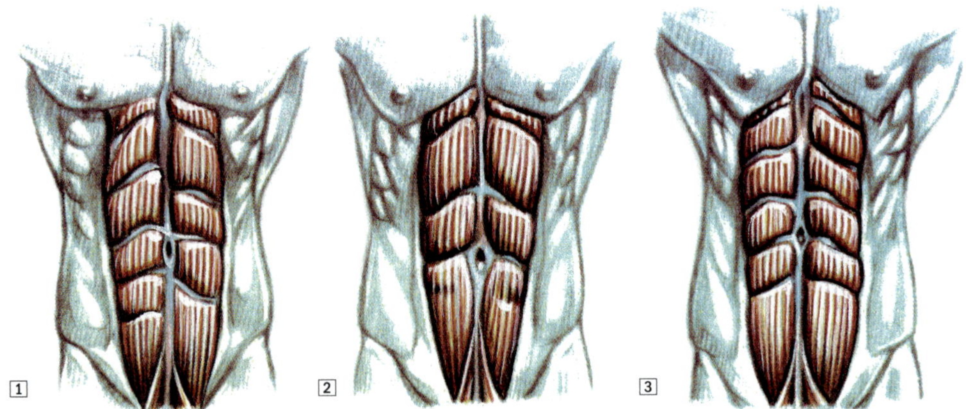

1 Asymmetric
2 Few tendinous intersections
3 Many tendinous intersections
The number of individual sections of the six-pack varies from one person to another, as does their symmetry.

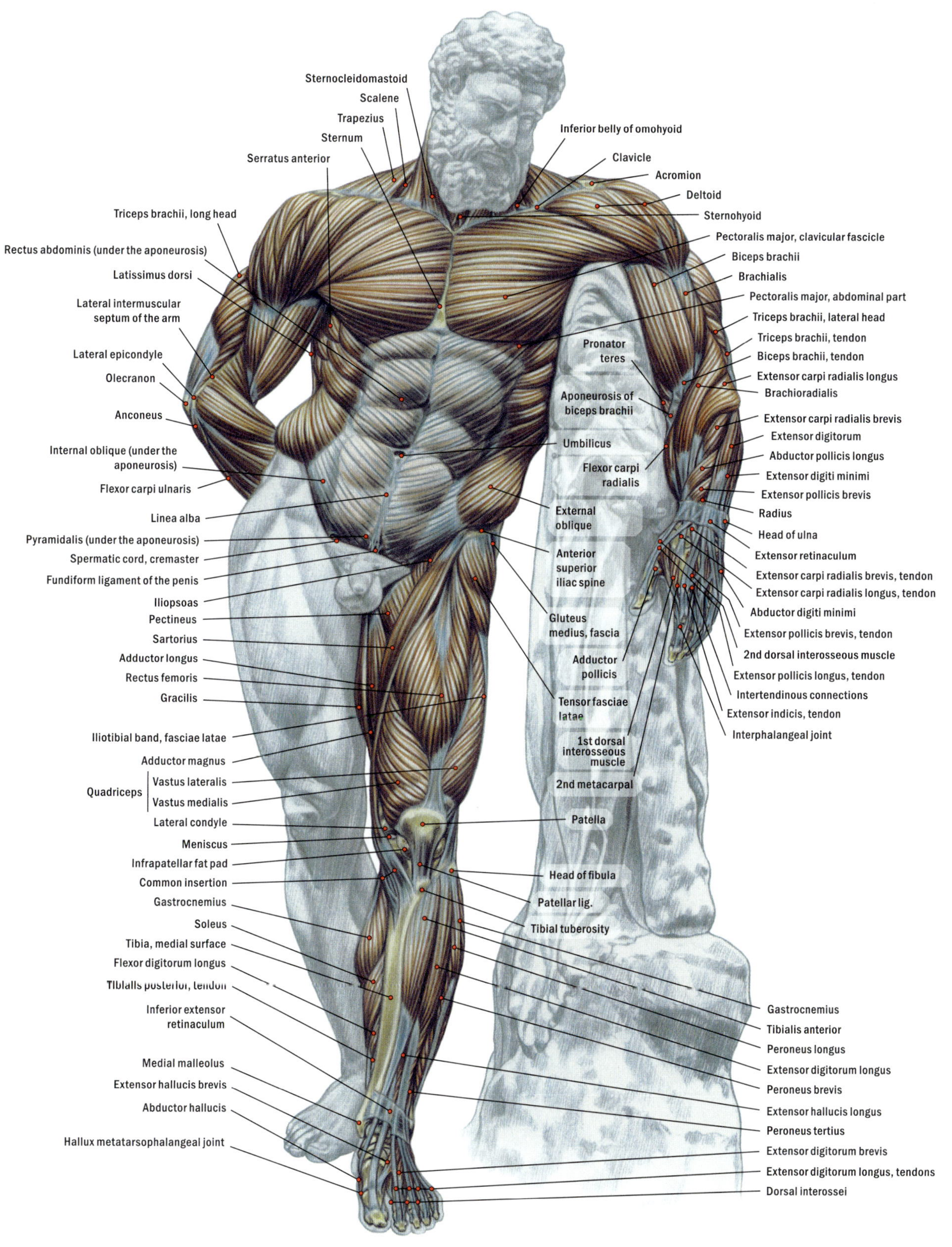

Sternocleidomastoid
Scalene
Trapezius
Sternum
Serratus anterior
Triceps brachii, long head
Rectus abdominis (under the aponeurosis)
Latissimus dorsi
Lateral intermuscular septum of the arm
Lateral epicondyle
Olecranon
Anconeus
Internal oblique (under the aponeurosis)
Flexor carpi ulnaris
Linea alba
Pyramidalis (under the aponeurosis)
Spermatic cord, cremaster
Fundiform ligament of the penis
Iliopsoas
Pectineus
Sartorius
Adductor longus
Rectus femoris
Gracilis
Iliotibial band, fasciae latae
Adductor magnus
Quadriceps
Vastus lateralis
Vastus medialis
Lateral condyle
Meniscus
Infrapatellar fat pad
Common insertion
Gastrocnemius
Soleus
Tibia, medial surface
Flexor digitorum longus
Tibialis posterior, tendon
Inferior extensor retinaculum
Medial malleolus
Extensor hallucis brevis
Abductor hallucis
Hallux metatarsophalangeal joint
Inferior belly of omohyoid
Clavicle
Acromion
Deltoid
Sternohyoid
Pectoralis major, clavicular fascicle
Biceps brachii
Brachialis
Pectoralis major, abdominal part
Triceps brachii, lateral head
Triceps brachii, tendon
Biceps brachii, tendon
Extensor carpi radialis longus
Brachioradialis
Extensor carpi radialis brevis
Extensor digitorum
Abductor pollicis longus
Extensor digiti minimi
Extensor pollicis brevis
Radius
Head of ulna
Extensor retinaculum
Extensor carpi radialis brevis, tendon
Extensor carpi radialis longus, tendon
Abductor digiti minimi
Extensor pollicis brevis, tendon
2nd dorsal interosseous muscle
Extensor pollicis longus, tendon
Intertendinous connections
Extensor indicis, tendon
Interphalangeal joint
Pronator teres
Aponeurosis of biceps brachii
Umbilicus
Flexor carpi radialis
External oblique
Anterior superior iliac spine
Gluteus medius, fascia
Adductor pollicis
Tensor fasciae latae
1st dorsal interosseous muscle
2nd metacarpal
Patella
Head of fibula
Patellar lig.
Tibial tuberosity
Gastrocnemius
Tibialis anterior
Peroneus longus
Extensor digitorum longus
Peroneus brevis
Extensor hallucis longus
Peroneus tertius
Extensor digitorum brevis
Extensor digitorum longus, tendons
Dorsal interossei

FARNESE HERCULES: SIDE VIEW

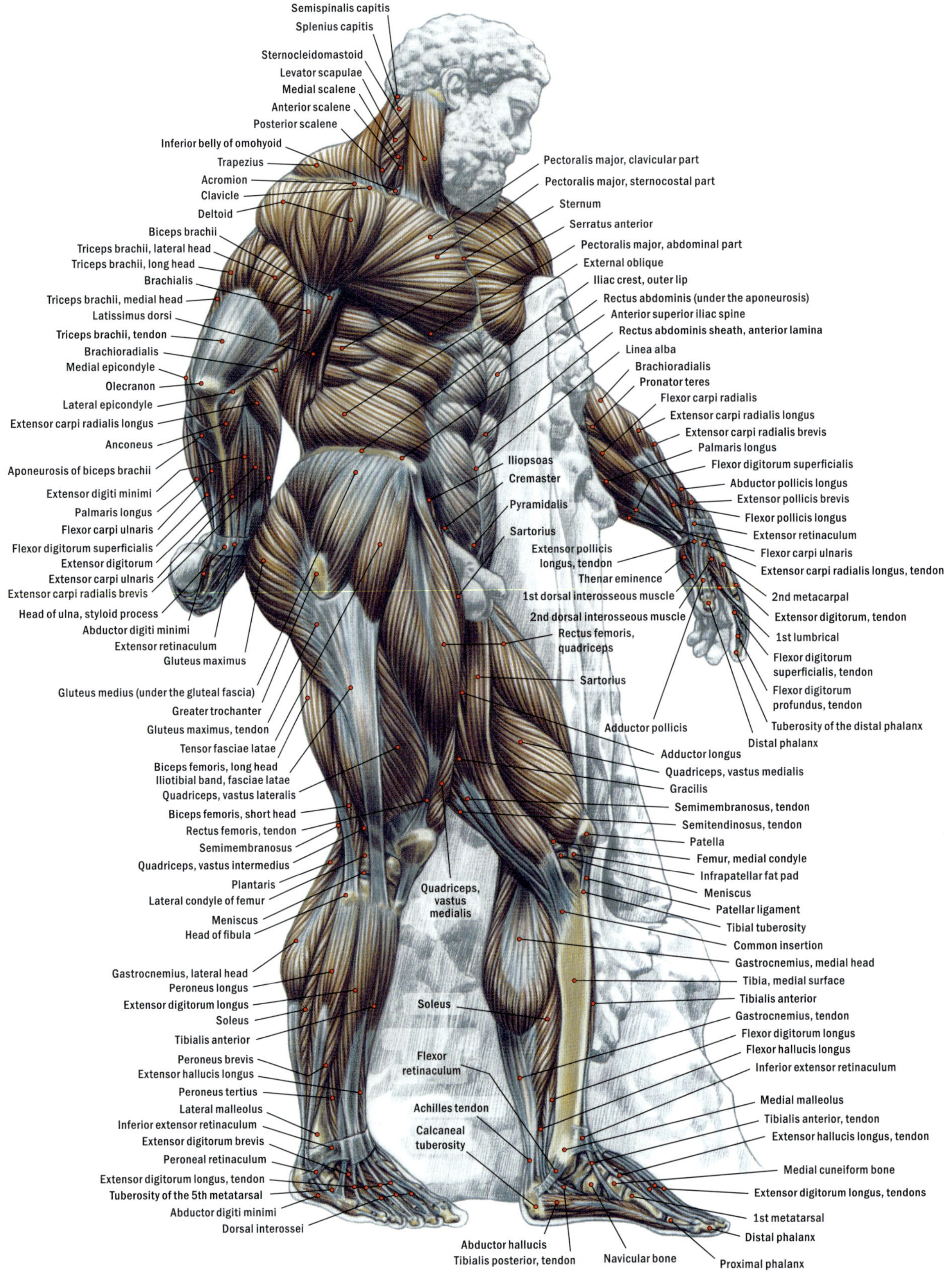

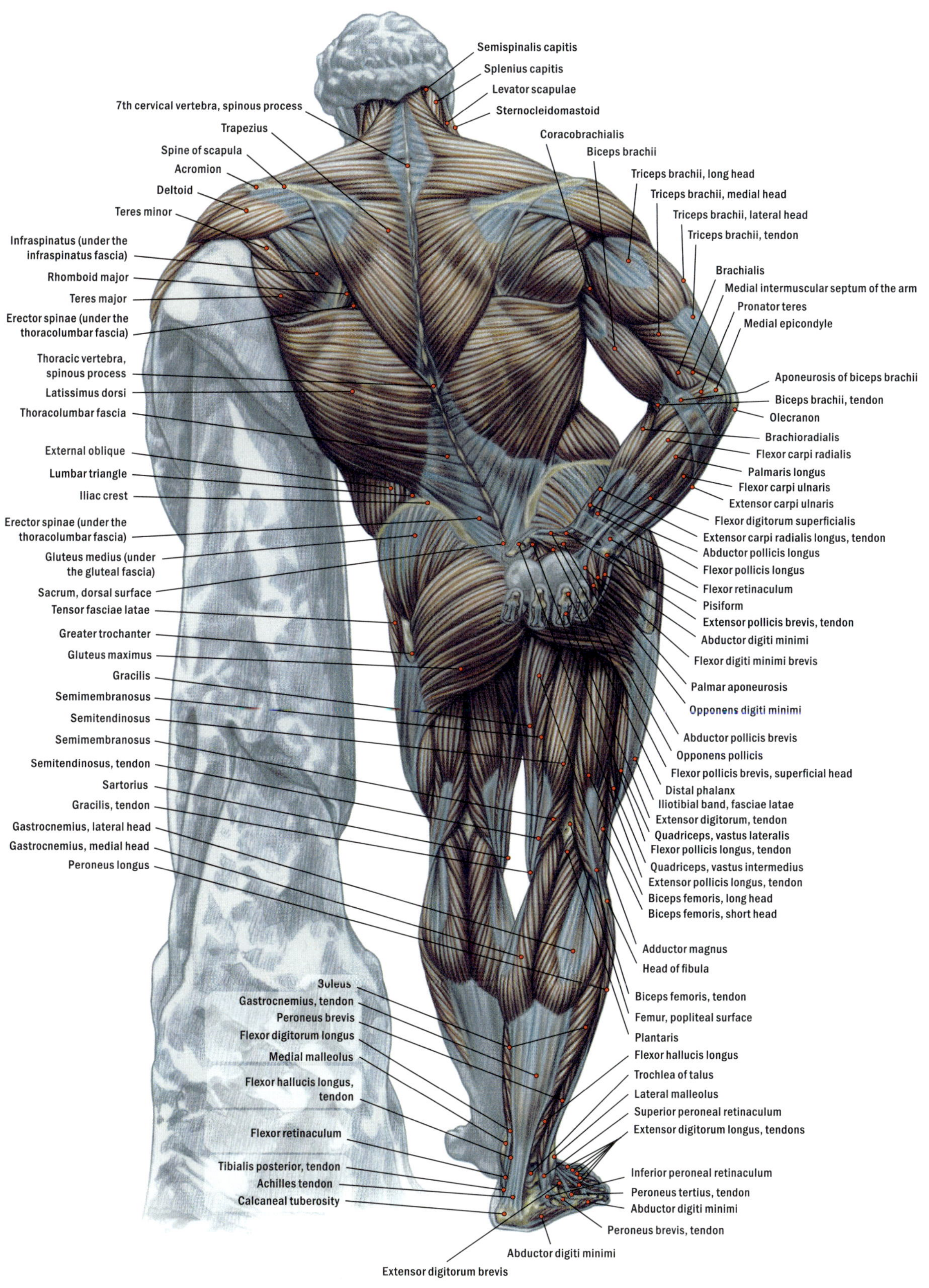

Semispinalis capitis
Splenius capitis
Levator scapulae
Sternocleidomastoid
Coracobrachialis
Biceps brachii
Triceps brachii, long head
Triceps brachii, medial head
Triceps brachii, lateral head
Triceps brachii, tendon
Brachialis
Medial intermuscular septum of the arm
Pronator teres
Medial epicondyle
Aponeurosis of biceps brachii
Biceps brachii, tendon
Olecranon
Brachioradialis
Flexor carpi radialis
Palmaris longus
Flexor carpi ulnaris
Extensor carpi ulnaris
Flexor digitorum superficialis
Extensor carpi radialis longus, tendon
Abductor pollicis longus
Flexor pollicis longus
Flexor retinaculum
Pisiform
Extensor pollicis brevis, tendon
Abductor digiti minimi
Flexor digiti minimi brevis
Palmar aponeurosis
Opponens digiti minimi
Abductor pollicis brevis
Opponens pollicis
Flexor pollicis brevis, superficial head
Distal phalanx
Iliotibial band, fasciae latae
Extensor digitorum, tendon
Quadriceps, vastus lateralis
Flexor pollicis longus, tendon
Quadriceps, vastus intermedius
Extensor pollicis longus, tendon
Biceps femoris, long head
Biceps femoris, short head
Adductor magnus
Head of fibula
Biceps femoris, tendon
Femur, popliteal surface
Plantaris
Flexor hallucis longus
Trochlea of talus
Lateral malleolus
Superior peroneal retinaculum
Extensor digitorum longus, tendons
Inferior peroneal retinaculum
Peroneus tertius, tendon
Abductor digiti minimi
Peroneus brevis, tendon
Abductor digiti minimi
Extensor digitorum brevis
7th cervical vertebra, spinous process
Trapezius
Spine of scapula
Acromion
Deltoid
Teres minor
Infraspinatus (under the infraspinatus fascia)
Rhomboid major
Teres major
Erector spinae (under the thoracolumbar fascia)
Thoracic vertebra, spinous process
Latissimus dorsi
Thoracolumbar fascia
External oblique
Lumbar triangle
Iliac crest
Erector spinae (under the thoracolumbar fascia)
Gluteus medius (under the gluteal fascia)
Sacrum, dorsal surface
Tensor fasciae latae
Greater trochanter
Gluteus maximus
Gracilis
Semimembranosus
Semitendinosus
Semimembranosus
Semitendinosus, tendon
Sartorius
Gracilis, tendon
Gastrocnemius, lateral head
Gastrocnemius, medial head
Peroneus longus
Soleus
Gastrocnemius, tendon
Peroneus brevis
Flexor digitorum longus
Medial malleolus
Flexor hallucis longus, tendon
Flexor retinaculum
Tibialis posterior, tendon
Achilles tendon
Calcaneal tuberosity

FEMALE ANATOMY, SUPERFICIAL AND DEEP MUSCLES: FRONT VIEW

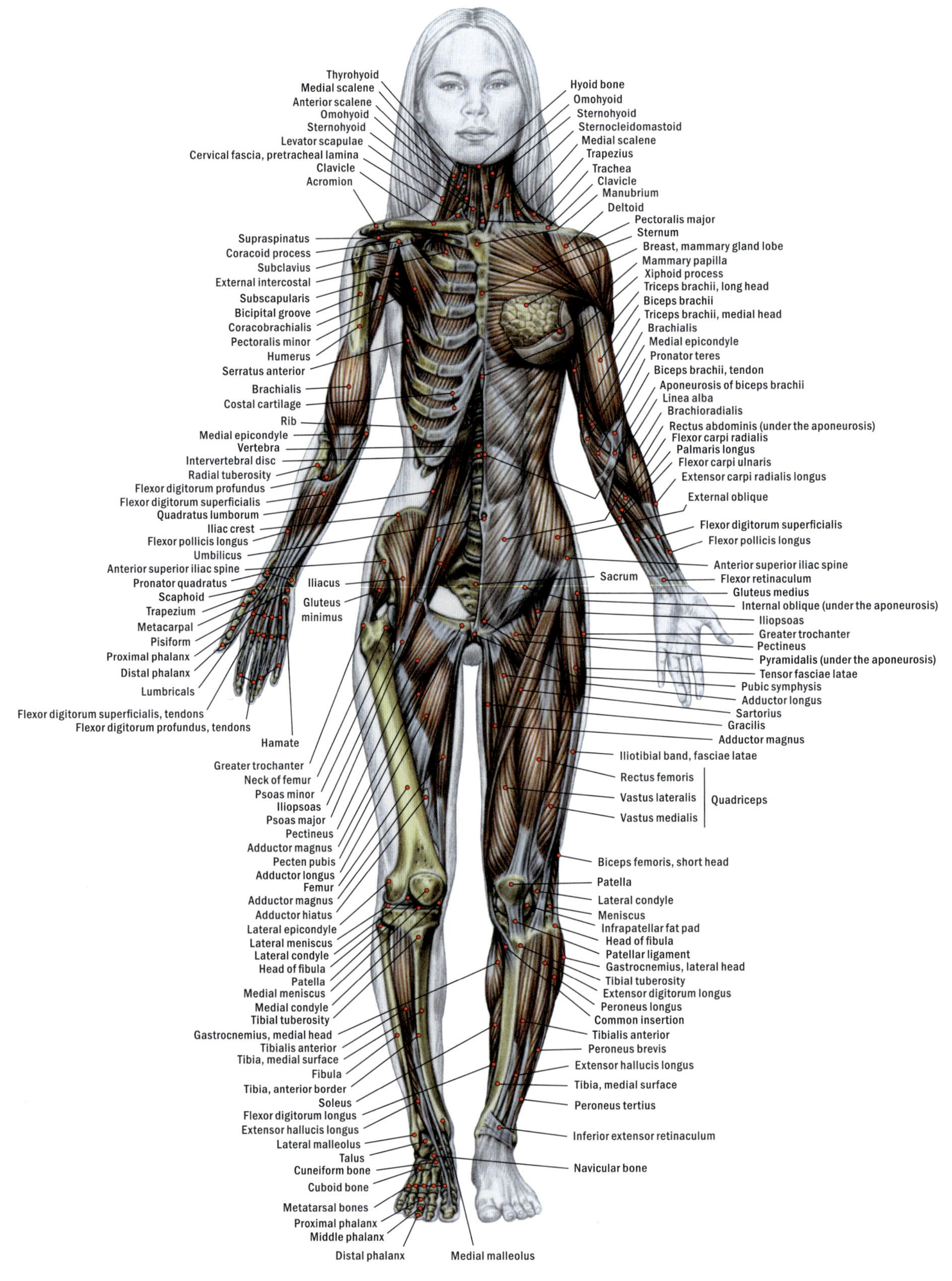

FEMALE ANATOMY, SUPERFICIAL AND DEEP MUSCLES: BACK VIEW

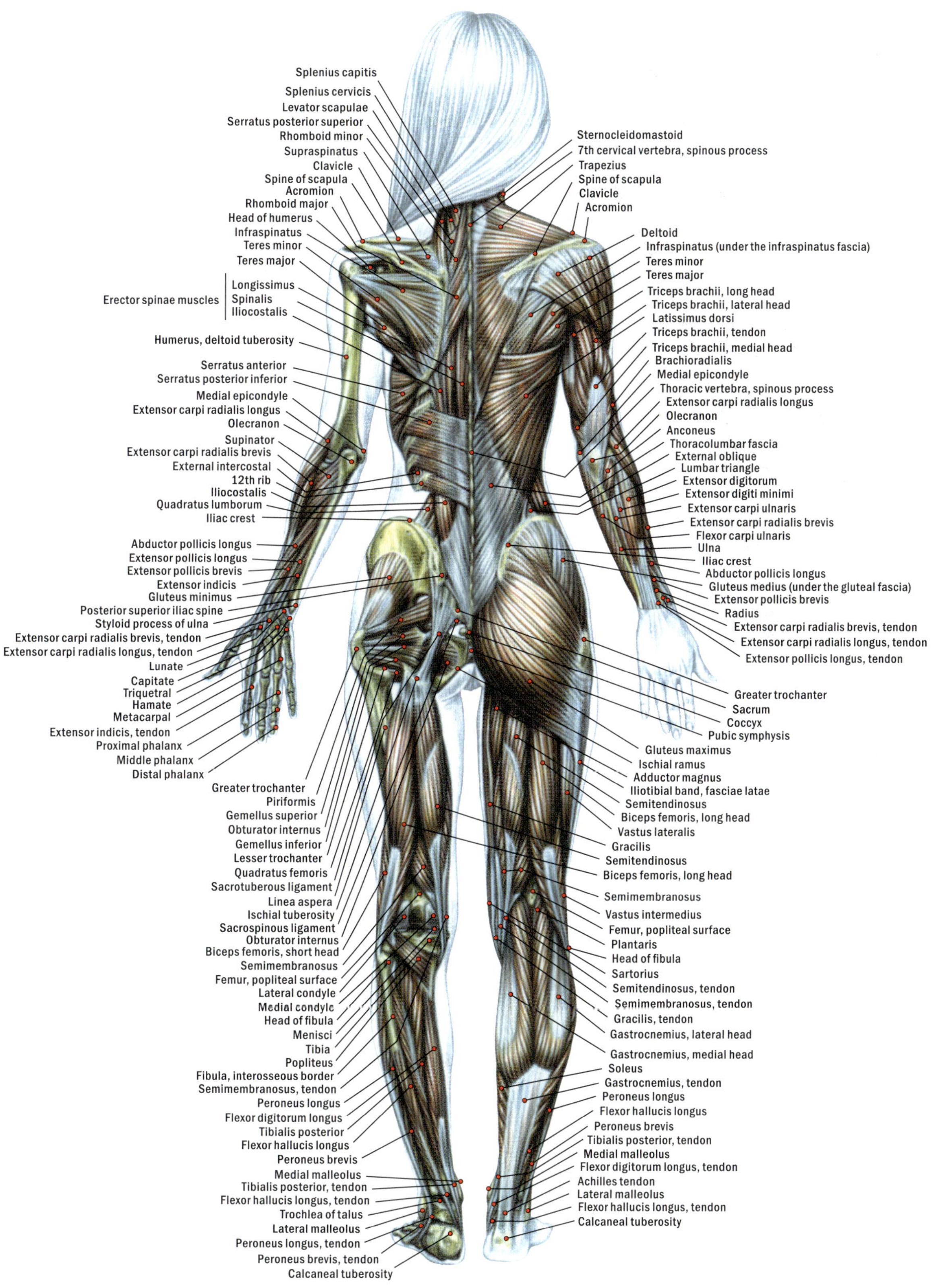

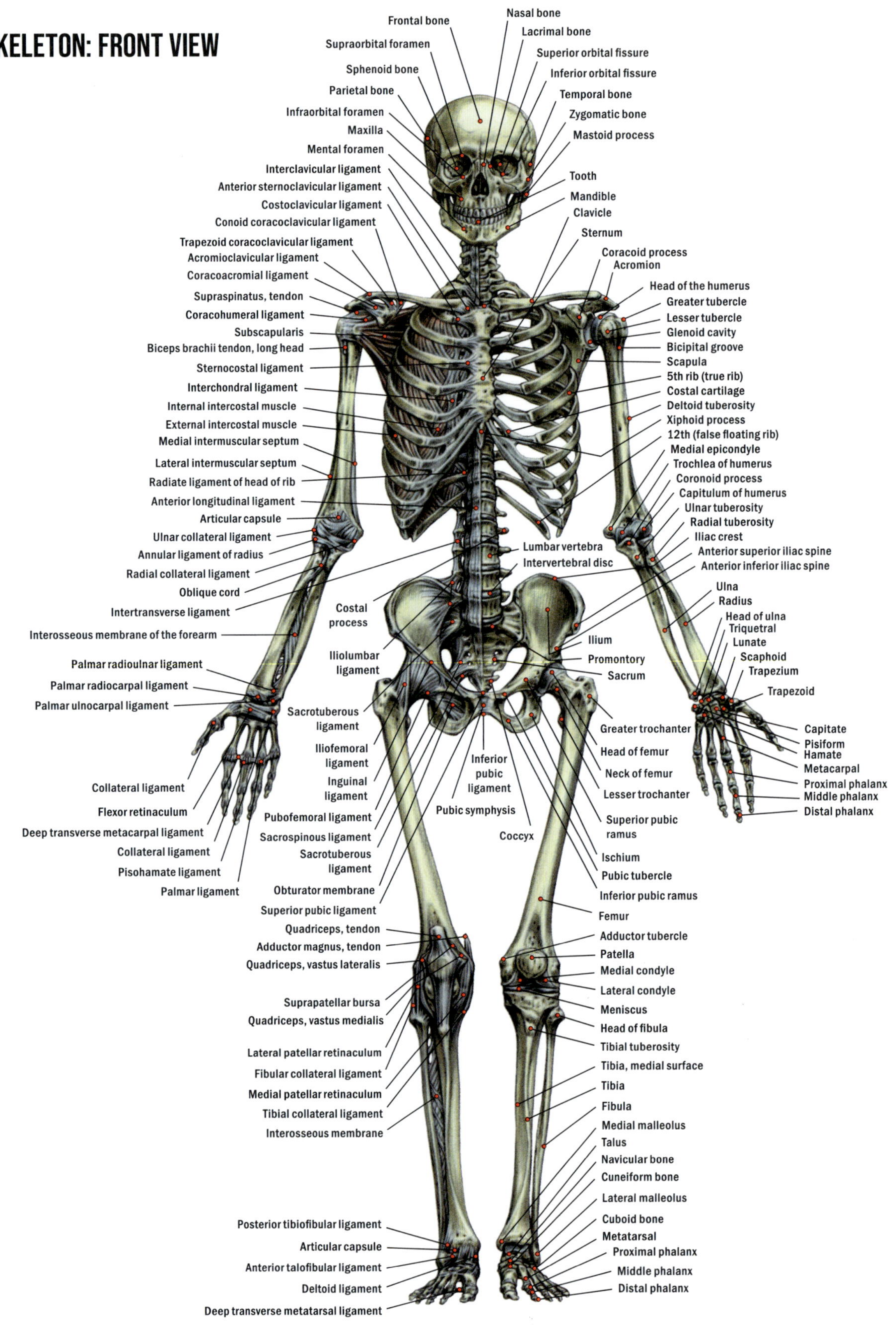

SKELETON: FRONT VIEW